7-55

Classic Descriptions
of Disease

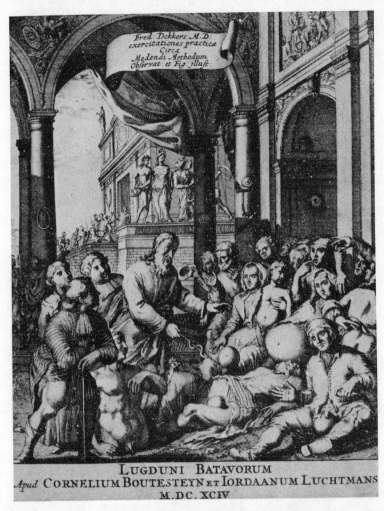

This is the FRONTISPIECE to the second edition of Dekkers' *Exercitationes practicae circa Medendi Methodum,* Leyden, 1694. Here the artist Joseph Mulder has depicted some of the gods of classical antiquity as well as diseases described and treated by the author. In the background we see an ancient temple. On the wall facing us stand Apollo, father of Asclepios, with his lyre, Aphrodite mother of the world, and Clotho, one of the Fates, holding the distaff in her left hand. Behind a column crouches Time, with a scythe in his right hand and an hour-glass in his left, ready to strike down the man who has lived his allotted span of years. In the foreground walks Asclepios touching the sick with his rod, around which a single serpent is coiled, the insignia since of the medical profession. Beside him the artist has placed a cock, since cocks were the favorite animals used in sacrifices to Asclepios. Among the various diseases shown are arthritis, rickets, abdominal cysts, hydrocele, and tumors of the legs and buttocks. On the pillars and walls hang various surgical instruments, including a cupping glass and a long tube for insufflating tobacco smoke into the rectum. The instruments, as well as the patients, are described and illustrated in the book.

Third Edition, Seventh Printing

Classic Descriptions *of* Disease

With Biographical Sketches of the Authors

By

Ralph H. Major, M.D.

Professor of Medicine

University of Kansas School of Medicine

Charles C Thomas, *Publisher · Springfield · Illinois · U.S.A.*

Published and Distributed Throughout the World by
CHARLES C THOMAS · PUBLISHER
BANNERSTONE HOUSE
301-327 East Lawrence Avenue, Springfield, Illinois, U.S.A.

© *1932, 1939, 1945, by* CHARLES C THOMAS · PUBLISHER
ISBN 0-398-01202-4

First Edition, 1932
Second Edition, 1939
Third Edition, First Printing, 1945
Third Edition, Second Printing, 1947
Third Edition, Third Printing, 1948
Third Edition, Fourth Printing, 1955
Third Edition, Fifth Printing, 1959
Third Edition, Sixth Printing, 1965
Third Edition, Seventh Printing, 1978

Printed in the United States of America

PREFACE TO THE SECOND EDITION

Every author is grateful for the opportunity which the preparation of the second edition affords him of correcting certain errors and omissions. I am deeply appreciative of the assistance rendered me by many friends in calling certain mistakes to my attention and in suggesting improvements.

In this second edition of *Classic Descriptions of Disease* new sections covering malaria and yellow fever have been included as well as additional readings and illustrations. Many of the biographical sketches have been rewritten and the index has been revised and enlarged. I hope these changes will commend themselves to the reader.

It is again a pleasure to express my appreciation of Mr. Thomas' assistance, encouragement and advice.

R.H.M.

PREFACE TO THE FIRST EDITION

The nucleus of this selection of classic accounts of disease was collected partly because of personal interest in the subject and partly for use in teaching. The value of referring students to classic accounts of disease has been stressed by many of our greatest clinicians, in our own generation notably by Sir William Osler. When, in the clinic, Corrigan's description of the pulse in aortic insufficiency is read while a patient suffering from this disease is presented, the pulse itself is no longer a mere name, but becomes endowed with a definite personality. When we read in our library Heberden's original description of angina pectoris, we cannot but have the thought that if physicians read this account more frequently fewer mistakes in the diagnosis of this condition would occur.

The appearance of Long's *Readings in Pathology* suggested the possibility of expanding my own selections until they attained the dimensions of a sizeable volume and after the later appearance of Fulton's *Selected Reading in the History of Physiology*, the idea took definite form. Mr. Thomas, to whom the manuscript was submitted, has not only undertaken the responsibility of its production but has been of the greatest possible assistance in the completion of the task. It is a great pleasure to acknowledge his cooperation and assistance and to express my appreciation of his interest, enthusiasm, and rare good taste.

My obligations are many to many, both books and persons. My greatest of the former is the assistance received from F. H. Garrison's *History of Medicine*. This mine of historical information, so replete with that accuracy and detail which we admire so much in our Teutonic colleagues, is now with American students the starting point of almost every investigation in the history of medicine. I have also obtained much aid from Professor Hermann Vierordt's *Medizin-Geschichliches Hilfsbuch*, a very valuable work which deserves a far wider use in this country. I have also consulted frequently Haeser's *Geschichte der Medizin*, Pagel and Neuburger's *Handbuch der Geschichte der Medizin*, Munk's *Roll of the Royal College of Physicians of London*, Bettany's *Eminent*

Doctors, Castiglioni's *Histoire de la médecine,* Sigerist's *Grosse Ärzte,* Camac's *Epoch-making Contributions,* Victor Robinson's *Pathfinders in Medicine,* Ruhräh's *Pediatrics of the Past* and Still's *History of the Paediatrics.* The biographical details have been obtained from the above works, from medical journals, from the *Dictionary of National Biography,* the *Allgemeine Deutsche Biographie,* the *Biographie Universelle,* the *Lexikon hervorragender Ärzte* and in many instances from biographical works which are mentioned in the text.

I am equally under deep personal obligations to certain individuals. Colonel F. H. Garrison, with whom I have discussed this book, has given me many invaluable suggestions, has supplied me with data and selections and shown me many other favors for which I am deeply grateful. Sir Humphry Rolleston has taken the pains to go over the plan and outline of this work and I wish to express my appreciation of his assistance and the splendid helpful suggestions he has made. Much additional aid also he has unconsciously given in his historical papers, particularly in the *Annals of Medical History,* from which much biographical data has been obtained. Dr. Arnold Klebs has aided me very materially in his helpful suggestions and his interest and encouragement are deeply appreciated. My old friend of Heidelberg days, the late Dr. Erich Ebstein, has aided me greatly in the preparation of this book. His unexpected death while at the height of his powers has been a great loss to medicine, and saddened his many friends who will long remember the genial doctor with his inexhaustible fund of medical anecdotes, his prodigious memory for events and his encyclopedic knowledge of medical history which was ever at the command of his colleagues. Dr. Ernest Wickersheimer has aided me materially in his suggestions and references to accounts worthy of inclusion, and I am also under obligations to Dr. Henry Barton Jacobs. To my friend Dr. Logan Clendening, I owe more than he would care to have me mention. He has supplied me with pictures, translations, biographies, and has had the rare courage to go over the manuscript in its unfinished state, and to give the most sane and constructive criticism. Finally I wish to express to Colonel P. M. Ashburn, librarian of the Surgeon General's Library, my sincere appreciation of his unfailing courtesy in supplying numerous selections and photographs and in guiding my path while visiting the library.

I am also under great obligations for the use of materials and pictures, to the editors of the *American Journal of Medical Sciences,* the *Boston Medical and Surgical Journal,* the *Bulletin of the Johns Hopkins Hospital,* the *British Medical Journal,* the *Edinburgh Medical Journal,* the *Lancet,* the *Münchener Medizinische Wochenschrift* and to the Royal College of Physicians in London, the Royal College of Physicians in Dublin, the University Press in Manchester, the Oxford Press, the British Museum, and Paul B. Hoeber, Inc. I wish also to make grateful acknowledgement to Miss Opal Woodruff, librarian of the University of Kansas School of Medicine, and to Mrs. Rose Hibbard, librarian of the Jackson County (Missouri) Medical Society who have aided me in many ways.

In collecting an anthology of this kind certain selections obviously are included and others omitted. The selections are chosen because of their interest in being either the first known, one of the earliest, or one of the most interesting accounts of the disease in question. Some sections of the book are so sparsely represented that they seem inadequate while others seem so fully represented as to be almost overdone. This is inevitable, however, since some diseases have more interesting and more extended histories than others and also because of personal taste, or bias, if you will, in the selection of authors.

In sections on infectious diseases one misses an account of the discoveries of Koch, Schaudinn, Kitasato, Bordet, Wassermann, and of that many-sided genius Edwin Klebs, who saw the typhoid bacillus before Eberth, the diphtheria bacillus before Löffler, and who inoculated monkeys with syphilis before Metchnikoff. Such discoveries belong, however, to the field of bacteriology, and these selections deal in the main with clinical medicine. The subject of therapeutics has not been included except in a few instances, where they seemed to round out unusually well the history of the disease in question. Neurological selections have been omitted for the reason that their interest and number are sufficient to form an independent series.

Unless otherwise indicated, I am responsible for the translations into English. In making translations from the Latin I have had in several instances the advantages of comparison with a French or German translation. Mistakes have probably crept in, since in many places it is difficult to be sure just what thought some Italian, Frenchman, or Spaniard writing in medieval Latin was trying to express, and at times a translator almost wonders if the author himself knew, particularly when he indulges in flights of speculation. In general, however, I believe the thought of the author has been reproduced with accuracy. Considerable liberty has been taken in paragraphing the accounts of the old authors since the modern reader is almost invariably appalled by the contemplation of a solid sheet of printed matter with no indentations or paragraphs. Such liberty, however, has not, I believe, interfered with the sense of the author or with his continuity of thought.

In conclusion I hope this book will not merit the reproof of Dr. Samuel Johnson, who is reported to have remarked after reading Cadogan's *Dissertation on the Gout,* that "all that is good he stole, all the nonsense is evidently his own."

PREFACE TO THE THIRD EDITION

Twelve years have passed since the first edition of this book appeared. Since then, many notable figures in the history of medicine have died, Professor Karl Sudhoff, Colonel Fielding Garrison, Doctor Arnold Klebs and Sir Humphry Rolleston, to mention only a few. From these men, all interested in the history of medicine have received much inspiration, and their passing leaves us with a sense of deep personal loss as well as with the realization of an irreparable loss to medicine. Their contributions to the history of medicine are a part of medical history itself, and as we look back over these years, they seem from the prospective of today to have been perhaps the golden age of medical history. The work of these men stimulated an interest in the history of medicine which has grown steadily from year to year. Fortunately, many stalwarts of this generation still remain to carry on the unfinished work of these men and a new generation is rising who will keep alive their enthusiasm and their love for this field of medicine.

In this third edition, several new selections have been added and the book has been provided with a bibliography which I hope may prove helpful. In the preparation of this edition I am deeply indebted to Dr. George Blumer, Dr. Henry Sigerist and Dr. Ludwig Edelstein. To my old friend and colleague, Dr. Logan Clendening, who patiently watched the gestation of this book, assisted at its birth and has thoughtfully and tenderly nursed its growing pains as it proceeded to later editions, my deepest gratitude!

CONTENTS

INTRODUCTION

HIPPOCRATES (460-370 B.C.).—*Hippocratic Facies. Carphologia. Hippocratic Fingers* 3

I. INFECTIOUS DISEASES

THE THEORY OF INFECTION

HIERONYMUS FRACASTORIUS (1484-1553).—*Concerning contagions and contagious diseases and their treatment* 7

ATHANASIUS KIRCHER (1602-1680).—*Physical and Medical Scrutiny of the pernicious contagious Disease and so-called Pestilence* 9

SYPHILIS

NICOLO LEONICENO (1428-1524).—*Concerning the epidemic which Italians call the Disease of the French but the French call Neapolitan* 13

FRANCISCO LOPEZ DE VILLALOBOS (1473).—*Treatise of the pestiferous Bubas* 16

JUAN ALMENAR (1502).—*A Treatise of the French Pocks* 19

GIOVANNI DI VIGO (1460-1520).—*Concerning the French Disease* 23

ULRICH VON HUTTEN (1488-1523).—*Of the wood called Guaiacum that healeth the French Pockes* 28

JACQUES DE BÉTHENCOURT (1527).—*New Litany of Penitence and Purgatory of Expiation* 35

HIERONYMUS FRACASTORIUS (1483-1553).—*Syphilis or the French Disease* .. 37

JOHN HUNTER (1728-1793).—*Experiments made to ascertain the Progress and Effects of the Venereal Poison* 42

JONATHAN HUTCHINSON (1828-1913).—*Heredito-Syphilitic Struma, and on the Teeth as a Means of Diagnosis* 46

TUBERCULOSIS

HIPPOCRATES (460-370 B.C.).—*The Epidemics* 52

RICHARD WISEMAN (1622-1676)—*A Treatise of the King's Evill* 53

FRANCISCUS SYLVIUS (1614-1672).—*Concerning Phthisis* 58

RICHARD MORTON (1637-1698).—*Of the Causes of an Original Consumption of the Lungs* 61

GASPARD-LAURENT BAYLE (1774-1816).—*Essential Character of Pulmonary Phthisis* 64

JEAN-ANTOINE VILLEMIN (1827-1892).—*Tuberculosis is Inoculable* 66

RENÉ-THÉOPHILE-HYACINTHE LAËNNEC (1781-1826).—*Physical Signs of Tubercles* 68

PLAGUE

THUCYDIDES (460-399 B.C.).—*History of the Peloponnesian War* 73

RUFUS OF EPHESUS (100 A.D.)—*On the Plague, from the Works of Ruffus* ... 76

MICHELE DI PIAZZA (1347).—*Historia Sicula ab anno 1337 ad annum 1361*.... 77

GUY DE CHAULIAC (1300-1368).—*The great Mortality* ....: 77

GIOVANNI BOCCACCIO (1313-1375).—*The Decameron* 80
BENGT KNUTSSON (1461).—*A litil boke the whiche traytied and reherced many gode thinges necessaries for the Pestilence* 82
ATHANASIUS KIRCHER (1601-1680).—*Physical and Medical Scrutiny of the Contagious Disease and so-called Pestilence* 84
NATHANIEL HODGES (1629-1688).—*Loimologia* 85
AMBROISE PARÉ (1510-1590).—*Of the Plague* 87
DANIEL DEFOE (1661-1731).—*A Journal of the Plague Year* 91

MALARIA

HIPPOCRATES (460-370 B.C.).—*Fevers* 94
ARISTOPHANES (450-380 B.C.).—*Agues and fevers* 95
MARCUS TERENTIUS VARRO (116-27 B.C.).—*Swamps breed certain animalculae* 96
AULUS CORNELIUS CELSUS (25 A.D.).—*Of the several kinds of fevers* 96
PLINY THE ELDER (23-79 A.D.).—*Remedies for Fevers* 97
MARTIAL (43-104 A.D.).—*Epigrams* 100
SIR ROBERT TABOR (1642-1681).—*The English Remedy* 100
ALBERT FREEMAN AFRICANUS KING (1841-1914).—*Mosquitoes and Malaria* 103
SIR RONALD ROSS (1857-1932).—*Pigmented Cells in Mosquitoes* 108

YELLOW FEVER

MATHEW CAREY (1760-1839).—*A Short Account of the Malignant Fever* 114
BENJAMIN RUSH (1745-1813).—*Bilious Remitting Yellow Fever* 118
JOSIAH C. NOTT (1804-1873).—*Yellow Fever contrasted with Bilious Fever* .. 121
CARLOS J. FINLAY (1833-1915).—*Yellow Fever: Its Transmission by Means of the Culex Mosquito* 125
WALTER REED (1851-1902).—*The Etiology of Yellow Fever* 130

TETANUS

HIPPOCRATES (460-370 B.C.).—*Tetanus* 134
ARETAEUS THE CAPPADOCIAN (Second or Third Century A.D.).—*On Tetanus* .. 134

DIPHTHERIA

ARETAEUS THE CAPPADOCIAN (Second or Third Century A.D.).—*On the ulcerations about the tonsils* 136
GUILLAUME DE BAILLOU (1538-1616).—*Constitutio Hiemalis Anni Domini 1576* 137
NICHOLAS TULP (1593-1674).—*Internal angina* 140
JOHN FOTHERGILL (1712-1780).—*An Account of the Sore Throat Attended with Ulcers* 142
JOHN HUXHAM (1692-1768).—*A Dissertation on the Malignant Ulcerous Sore-Throat* 146
FRANCIS HOME (1719-1813) 149
SAMUEL BARD (1742-1821).—*An Enquiry into the Nature, Cause and Cure of the Angina Suffocativa, etc.* 153
PIERRE BRETONNEAU (1778-1862).—*Treatise on diphtheria* 157

TYPHUS FEVER

JEROME CARDAN (1501-1576).—*The Bad Practice in Use among the Doctors* ..   161
HIERONYMUS FRACASTORIUS (1484-1553).—*Concerning a fever, which they call lenticular or punctate or petechial*   164
FRANCISCO BRAVO (1570).—*Opera Medicinalia*   165
TOBIAS COBER (-1625).—*The Hungarian Disease*   166
THOMAS WILLIS (1621-1675).—*Of Pestilential and Malignant Feavers in specie*   169
JAMES LIND (1716-1794).—*Of the Jail Distemper*   171
WILLIAM WOOD GERHARD (1809-1872).—*On the typhus fever*   173
CHARLES NICOLLE (1866-1936).—*Experimental transmission of typhus exanthematicus by the body louse*   177

TYPHOID FEVER

THOMAS WILLIS (1621-1675).—*Of a Putrid Feaver*   179
PIERRE BRETONNEAU (1778-1862).—*Concerning the disease to which M. Bretonneau . . . has given the name of dothinenteritis*   182
PIERRE CHARLES ALEXANDRE LOUIS (1787-1872).—*The Disease known under the Names of Gastro-enteritis, putrid, adynamic, ataxic, typhoid fever, etc.*   184

EPIDEMIC CEREBROSPINAL MENINGITIS

GASPARD VIEUSSEUX (1746-1814).—*Cerebral Malignant Non-contagious Fever*   188
ELISHA NORTH (1771-1843).—*Malignant Epidemic commonly called Spotted Fever*   189

SCARLET FEVER

DANIEL SENNERT (1572-1637).—*On Fevers*   192
THOMAS SYDENHAM (1624-1689).—*On the Scarlet Fever*, from *Processus Integri*   194

SMALLPOX AND MEASLES

RHAZES (860-932).—*Treatise on the Small-Pox and Measles*   196

MEASLES

THOMAS SYDENHAM (1624-1689).—*On the Measles*, from *Processus Integri* ..   198
HENRY KOPLIK (1858-1927).—*Spots pathognomonic of Measles*   199

MUMPS

HIPPOCRATES (460-370 B.C.).—*Mumps*   201

INFLUENZA

THOMAS SYDENHAM (1624-1689).—*Of the epidemic diseases*   201

SWEATING FEVER

JOHN CAIUS (1510-1573).—*A boke or counseile against the disease commonly called the sweate or sweatyng sickness*   202

CHICKENPOX

WILLIAM HEBERDEN (1710-1801).—*Variola Pusillae. The Chicken Pox*   206

GLANDULAR FEVER

EMIL PFEIFFER (1889).—*Drüsenfieber*   208

WHOOPING COUGH

GUILLAUME DE BAILLOU (1538-1616).—*Quinta seu Quintana* in the *Constitutio Aestiva Anni Domini 1578* 210

RHEUMATIC FEVER

GUILLAUME DE BAILLOU (1538-1616).—*Liber de rheumatismo* 212
THOMAS SYDENHAM (1624-1689).—*Rheumatism* from *Medical Observations* .. 213
RICHARD MORTON (1637-1698).—*Of a Consumption Proceeding from the Gout, and from a Rheumatism* 214
JOHN HAYGARTH (1740-1827).—*Of the Acute Rheumatism or Rheumatic Fever* 215
WILLIAM CHARLES WELLS (1757-1817).—*On Rheumatism of the Heart* 218
JEAN BAPTISTE BOUILLAUD (1796-1817).—*New Researches on Acute Articular Rheumatism* 220

RELAPSING FEVER

JOHN RUTTY (1698-1775).—*A Chronological History of the Weather and Seasons and of the Prevailing Diseases in Dublin* 223

SLEEPING SICKNESS

THOMAS WINTERBOTTOM (1766-1859).—*A Species of Lethargy* 224

SCHÖNLEIN'S DISEASE

JOHANN LUKAS SCHÖNLEIN (1793-1864).—*Peliosis Rheumatica* 225

FOCAL INFECTION

BENJAMIN RUSH (1745-1813).—*An Account of the Cure of Several Diseases by the Extraction of Teeth* 227

HODGKIN'S DISEASE

THOMAS HODGKIN (1798-1866).—*On Some Morbid Appearances of the Absorbent Glands and Spleen* 230

II. DISEASES OF METABOLISM

DIABETES MELLITUS

PAPYRUS EBERS (1500 B.C.).—*The passing of too much urine* 235
ARETAEUS THE CAPPADOCIAN (Second or Third Century A.D.).—*On Diabetes* .. 235
PARACELSUS (1493-1541).—*Concerning Diabetes* 237
THOMAS WILLIS (1621-1675).—*The Diabetes or Pissing Evil* 238
MATTHEW DOBSON (1776).—*Experiments and Observations on the Urine in a Diabetes* 242
THOMAS ADDISON (1793-1860).—*On a Certain Affection of the Skin* 245
ADOLF KUSSMAUL (1822-1902).—*A peculiar mode of death in diabetes* 245
OSKAR MINKOWSKI (1858-1931).—*Diabetes mellitus after extirpation of the pancreas* 249
EUGENE OPIE (1873-   ).—*Hyaline Degeneration of the Pancreas* 253
SIR FREDERICK BANTING (1892-1944).—*The Internal Secretion of the Pancreas* 256

THYROID DISEASE

MYXEDEMA

PARACELSUS (1493-1541).—*Concerning the Generation of Fools* 258

FELIX PLATTER (1536-1614).—*Concerning Alienation of the Mind* 263

WOLFGANG HOEFER (1614-1681).—*Affections of the Head. Foolishness* 264

THOMAS BLIZARD CURLING (1811-1888).—*Absence of the thyroid body* 266

SIR WILLIAM GULL (1816-1890).—*On a Cretinoid State Supervening in Adult Life in Women* 268

GEORGE R. MURRAY (1865-1939).—*The Life-History of the First Case of Myxoedema Treated by Thyroid Extract* 272

HYPERTHYROIDISM

CALEB HILLIER PARRY (1755-1822).—*Enlargement of the Thyroid gland in connection with Enlargement or palpitation of the Heart* 275

ROBERT JAMES GRAVES (1795-1853).—*Newly Observed Affection of the Thyroid Gland in Females* 279

CARL A. VON BASEDOW (1799-1854).—*Exophthalmos by Hypertrophy of the Cellular Tissue in the Orbital Cavity* 282

ALBRECHT VON GRAEFE (1828-1870).—*Concerning Basedow's Disease* 285

TETANY

JOHN CLARKE (1761-1815).—*On a peculiar species of convulsion* 287

GOUT

THOMAS SYDENHAM (1624-1689).—*A Treatise on Gout* 288

ADDISON'S DISEASE AND PERNICIOUS ANEMIA

THOMAS ADDISON (1793-1860).—*On the Constitutional and Local Effects of Disease of the Supra-Renal Capsules* 290

PAGET'S DISEASE

SIR JAMES PAGET (1814-1899).—*On a form of chronic inflammation of bones* 294

ACHONDROPLASIA

SAMUEL THOMAS VON SOEMMERRING (1755-1830).—*Pictures and Descriptions of some Monsters* 297

OSTEOMALACIA

THOMAS CADWALADER (1708-1779).—*An Extraordinary Case in Physick* 299

HENRY THOMAS (1776).—*A Remarkable Case of Softness of the Bones* 302

MYOSITIS OSSIFICANS PROGRESSIVA

JOHN FREKE (1688-1756).—*Extraordinary exostoses on the Back of a Boy* ... 303

HEBERDEN'S NODES

WILLIAM HEBERDEN (1710-1801).—*Digitorum Nodi* 304

ACROMEGALY

PIERRE MARIE (1853-1940).—*Two Cases of Acromegaly* 305

FRÖHLICH'S DISEASE

ALFRED FRÖHLICH (1901).—*A Case of Tumor of the Hypophysis Cerebri without Acromegaly* 307

PERSISTENT THYMUS

FELIX PLATTER (1536-1614).—*Suffocation from a concealed internal struma about the throat* 309

III. LEAD POISONING

NIKANDER (Second Century B.C.).—*Theriaca and Alexipharmaca* 312
PAUL OF AEGINA (629-690).—*A colicky affection* 312
FRANÇOIS CITOIS (1572-1652).—*The painful bilious Colic at Poitiers* 313
JOHN HUXHAM (1692-1768).—*On the Devonshire colic* 315
THÉODORE TRONCHIN (1709-1781).—*De colica Pictonum* 317
SIR GEORGE BAKER (1722-1809).—*An Inquiry concerning the Cause of the Endemial Colic of Devonshire* 320
HENRY BURTON (1840).—*Remarkable Effect upon the Human Gums produced by the Absorption of Lead* 324

IV. DISEASES OF THE CIRCULATORY SYSTEM
HEART-BLOCK

MARCUS GERBEZIUS (died 1718).—*Slow pulse* 326
GIOVANNI BATTISTA MORGAGNI (1682-1771).—*Letter the Ninth, Which Treats of Epilepsy* 327
THOMAS SPENS (1769-1842).—*A remarkable Slowness of the Pulse* 330
ROBERT ADAMS (1791-1875).—*Diseases of the Heart* 332
SIR WILLIAM BURNETT (1779-1861).—*A Case of Epilepsy attended with remarkable Slowness of the Pulse* 333
WILLIAM STOKES (1804-1878).—*Repeated pseudo-apoplectic attacks, not followed by paralysis, slow pulse* 335

AORTIC INSUFFICIENCY

WILLIAM COWPER (1666-1709).—*Of Ossifications or Petrifactions . . . in the Valves of the Great Artery* 339
RAYMOND VIEUSSENS (1641-1715).—*Treatise on the Heart* 344
GIOVANNI BATTISTA MORGAGNI (1682-1771).—*The Seats and Causes of Disease* 346
THOMAS HODGKIN (1798-1866).—*On Retroversion of the Valves of the Aorta* 348
JAMES HOPE (1801-1841).—*Signs of Disease of the Aortic Valves* 349
SIR DOMINIC JOHN CORRIGAN (1802-1880).—*On Permanent patency of the Mouth of the Aorta* 352
AUSTIN FLINT (1812-1886).—*On Cardiac Murmurs* 357
HEINRICH QUINCKE (1842-1922).—*Observations on Capillary and Venous Pulse* 361
PAUL-LOUIS DUROZIEZ (1826-1897).—*Double Intermittent Crural Souffle* 363

MITRAL STENOSIS

RAYMOND VIEUSSENS (1641-1715).—*Treatise on the Heart* 364
GIOVANNI BATTISTA MORGAGNI (1682-1771).—*The Seats and Causes of Disease* 367
JEAN NICHOLAS CORVISART (1755-1821).—*The Signs Characteristic of Stenosis of the Orifices* 368
RENÉ-THÉOPHILE-HYACINTHE LAËNNEC (1781-1826).—*Signs of cartilagenous or bony hardening of the valves* 371
R.-J.-H. BERTIN (1767-1828).—*Of the Symptoms and Diagnosis of Induration, and Vegetations of the Valves of the Heart* 372
JAMES HOPE (1801-1841).—*Signs of Disease of the Mitral Valve* 374
S.-A. FAUVEL (1813-1884).—*Stethoscopic Signs of Narrowing of the Left Auriculo-Ventricular Orifice of the Heart* 375
GRAHAM STEELL (1851-1942).—*The Murmur of High-Pressure in the Pulmonary Artery* 376

PULMONARY STENOSIS

JAMES HOPE (1801-1841).—*Signs of Disease of the Pulmonic Valves* 379

AORTIC STENOSIS

JAMES HOPE (1801-1841).—*Signs of Disease of the Aortic Valves* 380
WILLIAM STOKES (1804-1878).—*Extreme Ossific Disease of the Aortic Orifice* 380
JACOB MENDES DACOSTA (1833-1900).—*On Irritable Heart* 381

PULSUS ALTERNANS

LUDWIG TRAUBE (1818-1876).—*A Case of Pulsus bigeminus* 385

GALLOP RHYTHM

PIERRE-CARL POTAIN (1825-1901).—*Concerning the Cardiac Rhythm called Gallop Rhythm* 386

AURICULAR FIBRILLATION

HEINRICH EWALD HERING (1866-   ).—*Pulsus irregularis perpetuus* 390
JAMES MACKENZIE (1853-1925).—*Auricular Fibrillation* 392

EXTRA-SYSTOLES

JAMES MACKENZIE (1853-1925).—*The dropped beat* 397

PAROXYSMAL TACHYCARDIA

WILLIAM STOKES (1804-1878).—*Diseases of the Heart and the Aorta* 397
RICHARD COTTON (1820-1877).—*Unusually rapid action of the heart* 398
L. BOUVERET (1850-1929).—*Concerning essential paroxysmal tachycardia* ... 401

PERICARDITIS

GUILLAUME DE BAILLOU (1538-1616).—*Concerning palpitation of the heart* .. 404
RICHARD LOWER (1631-1691).—*Treatise of the Heart* 404
ALBRECHT VON HALLER (1708-1777).—*Stone in the Heart* 406

LEOPOLD AUENBRUGGER (1722-1809).—*Hydrops of the pericardium* 408
V. COLLIN (1824).—*Sound analogous to the creaking of new leather* 409
THOMAS ROTCH (1849-1914).—*Absence of resonance in the fifth right inter-costal space* 409
SIR WILLIAM BROADBENT (1835-1907).—*Adherent Pericardium* 411
WALTER BROADBENT (1895).—*An Unpublished Physical Sign* 413

ANGINA PECTORIS

EARL OF CLARENDON (1609-1674).—*Life of Edward, Earl of Clarendon* 416
WILLIAM HEBERDEN (1710-1801).—*Pectoris dolor* 418
JOHN FOTHERGILL (1710-1780).—*Farther Account of the Angina Pectoris* ... 422
JOHN HUNTER (1728-1793).—*Autopsy on Body of John Hunter* 423

CORONARY OCCLUSION

ADAM HAMMER (1818-1878).—*Thrombotic Occlusion of One of the Coronary Arteries* 424
GEORGE DOCK (1860-   ).—*Some notes on the Coronary Arteries* 428
WILLIAM OSLER (1849-1919).—*Angina pectoris* 431
JAMES B. HERRICK (1861-   ).—*Sudden obstruction of the coronary arteries* 434

DIGITALIS

WILLIAM WITHERING (1741-1799).—*An Account of the introduction of Fox-glove into Modern Practice* 437

ANEURYSM

JEAN FERNEL (1506-1588).—*Aneurysm* 443
AMBROSE PARÉ (1510-1590).—*Of an Aneurisma, that is, the dilatation or springing of an artery, veine or sinew* 443
RICHARD WISEMAN (1622-1676).—*Of an Aneurisma* 447
GIOVANNI MARIA LANCISI (1654-1720).—*On the Mode of Formation, the Causes and Symptoms of a Syphilitic Aneurism* 448
GIOVANNI BATTISTA MORGAGNI (1682-1771).—*The Seats and Causes of Diseases* 450
JEAN NICHOLAS CORVISART (1775-1821).—*Essay on the maladies and the organic lesions of the heart and of the great vessels* 455
W. S. OLIVER (1836-1908).—*Physical Diagnosis of Thoracic Aneurism* 456

ENDOCARDITIS

LAZARUS RIVERIUS (1589-1626).—*Caruncles resembling a Cluster of Hazelnuts* 458
GIOVANNI BATTISTA MORGAGNI (1682-1771).—*Excrescences on the Valves* ... 459
JEAN BAPTISTE BOUILLAUD (1796-1817).—*Confluent Vegetations on the Valves* 460
RUDOLF VIRCHOW (1821-1902).—*Concerning Acute Inflammation of the Arteries* 461
WILLIAM SENHOUSE KIRKES (1823-1864).—*Detachment of Fibrinous Deposits from the Interior of the Heart* 462
SIR SAMUEL WILKS (1824-1911).—*Pyaemia as a Result of Endocarditis* 467
E. F. H. WINGE (1827-1894).—*Mycosis endocardii* 471

APOPLEXY

JOHANN JAKOB WEPFER (1620-1695).—*Historiae apoplecticorum* 474
GIORGIO BAGLIVI (1668-1706).—*The History of the Sickness of Marcellus Malpighi, the Pope's Physician; with an Account of the Dissection of his Corps* 476

RAYNAUD'S DISEASE

MAURICE RAYNAUD (1834-1881).—*On local asphyxia and symmetrical gangrene of the extremities* 478

BUERGER'S DISEASE

LEO BUERGER (1879-1943).—*Thrombo-angiitis obliterans* 481

ERYTHROMELALGIA

S. WEIR MITCHELL (1830-1914).—*On a rare vaso-motor neurosis of the extremities* 483

V. DISEASES OF THE BLOOD

CHLOROSIS

JOHANNES LANGE (1485-1565).—*Concerning the Disease of the Virgins* 487

PERNICIOUS ANEMIA

JAMES SCARTH COMBE (1796-1883).—*History of a Case of Anæmia* 490
THOMAS ADDISON (1793-1860).—*Addison's Disease, Pernicious Anemia.*
                            See page 290
GEORGE R. MINOT (1885-   ).—*Observations of patients with pernicious anemia partaking of a special diet* 492

SICKLE-CELL ANEMIA

JAMES B. HERRICK (1861-   ).—*Peculiar elongated and sickle-shaped red blood corpuscles* 494

POLYCYTHEMIA

LOUIS HENRI VAQUEZ (1860-1936).—*A special form of cyanosis* 497
WILLIAM OSLER (1849-1919).—*Chronic cyanosis with polycythaemia and enlarged spleen* 500

LEUKEMIA

JOHN HUGHES BENNETT (1812-1875).—*Suppuration of the Blood* 505
RUDOLF VIRCHOW (1821-1902).—*White Blood* 508

PURPURA

AMATUS LUSITANUS (1511-?).—*The Seventieth Cure Which Has to Do with Exanthemata with a Disease Called Flea-Like without Fever Appearing in a Boy* 513
LAZARUS RIVERIUS (1589-1655).—*Of the Pestilential Feavers* 514
PAUL GOTTLIEB WERLHOF (1699-1767).—*Morbus maculosus haemorrhagicus* 517
EDUARD HENOCH (1820-1910).—*Concerning a Peculiar Form of Purpura* 518

HEMOPHILIA

JOHN C. OTTO (1774-1844).—*An Account of an Hemorrhagic Disposition Existing in Certain Families* 521

VI. KIDNEY DISEASES

CHRONIC NEPHRITIS

GUGLIELMO SALICETTI (1210-1280).—*Durities in renibus* 525
FREDERIK DEKKERS (1648-1720).—*Urine limpid, clear in phthisis* 527
DOMENICO COTUGNO (1736-1822).—*Commentary on Nervous Sciatica* 528
WILLIAM CHARLES WELLS (1757-1817).—*On the presence of the red Matter and Serum of Blood in the Urine of Dropsy* 529
JOHN BLACKALL (1771-1860).—*Observations on the Nature and Cure of Dropsies* 530
RICHARD BRIGHT (1789-1858).—*Reports of Medical Cases* 534

PAROXYSMAL HEMOGLOBINURIA

JOHANNIS ACTUARIUS (Thirteenth Century).—*Concerning Urines* 540
DR. DRESSLER (1854).—*A Case of intermittent Albuminuria and Chromaturia* 542
GEORGE HARLEY (1829-1896).—*Intermittent Haematuria* 543
WILLIAM H. DICKINSON (1832-1913).—*Intermittent Haematuria* 546

VII. RESPIRATORY DISEASES

CHEYNE-STOKES' RESPIRATION

HIPPOCRATES (460-370 B.C.).—*Philiscus, who lived by the wall* 548
JOHN CHEYNE (1777-1836).—*A Case of Apoplexy* 548
WILLIAM STOKES (1804-1878).—*Symptoms referrible to the respiratory function* 552

MOUNTAIN SICKNESS

JOSE D'ACOSTA (1590).—*The Naturall and Morall Historie of the East and West Indies* 553

BRONCHIAL CAST

NICHOLAS TULP (1593-1674).—*An Entire Vein Cast Up from the Lungs* 555
RICHARD WARREN (1731-1797).—*Of the Bronchial Polypus* 555

SKODAIC RESONANCE

JOSEF SKODA (1805-1881).—*Treatise on Percussion and Auscultation* 558

LOBAR PNEUMONIA

HIPPOCRATES (460-370 B.C.).—*Regimen in Acute Diseases* 561
ARETAEUS THE CAPPADOCIAN (Second or Third Century A.D.).—*On Pneumonia* 562
LEOPOLD AUENBRUGGER (1722-1809).—*Concerning scirrhus of the lungs and its signs* 563
RENÉ-THÉOPHILE-HYACINTHE LAËNNEC (1781-1826).—*Signs and Symptoms of Peripneumony* 565

PLEURISY AND EMPYEMA

HIPPOCRATES (460-370 B.C.).—*Concerning Diseases* 568
ARETAEUS THE CAPPADOCIAN (Second or Third Century A.D.).—*On Pleurisy* 569
AMBROISE PARÉ (1510-1590).—*Of the Pleurisie* 570
THOMAS WILLIS (1621-1675).—*Of a Pleurisie* 571
LEOPOLD AUENBRUGGER (1722-1809).—*Concerning hydrops of the chest* 573
RENÉ-THÉOPHILE-HYACINTHE LAËNNEC (1781-1826).—*Signs and Symptoms of Acute Pleurisy* 574

ASTHMA

ARETAEUS THE CAPPADOCIAN (Second or Third Century A.D.).—*On asthma* ... 576
THOMAS WILLIS (1621-1675).—*Of an asthma* 577

PNEUMOTHORAX

RENÉ-THÉOPHILE-HYACINTHE LAËNNEC (1781-1826).—*Of the exploration of pneumothorax with liquid effusion* 580

EMPHYSEMA

MATTHEW BAILLIE (1761-1823).—*Enlargement of the Cells of the Lung* 582
RENÉ-THÉOPHILE-HYACINTHE LAËNNEC (1781-1826).—*Of emphysema of the lungs* 583

VIII. DEFICIENCY DISEASES

SCURVY

JACQUES DE VITRY (? -1244).—*A Certain Pestilence* 585
JEAN, SIRE DE JOINVILLE (1224-1319).—*The Army Sickness* 586
JACQUES CARTIER (1491-1557).—From Hakluyt's *Voyages* 587
JAMES LIND (1716-1794).—*A Treatise of the Scurvy* 589
JOHN HUXHAM (1692-1768).—*A Method for preserving the Health of Seamen on long Cruises and Voyages* 592

RICKETS

DANIEL WHISTLER (1619-1684).—*Concerning the disease of English Children* 594
FRANCIS GLISSON (1597-1677).—*A Treatise of the Rickets* 596

SPRUE

ARETAEUS THE CAPPADOCIAN (Second or Third Century A.D.)—*On the Coeliae Affection* 600
VINCENT KETELAER (1669).—*Concerning native aphtha or Sprue of the Belgians* 601
WILLIAM HILLARY (1763).—*Aphthoides chronica, a new disease* 603

BERIBERI

JACOBUS BONTIUS (1592-1631).—*Concerning Paralysis of the type the natives call Beriberi* 604
NICHOLAS TULP (1593-1674.)—*Beriberi of the Indians* 606

PELLAGRA

GASPAR CASÁL (1679-1759).—*Natural and Medical History of the Principality of the Asturias* 607
FRANÇOIS THIÉRY (1755).—*Description of a Malady called Mal de la Rosa* 607
FRANCESCO FRAPOLLI.—*Observations on the Disease commonly called "Pelagra"* 612

NYCTALOPIA

WILLIAM HEBERDEN (1710-1801)—*Of the Nyctalopia or Night-Blindness* ... 615

IX. ALLERGIC DISEASES

HAY-FEVER

LEONARDO POTALLO (born 1530).—*Some have aversion to the odor of roses* .. 616
JOHANN NIKOLAUS BINNINGER (1628-1692).—*Concerning odors extraordinarily affecting & purging the body* 616
JOHN BOSTOCK (1773-1846).—*Case of a Periodical Affection of the Eyes and Chest* 618

ALLERGY IN INFECTIOUS DISEASES

EDWARD JENNER (1749-1823).—*An Inquiry into the Causes and Effects of the Variolae Vaccinae* 621

ANGIONEUROTIC EDEMA

ROBERT JAMES GRAVES (1795-1853).—*Fugitive Inflammation* 623
HEINRICH QUINCKE (1842-1922).—*Acute Localized Oedema of the Skin* 623

X. DISEASES OF THE DIGESTIVE TRACT

CARDIOSPASM

THOMAS WILLIS (1621-1675).—*Vomiting from the Mouth of the Ventricle being affected* 628

PEPTIC ULCER

JEAN CRUVEILHIER (1791-1874).—*Pathological anatomy of the human body* 628

CIRRHOSIS OF THE LIVER

JOHN BROWN (1642-1700).—*The Liver of an hydropical Person* 632
MATTHEW BAILLIE (1761-1823).—*Liver studded with tubercles* 634
RENÉ-THÉOPHILE-HYACINTHE LAËNNEC (1781-1826).—*Organic Diseases of the Liver* 635

GALLSTONES

GENTILE DA FOLIGNO (died 1348).—*Wonderful medical histories* 635
ANTONIO BENIVIENI (1443-1502).—*Stones found in the lining of the liver* 636
MATTEO REALDO COLOMBO (1516-1559).—*Autopsy on body of St. Ignatius of Loyola* 638
JEAN FERNEL (1506-1588).—*Some diseases in the gall bladder* 639
FELIX PLATTER (1536-1614).—*Calculus and sand in the liver* 640
WILHELM FABRY (1560-1634).—*Concerning two stones of enormous size found in the gall bladder* 640

DANIEL SENNERT (1572-1637).—*Concerning calculi, worms and hydatids arising in the liver* 642

FRANCIS GLISSON (1597-1677).—*Calculi in the biliary tract* 642

LORENZ HEISTER (1683-1758).—*Angular stones were found in the gall bladder* 643

GIOVANNI BATTISTA MORGAGNI (1682-1771).—*Concerning the Seats and Causes of Disease* 644

APPENDICITIS

JEAN FERNEL (1497-1558).—*The Causes and Signs of Diseases of the Intestines* 646

LORENZ HEISTER (1683-1758).—*Of an abscess in the vermiform process of the cœcum* 648

MESTIVIER (1757).—*On a tumor situated near the umbilical region* 650

JOUBERT DE LA MOTTE (1766).—*The Opening of the Cadaver of a Person dead of Tympanites* 650

JAMES PARKINSON (1755-1824).—*A Case of Diseased Appendix Vermiformis*.. 651

THOMAS HODGKIN (1798-1866).—*The Morbid Anatomy of the Serous and Mucous Membranes* 652

REGINALD H. FITZ (1843-1913).—*Perforating Inflammation of the Vermiform Appendix* 653

BIBLIOGRAPHY 657

INDEX 669

LIST OF ILLUSTRATIONS

Frontispiece: From Dekkers' *Exercitationes practicae Circa Medendi Methodum.* Leyden, 1694 ....*Frontispiece*

Statue of "Hippocrates" discovered on the island of Cos in 1933 by Professor Luciano Laurenzi 2

Hieronymus Fracastorius Veronensis (1484-1553). From Fracastorius' *Opera omnia.* Venice, 1584 7

Athanasius Kircher (1602-1680). An engraving of Kircher in 1664, age 62. From *Mundus subterraneus,* 1665 10

Nicolo Leoniceno (1428-1524). Portrait by Luigi Rossi. 14

Facsimile page from Juan Almenar's *A Treatise of the French Pocks* 22

Page from Traheron's translation of de Vigo's *Surgery,* first edition, 1543. This page describes the appearance of syphilis in Europe 24

Title page from Johannis de Vigo's *Practica in arte chirurgia copiosa,* 1514 ... 25

A page from the fifth book of de Vigo's *Chyrurgia: De Morbo Gallico* 27

Ulrich von Hutten (1488-1523). From a woodcut in von Hutten's *Gesprächbüchlein,* 1519 29

Title page from Jacques de Béthencourt's *Nova penitentialis quadragesima,* Paris, 1527 35

Statue of Fracastorius (1483-1553) by Danese Cattaneo, on the Piazza del Signori in Verona, erected in 1559. Kindness of Mr. R. Lier 38

First page of text from *Hieronymus Fracastorius, Syphilis, Sive Morbus Gallicus.* First Edition. Verona, 1530 40

John Hunter (1728-1793). Engraving from a painting by Sir Joshua Reynolds 43

Sir Jonathan Hutchinson (1828-1913). From a drawing by Walter Benington. 47

Richard Wiseman (1622-1676). From a miniature in the possession of His Grace the Duke of Rutland 53

Franciscus de le Boë Sylvius (1614-1672). An engraving by T. L. Durant. Frontispiece to *Opera medica.* Geneva, 1680 59

Richard Morton (1637-1698). From the frontispiece to *Phthisiologia: or a Treatise of Consumptions.* London, 1694 61

Jean-Antoine Villemin (1827-1892) 67

René-Théophile-Hyacinthe Laënnec (1781-1826). Lithograph by Formentin, published by Rosselin 69

Frontispiece of Thucydides' "Eight Bookes of the Peloponnesian Warre," translated by Thomas Hobbes, London, 1676 72

Guy de Chauliac (1300?-1368) 78

First page of "a litil boke" by the "Bisshop of Arusiens," Bengt Knutsson, published in London about 1485. Reproduced from the facsimile edition published by the University of Manchester Press in 1910 83

Frontispiece of Thomas Johnson's translation of Paré's works, published in London, 1644 89

Burying of the Dead in the Great Pit. A drawing by George Cruikshank from Defoe's *Journal of the Plague Year,* edition of 1876 92

Albert Freeman Africanus King (1841-1914) 104

Sir Ronald Ross (1857-1932). From *Ronald Ross* by R. L. Mégroz. (Allen & Unwin, London.) Photo by Haines 109

Josiah C. Nott (1804-1873). From *American Journal of Obstetrics* 122

Carlos J. Finlay (1833-1915) 125

Walter Reed (1851-1902) 130

Guillaume de Baillou (1538-1616). Etching by Jasper Isac from Baillou's de Morbis mulierum ac virginum liber. Paris, 1643 138

Nicholas Tulp (1593-1674). Engraving by L. Visscher. The frontispiece to *Observationes Medicae*. Leyden, 1716 140

John Fothergill (1712-1780). From the frontispiece to *A Sketch of the Life of John Fothergill* by James Hack Tuke, London, n.d. From the cameo by Wedgwood 143

John Huxham (1692-1768). Portrait by T. Rennell, engraved by J. Jenkins ... 147

Francis Home (1719-1813). From Comrie's *History of Scottish Medicine* 150

Samuel Bard (1742-1821). Drawing by McCleland. Etching by W. Main. From *American Medical Biography* by James Thacher. Boston, 1828 154

Pierre Bretonneau (1778-1862). Portrait by Moreau of Tours 158

Jerome Cardan (1501-1576). In his forty-ninth year. Woodcut from *De subtilitate libri XXI*. Basle, 1611 162

Tobias Cober (-1625). Frontispiece of *Observationum medicarum castrensium Hungaricarum decades tres*. Helmstad 1685 166

Pierre Charles Alexandre Louis (1787-1872) 185

Elisha North (1771-1843) 190

Daniel Sennert (1572-1637). Portrait of Sennert in 1627 drawn by August Buchner and engraved by Matthew Merian 192

Thomas Sydenham (1624-1689). From the portrait by Maria Beale and etched by Blooteling. Frontispiece to *Observationes Medicae* 1676 194

John Caius (1510-1573). From the portrait presented by Dr. Caius to the Gonville and Caius College. Artist unknown 203

John Haygarth (1740-1827). Frontispiece to *A clinical history of diseases*, London, 1805. From an etching by W. Cooke 216

Jean Bouillaud (1796-1881). Portrait by C. H. Lehman, 1875 221

Johann Lukas Schönlein (1793-1864). An engraving by Carl Mayer. Reproduced from the fifth edition of Schönlein's *Allgemeine und specielle Pathologie und Therapie* 226

Benjamin Rush (1745-1813). Portrait by Sully. From the engraving by Edwin. From *American Medical Biography* by James Thacher. Boston, 1828 228

Thomas Hodgkin (1798-1866). From the portrait in possession of Mrs. Lucy Hodgkin. Artist unknown 231

Facsimile of a page from the *Papyrus Ebers* 234

Thomas Willis (1621-1675). A copper engraving at the age of forty-five by Isabella Piccini. From the frontispiece of *Opera Omnia*. Geneva, 1694 ... 239

Title page of *Medical observations and inquiries by A Society of Physicians in London*. Volume V. London, 1776 243

Adolf Kussmaul (1822-1902). Portrait by Franz von Lenbach, 1895 246

Oskar Minkowski (1858-1931). From the *Münchener Medizinische Wochenschrift* 249

A plate from Opie's article on the Islands of Langerhans 255

Sir Frederick Grant Banting (1892-1944). Photograph by Ashley & Crippen 257

Paracelsus at the age of forty-seven. Reproduction of a woodcut from Paracelsus' *Operum Medico-Chimicorum sive Paradoxorum*, Frankfort, 1603. This is a variant of the engraving by Augustin Hirschvogel 259

A page from Paracelsus' *Opera Omnia*, Strassburg, 1603, describing cretinism and endemic goitre 261

Title-page from Felix Platter's *Praxeos medicae*. Basle, 1656 262

Felix Platter (1536-1614). From a painting by Hans Bock. In the Naturhistorisches Museum, Basle 263

Frontispiece from Wolfgang Hoefer's *Hercules Medicus*, first edition, 1657 265

Sir William Gull (1816-1890). From *A Collection of the Published Writings of William Withey Gull*, London, 1896 269

Caleb Hillier Parry (1755-1822). Engraving by Philip Audinet from a miniature sketch by John Hay Bell, 1804 275

Robert James Graves (1795-1853). From *Medical History of Meath Hospital* 279

Carl A. von Basedow (1799-1854). From *Münchener Medizinische Wochenschrift* 282

Albrecht von Graefe (1828-1870). Drawing by R. Lehman 285

Thomas Addison (1793-1860). Frontispiece to *A Collection of the Published Writings of Thomas Addison*. London, 1868 291

Sir James Paget (1814-1899). Portrait by George Richmond, 1867 295

Samuel Thomas von Soemmerring (1755-1830). Portrait by Thelot. Frontispiece to *Samuel Thomas von Soemmerring* by Wilhelm Stricker, Frankfurt am Main, 1862 297

Illustration of Achondroplasia. From Soemmerring's *Abbildungen und Beschreibungen einiger Misgeburten die sich ehemals auf dem anatomischen Theater zu Cassel befanden*, Mayence, 1791 298

Thomas Cadwalader (1708-1779). Portrait by Charles Wilson Peale (1770) in the College of Physicians, Philadelphia 300

A remarkable case of the softness of the bones by Henry Thomas. From the *Medical Observations and Inquiries*. Vol. v. London, 1776 303

Pierre Marie's first case of acromegaly 305

The patient in Fröhlich's article on *A Case of Tumor of the Hypophysis Cerebri without Acromegaly*. From the *Wiener Klinische Rundschau*, 1901 308

Title-page of Nikander's *Theriaca & Alexipharmaca*. From the translation by Euricius Cordus. Frankfort, 1532 311

Title-page from the Latin version of Paul of Aegina's works by Johannes von Andernach. Venice, 1542 313

Title-page of *De novo et populari apud Pictones dolore Colico bilioso Diatriba* by François Citois. Poitiers, 1616 314

Théodore Tronchin (1709-1781). After a pastel by Liotave 318

Title-page of *De colica pictonum* by Théodore Tronchin. Geneva, 1757 320

Sir George Baker (1722-1809). From G. P. Harding's drawing on stone of the miniature by Ozias Humphrey, Esq., R.A. 321

Giovanni Battista Morgagni (1682-1771). Drawing by Nathaniel Dance, Etched by Angelica Kauffman 328

William Stokes (1804-1878). Drawing by Sir Frederick Burton, 1849 336

William Cowper (1666-1709). Portrait by Closterman 340

Figures 1, 2, 3, 4, and 5 showing ossification in the coats of arteries. From Chapter xxiv of the *Philosophical Transactions of the Royal Society*, London, 1706. Engraver, M. Vander Gucht 342

Raymond Vieussens (1641-1715). Frontispiece to *Œuvres Françoises* de M. Vieussens. Toulouse, 1715 345

James Hope (1801-1841). From the biography, *Memoir of the late James Hope, M.D.*—written by Mrs. Hope and published in London in 1848 350

Sir Dominic John Corrigan (1802-1880). The portrait by W. Catterson Smith which hangs in the Royal College of Physicians, Dublin 353

Austin Flint (1812-1886). From William B. Atkinson's *Physicians and Surgeons of the United States*, Charles Robson. Philadelphia, 1878 358

An illustration of mitral stenosis from Vieussens' *Traité nouveau de la structure et des causes du mouvement naturel du cœur*. Toulouse, 1715 367

Jean Nicholas Corvisart (1755-1821). Portrait by Charles Bazin. Etching by Delpech 369

Jacob M. Da Costa (1833-1900). From *Memoir of Da Costa* by J. C. Wilson, 1902 382

Curve of Pulsus alternans from Traube's article on *A case of pulsus bigeminus* in the *Berliner Klinische Wochenschrift*, 1872 386

Pierre-Carl Potain (1829-1901). From *Bulletin de l'Academie de Médicine*, 1927, xcviii, 569 387

Heinrich Ewald Hering (1866-   ), from the *Münchener Medizinsche Wochenschrift* 391

Sir James Mackenzie (1853-1925). Photograph by Emery Walker 393

Richard Lower (1631-1691). Portrait of Lower at the age of 55 years 405

Albrecht von Haller (1708-1777). Portrait by E. J. Handemann, engraved by P. F. Tardieu 407

Sir William H. Broadbent (1835-1907). Photograph by Elliot and Fry 412

The Earl of Clarendon. Frontispiece to *The Life of Edward Earl of Clarendon* (Oxford 1759). Drawn by P. Lely. Etched by R. White 417

William Heberden (1710-1801). Reproduced from a portrait by Sir William Beechey, R.A. 419

Adam Hammer (1818-1878). From a painting by Dr. Adolf Neubert 425

George Dock (1806-   ) 429

James B. Herrick (1861-   ). Photograph by Walinger, Chicago 435

William Withering (1741-1799) 438

Ambroise Paré (1510-1590). A portrait of Paré at the age of 75. From *Les œuvres d'Ambroise Paré*. Lyon, 1633 444

Giovanni Maria Lancisi (1654-1720). Etching by Sebastian Conra 449

Giovanni Battista Morgagni (1682-1771). From the frontispiece to *De sedibus et causis morborum*, 1761 451

William Senhouse Kirkes (1823-1864) 463

Sir Samuel Wilks (1824-1911) 468

Emanuel Fredrik Hagbarth Winge (1827-1894) 472

Johann Jakob Wepfer (1620-1693). From *Historiae apoplecticorum*. Amsterdam, 1724 475

An illustration of gangrene of the extremities from Maurice Raynaud's *De l'asphyxie locale et de la gangrène symétrique des extrémités*, Paris, 1862 478

Leo Buerger (1879-1943). Photograph by Marceau, New York 482

S. Weir Mitchell (1830-1914) 484

Johannes Lange (1485-1565). Frontispiece to Lange's *Epistolarum medicinalium*. Frankfort, 1589 489

George Richards Minot (1885-   ). Photograph by Alfred Brown, Brookline,
    Massachusetts 492
Louis Henri Vaquez (1860-1936) 498
Sir William Osler (1849-1919). The head of Osler from Sargent's famous paint-
    ing *The Four Doctors* in the Welch Library of the Johns Hopkins Univer-
    sity 501
Rudolf Virchow (1821-1902) 509
Title page of the *Curationum Medicinalium* of Amatus Lusitanus. Lyons, 1580   513
Lazarus Riverius (1589-1655). Frontispiece to *The Practice of Physick* trans-
    lated by Nicholas Culpepper, London, 1668 515
Paul Gottlieb Werlhof (1699-1767). From Werlhof's *Opera Omnia*. Hanover,
    1775 517
Eduard Henoch (1820-1910). From the *Münchener Medizinische Wochen-
    schrift* 519
John C. Otto (1774-1844). From lithograph in College of Physicians, Phila-
    delphia 522
William de Saliceto (1210-1280). From the bas-relief of Ferranini at Piacenza   525
A page from Saliceto's chapter on *Sclerosis of the Kidneys* 526
Sir Richard Bright (1789-1858). Portrait by T. R. Say 534
Page from *De urinis* by Joannes Actuarius. Basle, 1529 541
George Harley (1829-1896). 544
John Cheyne (1777-1836). Engraving by F. C. Lewis. From *Essays on partial
    derangement of the mind in supposed connection with religion*. Dublin, 1843   549
Tulp's illustration of bronchial cast 556
Warren's illustration of bronchial cast 557
Joseph Skoda (1805-1881). From Sternberg's *Josef Skoda*, Vienna, 1924   559
Leopold Auenbrugger (1722-1809). Painted in 1770. Artist unknown. Restored
    by Kurt von Goldenstein 563
A plate from Matthew Baillie's *Morbid Anatomy* of a lung showing emphysema   582
James Lind (1716-1794). Portrait by Sir George Chalmers 590
Daniel Whistler (1619-1684). Portrait in the Royal College of Physicians, Lon-
    don 594
Francis Glisson (1597-1677). Glisson at the age of 30. From the drawing by
    W. Faithorne 596
Frontispiece from Glisson's *De rachitide*. Leyden, 1671 598
Title page of Ketelaer's *de Aphthis*, 1672 602
A patient suffering from pellagra. From Casal's *Historia natural y medica de el
    principado de Asturias*, Madrid, 1762 608
Frontispiece to Botalli's *Opera Omnia*. Leyden, 1660 614
Johann Nikolaus Binninger (1628-1692). From a portrait appearing in Bin-
    ninger's *Observationum et curationum medicinalium*. Montbéliard, 1673 ..   617
John Bostock (1733-1846). From Jenkins' engraving of a portrait of Bostock
    by Partridge 619
Edward Jenner (1749-1823). From a portrait by J. R. Smith, 1801 621
Heinrich Quincke (1842-1922) 624
Title page of *Pharmaceutice rationalis*, by Thomas Willis, London, 1679   626
Jean Cruveilhier (1791-1874). Engraving by Lasnier, 1865 629
Illustrations of ulcer of the stomach. From Cruveilhier's *Anatomie Patholo-
    gique du corps humain*. Paris, 1835-1842 630

John Brown (1642-1700). Brown at the age of 35. From the frontispiece to
   A complete treatise of preternatural tumours. London, 1678 633
An illustration of cirrhosis of the liver from Brown's article in the *Philosophical
   Transactions of the Royal Society*. London, 1685 634
Cirrhosis of the liver. A plate from Matthew Baillie's *Morbid Anatomy* 634
Picture of Gentile da Foligno from Avicenna's *Canonis libri*, Venice, 1520 636
Introduction to Benivieni's *de abditis*. Basle, 1529 637
Illustrations of gallstones from Guilhelmi Fabricii Hildani *Opera Observationum
   et Curationum Medico-Chirurgicarum Quae Extant Omnia*, Francofurto
   MDCLXXXII 640
Wilhelm Fabry von Hilden (1560-1634) 641
Jean Fernel (1497?-1558). From his *Therapeutics Universalis*. Frankfort, 1581   647
Lorenz Heister (1683-1758). From the frontispiece to Heister's *Medicinische
   Chirurgische und Anatomische Wahrnehmungen*. Rostock, 1753 649
Reginald H. Fitz (1843-1913). From a photograph in the Library of the Jackson
   County (Mo.) Medical Society 653

Classic Descriptions
of Disease

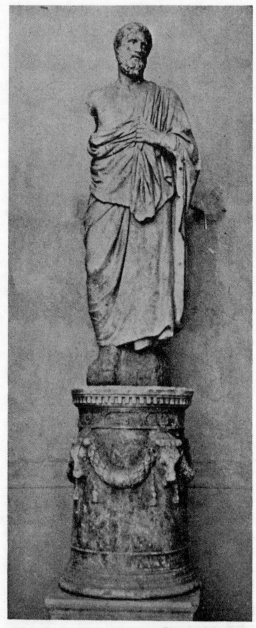

Statue of "Hippocrates" discovered on the Island of
Cos in 1933 by Professor Luciano Laurenzi.

INTRODUCTION

Hippocrates

"Life is short, and the Art long; the occasion fleeting; experience fallacious, and judgment difficult. The physician must not only be prepared to do what is right himself, but also to make the patient, the attendants and the externals cooperate." Thus runs the first aphorism of Hippocrates on whom history has bestowed the title of the "Father of Medicine." His countrymen believed he was descended from Aesculapius, the God of Healing and most of the stories we possess concerning his life are legends and not historical facts. He was born about 460 B.C. on the island of Cos and had as contemporaries some of the greatest men of all time: Pericles the statesman; the poets Aeschylus, Sophocles, Euripides, Aristophanes, and Pindar; the philosophers Socrates and Plato; the historians Herodotus, Xenophon, and Thucydides; and the unrivalled sculptor Phidias. He inherited a distinguished position in the Temple of Aesculapius at Cos and began the study of medicine there. He studied for a time at the neighboring school of Cnidos and then returned to Cos. Later he travelled extensively and practised in Thrace, Delos, and Thessaly. According to a tradition he stamped out the great plague of Athens by the expedient of building fires. Thucydides however, an eye-witness of that plague, does not mention Hippocrates and further states that all measures employed in combatting the plague were unsuccessful. Hippocrates died in Thessaly, circa 375 B.C. His sons Thessalus and Draco and his son-in-law Polybus were famous and successful physicians.

Hippocrates was primarily a physician, endowed with remarkable powers of observation and with an unusual store of common sense. Instead of attributing disease to the gods and speculating as to why man was punished, Hippocrates, unlike the generations of philosopher-physicians who had preceded him, avoided all speculation. "Some say," he wrote, "both physicians and sophists, that it is impossible to understand medicine, unless we know what man is, how he originated, and how he became, in the beginning an actual body ... but for myself, I believe, that all these forms of speech of sophists and physicians, and all that they write on nature belongs to the business of writing and not to medicine itself." Hippocrates stressed the study of patients and the symptoms they presented. He founded the bedside method of study, neglected for centuries and then revived with such signal success. His forty-two clinical cases were almost the only record of the kind for the next 1700 years. He recorded his failures as well as his successes. "I have written this down deliberately," he says, "believing it to be valuable to learn of unsuccessful experiences and to know the cause of their failure."

Many of the oldest known descriptions of disease are from Hippocrates. "It has often been remarked that his clinical pictures of phthisis, puerperal septicaemia, epilepsy, epidemic parotitis, the quotidian, tertian, and quartan varieties of remittent fever, and some other diseases, might, with a few changes and additions, take their place in any modern text-book" (Garrison). He was a

precursor of Laënnec in the discovery of auscultation. In his Second Book on
Diseases, he notes that in pleurisy one hears "a sound like that made by
leather." In the same book, when discussing hydrothorax, he notes "if one
places his ear against the chest and listens for a long time, he hears it bubbling
inside like vinegar." The terms "Hippocratic facies," "Hippocratic fingers," and
"Hippocratic succussion" are familiar to every medical student. The first selection describes the Hippocratic facies and the second the curved nails. Later
selections describe the pleural friction rub and râles. Since Hippocrates mentions specifically placing the ear against the chest, he was apparently familiar
with immediate auscultation and, it is probable, that he employed this method
when he heard râles, the pleural friction rub and the succussion splash.

Many translations of Hippocrates' works have been made. The English
translation by Francis Adams ranks among the best. Adams was a country
physician in the little Scotch village of Banchory, where, in the midst of an
arduous and extensive practice, he found time to read "almost every Greek work
which has come down to us from antiquity except the ecclesiastical writers." His
translation of Hippocrates appeared in 1849. In addition to this translation, he
also translated the works of Paulus Aegineta and of Aretaeus.

The familiar bust in the British Museum so frequently reproduced as the
bust of Hippocrates, is not that of the great physician but represents the stoic
philosopher Chrysippus. In 1933, Professor Luciano Laurenzi, in the course of
his excavations on the island of Cos, discovered a statue which many believe
to be of Hippocrates. This statue, which is the work of a Greek sculptor and
dates from the third century B.C., is reproduced on *page 2*.

THE BOOK OF PROGNOSTICS*

1. It appears to me a most excellent thing
for the physician to cultivate Prognosis; for
by foreseeing and foretelling, in the presence
of the sick, the present, the past, and the
future, and explaining the omissions which
patients have been guilty of, he will be the
more readily believed to be acquainted with
the circumstances of the sick; so that men
will have confidence to entrust themselves to
such a physician. And he will manage the
cure best who has foreseen what is to happen
from the present state of matters. For it is
impossible to make all the sick well; this
indeed, would have been better than to be
able to foretell what is going to happen; but
since men die, some even before calling the
physician, from the violence of the disease,
and some die immediately after calling him,
having lived, perhaps, only one day or a
little longer, and before the physician could

bring his art to counteract the disease; it
therefore becomes necessary to know the
nature of such affections, how far they are
above the powers of the constitution; and,
moreover, if there is anything divine in the
diseases, and to learn a foreknowledge of
this also. Thus a man will be the more
esteemed to be a good physician, for he will
be the better able to treat those aright who
can be saved, from having anticipated everything; and by seeing and announcing beforehand those who will live and those who will
die, he will thus escape censure.

2. He would observe thus in acute diseases: first, the countenance of the patient,
if it be like those of persons in health, and
more so, if like itself, for this is the best of
all; thereas the most opposite to it is the
worst, such as the following: *a sharp nose,
hollow eyes, collapsed temples; the ears cold,
contracted, and their lobes turned out; the
skin about the forehead being rough, distended, and parched; the color of the whole*

* *The Genuine Works of Hippocrates,* translated by Francis Adams, New York, Wm. Wood,
n.d., I, p. 194.

face being green, black, livid, or lead-colored. If the countenance be such at the commencement of the disease, and if this cannot be accounted for from the other symptoms, inquiry must be made whether the patient has long wanted sleep; whether his bowels have been very loose; and whether he has suffered from want of food; and if any of these causes be confessed to, the danger is to be reckoned so far less; and it becomes obvious, in the course of a day and a night, whether or not the appearance of the countenance proceeded from these causes. But if none of these be said to exist, and if the symptoms do not subside in the aforesaid time, it is to be known that certain death is at hand. And, also, if the disease be in a more advanced stage either on the third or fourth day, and the countenance be such, the same inquiries as formerly directed are to be made, and the other symptoms are to be noted, those in the whole countenance, those on the body, and those in the eyes; for if they shun the light, or weep involuntarily, or squint, or if the one be less than the other, or if the white of them be red, livid, or has black veins in it; if there be a gum upon the eyes, if they are restless, protruding, or are become very hollow; and if the countenance be squalid and dark, or the color of the whole face be changed—all these are to be reckoned bad and fatal symptoms. The physician should also observe the appearance of the eyes from below the eyelids in sleep; for when a portion of the white appears, owing to the eyelids not being closed together, and when this is not connected with diarrhoea or purgation from medicine, or when the patient does not sleep thus from habit, it is to be reckoned an unfavorable and very deadly symptom; but if the eyelid be contracted, livid, or pale, or also the lip or nose, along with some of the other symptoms, one may know for certain that death is close at hand. It is a mortal symptom, also, when the lips are relaxed, pendent, cold, and blanched.

3. It is well when the patient is found by his physician reclining upon either his right or his left side, having his hands, neck, and legs slightly bent, and the whole body lying in a relaxed state, for thus the most of persons in health recline, and these are the best postures which most resemble those of healthy persons. But to lie upon one's back, with the hands, neck, and legs extended, is far less favorable. And if the patient incline forward, and sink down to the foot of the bed, it is a still more dangerous symptom; but if he be found with his feet naked and not sufficiently warm, and the hands, neck and legs tossed about in a disorderly manner and naked, it is bad, for it indicates aberration of intellect. It is a deadly symptom, also, when the patient sleeps constantly with his mouth open, having his legs strongly bent and plaited together, when he lies upon his back; and to lie upon one's belly, when not habitual to the patient to sleep thus while in good health, indicates delirium, or pain in the abdominal regions. And for the patient to wish to sit erect at the acme of a disease is a bad symptom in all acute diseases, but particularly so in pneumonia. To grind the teeth in fever, when such has not been the custom of the patient from childhood, indicates madness and death, both which dangers are to be announced beforehand as likely to happen; and if a person in delirium do this, it is a deadly symptom. And if the patient had an ulcer previously, or if one has occurred in the course of the disease, it is to be observed; for if the man be about to die the sore will become livid and dry, or yellow and dry before death.

4. Respecting the movement of the hands I have these observations to make: When in acute fevers, pneumonia, phrenitis, or headache, the hands are waved before the face, hunting through empty space, as if gathering bits of straw, picking the nap from the coverlet, or beating chaff from the wall—all such symptoms are bad and deadly.

5. Respiration, when frequent, indicates pain or inflammation in the parts above the diaphragm: a large respiration performed at a great interval announces delirium; but a cold respiration at nose or mouth is a very fatal symptom. Free respiration is to be looked upon as contributing much to the safety of the patient in all acute diseases, such as fevers, and those complaints which come to a crisis in forty days.

* * *

17. Empyema may be recognized in all cases by the following symptoms: In the first place, the fever does not go off, but is slight during the day, and increases at night, and copious sweats supervene, there is a desire to cough, and the patients expectorate

nothing worth mentioning, the eyes become hollow, the cheeks have red spots on them, the nails of the hands are bent, the fingers are hot, especially their extremities, there are swellings in the feet, they have no desire for food, and small blisters (phlyctaenae) occur over the body. These symptoms attend

chronic empyemata, and may be much trusted to; and such as are of short standing are indicated by the same, provided they be accompanied by those signs which occur at the commencement, and if at the same time the patient has some difficulty of breathing.

I. INFECTIOUS DISEASES

THE THEORY OF INFECTION
Hieronymus Fracastorius Veronensis

CHAPTER I*
WHAT IS CONTAGION?

Now we will speak of contagion, on account of which there are so many questions concerning the sympathy and antipathy of things, and we will begin with general questions and then other principles.

According therefore as the name indicates, contagion is an infection passing from one individual to another. For a contagion there must be two factors, either two different individuals or two contiguous parts of the same individual: indeed of that between different individuals we speak as simply and properly contagion, of that between two parts of the same person, we do not speak of as a true contagion but of a sort of contagion. Moreover the infection is seen to be the same for him who has received or has given the infection: also we speak of infection when the same virus has touched one or the other. Also as to those who die from having imbibed poison, we say perhaps they are infected but not that they have suffered from contagion. And in the air where milk, meat and other things normally become putrid, we say there has been a corruption but not that they have suffered a contagion, nor that the air itself was similarly corrupted: and we will investigate this diligently in the subsequent chapters.

Every action and occurrence takes place upon the substance of bodies or their appendages: therefore we do not say anyone has received contagion, who was vexed or corrupted by another, for it is seen that contagion is an infection of the substance itself of bodies.

Now therefore, when a burning house destroys its neighbors, do we call it contagion? Certainly not, this is not called contagion, not in general because the house has been destroyed first and then destroys everything but because infection itself is composed of minute and insensible particles and proceeds

* Hieronymus Fracastorius Veronensis, *Opera omnia*, Venice, Junta, 1584, pp. 77-78.

from them; and which the term infection indicates, for we do not call infection a destruction that is total, but only to a certain degree, and from insensible particles.

For I call the whole composite picture, indeed the small and insensible particles, of

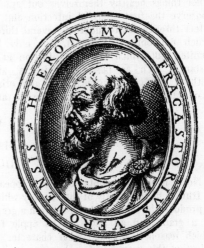

HIERONYMUS FRACASTORIUS VERONENSIS
(1484-1553)

From Fracastorius' *Opera omnia*.
Venice, 1584

which the whole is composed, contagion. A fire is seen therefore to act on the whole, a contagion on the component parts, but the whole may be destroyed soon by them, therefore contagion is considered as a condition produced by the mixing. But as mixtures can be destroyed or damaged in two fashions, one method by the advent of a contrary element, so that they do not preserve their form, the other method by a dissolution of the mixture, as happens in putrefaction, so perhaps the doubt arises whether contagion is only caused by infection brought by small particles, and this indeed be infection, or whether by a corruption of these particles, or rather only by a change, and which indeed may happen: wherefore it may be questioned whether all contagion may not be a putrefaction. More-over all these questions are clearer, if we seek diligently first the fundamental differences and the causes of contagions.

* * *

CHAPTER II
CONCERNING THE FUNDAMENTAL DIFFERENCES OF CONTAGIONS

The fundamental differences of all contagions are seen to be three in number: those infecting by contact alone, those only by contact and leaving fomites by which they are contagious such as scabies, phthisis, itch, baldness, elephantiasis and others of this sort, I call fomites, clothing, screens and other things healthy themselves but apt to conserve the first seeds of infection and to infect through them and then several things which not only by contact, not only by fomites, but which transfer infection at a distance, such as pestilential fevers, and phthisis and certain ophthalmia and other exanthemata, which are called variola and the like. And these are seen to follow a certain rule, those which produce contagion from a distance are accustomed to infect both by fomites and by contact, those which are contagious through fomites are also contagious by contact. At a distance all are not contagious but all are by contact, thus it is most simple that we occupy ourselves with studying first that contagion. which infects solely by contact, and its cause inquiring in what manner it takes place and of what origin soon then studying other questions so that we may see whether there be any character common to all or differing in certain instances and what characteristic each one may have.

* * *

CHAPTER III
CONCERNING CONTAGION WHICH IS PRODUCED BY CONTACT ALONE

Not it is observed contagion which appears in fruit to be the mostly of that variety which is produced by contact alone, as from a grape to a grape and an apple to an apple for which reason it is asked what character of infection this may be: for they are spoiled by contact first with one of them which became rotten that is evident, but from what cause it is not evident. But the first one from whom all the infection passed to the others became putrid, and it would be agreed that the second received a similar putrefaction if indeed contagion and infection are. similar to each other. For putrefaction is a dissolution of this mixture by the evaporation of the innate heat and moisture, indeed the cause of this evaporation is always a strange heat, whether it be in the air, whether in the surrounding humidity: therefore although the cause of the putrefaction is one or the other, the cause of the contagion is identical, that is external heat.

But this heat in the first place comes either from the air or from somewhere else and is not yet called infection, in the second place it comes from those insensible particles which evaporate from the first one. and now there is contagion because the infection is similar in both cases. Moreover the heat evaporating from the first could produce in the second, that which the air produced in the first, and in like manner cause putrefaction, indeed more likely because of the resemblance.

Now, moreover, among the particles which evaporate from the first cause are some which are hot and dry, either of themselves or from mixing, others are hot and humid, either of themselves or from mixing. Those hot and dry are seen to be more apt to burn. but less apt to cause putrefaction. Indeed those which are hot and humid, are on the contrary more likely to cause putrefaction, indeed less likely to burn. For humidity softens and loosens and renders easily separable the parts it touches. but heat raises them up and separates them. Hence a dissolution of the mixture was caused by the evaporating heat and the innate humidity, which dissolution was putrefaction.

Wherefore it should be considered that the hot and humid particles, either by themselves, or from the humid mixture, which evaporate from the first fruit, are the active principle and seeds of this putrefaction, which it produces in the second fruit. I say moreover the humidity from the mixture, because in the evaporations, which take place in putrefying things, it happens that small particles are mixed as much as possible, and thus the active principle is formed now of some generations now of new corruptions. And this mixture, which is made from heat with humidity, is moreover most suited to the production of putrefactions and contagions. In fruits therefore which contagion strikes, it is considered to be caused by this principle, and also in all other fruit too, which the putrefying fruit itself touches, if conditions be similar the same thing happens and it is right to consider it due to the same cause: moreover this principle consists of those small insensible particles which evaporate, indeed hot and acrid but of a humid mixture which henceforth are called seeds of contagion.

Athanasius Kircher

Athanasius Kircher was born at Geisa in 1602 and received his preliminary education at the Jesuit College of Fulda. In 1618 he entered the Jesuit order at Paderborn and remained there until 1622, when the seminary was dissolved and its inmates forced to flee before the army of the warlike Lutheran Bishop of Halberstadt. He completed his studies at Cologne, Coblence and Heiligenstadt, and then became professor of philosophy, mathematics and Oriental languages at Würzburg. The approach of the Swedish army under Gustavus Adolphus led to the abandonment of the college and both teachers and pupils sought safety in flight. "As everything in Germany," he wrote, "was topsy-turvy and there was no hope of returning or remaining," he proceeded to Avignon where he taught mathematics and began his studies of Egyptian hieroglyphics, a study which remained one of his major interests throughout his life. In 1635 he went to Rome at the command of Pope Urban VIII and was made professor of mathematics at the Collegium Romanum. He held this chair for forty-five years, until his death in 1680.

Kircher was a man of wide and varied learning and enjoyed a tremendous reputation during his life-time. He was the author of more than forty books on magnetism, optics, sun-dials, acoustics, music, astronomy, mechanics, arithmetic, natural history, medicine, philosophy, theology, philology, universal language, archeology, history, geography, prestidigitation, and magic. A man of prodigious memory and of a remarkable industry, he was profoundly lacking in judgment and in critical sense. One of his biographers, Brischar, links his name with those of Galileo and Newton, while another Erman, describes him bluntly as a charlatan, and adds that "he was not an investigator, who was satisfied, when the few experts understood his works; what his nature needed was the empty admiration of the so-called 'wide circles' and in order not to lose this he didn't stop at forgeries."

He was probably the first investigator to employ the microscope in the study of disease. He described animaliculae in putrefying meat, in sour milk and in rotten wood. While he could not possibly have seen the plague bacillus with the microscope he employed, he may possibly have seen larger bacilli. He was undoubtedly the first to express the doctrine that contagious diseases were spread by small living animals invisible to the naked eye, although

Fracastorius had previously expressed a similar idea "as if in terms of physical chemistry" (Garrison). Kircher, who was interested in all natural phenomena, was an eye-witness of the epidemic of plague which raged in Rome during the

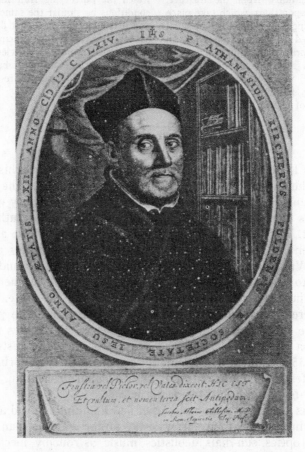

ATHANASIUS KIRCHER (1602-1680)
An engraving of Kircher in 1664, age 62. From *Mundus subterraneus*. Amsterdam, 1665

years 1656 and 1657. His *Scrutinium physico-medicum Contagiosae Luis, quae Pestis dicitur* appeared in Rome in 1658 and was dedicated to Pope Alexander VII.

§II

CONFIRMING EXPERIMENTS*

Everything putrid filled with worms.

Therefore it is certain that the air, water and earth are filled with innumerable small animals; and furthermore that they can be

* Kircher, Athanasius, *Scrutinium physico-medicum contagiosae luis quae pestis dicitur*, Rome, Mascardi, 1658, pp. 43, 50, and 140-142.

demonstrated. It has been moreover known to everyone that worms grow from putrefying corpses; but since that admirable invention the microscope, it is known that everything putrid is filled with innumerable worms, invisible to the naked eye; which moreover I would not have believed had I not proved it by the experiments of many years. In order to demonstrate this, note

Experiment I

Spoiled meat filled with worms

Take a piece of meat, leave it exposed at night to a wet moon until early the following morning, then study it with the microscope, and you will find, that through the corruption contracted from the moon it has been filled with innumerable worms of different sizes which cannot be seen without the microscope, except those which have grown large and are visible. The same you will find in cheese, milk and vinegar and in numerous similar spoiled substances. But the microscope must not be carelessly set up, but by a hand not only diligent but expert; my own is such that objects appear a thousand times larger than they really are.

Milk, cheese, vinegar filled with worms.

* * *

CHAPTER VIII

THE PUTRID CADAVERS OF THOSE INFECTED WITH THE PLAGUE FROM AN OUTPOURING OF ANIMATE AND INANIMATE CORPUSCULA ARE THE CAUSE OF CONTAGION

The pestilential poison attracted and inhaled by man soon destroys the internal spirits together with the native heat, immediately changes by its virulence the latent humor into a putrid one, from which condition a pestiferous odor follows which corrupts those who are near the patient and

What is the pestilential exhalation?

infects their clothes with the exhalation. This exhalation is nothing else than the evaporation of the putrid humor; an evaporation indeed composed of innumerable and invisible corpuscula, which, when they reach the free air, soon spreading out infect everything around with a virulent contagion; which with the same lethal and putrid power persist, are either received into the body by the breath, or introduced through secret hiding-places in the clothes, soon they affect him and then spread out further. In cadavers, indeed in every body with this plague this exhalation of the corpuscles is scattered and not only infect those near, but also are transformed into an animated progeny of most minute and invisible animalculae, which invade first linen, clothing, wood or anything of a porous and loose texture, then inspired in-

By what method the corpuscles are propagated

wardly they contaminate the innermost humors; then at the first contact, like touching oil, they communicate the contagion to the pores of the hands and fingers by contact; also in clothes contaminated by the poison, the poison excited by the heat gets in through the pores of the skin just as when breathed in by the breath, and affects them, which plague patients know to their own great sorrow.

Indeed that this living effluvia is composed of invisible living corpuscula, is obvious from the innumerable worms which abound in such bodies, some of which grow large enough to be visible, while others remain of a size which is invisible, these corpuscles or particles multiply in such numbers, become innumerable and constitute the effluvia. Some when they are most minute thin and light are tossed about by the slightest current of air; since also they are sticky and like glue they attach themselves easily to the inner portions of the clothing, cords, linen and fibers; and indeed to anything porous such as wood, bone or cork and by their minuteness penetrate metals, where they scatter new seeds of contagion; and since they are so tenacious they live a long time from the moisture alone drawn from the humid air about, and which they soon convert into a virulent substance.

The effluvia is a living stench of worms.

The manner in which the pestilential foetor persists.

Thus it is very difficult to wash the poison from such things either by long washing or frequent washing with vinegar and lye, therefore the most effective of all remedies is to consume them in the fire; thus clothing and household goods infected with the same contagion when carried somewhere else, in a short time produce tragic catastrophes; indeed not only whole cities are attacked by the sudden and unexpected contagion but also provinces and entire kingdoms. We see the method and manner by which contagion is wont to be propagated; now we will confirm what we have said above by examples.

CHAPTER IV

CONCERNING THE REMARKABLE EFFECTS OF CONTAGION OR PESTILENTIAL FOMITES AND THE POWERS OF THESE CONTAGIOUS THINGS

It should be asked therefore, in what manner and in what ways the plague is acquired by direct contact. I answer, it can spread in many ways, and how, is quite evident. Some of the explanations above are recalled by a few. Therefore, I say first; either the pestiferous exhalations of the earth, or the contaminated air or the infected man are the origin of all infections: for the pestilential exhalations from the bowels of the earth first infect the air; the air inhaled then infects man; this overwhelms nu-
The plague is acquired by touch of things merous others with the acquired evil. I say secondly not so much by immediate contact the infected acquire the plague, but by the contact of all those things, which are in the place, where the patient lies, one can contract the infirmity. These act in this same manner since, as I explain above, the plague is living: for a patient infected with the fierce plague, soon contracts a terrible putrefaction, which we teach, moreover, to be from the generated worms. For these worms are the propagators of the plague, so small, so fine, and subtle that they elude all discernment by the sense,

and also are perceived only with a most excellent microscope, you may call them atoms. Indeed, similarly, they multiply in such numbers that they cannot be
Small, invisible worms are the propagators of the plague counted; these thus are conceived and generated from putrefaction, thus are extruded easily by all openings and pores of the body with the sweaty exhalations; moreover are scattered, indeed, by the lightest agitation of the air, just as particles in a dark place are agitated in the rays of the sun; and thence they scatter, so that they attack whatever they meet. They then adhere most tenaciously and penetrate deeply into the innermost pores. This thing, moreover is not different, as I said, the putrid blood of sufferers from fevers, as I taught above, which an hour or so after venesection was found full of worms so that it almost astonished me, and, indeed, the man was still living; when dead, innumerable, invisible worms abounded, then I convinced myself that Job was right, "I have said to corruption, Thou art my father: to the worm, Thou art my mother, and my sister."

SYPHILIS

The origin of syphilis, in spite of centuries of patient research, seems shrouded in ever-increasing mystery. The theory that syphilis was introduced into Europe by the sailors of Columbus who had contracted the disease in America, was soon accepted by the medical writers of the sixteenth and seventeenth centuries. All have stressed its appearance in the army of Charles in Naples in 1495. Sudhoff holds, however, that this was an outbreak of typhoid or paratyphoid fever and dismisses the story of the high mortality at Naples, as an "Ammenmärchen" (nursery tale).

In 1863 Captain Dabry in his book *La Médecine chez les Chinois,* gave a striking account of syphilis, taken presumably from the writings of Huang-Ti 2637 B.C. Okamura, however, states he has studied these ancient books with great care, that they contain no description of syphilis, and that syphilis did not appear in China until after its introduction from Europe, early in the sixteenth century. Dohi, in his scholarly *Beiträge zur Geschichte der Syphilis* presents strong evidence that the disease was unknown in China or in Japan until the end of the fifteenth or the beginning of the sixteenth century. Whether or not syphilis was introduced from America or had existed previously in

Europe, it certainly attracted no general attention until at the close of the fifteenth and the beginning of the sixteenth century.

From the innumerable accounts of syphilis in the fifteenth and sixteenth centuries, seven selections have been chosen. Leoniceno, at the height of his reputation, when the outbreak of syphilis in Europe occurred, wrote a small treatise on the "French Disease" which remains a classic. Béthencourt's account is of especial interest, since he as a French physician, resented the term "French Disease" and proposed the name "Venereal Disease." Almenar the Spaniard, a favorite author in his day and a loyal son of the Church, did not believe the clergy contracted the disease in the same manner as did other people. Di Vigo's account of syphilis is in many ways the best of the group and is a striking proof of the great powers of clinical observation he possessed. Von Hutten, a picturesque figure in the intellectual life of his time, devoted most of his energies to the popularization of guaiac as a cure for syphilis. Villalobos sang of syphilis in verse and Fracastor, who composed the most famous medical poem of all time, gave the disease its present name. John Hunter's unfortunate self inoculation added confusion to the subject but gave us a remarkably vivid account of the symptoms following infection. Among the moderns Jonathan Hutchinson is included, a manysided genius, who probably knew more of clinical syphilis than any man who has ever lived.

Nicolo Leoniceno

Few physicians have been more prominent or influential in their age than Nicolo Leoniceno of Ferrara. Leoniceno was born in 1428, in Lonigo near Vicenza, studied at Vicenza and Padua, and then travelled extensively over Europe spending some time in England. After his return to Italy, he became professor at Padua, then at Bologna, and finally in 1464 at Ferrara. He was professor at Ferrara for sixty years and died in 1524 at the advanced age of ninety-six. His remarkable vitality became almost lengendary for he was active in his professional duties and lectured regularly while more than ninety-five years of age.

Leoniceno was a great humanist and a profound Greek scholar. He was the first to translate Hippocrates and Galen into Latin and he was a champion of the teachings of Hippocrates against the innovations of the Arabian physicians, who were much in vogue during his time. His great admiration for the clinical genius of Hippocrates is expressed repeatedly in his medical writings. While he repeatedly criticizes Avicenna and other Arabian physicians, he often praises the remarkable clinical acumen of Rhazes. He was a good botanist and in his tract on the errors of Pliny enumerated the many botanical mistakes in the *Natural History* of Pliny. This exposé required rare courage on the part of Leoniceno and its publication loosed a stream of invective at its author for daring to question the accuracy of an authority who was regarded with an almost sacred veneration.

Leoniceno's treatise on syphilis *Libellus de Epidemia, quam vulgo morbum Gallicum vocant,* was published first at Venice by the great humanist printer

Aldus Manutius in 1497. Leoniceno was at this time almost seventy years old and at the height of his reputation. His little book attracted immediate attention and was reprinted many times. He insists that syphilis is a disease of great antiquity and was known to Hippocrates and to the ancients. He notes the

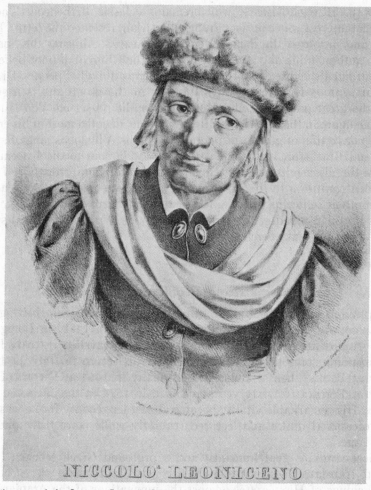

NICCOLO' LEONICENO

Courtesy of the Surgeon General's Library
NICOLO LEONICENO (1428-1524)
Portrait by Luigi Rossi

appearance of the primary lesions on the genitalia, followed by pustules in other parts of the bodies. He describes eye lesions, buboes, and joint pains and notes that patients at autopsy show lesions of the internal organs; however, he does not seem to stress the importance of sexual contact, although he clearly recognizes the contagiousness of the disease.

The following translation of Leoniceno's treatise is from the so-called "Collectio Veneta II," *Liber de Morbo Gallico* published at Venice in 1535.

CONCERNING THE EPIDEMIC WHICH THE ITALIANS CALL THE FRENCH DISEASE BUT THE FRENCH CALL NEAPOLITAN*

A former age believed new diseases, unknown to previous generations, to have come to Italy, although Pliny, a most erudite man not only of Italy but of almost all Europe, relates in the twenty-sixth book of his natural history that lichens were unknown before the reign of Claudius. Indeed I hold I may consider as a fact for other parts of Europe as well. I may dare affirm for certain, that lichens were familiar to the Greeks years before Claudius reigned, because Hippocrates, the most ancient Greek author with many others in places, especially in the third part of the Aphorisms, in the discussion of summer diseases makes mention of lichen, so it seems highly probable to me that this disease infested Italy, although perhaps for a long interval of time before Claudius, it was not yet propagated by the Roman Empire to the other nations, and indeed therefore among the Greek physicians frequenting Rome there were less namers for this disease. For this reason while it continued without name, it was poorly understood but after Claudius' reign, with the Greek arts and especially medicine now blooming in the city, naming lichen as well as mentagra made one more illustrious.

Likewise in a measure this happens in our time, for now a disease of an unusual nature has invaded Italy & many other regions. In the beginning pustules are on the private parts, soon on the whole body and frequently located on the face itself besides causing great hideousness as well as a great deal of pain. Moreover to this disease the physicians of our time do not yet give a name, but is called by the common name of French disease, as if this contagion were imported from France into Italy or because Italy was invaded at the same time both by the disease itself & the armies of the French.

* * *

Who likewise may not recognize similarly the epidemic of our time from the words of Hippocrates for they were so many which appearing at some time with both ulcers of the mouth & sores on the lips, & black pustules like carbuncles, always causing intolerable

itching & many other tubercles, at one time moreover to suffer from injury to the eyes. it is not profitable to recall, since these were so remarkable as to need description. So that therefore we may understand briefly the nature of the French disease. This exists not in one kind but in many types, and we can describe it in this fashion. The French disease has pustules, generated from the diverse corruption of the humors, because of too much air in the heat and humidity especially intemperate, at first on the privates, then the rest of the body and commonly accompanied with great pain. Why do they attack the private parts first, then the rest of the body? The cause we explained from the exposition of Galen. But neither is it difficult also why there may have been pain in the diseases themselves? To arrive at a reason, particularly when before that, it was observed they had suffered great pain, those in whom either none, or very few pustules appeared on the outer skin. For the noxious humor which nature makes more feeble, which nevertheless is able to come to the surface, also settles in the nerves of the joints, and there it produces great pain, besides among other things, in two ways, as Galen says, in the exposition of aphorisms, third part, which begins thus. In truth in those sick from black bile, as well as mad, & epileptics, oppressed nature is accustomed to relieve itself by sending the useless material from the internal and important organs to the external skin or to the private parts, so they are full of kernels & pushing into the structure of the joints, for these are especially liable to bad effusions, as is seen from Galen's exposition of the aphorisms, fourth part, saying thus. Whoever have lassitude in fever, have abscesses in the joints as well as in the jaws. Hippocrates suggests the first type, when in another aphorism he enumerates lichens, leprosy & ulcerous pustules among the diseases of spring, many of which according to the same Hippocrates are shared with summer. Now the second when phymata, which are properly tubercles, arise in the glandular parts (as Paul as well as Galen knew) and soon cause pain of the joints. For this reason it is thought in the french disease, it produces at one time the same material & pustules & it is believed to excite pain in the joints, and as

---

*Leonicenus, Nicolaus, *Liber de Morbo Gallico*, Venice, Patavino and Ruffinelli, 1535, p. **Aiii.**

far as this is concerned it is believed it may belong not to two diseases, but to one alone, of which pain is a symptom. For those, who themselves have no pustules on the external surface, nevertheless can have similar abscesses on the inside, with sometimes (as they say) a greater pain. Certainly many physicians have discovered this to be so in certain dead persons, whom the french disease infected while living, their diseases investigated, thanks to dissections, indeed also the meaning as well as the reason of this thing is set forth, since (as Galen says) in the book which was written concerning black cholera, also it is not believed anywhere that the internal organs are extremely hard, so that they are not exposed to the same poisons, with which we see the externals affected. This I hold regarding the nature of the french disease and the causes of the disease itself, while I may describe next the accidents attending the disease itself. Even if I believe firmly, that the french disease under another name was common to the ancients, and that I should have described a simple type, yet it would not have been possible for me for the multiplex nature of the disease itself demands explanation. Finally it is seen that Hippocrates had regarded in his teaching of viruses that a similar epidemic happening in his time was from a similar cause and described completely various types of ulcers as well as tumors. Because if anything is supposed to be known by Hippocrates himself he would attempt to define better the french disease.

Villalobos

The 'Tratado sobre las pestiferas Bubas' of Francisco Lopez de Villalobos, which was printed at Salamanca in 1498, was the first treatise on syphilis to appear in Spain, and one of the earliest in all Europe. Francisco Lopez was born in Villalobos in either 1473 or 1474 and studied medicine in Salamanca and was still a student there in his twenty-fourth year when he wrote his *Treatise on the pestilential Bubas*. The primary lesion of this disease was called a Buba or a pimple and from this work was derived the name of the disease.

Villalobos, in 1514, became physician to King Ferdinand and travelled over a large part of Spain in the course of his attendance on the monarch. He remained at Court for many years and seemed to have been held in high esteem. In the letters which have been preserved, he refers frequently to his dissatisfaction at Court life. He was later physician to Charles I, King of Spain, who became Charles V, Emperor of Germany, and was in Italy during the wars which Charles waged against the French. In his later years he devoted himself almost exclusively to literature and achieved great reputation in his native land. The date of his death is unknown. His 'Tratado sobre las pestiferas Bubas' was written in verse in the Castillian tongue because, as the author remarks in the preface, "the physicians of these domains being little familiar with Greek and Latin, the common tongue will popularize more easily the knowledge of scientific works." Only four copies of the first edition are known. The following extracts are from the translation of George Gaskoin, London, 1870.

Villalobos makes no mention of a possible American origin of the disease, but he has great faith in astrology. He points out in stanza XXXVII the important fact that the small ulcer on the penis preceded by many days the eruption of the disease elsewhere. In stanza LXIII, Villalobos praises an ointment containing mercury.

By the licentiate de Villalobos.
On the contagious and accursed bubas.*
History and medicine.

I

What time ruled those princes wise and glorious,
How great and loved and how allied is here no need to tell.
Blest of God, and made by Him so victorious,
In the blason of their power so notorious,
The kings don Fernando and donna Isabel;
Through all the whole universe their fame now was spread,
Where men and laws are found, and aught of culture springs,
Now all of blighting arrogance was captive led;
At this time all their land in peace was swayed,
All tyrants were destroyed, whether vassals or kings.

II

Even thus as they dwelt in fair and stately show,
In the which they continue wherever they are found,
Having God for their aid, and the people's love also,
With great store of blessings in the world below,
And far more of promise in the realms beyond.
Being then in Madrid at that time and season,
For new kind of sin as soon we shall relate,
There came forth from God a gen'ral malison,
That fell on all the land, each province and nation,
All countries that we know or where we penetrate.

III

It was a pestilence ne'er to be found at all
In verse or in prose, in science or in story,
So evil and perverse and cruel past control,
Exceedingly contagious, and in filth so prodigal,
So strong to hold its own, there is little got of glory;
And it makes one dark in feature and obscure in countenance,
Hunchback'd and indisposed, and seldom much at ease,
And it makes one pained and crippled in such sort as never was,
A scoundrel sort of thing, which also doth commence
In the rascalliest place that a man has.

IV

He states the opinion of theologians as to the superven-
tion of this malady.

Theologians pretend the cause of it doth lie
In certain new-found sins that are rife in Christendom.
Oh! Providence divine, oh! judgment from on high!
Which ever hast in store a perfect penalty.
Howe'er we go astray, our folly is brought home.
Out of heaven Thou hast seen all this schism and dissension,
In thy sons and thy servants, both churchmen and lay,
How for mere opinion's sake and the lust of contention,
With shrewd swelling taunts and vehement intention,
They make appeal to arms in disorderly array.

* * *

* *The Medical Works of Villalobos,* translated by George Gaskoin, London, Churchill, 1870, p. 93.

VIII

Second theological opinion.

But some to luxury, and all of wanton sense,
To which the world is giv'n do refer the same.
The ailment, say they, is a just and proper sentence;
According to the sin so is the repentance,
And the part that suffers most is the part most to blame.
And this seems borne out by a passage in Scripture,
Chapter XII, Genesis, where we read of Egypt's king,
Pharaoh, engrossed by excellence of feature
In Sarah. God struck him in his nature
With this same disease, or some such other thing.

*   *   *

X

*He cites the opinion of the astrologers as to the advent
of this malady.*

Astrologers say by their computation
It is due to conjunction of Saturn and Mars,
For Saturn he is lord of the adust passion,
And Mars of the members of generation,
From which of this infirmity the first proceeding was;
But if so be that Mars is tormented in his place
By that restless fellow Saturn, his determined adversary,
How with Venus then and Mars; if we seek our solace
In the using of their acts, must we study heaven's face,
To see if Saturn's there? it behooves us to be wary.

XI

*He gives the opinion of the physicians about the
aforesaid.*

Physicians say the secret of its power
In melancholy humour and salt phlegm doth lie,
Which occasion in all organs what obstructions do occur,
Proceeding from a mighty distemperature
Of the liver, which is turned to hot and dry;
And this from something baneful in the air is bred,
And also from bad habits and from sustenance,
And joined along with this the aforementioned;
Even so the mischief works, and gets so far ahead,
That neither cure nor regimen can check its insolence.

*   *   *

XXVII

*He begins to speak of the passion and the name
it should have.*

And having now declared on what my view is based,
All ground of altercation I would readily abjure,
And whether with sarna it is well or ill placed,
Concerning the disease with so much prefaced,
Let us speak of the name, the passion and the cure.
And in my poor conceit as a fitting name for this
Which coming out of sin shows exceeding cruelty,
Sarna egypciaca will not be amiss,

For it's loathsome and perverse just as sarna is
And it's surely sent by God as pain and penalty.

* * *

XXIX

The causes that bring this complaint, and first of the universal and equivocal.

The cause first in order that brings this complaint
Is hurtful impression of bodies celestial,
Which produces in the air an infectious taint,
Corruption in our flesh is thereon consequent
If thereunto concur some causes terrestrial.
A very complex harm is the primal cause thereof,
And constellations of unfortunate planets,
And this from astrology derives its proof,
By voice of all well versed in it the thing is plain enough
Our art itself to theirs in this subordinates.

* * *

XXXVII

He goes on to state why the ailment shows itself in these organs many days before its coming.

With this kind of ailment in the very first place,
The liver is distempered in the sense of dry and hot,
And gross and adust humours grow therein apace,
(But in the first beginning this is not so much the case)
And the strength to void it forth the liver will have got.
By all this noisome stuff diseased and much tormented.
Through its conduits forthwith some more or less it chases,
And this ere any portion in the veins is spread,
Thus 'tis that the passion on these members is presented
Many days before it yet hath appeared in other places.

* * *

LXIII

Another ointment of a stronger sort.

If something shall seem needed of a character more fine,
And stronger than the last, take both the arsenics
And bright yellow sulphur, with which you will combine
The black hellebore and the resin of pine,
All of these in the like proportion you mix;
With garlic ash rub, and after you will add
Some incense and myrrh, aloes and Negilla;
Hog's lard and kill'd quicksilver next should be had.
And oil, juice of lemon, or cider instead.
Make your ointment and lay it upon the pustilla.

Juan Almenar

Juan Almenar, a Spanish physician of the fifteenth century is one of the first who wrote on the venereal disease. He indicated a good method for employing mercury in his treatise *De Morbo Gallico,* Venice, 1502, in 4°; reprinted at Paris, 1516, in-folio, at Lyon, 1528 and 1539 8°, and at Basle, 1536, in 4°. This deserves still to be consulted for its findings, and especially for the history of this disease, whose sudden apparition in Europe will always be for the philosophizing physician an interesting subject for research. It is singular that Almenar, deceived by a blind attachment to the ecclesiastical order, could not conceive of venereal disease in priests being caused in the same way as in other men. He prefers to ascribe it hypothetically and gratuitously to the influence and corruption of the air. (Translated from *Biographie Universelle, Ancienne et Moderne* (Paris, 1811), i, p. 605.)

The following selections from Almenar's book were taken from William Clowes' *A prooved practise for all young Chirurgians** and were presumably translated by Clowes from the Latin. Later editions of Clowes' work do not contain this translation of Almenar's treatise but instead Clowes' own book on the French Disease. William Clowes was a London surgeon during the reign of Queen Elizabeth and ranks as the greatest English surgeon of his time.

A TREATISE OF THE FRENCH POCKS, WRITTEN BY JOHN ALMENAR A SPANISH PHISITION

Chap. I

OF THE BEGINNING AND DEFINITION OF THIS DISEASE

It is concluded by certain wise men, that this disease which amongst the Italians is called *Gallicus,* that is to say, the French disease, should now be named *Patursa,* which is by interpretation, a disease filthie and Saturnall. It is a filthie disease, because it maketh women to bee esteemed unchast and irreligious. It is *Saturnall,* because it took the beginning from Saturne when he entered into Aries, having the rest of the heavenly aspects helping thereunto. And albeit that influence have ceassed, it is not necessarie that the disease should ceasse, because many infected bodies remayned, whereby others have bene infected: Hereof it may be concluded, that this disease shall continue many yeeres, and therefore let men take heede that by other mens example it may bee sayd of them: Happie is he whom others danger make warie. The disposition which proceeded of the celestiall influence making impression into the bodies, did burne the humours in respect of Aries, which signe is hot and drie, and after this burning cold and drie humours were engendered on Saturnes part, which signe is by nature colde and drie. These colde and drie or melancholike humours caried to divers places bring divers paines, and in the skinne bring forth divers kinds of pustles or wheales. It may be thus defined. The French Pockes or Patursa is an universall or popular ill disposition in the parts of the bodie, consisting principally in the liver and veynes, and their humors, whereof ensue these accidents, to wit, paynes and wheales in all the bodie. The efficient cause is touched, when it is called universall or popular, that is, proceeding from the influence of the heavens: the formall, when it is called an evill disposition: the materiall, when it is sayd to be in the parts. Also the difference is touched, when it is sayd that paynes doe ensue it, & Concerning the ende, the bodily Phisition intermedleth not; but the spirituall Phisitions affirme them to bee sent for the punishment of sinne. Wherefore they which would bee delivered, and escape this, let them take heede of sinne, and applye thier mindes to God: for only God cureth infirmities, as Mesus sayth in his treatise de Appropriatis. Of this definition doe followe many and profitable consequences. First, that this disease is one, and not many, as some have insufficiently affirmed, because they could not be given one definition of it, neither had it alwaies one only efficient cause, neither would one kinde of cure agree, neither had it one name; which is absurd as partly hath appeared alreadie, and shall more plainly be shewed hereafter. The second consequence is, that they are deceived, which think they have found the head or fountaines of this disease,

---

* Clowes, Wylliam, *A prooved practise for all young Chirurgians* (London, 1588). Printed by Thomas Orwyn for Thomas Cadman. P. 97.

to bee the paine in the joynts and pustles in the face, because the former definition agreeth not unto them. Moreover, all the paynes are not in the joynts, neither are all the wheales like red pustles in the face. Therefore neither this disease nor the cure of it can be referred unto them, as it shall be hereafter shewed. The third consequence, that they which cure onely wheales, or onely looke to the paynes, doe cure imperfectly. For who can cure perfectly the headach, or the drinesse of the tongue, or thirst, which come from a Feaver, unless he first cure the Feaver. For the accident followeth the disease, as the shadow doth the bodie. *Gal. lib. 3. de accident.* And therefore the paynes cannot bee cured as the pustles, except the disease be first cured, because these are either accidents, or conioyned sickness, which follow the principall, and doe presuppose, it must be first cured, as Evicen testifieth *tract. 1. fen. 3.* and in many places. The fourth consequence, if any doe joyne the cure of the Empiricks with those which think they cure orderly, as the annoynting of the Empiricks, and the purging of the Phisitions, yet the cure is insufficient, because by those medicines the il complexion which is fixed in the parts cannot be removed. And this was the cause, that many have thought themselves cured when they were not. And if any have bene cured, it was, be reason that the humors were thorughly purged by solutine medicines and unctions: which avoyded, nature was stronger and superior to the disease and that evill complexion, and expelled it. This had not so fallen out, except the nature had bin strong, and the impression little, but where the strength was weake, and the impression strong, this disease could not be expelled. This difference in the strength of nature, and the impression hath bene the cause, that some have bene cured without medicines, some with medicines, others could not by any meanes be cured. Now wee will shewe that way which both reason and experience hath taught to hale all, not onely by removing with medicines the humor which procureth actual payne and pustles, and hath abilite prepared to the same, but also that evill complexion which in infecteth the humors (they being first purged) as order requireth, wherein the treasure of this cure consisteth. I could inferre many other consequences, but because it is tedious to use many words in

things not available to the cure (as **Galen** sayeth) *1. de regim. acut.* This shalbe sufficient. It remayneth to determine of the causes.

CHAP. 2

OF THE CAUSES OF THE FRENCH POCKES

There is a twofold kinde of causes, because some are first, some corporall: and those of two sorts, partly antecedent, partly conioyed. That which is first, or originall in this disease, is twofold, whereof the first is the only influence or corruption of the aire, from whence we must charitably thinke, that it infected those which were religious. The second is conversation, as by kissing and sucking, as appeareth in children, or by carnall copulation, as it hath happened to many & very often, but by other meanes, and chiefly by the influence of corruption of the aire, very seldome. It may also be caused by other means of conversation, which I leave to thy consideration. It is sufficient to knowe by experience, that this disease is contagious and by probabilitie of reason wherein it is like to other contagious diseases, it may be so accepted. Hereupon Avicen saith in p. *2* of his 1. concluding his treatise of the dispositions of sicknesses. Some there are which pass from one to another, as the Leprosye, Scabs, Pocks, pestilent Fevers, rotten apostemes. Now of the antecedent causes, there are foure kindes, as there are foure humors, which may be the matter of this disease through their ill disposition, whereby they are apt to receive the impression heerof: to wit, blood, choler, fleame, melancholy. The conioyned cause is double, one is the cause of the disease, and it is the humor which being first infected or altered by the originall causes, infecteth the partes and other humors, and therefore it is sayd, the first originall causes move the antecedent. But the conioyned cause of the accidents is that humor which immediately procureth paynes and wheales. But here it may be demanded whether the evill qualitie in the humor, which is the antecedent cause, may be a disease. It seemeth it cannot, sith a disease affecteth a living thing, but the humor liveth not. Whereto it may be answered, that the humor which is in the lyver and veynes infected with this evill quality may be the subject of a disease, so it be graunted that that ill qualitie have not attayned the part, because it may hinder digestion in the liver and veines, and ingender corrupt humors: therefore by the definition of a disease, it appeareth to be a disease. Now to the argument, it is answered, that it is sufficient

disease be in it as in a subject, I answere, it is an antecedent cause in respect of the paynes and pustles, because it is apt to flowe to the places of paine and pustles: It is a conioyned cause, in as much as it causeth an

97

A TREATISE OF THE
FRENCH POCKS, WRITTEN·
by *Iohn Almenar* a Spanish Phisition.

Chap. 1.
Of the beginning and definition of this diseafe.

I is concluded by certaine wise men, that this disease which amongst the Italians is called *Gallicus*, that is to say, the French disease, should now bee named *Patursa*, which is by interpretation, a disease filthie and Saturnall. It is a filthie disease, because it maketh women to bee esteemed vnchast, and irreligious. It is *Saturnall*, because it tooke the beginning from Saturne when he entred into Aries, hauing the rest of the heauenly aspects helping thereunto. And albeit that influence haue ceassed, it is not necessarie that the disease should ceasse, because many infected bodies remayned, whereby others haue bene infected: Thereof it may be concluded, that this disease shall continue many yeeres, and therefore let men take heede that by other mens example it may bee sayd of them: Happie is he whom others daunger make warie. The disposition which proceeded of the celestiall influence making impression into the bodies, did burne the humours in respect of Aries, which signe is hot and drie, and after this burning cold and drie humours were engendred on Saturnes part, which signe is by nature colde and drie. These colde and drie or melancholike

Facsimile page from Juan Almenar's A Treatise of the French Pocks

that a living thing be the subject of denomination or be that which is named diseased, it must not be that wherein the disease is settled, yea that is most stable, that the humor is the subject wherein the disease is settled. And if it be sayd, how can the humor be an antecedent cause, and yet a

ill complexion in the member: it is the subject of a disease, in respect it hath a disposition, whereby the action of the member is hurt, whereupon it is called diseased. If you consider these things well, you shall comprehend all the difficulties which may be incident to the definition.

CHAP. 3

OF THE SIGNES OF THE FRENCH POCKS

The signes are, hurt in the yard, especially corroding, heaviness of the head, and payne in the necke, which little by little are spread towards the shoulders and spade bones to the joynts, first in the armes, then in the legges, and sometime in the muscles and sinewes which are in those parts, the payne increaseth in the night, and decreaseth in the day. The cause is, that nature is then retyred home and stronger, as also in regard of the moistnesse and coldnesse of the night, the matter is increased. In the day, nature is drawne from the sense hereof, and doth not so much move the humors, partly being weake, partly occupied in other actions. I will shew the signes of the causes respecting the payne and pustles, as others also in the tree of signes heereafter set downe. If the payne be sharpe, and quickly arising, and the pustles little, of a citron colour, ulcerated and the skinne rough, they come of choller. If the payne do slowly come forth, the pustles broade & whitish, they are of fleame. If they have great itching, and some heate, they proceed of salt flegme. If they be black and small, not paynefull, they are of meloncholy. If they be red, and not paynefull, they are of blood. You shall find these signes intermedled if you view others: for as corruption seldome happeneth in one onely humor (sayth *Galen 1. regim. accut.*) even so you shall seldome finde the signes foretelling one onely humor. Therefore you must gather all the signes in your minde, and comparing them together, attayne to that which is principall, and according to that humor dispose your cure.

Johannis de Vigo

Johannis de Vigo or Giovanni di Vigo (1460-1520) became surgeon to Pope Julius II in 1503. He was born near Genoa and for this reason was often referred to as Johannis de Vigo, Genuensis. He came to Rome just at the time when Michelangelo was painting the ceiling of the Sistine Chapel and Raphael was finishing his marvelous frescoes in the Vatican. He seems to have been a very amiable and attractive man. His *Practica in arte chirurgica copiosa* first appeared in 1514 and had such success that it ran through fifty-two editions. He was an eyewitness of the first great European epidemic of syphilis and his account of this disease, as the reader will see, is quite accurate.

In the selection which follows, he stresses the contagiousness of the disease, its origin from sexual intercourse with an infected person, and its rapid dissemination throughout the body. He described quite accurately the primary lesion, the indurated chancre, the secondary eruptions, the formation of gummata, and emphasizes the fact that the pains are worse at night and may subside during the day. He also refers to the specific action of mercury, both upon the lesions and upon the pains so common in this disease. He describes eye lesions, possibly iritis, and ulcerations of the nose. He believed that cauterization of the initial sore was a very effective treatment, an idea which persisted for centuries. de Vigo employed a plaster in the treatment of syphilis, the most important ingredient of which was mercury. This plaster is still found in the pharmacopoeia. de Vigo, in the passage selected, expressed his belief that the disease was quite new and unknown until his time, with the possible exception of the passage referred to in the Celsus and the history of the disease of the Emperor Augustus. Fournier, who has studied these two accounts, assures us that they do not describe any disease remotely resembling syphilis.

At the end of the ninth book of his *Chirurgia*, he writes:

We have completed and sealed and brought to an end, with the approval of God, the whole work of our surgery at Rome, in the year of our Lord MDXIII, on the first day of January, Julius II reigning, in the tenth year of his pontificate, at which time also we were assisting His Holiness by discharging the duty of surgeon to him. Praise be to God and to the most glorious Virgin Mary, blessed by whose name.

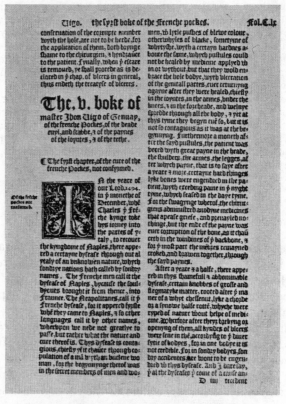

Page from Traheron's translation of de Vigo's *Surgery*,
first edition, 1543. This page describes the appearance of syphilis in Europe.

The fifth book of his Chirurgia *De Morbo Gallico* begins, using the quaint translation of Traheron:

In the yeare of our Lord, 1494, in ye monethe of December, when Charles ye Frenche kynge toke hys iorney into the partes of Ytaly, to recouer the kyngdome of Naples, there appered a certayne dyseasse through out al Ytaly of an unknowen nature, whych sondrye nations hath called by sondry names. The Frenche men call it the dyseasse of Naples, bycause the souldyours brought it from thence, into Fraunce. The Neapolitanes, call it ye Frenche dyseasse, for it appered fyrste when they came to Naples, and so other languages call it by other names, wheruppon we nede not greatlye to passe, but rather what the nature and cure therof is. Thys dyseasse is contagious, chiefly yf it chaunce through copulation of a man wyth an unclene woman, for the begynnynge therof was in the secret members of men and women, with lytle pushes of blewe colour, otherwhyles of blacke, sometyme of whytyshe, wyth a certayn hardnes aboute the same, whych pustules could not be healed by medicine applyed with in or wythout, but that they wold enbrace the hole bodye, wyth ulceration of the genitall partes, euer returnyng agayne after they were healed, chiefly in the ioyntes, in the armes, under the knees, & in the foreheade, and welnye spredde through all the body, & yet at thys tyme they begyn euen so, but it is not so contagious as it was at the begynnyng.

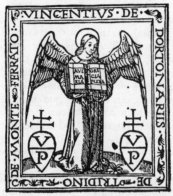

Title page from Johannis de Vigo's *Practica in arte chirurgia copiosa*, 1514

For the sake of easier reading a translation into modern English has been made.

LIBER QUINTUS. DE MORBO GALLICO*

In the year 1494, in the month of December, the year when King Charles VIII passed into Italy with the French army to recover the Kingdom of Naples, there appeared this same year, throughout almost all Italy, a malady of a nature unknown up to that time.

This malady received from different peoples whom it affected different names. It was called the Disease of Naples by the

* *Opera Domini Joannis de Vigo in Chyrurgia,* Lyon, J. Moilin, 1534.

French, who claimed that they got it at Naples and took it from there to their own country. The Neapolitans, for their part, gave it the name of the French disease, because it appeared and was seen for the first time in Italy at the time of the French expedition. The Genoans called it "lo malo de le tavelle"; the Tuscans called it "lo male de le bulle"; the Lombards, "lo male de le brosule"; the Spaniards, "labones." Every people gave it whatever name it liked. After all, such a name makes little difference; the essential thing for us is to know how to treat and cure this malady.

It was and it is still a contagious disease.

The contagion which gives rise to it comes particularly from coitus; that is, sexual commerce of a healthy man with a sick woman or the contrary.

The first symptoms of this malady appear almost invariably upon the genital organs, that is, upon the penis or the vulva. They consist of small ulcerated pimples of a color especially brownish and livid, sometimes black, sometimes slightly pale. These pimples are circumscribed by a ridge of callous-like hardness. These first lesions have been combatted by all sorts of tonics and internal remedies, but one succeeds only rarely in preventing them from scattering their venom throughout the entire organism. There then appear a series of new ulcerations on the genitalia, which are just as difficult to cure and quite as prompt to reappear after cure. Then the skin becomes covered with scabby pimples or with elevated papules resembling small warts. These eruptions appear especially on the forehead, the skull, the neck, the arms, the legs, and they spread sometimes over the entire surface of the body. Such was the course which the disease pursued at the time of its first appearance and such it is still to those it affects today.

That is not all. A month and a half, about, after the appearance of the first symptoms, the patients are afflicted with pains sufficiently severe to draw from them cries of anguish. These pains are situated particularly in the frontal region, then in the shoulder blades, shoulders and arms, often the tibias, thighs and hips.

Still very much later (a year or even longer after the above complication) there appear certain tumors of a scirrhus hardness, which provoke terrible suffering. The pain which they produce is characteristic in being aggravated during the night and diminishing during the day. Then, in vain the entire armament of sedatives and remedies with an old reputation are given these patients, with no sedative effect upon the pains of the patient. In the end, these horrible sufferings terminate most commonly in lesions of the bones or the enveloping membranes of the bones, such as are produced in spina ventosa. Very often, too, the healed members remain retracted.

About a year and a half after the appearance of this base and detestable disease, certain tumors appear on the body, constituted of a viscous phlegmatic matter, about as large as a medium size chestnut, of a white color and soft like a tendon or a nerve becomes semi-putrefied. These tumors mature without any abscess and a cure is effected by many remedies.

As to these secondary ulcers, they vary in form to infinity. To tell the truth, they assume all appearances, they take all kinds of masks, because their characters harmonize themselves in some way with the complexion and temperament of each patient.

In fact, the multiple manifestations of this odious malady vary in an incredible manner from one subject to another. At this point one would add to his list the majority, I would almost dare say all, of the constitutional diseases described by physicians ancient and modern. Think of it! Now, for the apostemes (tumors), in the first place, one never finds in the French disease all the well known varieties, warm aposteme, aposteme which is a mixture of cold material such as phlegm or atrabile, bloody aposteme mixed with phlegm or phlegmon undimiades (edematous phlegmon) aposteme finally of all kinds and every form. Do we not observe also in this same disease all the different possible kinds of cold apostemes or of tumors, as glandular engorgements, scrofulae, nodi, tumors leading to caries of the bones of the skull, scirrhous, cancerous or non-cancerous, etc.? Do we not see included in it the different kinds of formica, of eruptions—bloody, suppurative, herpetic, carbuncular, etc.—without speaking of gangrene or noma? As far as the ulcers which come from this disease are concerned, they vary in appearance almost to infinity, modifying their character according to the complexion of the patient; and one can say without exaggeration that a tentative examination reveals in this malady all the forms of ulcers described up to our day. Ulcers corrosive, putrid, serpiginous (a variety especially common), cancerous, gangrenous, virulent, malignant, biting, painful, purulent, cavernous, fistulous, bony, callous and encrusted; and more especially still all the chronic and rebellious types in which a sort of evil spirit seems to hinder the cicatrization. Also, these ulcers might be said incidentally to show a double character in the difficulty in obtaining a cure and in a singular tendency to recur.

It is the same for the pain, all forms of which possible and imaginable are met in this malady in a common fashion: generalized cold ophthalmia with obscuring of vision!

How many other lesions also issue from the same source—lesions as diverse as they are multiple! To enumerate and cite incidentally all the morbid manifestations of this disease would be a long labor. I will not mention more. I will mention only one to close: There is a little fever (febricula) which coming, adds itself to all the preced-

A page from the fifth book of de Vigo's *Chyrurgia: De Morbo Gallico*

arthritic pains, sciatica, podagra, chiragra, gonagra, etc.

On the other hand, one does not observe as manifestations of this disease every kind of psorasis or unsightly eruptions, ringworm, or see indeed any kind of leprosy, without speaking of scalp eruptions, vitiligo, serpigo, lupus or dirty ulcerations of the feet and hands.

How often, too, do we not have to treat different ocular diseases coming from the same origin: notably a particular kind of

ing symptoms, which insensibly carries the unhappy patients to consumption, progressive decline and death.

Also, as I have said, the French disease always takes its origin from sexual intercourse of a healthy man with an infected woman or reciprocally, of a healthy woman with an infected man, but later the virus which is characteristic of it or the virus of the initial lesion which has developed on the genital organ, becomes scattered throughout the entire body and is disseminated in all parts of the organism, from the highest to the lowest; it begins then to infect the entire mass of the blood.

It is at the period when this morbid virus has impregnated the body, that one sees symptoms which are outspoken—notably the eruptions and pains. These eruptions cover the skin with patches and numerous scabs similar in appearance to those of scabies. So far as the pains are concerned, they are situated sometimes in the forehead, sometimes in the shoulders, sometimes in the legs, the hips, the arms. I stress again the fact that the pains are worse during the night and become calm during the day. We note also that they are located more commonly outside rather than in the joints themselves. They are more periarticular than articular, to speak correctly. Finally, the curious peculiarity already mentioned above—they are relieved not at all or they are relieved only very slightly by a long series of calming remedies which, according to unanimous opinion of physicians, both ancient as well as modern, constitute infallible specifics for pain in disease. They are not modified at all by all of these remedies. Sometimes, indeed, under their influence, they do nothing but increase in intensity.

This last fact has its significance. It demonstrates clearly that the French disease was never observed by the ancients and that it constitutes a disease of quite a recent origin.

It appears however that an affection something like the French disease was indicated by Celsus in his chapter *De cura morbi elephantiae* and by Ugo de Sienna in his LV. *Consultation* It is possible also, at least according to the testimony of Suetonius, that the Emperor Augustus was afflicted with a similar malady. "This prince," says the historian whom we have just cited, "was contin-

ually exposed during his entire life to grave and dangerous diseases. . . . His body was covered with spots." It says also, "that the skin of his chest and of his stomach was sprinkled with birthmarks which by their location, as well as by their number, called to mind exactly the constellations of the Great Bear, etc." Also, this prince owed his cure to the employment of remedies and treatment up to that time unknown, which received with him a first application.

To return to our subject, as well as to the disease of the Emperor Augustus; the French disease of our day cannot be combatted in efficient fashion, except by the use of remedies up to this time unknown. It we are going to succeed in procuring some relief to our patients, it is due solely to the invention of new therapeutic matters and all the old treatments, indeed the best proved, indeed those which have received the sanction of experience and of time, give us no succor. According to Galen and Avicenna, resolving and anodyne agents have the power of dispelling almost at a blow every kind of pain. Well, what is the action of these remedies upon the pain of the French disease? It is nothing, absolutely nothing. We have convinced ourselves of that by experience and we are completely convinced of the absolute impotence of all the anodyne oils, of all the calming salves, of all the consoling unctions, baths of water, fumigations, etc. On the contrary, what striking relief follows the simple unction to which a small dose of mercury communicates a virtue practically marvelous. I have often seen, for my part, after a single week of treatment by mercurial unction practiced upon the ailment, the pains of the French disease disappear entirely, the ulcerations heal, the eruptions disappear and the skin clear of all its spots.

Ulrich von Hutten

One of the most picturesque figures to contribute to medical literature is Ulrich von Hutten, poet and reformer. He was born near Fulda in 1488, the member of a poor but distinguished knightly family. Because he was sickly and of poor physique his father felt he was destined for the cloister and sent him to the Benedictine house near Fulda. Here he became inspired with a great zeal for learning, but finding the dull monastic life unbearable, he fled from the monastery, losing thereby all chance for preferment at the hands of the Church and earning the undying wrath of his father. For nine years he wandered through Germany and Italy, being warmly received by the Humanists, but eventually quarreled with his friends and at one time was forced by poverty to enlist as a common soldier in the army of the Emperor Maximilian.

In 1514, because of his poetic gifts, he won the favor of Albert, Elector of Mayence and Archbishop of Brandenburg, and had dreams of a long and happy career in letters under the protection of this patron. Later however, his

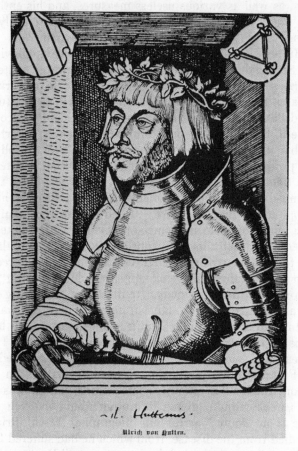

Ulrich von Hutten.

ULRICH VON HUTTEN (1488-1523)
From a woodcut in von Hutten's *Gesprächbüchlein*, 1519

attacks upon the Duke of Württemberg (who murdered his cousin), his espousal of the Lutheran cause and his attacks upon the papal claims in Germany so frightened Albert that he dismissed Hutten from his court. Pope Leo X ordered him to be arrested and sent to Rome, and assassins followed him everywhere. He fled to Basle, where Erasmus, fearing his loathsome disease and knowing his habit of borrowing money, refused to see him. Finally he went to Zürich, where he was received kindly by the reformer Zwingli. With him he found refuge on the Island of Ufnau in the Lake of Zürich. Here he died in 1523 at the age of thirty-five, penniless, possessing not a single book, and owning only the clothes on his back and his pen, which while it had brought him great misfortunes, had also assured him of a permanent place in literature.

Hutten's *De morbo Gallico* first published in 1519, was very widely read, was translated into English, French, and German and had a great influence upon the development of the therapeutics of syphilis. "The vociferous protest against the eleven courses of inunctions to which the unlucky knight submitted for nine years, as well as various useless measures, and his enthusiastic praise of guaiac by which, he believed erroneously, he was promptly healed, could not be brushed aside and coming from such a man was also believed" (Proksch). Hutten's book was widely read and there is convincing evidence presented by Sticker that Palmarius and Fernel borrowed sentences and complete paragraphs for their books on syphilis. As Sticker remarks, "they quote all the Greeks on syphilis, but secretly copy from Hutten." Hutten's work on syphilis was dedicated to his patron Albert, who, history records, played an important rôle in the history of the Reformation. It was Albert, who, in order to pay his debts, obtained the permission of Pope Leo X to sell indulgences in his diocese, a proceeding which aroused the ire of Luther. Hutten's works were placed on the Index and in some editions of *De morbo Gallico* the name of the author is stamped out. At the close of his book he addresses himself again to the Archbishop, noting that this work: "I dedicate to your Eminence, not that I intend these things for your use, since our saviour Christ takes care that you may never need it, but that this be in your library, available to the needs of all."

We know from other writings of Hutten that he had suffered from syphilis for about ten years before his book appeared. Hutten after trying various methods of treatment took the guaiac treatment at Augsburg in the autumn of 1518 and, after its completion, fancied himself cured. He was urged by Dr. Paul Ricius to write a book on the subject and immediately began the composition of his treatise which was finished early in the year 1519. The book was widely read and soon after its appearance was translated into German, English and French. Many physicians of the time writing on the disease, as Professor Georg Sticker has shown, copied entire paragraphs or even pages from Hutten's book without giving its author credit or even mentioning his name. "There is no doubt," writes his biographer David Friedrich Strauss, "that Hutten died from the disease, from which he had suffered for many years, and which, after apparently healed, broke out anew." Hutten's infirmities were the subject of many jibes from his political and theological opponents and subsequent historians have never failed to stress his moral shortcomings. However, as Ernest Zimmermann has remarked, "In judging Hutten we must bear in mind that he lived at a time when a Borgia assumed the Papal throne, when it was no secret that the latter's successor died of syphilis, when Cellini was writing his autobiography and relating of the pretty wench who made him a present of a pox, costing him his eyesight for a spell. Modesty did not compel men to lock fast in secrecy, sexual indiscretions with resulting venereal infections."

CHAP. I

Of the beginning of the FRENCH POX, and the several Names by which it has been called*

It hath pleased God, that in our time, Sicknesses should arise, unknown to our Forefathers, as we have Cause to surmise.

In the Year of Christ 1493, or thereabout, this Evil began amongst the People, not only of *France*, but originally at *Naples* in the *French* Camp, who under King *Charles* were set down before that Place, and where it was taken notice of, before it came elsewhere; upon which account the French, disdaining that it should be called of their Country, gave it the Name of *Neopolitane*, or the *Evil* of *Naples;* reckoning, it is before observed, a Scandal to them to have it called by that of the *French Pox.* However the Consent of all Nations hath obtained, and we also in this Book, shall so call it, not out of Envy to that noble and courteous People, but to prevent a Misunderstanding among some, should we give it any other Appellation.

At the time of its first Appearance, some Men superstitiously named it the Sickness of *Mevin,* from I know not what holy Man of that Name. Some again accounted it of kin to *Job's* Scab, whom this Likeness I think also hath brought into the Number of *Saints.*

Some took upon them to declare it the same Infirmity, wherewith the Monk *Evager* was grieved, through immoderate Cold, and feeding upon raw Meats, when he was in the Desert; and therefore he also was sought from afar, by great resort of Men, offering abundant Gifts at his Chapel, which is in *Vestrike.* And because the Name of this Saint was not only rightly known among the Common People of *Almayn,* they called it incorrectly *Fiacre's Sickness,* for *Evager's;* not so much inquiring after the Lives of these, but merely believing that they should have Help by their Means; Such was the Opinion of the People, and hence arose the same.

There were Images offered also and hung up before St. *Roch,* and his old Sores were

A Treatise of the French Disease, Published about 200 years past by Sir Ulrich Hutten, Kt. of Almayn in Germany, Translated soon after into English by a Canon of Marten-Abbye, now again revised . . . by Daniel Turner of the College of Physicians in London, London; Printed for John Clarke, 1730, p. 1.

afresh remember'd, which thing, if it were done of a godly Mind, I do not reprove; but if for Advantage and filthy Lucre in the Inventors thereof, 'tis strange that so great Iniquity should have place at a time of so great Calamity and miserable Destruction of Mankind.

The *Divines* imputed this disease to the Wrath of God, sent from Heaven as a Scourge for our Wickedness, and took upon them thus to preach openly, as if they had been admitted of Council with God, and came to understand thereby, that Men never lived worse, or so bad as we; or as if in the Golden Age of *Augustus* and *Tiberius,* when Christ was here on Earth, no such Evil could have happened; as if Nature had no Power to usher in any new Diseases, which in all other things bringeth forth great Changes and Alterations. As well may they prattle that of late in our times, because Men are grown better in their Lives, therefore is the Remedy of *Guajacum* found out as a Cure for this Sickness: So well do these things accord, which these Pretenders to the Oracles of God do thus deliver to us.

Now also began the Enquiry of the Physicians, who searched not so much for proper Remedy, as for the Cause; for they cared not even to behold it, much less at the first to touch the infected; for truly when it first began, it was so horrible to behold, that one would scarce think the Disease that now reigneth to be of the same kind. They had *Boils* that stood out like Acorns, from whence issued such filthy stinking Matter, that whosoever came within the Scent, believed himself infected. The Colour of these was of a dark Green and the very Aspect as shocking as the Pain itself, which yet was as if the Sick had laid upon a Fire.

Not long after its beginning, it made a Progress into *Germany*, where it hath wander'd more largely than in any other Place; which I ascribe to our greater intemperance than that of other Nations.

There were some who having taken Counsel of the Stars, prophesy'd that this Sickness should not endure more than seven Years, in which they were out, if they meant the same of the Evil in general, and all the subsequent Symptoms; but if they interpreted concerning the foresaid most outragious kind thereof, which cometh of itself, and not barely by Infection, Corruption of the Atmosphere, or of divine Appointment, they were then, I say, not deceived; for it tarried not long above the seventh Year before the Disease abated of its Fierceness, and that the succeeding one, which yet remaineth, became not so filthy. The Soars being now less, neither so high, nor yet so hard, though there is often a broad creeping Scab, under which the Poison lurketh, and bringeth forth farther Mischiefs; and it is thought this Disease in our Days ariseth not, unless by infection from carnal Contact, as in copulating with a diseased Person, since it appears now that young Children, old Men and others, not given to Fornication or bodily lust, are very rarely diseased: Also the more a Man is addicted to these Pleasures, the sooner he catcheth it, and as they manage themselves after, either temperately or otherwise, so it the sooner leaves them, holds them a long time, or utterly consumes them. Thus is it more easy to the *Italians* and *Spaniards* as well as others, living soberly, but through our surfeiting and Intemperance it doth longer hold, and more grievously vex us.

* * *

CHAP. II

Of the Causes of this Disease

The Physicians have not yet certainly discovered the secret Cause of this Disease, although they have long and diligently enquired after the same. In this all agree, which is very evident, that through some unwholesome Blasts of Air, which happen about that time, the Lakes, Fountains, and even the Waters of the Sea were corrupted, and the Earth for a large Tract, as it were poisoned thereby: The Pastures were infected, and venomous, Streams filled the whole Air, which living Creatures took in with their Breath; for this Distemper at first was found among the Cattle as well as among Men.

The *Astrologers* deriving the Cause from the Stars, said, That it proceeded from the Conjunction of *Saturn* and *Mars,* which happened not long before, and of two Eclipses of the Sun; affirming, that hence they perceived were like to ensue many *cholerick* as well as *phlegmatick* Distempers, which would long contiue, and slowly depart; such as *Elephantiasis, Lepra, Impetigo,* and all kinds of Scabs and Boils, with whatever could afflict Man's Body, as the *Gout, Palsy, Sciatica* or *Joynt-Ach,* and the like Infirmities; and that these should chance rather in the North, by reason of the Sign *Aquarius,* wherein fell the first Eclipse, and in the West from *Piscis,* in which happened the last.

But the Physicians concluded this to arise from ill Humours abounding in Men's Bodies, as black, adust or yellow Choler; salt Phlegm; of one of these alone, or mix'd together with the rest, and thrown out to the Skin, which is covered over with Scabs; whilst that which proceedeth of raw, heavy and gross Humour, is cast upon the Joints, causing great Pain therein, raising also Swellings with hard Knobs, or Knots, and shriveling of the Skin; with stubborn Headaches also, strangely altering the Complection of the Sick. Some briefly concluding say, it arose from a corrupt, burnt or adust, and infected Blood, and these Disputes held doubtful for a long time, the Nature of the Disease not rightly known; but now it is generally believed, and my self do verily think it to be no other, than the Effect of an aprostemated, rotten or corrupted Blood, which beginning to dry, turneth into these hard Swellings or Knobs, the Spring or Source of which is in the Liver corrupted.

To enquire farther after the Nature and Quality of this sickness would be tiresome and uncertain; for we see in our times diverse Opinions very confidently held forth, and much Pains in the Physicians have taken therein, since it came among us. Those of *Germany,* for the Space of two Years, were employed in such like Disputations; and when I was yet a Child, they undertook to heal me: But what Profit came thereof, the End did shew; notwithstanding they were bold enough to tamper with their foreign Drugs and Spices, and to mingle and administer many things to little purpose. I remember among others, they forbid me to eat Peas, for in some Places, there were found certain Worms therein, which had Wings; of the which Hogs Flesh also was thought to be infected, because that Creature especially was found diseased, either with this, or some other like it.

CHAP. III

Of the SYMPTOMS *Attending This Disease*

Though this Distemper singly may be lightly accounted, yet doth it soon convert itself into many others; and indeed whatever Pains affect a Man's Joints, may seem to arise hence; for first there is a sharp Ach in these Parts, and yet nothing to be seen; but afterwards a Flux of Humours falls down, occasioning a Swelling, which beginning to harden about the Part, a most vehement Pain ariseth: which is the first Appearance of the Distemper when it begins to fortify itself as in a Castle, there resting for a long time, and thence to disperse its Emissaries into every part of the Body, kindling therein all sorts of Aches and Dolors; when the longer the Swellings are before they ripen, the more Pain is the Patient to suffer, and truly of all others, this is the most intolerable. I myself had such a Knob or hard Swelling above my left heel on the inside, the which after it was indurated for the Space of Seven Years, could by no Applications be softened or brought to Matter, but still continued like a Bone, till by the help of *Guajacum* it gradually vanished.

In Women the Disease resteth in their secret Places, wherein are little pretty Sores, full of venomous Poison, being very dangerous for such as unknowingly meddle with them; the which Sickness, when contracted from these infected Women, is so much the more grievous, by how much they are more inwardly corrupted and polluted therewith. By this a Man's Sinews are sometimes relaxed, and again grow hard, and contract themselves. Sometimes the Disease transforms itself into the *Gout;* at others, into a *Palsy* and *Apoplexy*, and infecteth many also with a *Leprosy;* for it is thought these Diseases are Neighbours each to the other by reason of some Affinity there appears between them; those which are seized with the *Pox,* frequently becoming *Lepers,* and through the acuteness of the Pain, Men will shake and quiver as in a Fever.

After this there will appear small Holes and Sores, turning *cankerous* and *fistulous,* which the more putrid they grow, the more they will eat into the Bones, and when they have been long corrupted the Sick grows lean, his Flesh wasting away, so that there remaineth only the Skin as a Cover for them: And by this many fall into Consumption, having their inward Parts corrupted.

Besides all which, from this Disease floweth another called *Cachexy,* which renders the Body bloated, as if the Flesh and Skin were filled with Water. Some have Sores in their Bladder, and oftentimes the Stomach and Liver is quite spoiled by the sickness; and in this their Opinion is false, who say, that these Humours, Swellings and Knobs, are not the proper Symptoms of this Disease, but happen only by the Use of the *Quick-Silver Ointments,* of which Opinion are most part of our physicians in *Almayn;* but they are deceived in this thing as they are in many others; for I know it of a Certainty, that there are some who have had these Appearances which were never anointed with *Quick-Silver;* as among others I could here name, I have had certain Knowledge and Experience in my Father *Ulrich de Hutten.*

CHAP. IV

How Men at first attempted the Cure of this Disease

Whilst the Physicians were thus confounded like Men amazed, the Surgeons as wretchedly lent a helping Hand to the same Error, and first began to burn the Sores with hot Irons. But for as much, as there seemed no end of this Cruelty, they endeavoured now to avoid the same with their *Ointments*, but all in vain, unless they added *Quick-Silver* thereunto. To this purpose they used the Powders of *Myrrh, Mastich, Ceruse, Bayberries, Allum, Bole Armoniac, Cinnabar, Vermillion, Coral, burnt Salt, Rust of Brass, Litharge, Rust of Iron, Refine of Turpentine,* and all manner of the best Oils, as of *Bay, Roses, Turpentine, Juniper,* [and of yet greater Power] the Oil of *Spike;* also *Hogs-Lard, Neats-Foot Oil, May Butter, Goats* and *Deers Suet, Virgin Honey, red Worms dried to Powder or boiled up with Oil, Camphire, Euphorbium, Castor.*

With these, fewer or more, they anointed the sick Man's Joints, his Arms, Thighs, his Neck and Back, with other parts of his Body. Some using these Anointings once a Day, some twice, others three times, and four times, others; the Patient being shut up in a Stove, with continual and fervent Heat, some twenty, some thirty, whole Days. Some lying in Bed within the Stove were thus anointed, and covered with many Clothes, being compelled to sweat; Part at the second anointing began to faint; yet was the Ointment of such Strength, that whatsoever Distemper was in the upper Parts it drew it into the Stomach, and thence to the Brain; and so the Disease was voided both by the Nose and Mouth, and put the Patient to so great Pain, that except they took good heed, their Teeth fell out, and their Throats, their Lungs, with the Roofs of their Mouths, were full of Sores; their Jaws did swell, their Teeth loosen'd, and a stinking Matter continually was voided from these places. What Part soever it touched, the same was strait corrupted thereby, so that not only their Lips, but the inside of their Cheeks, were grievously pained, and made the Place where they were, stink most abominably; which sort of Cure was indeed so terrible, that many chose rather to die than to be eased thus of their Sickness. Howeveit, scarce one Sick Person in a hundred could be cured in this Way, but quickly after relapsed, so that the Cure held but for a few Days. Whereby may be infer'd what I suffered in the same Disease, who underwent the same in this Fashion for eleven times, with great Peril and Jeopardy of Life, struggling with the Disease nine Years together, taking all the time whatever was thought proper to withstand the Disease; such as *Baths* with *Herbs, Drinks* and *Cor-*

rosives, of which kind we had *Arsnick, Ink Calcantum, Verdegrease* and *Aquafortis,* which occasioned such bitter Pains, that those might be thought very desirous of Life, who had not rather die than thus prolong it. For these Curings were exceedingly painful that were set upon by these Ointments, and the more so, being set about by ignorant Men, who knew nothing of their Operation; for not only the Surgeons, but every bold Fellow played the Physician in this Business, using to all manner of Sick People the same Ointment, either as he had seen used by others, or as he had undergone it himself. And so they undertook to cure all with one Medicine; or as the Proverb says, *The same Shoe for every Foot.* If any thing happened wrong for want of good Advice, they knew not what to do or say; and these *Men Tormentors* were suffered thus to practice on all Persons as they were minded. whilst the Physicians were as Men struck dumb, not knowing what Course to take; and thus without Rule or Order, with torment of Heat, and plenty of Sweat, all were set upon after one Fashion, without regard of Time, Habit or Complection. Neither had these wretched *Anointers* so much Sense as to prepare the Body with Laxatives, to abate something of the Matter which occasioned this Evil; or to diet them properly, so that at last the Matter came to this, that most of them lost their Teeth, their mouths being all in a Sore, and through Coldness of their Stomachs and filthy Stench their Appetites were destroyed; and although their Thirst was most intolerable, yet they found no Liquor to help them. Many were so light and giddy that they could not stand: Some run mad, and not only their Hands and Feet, but their whole Bodies trembling: Some also were forced to mumble and stammer in their Speech as long as they lived, without any Remedy. Many I have seen die in the midst of these Curations; and one I knew who did his Cures in such manner, that in one Day he killed three Husbandmen, through excessive Heat, which they patiently underwent, being shut up in a close Stove, trusting thereby only, they should gain Health the sooner, till through such excessive Heat their Hearts failed them, not perceiving themselves to die, while they were thus miserably suffocated. Others I beheld whose Throats were swelled up, that there was not room for the filthy Matter to be voided; so that they were strangled and their Breath stopped up. Another sort there were, who could make no Water, very few were they who could get their Health after all these Pains and Perils of Life.

Jacques de Béthencourt

Jacques de Béthencourt, a physician at Rouen, was one of the earliest French physicians to write an account of syphilis. His *New Litany of Penitence* was published at Paris in 1527 and is especially noteworthy for the introduction

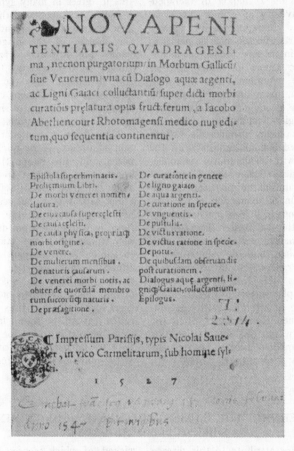

Title page from Jacques de Béthencourt's *Nova penitentialis quadragesima.* Paris, 1527

of the term "Morbus venereus" or "venereal disease" into the nomenclature of syphilis. Béthencourt rejects the common term "Morbus Gallicus" (French disease) and suggests that since the disease arises from illicit love it should be called the malady of Venus or venereal disease. Béthencourt affirms that syphilis is a new disease, unknown to the ancients and that it did not appear in Europe until towards the end of the fifteenth century. He states that it arises from sexual contact and that it can be transmitted to the offspring. He fell, however, into the serious error of confusing syphilis with gonorrhoea.

The following selections are from the *Nova penitentialis quadragesima, nec non purgatorium in Morbum Gallicum sive Venereum,* . . . a Jacobo Abethencourt, Paris, 1527.

CONCERNING THE NAME OF THE VENEREAL DISEASE; AND WHY THE NAME OF A SAINT SHOULD BE BY NO MEANS SELECTED*

Galen says in his 2 chapter of therapeutics that the diversity of names should be carefully studied. Some names of diseases are from the parts affected such as pleuritis, which is a pain in the side, ischias, nephritis, cephalalgia. The names of other diseases come from the symptoms, thus volvulus, apepsia, apnoea, paraphrosine; frequently from both such as otalgia, cephalia, odontalgia, hysteralgia; commonly from the cause, as white phlegm melancholia (which the Greeks called leukophlegmosia). In the same manner with elephantiasis, staphila, atheroma, mellideris. Galen says Chapter 3 de morbo, the fame of the physician is seen to depend not on the name but in the carrying out of things. Still it is not necessary. Galen says in the 1 Chapter Therapeutics is betrayed by names, certainly names with the same meaning; and the similarity of names produces raillery. For indeed the year in which Charles VIII King of the French laid siege to Naples, a certain disease broke out among some of our men both foot-soldiers and horsemen. The Italians call it the French disease, we on this side of the Alps call it the Neapolitan disease, others the great pox, many elephantiasis, indeed with this it agrees in many symptoms. Some call it lichen or impetigo. Others from its location mentagra or pudendagra. And many, the disease of the magnates. Plato says names are introduced for things not by choice: or otherwise by the instinct of nature. If named from the cause (which according to my judgment certainly should be done) the disease justly should be called the venereal disease (morbus venerus).

Many have attributed the disease to certain saints, as to the mighty Saint Sement, perhaps for this reason that the disease we know to be abundant and widespread. Not a few call it the disease of Saint Job: which (they say) was a foul scabies. Hippocrates says in his book on the sacred disease, if those in bed suffer from dreams, terrors and such things they are said to be deceitful enchanters and repugnant to an honest man, although they practice atonements and charms, so they do not make a wicked divinity holy; and their piety is wicked. And since such a disease arises from sexual intercourse (as will be shown in what follows) it seems unworthy to ascribe it to these saints, since we do not wish to attribute it to men of the most exemplary life.

* * *

CONCERNING THE CAUSES AND FIRSTLY CONCERNING THE SUPER-CELESTIAL CAUSES

The Theologians attribute to this disease a divine (super-celestial) cause; & to be a scourge of God for the punishment of the wicked, of which scourge the Psalmist with an iron rod punishes their iniquities. Moses said in the 28th chapter of Deuteronomy: "If you will not hear the voice of the Lord your God, you will be struck by the botch of Egypt and with the emerods."

* de Béthencourt, Jacques, *Nova penitentialis quadragesima, nec non purgatorium in morbum Gallicum sive Venereum,* Paris, Saveler, 1527, p. B ii.

* * *

CONCERNING THE SIGNS OF VENEREAL DISEASE, AND INCIDENTALLY CONCERNING THE NATURE OF CERTAIN MEMBERS AS WELL AS FLUIDS

I should like certainly the treatment of this venereal disease to be evident to us as well as its striking characteristics. There is no doubt but that it takes its primary origin from venery. From this venereal contagion it has arisen. With small body and certain adults (though more rarely) it can arise both from chaste and from sexual contact. And it happens to those persons of great piety in visiting through human charity the unfortunate, and indigent (which is to be piously believed). If by venereal contact (for at this time it is scarcely by any other method) it breaks out on the skin of the penis and the cervix of the womb. Indeed they are the organs of propagation & if grisly (as Galen says) the neck of the womb as well as the penis becomes cartilagenous. . . . Therefore virulent, bloody ulcerations appear on these parts. But if this disease was contracted otherwise, that is without sexual intercourse, such ulcers appear on the parts exposed to contagions; for example it appears on the mouth of babies from nursing women infected with the venereal disease. Such ulcers and pustules appear on the legs and head. Besides indeed the principal member, from which nature is much disturbed, sends juices chiefly mixed phlegm to the other juices, to the forehead, cervis, temples, arms and not to many other parts: these things are followed by pustules, a severe pain appears in the said parts but not in the nerves and muscles. Therefore the senses are not affected nor obviously the power of motion. And if the disease proceeds further on account of the flow of vicious humors in this disease from the head ulcers can be formed in the trachea, or throat, or esophagus, palate or fauces. If it proceeds further than this, the nose is damaged, then it shows its malignity in other places.

* * *

DEFINITION OF THE VENEREAL DISEASE

The venereal disease is a condition of the body proceeding from sexual intercourse and contagion: at the onset causing ulcers on the genitalia or the point of contagion: then corrupting the humors especially the phlegm, the organs of generation: by which postules, tumors, ulcers and pains are produced.

Hieronymus Fracastorius

Hieronymus Fracastorius was born in Verona in 1483, the son of a noble family. Two circumstances of his infancy were remarkable. He was born with such a small mouth that it was necessary to enlarge it with a surgical instrument so that the infant could nurse and one day while in the arms of his mother, she was struck by a thunderbolt and killed, while the infant was unharmed. He went to the renowned University of Padua, where he studied philosophy, mathematics, *belles-lettres* and medicine. He practiced medicine, after graduation, at Verona, and rapidly acquired a reputation that spread not only throughout Italy, but throughout Europe as well. Medicine was his chief passion, but he also found time to study mathematics, music, geography, and botany, and to write poetry.

Fracastorius' *'Treatise on Contagion,'* which appeared in 1546, comes very near to expressing the modern conception of bacterial infections. He recognizes infection by contact, through an intermediary and by means of fomites. He describes contagion as a sort of putrefaction, caused by particles not perceived by our senses (*insensibilibus particulis*) and he recognized the contagiousness of smallpox, measles, tuberculosis, rabies, and syphilis. He gave the first clear

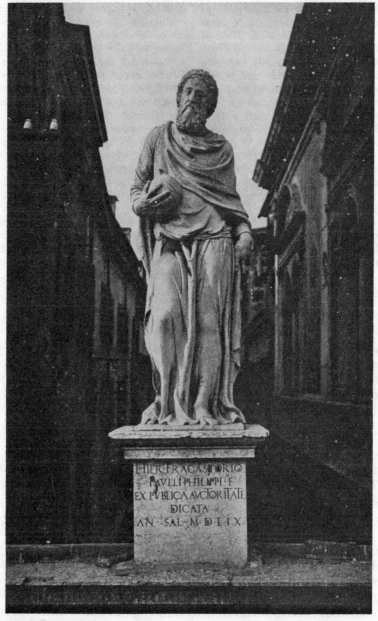

Kindness of Mr. R. Lier

STATUE OF FRACASTORIUS (1483-1553) BY DANESE CATTANEO, ON THE PIAZZA
DEL SIGNORI IN VERONA, ERECTED IN 1559

account of typhus fever, a translation of which appears later in this book (page 164). The Venetian ambassador, Andrea Navagiero, whose tragic death he describes, was a lifelong friend and an old fellow student at Padua. His eulogy of Navagiero, which fills an entire page, is omitted from the translation.

Fracastorius was not only a physician, poet, mathematician, physicist, and astronomer, but also a geologist who saw fossil remains as the bodies of pre-historic plants. He died in 1553 of apoplexy. In 1559 a statue was erected in his memory at Verona with an eulogy of the author of "that divine Poem Syphilis." This poem, written, as he says, in his lighter moments, brought him more fame than all of his scientific writings. It appeared first in 1530 and was dedicated to the illustrious Cardinal Bembo, his old friend and classmate at Padua. The following selections from the third book relates the legend of the shepherd Syphilis, who, for an act of impiety, was struck with the French disease. This poem became so famous that the word *syphilis* soon became the universal term for this disease and displaced all other designations. The translation in English verse, in the Surgeon General's Library, is by Mr. Tate and bears no date or place of publication. This Mr. Tate was Nahum Tate, English poet and playwright, who was born in Dublin in 1652 and became poet laureate in 1692. He wrote several plays, but is best known for his version of the Psalms of David and his hymns "As pants the hart" and "While shepherds watched." He died in 1717 in the Mint, Southwark, where he had fled to escape his creditors. The British Museum has a copy of his *Poetical History of the French Disease* published in London in 1685. In the biographical sketch of Fracastorius preceding Tate's translation, the statement is made that Fracastorius during an epidemic of the plague withdrew from Verona to his country estate and employed his leisure in writing the poem that later brought him fame.

This poem describes a visit of the Spanish to one of the isles in the West Indies where they witnessed a strange religious ceremony. They observed the worshippers were all suffering from a loathsome disease. The Spanish general, inquiring of the native prince the meaning of the religious rites and the infected throng of worshippers, heard from him an account of a new disease and its origin. The following selection is the speech of the native prince and is only a fragment of the poem.

A POETICAL HISTORY OF THE FRENCH DISEASE

Perhaps you may have heard of *Atlas* name,
From whom in long descent great Nations came;
From him we sprang, and once a happy Race,
Belov'd of Heav'n while Piety had place
While to the Gods our Ancestours did Pray,
And grateful Off'rings on their Altars lay.
But when the Powers to be dispis'd began,
When to leud Luxury our Nation ran;
Who can express the Mis'ries that ensu'd,
And Plagues with each returning Day renew'd.
Then fair *Atlantia* once an Isle of fame;
(That from the mighty *Atlas* took its Name,

Who there had govern'd long with upright Sway)
Was gorg'd entire, and swallowed by the Sea
With which our Flocks and Herds were wholly drown'd,
Not one preserv'd or ever after found.
Since when outlandish Cattle here are slain,
And Bulls of foreign Breed our Altars stain,
In that dire Season this Disease was bred,
That thus o'er all our tortur'd Limbs is spread:
Most universal from its Birth it grew,
And none have since escap'd or very few;
Sent from above to scourge that vicious Age,

And chiefly by incens'd Apollo's Rage,
For which these annual Rites were first
  ordain'd,
Whereof this firm, Tradition is retain'd.
  A shepherd once (distrust not ancient
    Fame)
Possest these Downs, and *Syphilus* his Name.
A thousand Heifers in these Vales he fed.

But to the Noon-day Sun with up-cast Eyes,
In rage threw these reproaching Blasphemies.
Is it for this O *Sol*, that thou art styl'd
Our God and Parent? how are we beguil'd
Dull Bigots to pay Homage to thy Name?
And with rich Spices feed thy Altar's flame:
Why do we yearly Rites for thee prepare,
Who tak'st of our affairs so little Care?

HIERONYMI FRACASTORII
SYPHILIS,
SIVE MORBVS GALLICVS
AD P. BEMBVM.

Vi casus rerum uary, quæ semi-
  na morbum
q   *I nsuetum, nec longa ulli per se-*
  cula uisum
  A ttulerint : nostra qui tempesta-
  te per omnem

E uropam, partim'q, Asiæ, Libyeq, per urbes
S æuyt : in Latium uero per tristia bella
G allorum irrupit : nomen'q, à gente recepit.
N ec non et quæ cura : et opis quid comperit usus,
M agnaq, in angustis hominum sollertia rebus :
E t monstrata Deum auxilia, et data munera cœli,
H inc canere, et longe secretas quærere causas
A era per liquidum, et uasti per sudera olympi
I ncipiam, dulci quando nouitatis amore
                              a   ij

First page of text from *Hieronymus Fracastorius,
Syphilis, Sive Morbus Gallicus.* First
Edition (Verona, 1530)

A thousand Ews to those fair Rivers led:
For King *Alcithoüs* he rais'd this Stock,
And shaded in the Covert of a Rock
For now 'twas *Solstice,* and the *Syrian* Star
Increast the Heat and shot his Beams afar;
The Fields were burnt to ashes, and the
  Swain
Repair'd for shade to thickest Woods in vain,
No Wind to fan the scorching Air was found,
No nightly Dew refresht the thirsty Ground;
This Drought our *Syphilus* beheld with pain,
Nor could the suff'rings of his Flock sustain,

At least thou might'st between the Rabble
  Kine
Distinguish, and these royal Herds of Mine.
These to the great *Alcithoüs* belong,
Nor ought to perish with the Vulgar throng.
Or shall I rather think your Diety
With envious Eyes our thriving Stock did
  see?
I grant you had sufficient cause indeed,
A thousand Heifers of the snowy Breed,
A thousand Ews of mine these Downs did
  feed;

Whilst one Etherial Bull was all your flock,
One Ram, and to preserve this mighty Flock,
You must forsooth your *Syrian* Dog
maintain,
Why do I worship then a Pow'r so Vain?
Henceforth I to *Alcithoüs* will bring
My off'rings and Adore my greater King,
Who do such spacious Tracts of Land
possess,
And whose vast Pow'r the conquer'd Seas
confess.
Him I'll invoke my Suff'rings to redress.
He'll streight command the cooling Winds to
blow.
Refreshing Show'rs on Trees and Herbs
bestow.
Nor suffer Thirst, both Flock and Swain to
kill:
He said, and forthwith on a neighbouring
Hill
Erects an Altar to his Monarch's name,
The Swains from far bring Incense to the
Flame;
At length to greater Victims they proceed,
Till Swine and Heifers too by hundreds
Bleed,
On whole half roasted Flesh the impious
Wretches feed,
All quarters soon were fill'd with the Report,
That ceas'd not till it reacht the Monarch's
Court;
Th' aspiring Prince with Godlike Rites o'er
joy'd,
Commands all Altars else to be destroy'd,
Proclaims Himself in Earth's low sphere
to be
The onely and sufficient Deity;
That Heav'nly Pow'rs liv'd too remote and
high,
And had enough to do to Rule the Sky.
Th' all-seeing Sun no longer could sustain
These practices, but with enrag'd Disdain
Darts forth such pestilent malignant Beams,
As shed Infection on Air, Earth and Streams;
From whence this Malady its birth receiv'd,
And first th' offending *Syphilus* was griev'd,
Who rais'd forbidden Altars on the Hill,
And Victims bloud with impious Hands did
spill;
He first wore Buboes dreadful to the sight,
First felt strange Pains and sleepless past
the Night:
From him the Malady receiv'd its name,
The neighbouring Shepherds catcht the
spreading Flame:

At last in City and in Court 'twas known,
And seiz'd the ambitious Monarch on his
Throne;
In this distress the wretched Tribes repair
To *Ammerice* the Gods Interpreter,
Chief Priestess of the consecrated Wood,
In whose Retreats the awful Tripod stood
From whence the Gods responsal she exprest;
The Crowd enquire what Cause produc'd
this Pest,
What God enrag'd? and how to be appeas'd,
And last what Cure remain'd for the
Diseas'd?
To whom the Nymph reply'd—the Sun
incens'd,
With just revenge these Torments has
commenc'd.
What man can with immortal Pow'rs com-
pare?
Fly, wretches, fly, his Altars soon repair,
Load them with Incense, Him with Pray'rs
invade,
His Anger will not easily be laid;
Your Doom is past, black Styx has heard
him swear,
This Plague should never be extinguisht here,
Since then your Soil must ne'er be wholly
free,
Beg Heav'n at least to yield some Remedy:
A milk white Cow on Juno's Altar lay,
To Mother Earth a jet-black Heifer slay;
One from above the happy Seeds shall shed,
The other rear the Grove and make it
Spread,
That onely for your Grief a Cure shall yield.
She said: the Croud return'd to th' open'd
Field,
Rais'd Altars to the Sun without delay,
To Mother Earth, and *Juno* Victims slay.
'Twill seem most strange what now I shall
declare,
But by our Gods and Ancestours I swear,
'Tis sacred Truth . . .
These Groves that spread so wide and look
so green
Within this Isle, till then, were never seen,
But now before their Eyes the Plants were
found
To spring and in an instant Shade the
ground,
The Priest forthwith bids Sacrifice be done,
And Justice paid to the offended Sun;
Some destin'd Hetd t' attone the Crimes of
all,
On *Syphilus* the dreadful Lot did fall,

Who now was plac'd before the Altar bound,
His head with sacrificial Garlands crown'd,
His Throat laid open to the lifted Knife,
But interceding *Juno* spar'd his Life,
Commands them in his stead a Heifer slay,
For *Phoebus* Rage was now remov'd away.
This made our grateful Ancestours enjoin,
When first these annual Rites they did assign,
That to the Altar bound a Swine each time
Should stand, to witness *Syphilus* his Crime.
All this infected Throng whom you behold,
Smart for their Ancestours Offence of old:
To heal their Plague this Sacrifice is done,
And reconcile them to th' offended Sun.
The Rites perform'd, the hallow'd Boughs
    they seize,
The speedy certain Cure for their Disease.
    With such discourse the Chiefs their Cares
    deceive
Whose Tribes of different Worlds united live,
Till now the Ships sent back to *Europes*
    shore,
Return and bring prodigious Tidings o'er.
That this Disease did now through Europe
    rage,
Nor any Medicine found that cou'd assuage,
That in their Ships no slender Number
    mourn'd,
With Boils without and inward Ulcers burn'd.
Then call'd to mind the Bird's prophetick
    sound,
That in these Groves Relief was to be found.
Then each with solemn Vows the Sun
    entreats,
And gentle Nymphs the Gardians of those
    Seats.
With lusty Strokes the Grove they next
    invade,
Whose weighty Boughs are on their Shoulders
    laid,

Which with the Natives Methods they
    prepare,
And with the healing Draughts their Health
    repair,
But not forgetful of their Country's good,
They fraight their largest Ships with this
    rich Wood,
To try if in our Climate it would be
Of equal use, for the same Malady:
The years mild Season seconds their desire,
And western Winds their willing Sails inspire.
Iberian Coasts you first were happy made
With this rich Plant, and wonder'd at its Aid;
Known now to *France* and neighbouring
    Germany
Cold *Scythian* Coasts and temp'rate *Italy*,
To *Europe's* Bounds all bless the vial Tree.
    Hail heav'n-born Plant whose Rival ne'er
    was seen,
Whose Virtues like thy Leaves are ever
    green;
Hope of Mankind and Comfort of their Eyes,
Of new discover'd Worlds the richest Prize.
Too happy would Indulgent Gods allow,
Thy Groves in Europe's nobler Clime to
    grow:
Yet if my Streins have any force, thy Name
Shall flourish here, and *Europe* sing thy
    Fame.
If not remoter Lands with Winter bound,
Eternal   Snows,   nor   *Libya's*   scorching
    Ground:
Yet *Latium* and *Benacus* cool Retreats,
Shall thee resound, with *Athesis* fair Seats.
Too, blest if *Bembus* live thy Growth to see,
And on the Banks of *Tyber* gather thee,
If he thy matchless Virtues once rehearse,
And crown their Praises with eternal Verse.

FINIS

John Hunter

The career of John Hunter is one of the most amazing in medical history. Although hampered by a defective education, unable usually to express himself clearly by either written or spoken word, confessedly ignorant of the work of his surgical colleagues at home and that of his foreign contemporaries, yet by sheer force of industry and an irrepressible curiosity to examine the workings of Nature in all her forms, he became the foremost surgical investigator of his age, the leading surgeon in the world's metropolis, the founder of the greatest tradition in the annals of British surgery. He towers above his contemporaries, his predecessors and his successors, and, as Ambroise Paré is the greatest figure in the history of French surgery, so John Hunter is by common agreement the greatest in the history of British surgery.

John Hunter was born on July 14, 1728 at Long Calderwood in Lanarkshire, Scotland, the youngest of ten children. His father, who was nearly seventy years of age at the time of his birth died when John was only ten. He was an

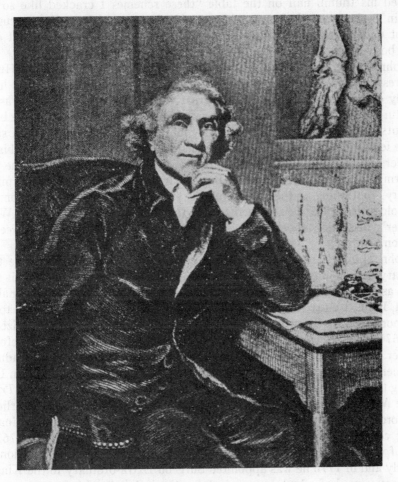

JOHN HUNTER (1728-1793)
Engraving from a painting by Sir Joshua Reynolds

idle youth, a very poor student and left the grammar school quite ignorant of the learning it was supposed to impart. Tiring after a few years of his idle life in Long Calderwood, he wrote to his brother William, who had become a celebrated teacher of anatomy, expressing a desire to assist him in his dissections. Receiving a kind invitation from his brother to come to London, John Hunter arrived there in 1748, aged twenty-one years. He immediately began to dissect under the eyes of his elder brother and for eleven successive winters his life was passed in the dissecting room. He attended the lectures of Cheselden at

Chelsea and in 1754 became a pupil at St. Bartholomew's Hospital where Percival Pott was the leading surgeon.

In 1755, he entered Oxford University but remained there less than two months. "They tried to make an old woman of me," he said in later years, "they wanted to stuff me with Greek and Latin at the University, but" and he pressed his thumb nail on the table "these schemes I cracked like so many vermin as they came before me." Long after he wrote, "Jesse Foot accuses me of not understanding the dead languages; but I could teach him that on the dead body which he never knew in any language dead or living."

John Hunter was soon admitted to a partnership in Dr. William Hunter's lectures but here his defective education and his inability to express himself clearly or properly was a source of great embarrassment. On one occasion in a lecture, after a vain attempt to express himself clearly, he said, "the ball hit the guts such a damned thump that they mortified." Despite his lack of success in the lecture room John Hunter continued to be of great assistance to his elder brother and began to make important anatomical discoveries. In 1760 he joined the army as a staff surgeon and for three years was deep in the study of military surgery, continuing at the same time his studies in comparative anatomy and physiology. In 1763 he returned to London, but finding his place in William Hunter's dissection room occupied by another, he started in practice as a surgeon.

John Hunter's success in practice came very slowly. His attitude to the ordinary patient was probably well expressed in his classic remark to his friend Lynn as he laid aside his dissecting instruments to answer a professional call: "Well, Lynn, I must go and earn this damned guinea, or I shall be sure to want it tomorrow." His scientific achievements were, however, soon recognized and in 1767 he was elected a Fellow of the Royal Society, three months before his brother was similarly honored. The following year John Hunter was admitted as a member of the Corporation of Surgeons and in 1771 he married Ann Home, paying the expenses of the wedding from the sale of the first part of his *Treatise of the Natural History of the Teeth*. Hunter had expected to marry earlier but was forced to postpone the marriage because of the infection he had inadvertently contracted in the course of his experiments upon himself in 1767, the cure of which he says occupied three years. Hunter's fame and reputation grew steadily and in 1776 he was appointed Surgeon Extra-ordinary to the King and for many years he had a large surgical practice in London, his income exceeding six thousand pounds a year.

Hunter's health, which had been excellent until his unfortunate inoculation in 1767, began to fail in 1773. He had frequent attacks of dizziness and of angina. His old friend and pupil Edward Jenner, who saw him in Bath in 1777, was so shocked at his appearance that he wrote Heberden: "I thought he was affected with many symptoms of angina pectoris." In 1788 Hunter wrote Jenner that a severe indisposition had prevented him from writing although he added jestingly, "when two guineas rouse me I cannot resist." In 1793 Hunter attended a meeting of the Board at St. George's Hospital and following a heated discussion, "he withheld his sentiments, in which state of restraint he went into the next room, and turning round to Dr. Robinson, one of the physiciar.s of the hospital, he gave a deep groan and dropt down dead." John Hunter was buried quietly in the vaults of St. Martin-in-the-Fields on the 22nd of October, 1793. In 1859 the body was reinterred in Westminster Abbey between the graves of Wilkie and Ben Jonson.

John Hunter was remarkable both for his achievements and his personality. One who reads his career is filled with admiration for his genius, entertained by the shrewd, witty remarks which enliven all his correspondence and often convulsed with laughter at the amusing adventures which mark his pursuit of knowledge. His unfortunate experience with his ill fated inoculation with syphilis has been immortalized by the name of "Hunterian chancre" to describe the primary lesion of lues venerea. The experiment described in the following selection was carried out on himself and, unfortunately, the subject from whom the gonorrhoeal pus was obtained also suffered from syphilis. This led Hunter into the grave error of assuming that gonorrhoea and syphilis were the same disease, an error which persisted in medicine for a century.

SECTION II

EXPERIMENTS MADE TO ASCERTAIN THE PROGRESS AND EFFECTS OF THE VENEREAL POISON*

To ascertain several facts relative to the venereal disease, the following experiments were made. They were begun in May, 1767.

Two punctures were made on the penis with a lancet dipped in venereal matter from a gonorrhoea; one puncture was on the glans, the other on the prepuce.

This was on a Friday; on the Sunday following there was a teazing itching in those parts, which lasted till the Tuesday following. In the mean time, these parts being often examined, there seemed to be a greater redness and moisture than usual, which was imputed to the parts being rubbed. Upon the Tuesday morning, the parts of the prepuce where the puncture had been made were redder, thickened, and had formed a speck; by the Tuesday following, the speck had increased and discharged some matter, and there seemed to be a little pouting of the lips of the urethra, also a sensation in it in making water, so that a discharge was expected from it. The speck was now touched with lunar caustic, and afterwards dressed with calomel ointment. On Saturday morning, the slough came off; and was again touched, and another slough came off on the Monday following. The preceding night the glans had

* Hunter, John, *A Treatise on the Venereal Disease*, London, Sherwood, Neely and Jones, 1818, p. 449.

itched a good deal, and on Tuesday a white speck was observed where the puncture had been made; this speck, when examined, was found to be a pimple full of yellowish matter. This was now touched with the caustic, and dressed as the former. On the Wednesday, the sore on the prepuce was yellow, and therefore was again touched wth caustic. On the Friday both sloughs came off: and the sore on the prepuce looked red, and its basis not so hard; but on Saturday it did not look quite so well, and was touched again; and, when that went off, it was allowed to heal, as also the other, which left a dent in the glans. This dent on the glans was filled up in some months, but for a considerable time it had a bluish cast.

Four months afterwards the chancre on the prepuce broke out again; and very stimulating applications were tried; but these seemed not to agree with it, and nothing being applied, it healed up. This it did several times afterwards, but always healed up without any application to it. That on the glans never did break out; and herein also it differed from the other.

While the sores remained on the prepuce and glans, a swelling took place in one of the glands of the right groin. I had for some time conceived an idea that the most effectual way to put back a bubo was to rub in mercury on that leg and thigh, that thus a current of mercury would pass through the inflamed gland. There was a good opportunity of making the experiment. I had often succeeded in this way, but now wanted to put it more critically to the test.* The sores upon the penis were healed before the reduction of the bubo was attempted. A few days after beginning the mercury in this method, the gland subsided considerably. It was then left off; for the intention was not to cure it completely at present. The gland some time after began to swell again, and as much mercury was rubbed in as appeared to be sufficient for the entire reduction of the gland; but it was meant to do more than to cure the gland locally, without giving enough to prevent the constitution from being contaminated.

About two months after the last attack of the bubo, a little sharp pricking pain was felt in one of the tonsils in swallowing any thing; and, on inspection, a small ulcer was found, which was allowed to go on till the nature of it was ascertained, and then recourse was had to mercury. The mercury was thrown in by the same leg and thigh as before, to secure the gland more effectually, although that was not now probably necessary.

As soon as the ulcer was skinned over, the mercury was left off, it not being intended to destroy the poison, but to observe what parts it would next affect. About three months after, copper-coloured blotches broke out on the skin, and the former ulcer returned in the tonsil. Mercury was now applied the second time for those effects of the poison from the constitution, but still only with a view to palliate.

It was left off a second time, and the attention was given to mark where it would break out next; but it returned again in the same parts. It not appearing that any fur-

ther knowledge was to be procured by only palliating the disease a fourth time in the tonsil, and a third time in the skin, mercury was now taken in a sufficient quantity, and for a proper time, to complete the cure.

The time the experiments took up, from the first insertion to the complete cure, was about three years.

The above case is only uncommon in the mode of contracting the disease, and the particular views with which some parts of the treatment were directed; but as it was meant to prove many things, which, though not uncommon, are yet not attended to, attention was paid to all the circumstances. It proves many things, and opens a field for further conjectures.

It proves first, that matter from a gonorrhoea will produce chancres.

It makes it probable that the glans does not admit the venereal irritation so quickly as the prepuce. The chancre, on the prepuce, inflamed and suppurated in somewhat more than three days, and that oɪ the glans in about ten. This is probably the reason why the glans did not throw off its sloughts so soon.

It renders it highly probable, that to apply mercury to the legs and thighs, is the best method of resolving bubo; and therefore also the best method of applying mercury to assist in the cure, even when the bubo suppurates.

It also shows that buboes may be resolved in this way, and yet the constitution not safe: and therefore that more mercury should be thrown in especially in cases of easy resolution, than what simply resolves the bubo.

It shows that parts may be contaminated, and may have the poison kept dormant in them while under a course of mercury for other symptoms, but break out afterwards.

It also shows that the poison, having originally only contaminated certain parts, when not completely cured, can break out again only in those parts.

* The practice in 1767 was to apply a mercurial plaster on the part, or to rub in mercurial ointment on the part, which could hardly act by any other power than sympathy.

Sir Jonathan Hutchinson

Jonathan Hutchinson was born at Selby, Yorkshire, in 1828. He studied medicine first at the York School of Medicine and Surgery, a small school, in which, Hutchinson later remarked, he was the only pupil in some of the classes and so received the undivided attention of the lecturers. In 1849 he proceeded to London, where he studied at St. Bartholomew's Hospital and obtained the diplomas of M.R. C.S. and L.S.A. in 1850. Hutchinson was soon appointed to the staffs of several hospitals, and in 1862 became lecturer on surgery at the London Hospital Medical College. He was quite active in the Royal College of Surgeons, was elected to F.R.S. in 1882, and received honorary degrees from the universities of Glasgow, Cambridge, Edinburgh, Ox-

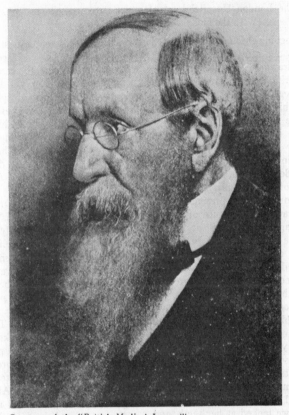

Courtesy of the "British Medical Journal"

SIR JONATHAN HUTCHINSON (1828-1913)
From a drawing by Walter Benington

ford, Dublin, and Leeds. In 1908 he was knighted for his distinguished services to medicine. His death occurred in 1913.

Sir Jonathan Hutchinson was a member of the Society of Friends and when residing at his home in *Haslemere* was accustomed to lecture every Sunday afternoon at a Quaker meetinghouse, his topics varying from "Wordsworth's Poetry" to "Leprosy." He had a large museum and library at his home, one exhibit showing the history of the centuries from ancient Egypt to Queen Victoria. Few medical men have been so versatile in their own fields. Hutchinson was a general surgeon, an ophthalmologist, a dermatologist, a syphilologist, and a neurologist. Syphilis interested him perhaps more than anything else and during his lifetime he saw more than one million patient's suffering from this disease. Hutchinson's contributions to medical science were very numerous and important but he is perhaps best remembered for his description of a certain deformity of teeth characteristic of hereditary syphilis.

CLINICAL LECTURE ON HEREDITO-SYPHILITIC STRUMA: AND ON THE TEETH AS A MEANS OF DIAGNOSIS*

Delivered at the London Hospital by JONATHAN HUTCHINSON, ESQ., Assistant Surgeon to the Hospital, and Lecturer on Surgery.

Gentlemen: In going through Sophia Ward on Monday last, our attention was, as you will remember, drawn to the case of a little girl who is suffering from a large ulcer on the front of her leg.

Sarah W. is a child of fairly healthy aspect, aged eleven. The disease for which she is under treatment is a large oval ulcer on the front of her right leg, which has laid bare about two inches of her tibia. The ulceration has evidently been, indeed it still is, of the type of chronic phagedena. The edges are undermined; they present a livid or gray surface, and are destitute of granulations. A week ago, Mr. Powell, at my request, applied the strong nitric acid to certain parts of the edge, where the ulceration was most inclined to spread, and with decidedly good effect; although the sore did not take on healthy action.

On two occasions, as you are aware, we had passed this child without arriving at anything definite as to the diagnosis of her affection. On Monday, however, my attention was drawn to the very unusual features which the ulcer presents; and the question suggested itself to my mind—Could it depend upon an inherited taint of syphilis? Following up this idea, we looked at her teeth, and found that her upper incisors were of very peculiar shape, and in fact, of the type most characteristic of the taint in question. We learnt, on inquiry, that she is the eldest, and, indeed, the only living child, of her parents. He mother is stated to have had several others, but they are all dead. Further than this we had no opportunity for pursuing the family history, as neither her father nor mother was present.

On looking into her throat, we found that her uvula and soft palate had been extensively destroyed by ulceration; a condition of things

Brit. M. J., 1861, I, 515-517.

which, I need not say, strongly confirmed my opinion. These discoveries at once changed my view of the case; and, instead of considering it as simply a disease of debility, I regarded it as one of specific taint to be treated by specific remedies. The quinine and codliver oil which she had been taking were discontinued, the iodide of potassium in full doses was prescribed. The result of this change was that, in a few days, the edges of the sore have assumed a freely granulating condition.

In this instance, the usefulness of the teeth as a means of diagnosis was very forcibly illustrated. Usually, the subjects of inherited syphilis display in their physiognomy peculiarities sufficiently well marked to lead, if not to a positive opinion, at least to a strong suspicion. They show, in nine cases out of ten, a very pasty, pallid skin, and a drawn, haggard expression of face, as of premature old age. The bridge of the nose is almost always sunken and broad and there are frequent little pits or cicatrices about the cheeks and forehead, and symmetrical linear scars extending from the angles of the mouth. In Abigail Hammond, a girl who occupies a bed in the next ward, suffering from disease of the knee-joint, all these peculiarities are very noticeable; and the *tout ensemble* of her visage would attract the attention of even a careless observer. She has also suffered from interstitial keratitis, which has left both her corneae hazy; whilst both pupils are notched and irregular, from the effects of a bygone attack of iritis.

Sarah W., however, although not robust looking, does not differ materially in appearance from hundreds of other children of her age. We have, as I have said, prescribed for her on two occasions without suspecting the true nature of her disease. It was her teeth, and her teeth only, which led me to give a confident opinion as to her diathesis, and to alter the treatment of her case. Now, however, that we have gained this knowledge, it is easy to see that there are suspicious features in the ulcer itself. Notice the surface of the exposed bone. Instead of being smooth and even as that of a healthy tibia should be, it is raised, worm-eaten, and like pummice-stone, remarkably resembling what we often see on the skull when exposed by the ulceration of syphilitic node. It is clear that the disease has begun in chronic periostitis, and that the thickening of the exterior of the bone has preceded the phagedenic ulceration by which the surface has been exposed.

We will, however, for the present, restrict our attention to the teeth as a means of diagnosis of hereditary taint. On this important symptom, I will offer for your guidance the following observations:

1. Remember that it is the permanent set only which show any peculiarities. The milk teeth of syphilitic infants, although liable to premature caries, show no peculiarities of form.

2. *The central upper incisors are the test-teeth.* You may neglect all the others; for, although malformations are often observed in them also, as, for instance, a rounded peg-like form in the lower incisors, yet there is nothing that is trustworthy, and much that is liable to mislead. Look at once at the two upper central incisors; and if they be broad, well-made teeth, you may throw away suspicion as far as dental indications are concerned.

3. The peculiarities of the central upper incisors which denote hereditary syphilis are well shewn in the two patients to whom I have referred, and in the sketches which I now exhibit. The teeth are short and narrow. Instead of becoming wider as they descend from the gum, they are narrower at their free edge than at their crowns, their angles having been, as it were, rounded off. In the centre of their free edge is a deep verticle notch made by the breaking away *or* non-development of the middle lobe of the tooth-crown. This notch, taken together with the narrowness and shortness of the tooth, is the main peculiarity; but you will observe also that the colour of these teeth is not good. Instead of looking like ivory with a

thin coating of pearl, they present a semi-translucent appearance, not unlike that of bad size, as we see it displayed in the oil-men's shops.

In respect to the value of this symptom, I may express the utmost confidence in it. I frequently see sets of teeth so characteristic that, without asking for any other knowledge, I would venture a positive opinion as to their possessor having suffered in infancy from inherited syphilis. In the majority, of course, the peculiar features are less well marked, and furnish only one among many symptoms on which to base a diagnosis. It is only by long practice in the observation of the malformations of teeth, that dexterity in using them as a means of diagnosis can be obtained. You must at first exercise the utmost caution, or you may be misled into great errors. Remembering that it is not all irregular or misshapen teeth which indicate hereditary syphilis. *The commoner and more conspicuous varieties of malformation have, indeed, nothing to do with that disease.* Craggy or "rocky" teeth are not syphilitic; "honey-combed" teeth (eaten into little pits on their surfaces) are not syphilitic; as a rough rule, teeth which are much broken have nothing to do with the syphilitic type. Whenever you see a whole row of front teeth marked by a horizontal line or furrow, which crosses them midway between the neck and the edge (or nearer to the latter), and at the same level on all, you may, for the most part, dismiss the suspicion of syphilis. It is the notching and dwarfing of the upper central incisors which constitutes the only condition to which suspicion ought to attach. As I have stated, this condition is, as compared with certain others ("honey-combed," "rocky teeth," etc.), but rarely met with. The great usefulness of this symptom consists in the fact that it is objective and indelible. You need ask no questions; but have simply to observe and draw your own conclusions. In many, indeed in the majority, of the cases in which hereditary syphilis is suspected, you are precluded, by the fear of causing family mistrust, from putting any direct questions. In most instances, the taint has been derived from the father, who had suffered from syphilis before marriage. The mother of the child is not unfrequently in entire ignorance of the nature of its malady; and it would be unkind and very wrong to excite her suspicions. In seeking for corroborative testimony, after having inspected the teeth, you will proceed with great circumspection. It is a good plan to ask if the child suffered much when cutting its first teeth, if measles, scarlet feaver, etc., occurred in infancy. Such questions will generally elicit what you want to know, without conveying any hint whatever as to your own view of the case. If you are told that when a baby the child was very ailing and puny, suffered from rash, had "thrush" badly, and was much troubled with snuffles, it will not be needful to push the investigation much further. You may ask if the "thrush went through it"; and the answer you will receive will often inform you as to whether the child had condylomata of the anus. The children who suffered severely from hereditary syphilis are usually the eldest in the family. Almost always those who present well-characterized teeth are the eldest living. Very often there have been either stillbirths, or several have died in infancy, who, if they had lived, would have been older than the patient; but still, almost always, the latter is the oldest living. This circumstance is, of course, easily explained by reference to the fact that the parental taint has usually been acquired before marriage, and is, with the lapse of years, gradually wearing out. I have, in many instances, found the eldest child of a syphilitic family with notched teeth and senile physiognomy; the second child presenting similar features in a less marked degree; the third less still; and the fourth or fifth appearing to be in good health, and free from any peculiarity either in teeth or features.

That the syphilitic taint existing in the parents is peculiarly fatal to the life of the offspring, is an undoubted fact. In many cases a syphilitic husband is not fecund, and no conceptions occur. In others, two or three miscarriages happen soon after marriage, and then the woman ceases to conceive; whilst in others, and the larger proportion, a succession either of premature births, or of tainted infants destined to die within a few months, occurs. The number of infants inheriting the syphilitic taint in a severe form who are ultimately reared is, I suspect, but small. I shall bring before you this afternoon three patients, the undoubted subjects of inherited syphilis, and you will notice that in each instance the patient is an only child. All of them are girls, another fact worthy of notice. To whatever cause it may be assigned, there is no doubt that a larger proportion of our patients with this form of disease are females. I suspect that this is so because a larger number of male conceptions end in abortion.

I will now ask your attention to the case of Ann Inkpenn, a little girl aged seven, whom we admitted yesterday. She comes on account of angular curvature of the dorsal spine, attended with iliac abscess, which has opened in the right groin. Her physiognomy is markedly syphilitic, the skin being thick and sallow, the bridge of the nose flat, and the lips puckered by cicatrices. She has as yet not cut any of her permanent teeth. Let us look at the state of things in her mouth. You will observe that she has lost all her upper incisors and her two lower central ones; the gums are quite sound, and look as if the teeth had been out for a long time, her mother tells me that it is more than four years since they fell. I told you just now that the milk-teeth are not affected, as regards their form, by hereditary syphilis, but that they are liable to premature caries. This early caries, I may add, usually affects the upper incisors; that is, the same teeth which, in the permanent set, shew the most characteristic deviations from the normal form. It is very common, indeed, for these patients to lose their front teeth several years before those of the second set appear.

The history of the patient now before us (Inkpenn) we obtained very easily. Having first mentioned to those of you who were then present my opinion as to the nature of the case, I simply asked her mother whether the child was very healthy as a baby, and was at once told that she had suffered most severely "from the disease from her father." It appears that for years she was puny and very ailing, that she had snuffles, a bad rash over the body, and "thrush in the mouth," which, if we interpret, probably means syphilitic stomatitis. You will notice that she has a divergent strabismus, her right eye looking outwards.

Ann Inkpenn is the subject of caries of the dorsal vertebrae; Sarah W. has disease of her tibia; and in the case of the third patient, Abigail Hammond, there is chronic disease of the knee-joint. All three would, a few years ago, have been considered "strumous" in a marked degree; indeed, the form of ophthalmia from which Hammond has suffered is designated in most ophthalmic treatises as *par excellence "strumous* corneitis."* Very vague, as you know, is the meaning usually attached to this word "struma." If, however, names are to be of any use as indicative of a knowledge of the causes of the malady designated, we must insist upon its receiving a modifying addition in the present instances. These patients are not "strumous" in the sense of being liable to tuberculous affections, or likely to die of phthisis, nor do any of them show tendency to disease of the lymphatic glands. There is no reason for believing that the diseases from which they suffer are other than the direct consequences of the specific taint derived from their parents. The treatment likely to be most useful in each instance is that of tertiary syphilis, namely, full doses of iodides and small ones of mercurials, whilst comparatively little good would come of the use of tonics and cod-liver oil. The distinction between tubercular struma and heredito-syphilitic struma* is, therefore, one of the utmost importance.

TUBERCULOSIS

Tuberculosis, one of the most ancient of diseases, has been described by a host of writers. Hippocrates delineated the clinical picture of this malady with an accuracy which has been rarely equalled and never surpassed. Wiseman, by general consent, has left us the classical account of scrofula which even his belief in the efficacy of the King's Touch has failed to mar. In stressing the importance of the anatomical tubercle in the lungs, Sylvius introduced a new concept into medical thought. This idea was elaborated by Morton, who, however, included many wasting diseases not due to tuberculosis in the group of consumptions. Bayles' pathological studies initiated the modern era in the study of disease and his friend Laënnec, by his discovery of auscultation, pointed out the physical findings in tuberculosis and created a new vocabulary which the modern physician still employs. Most of Laënnec's treatise on auscultation describes the physical changes produced by this disease.

Villemin in a series of carefully planned and skillfully executed experiments established the contagiousness of tuberculosis. This epochal piece of research which foreshadowed the discovery of the tubercle bacillus, marks the introduction of a method into medicine, without which we cannot visualize modern bacteriology.

* The word "struma," to which some may object in the sense here used, has been retained after much consideration. We have no other word by which to designate the state of constitutional peculiarity to which reference is made. There is no doubt but that the various affections incident chiefly to childhood and the preadult period, which have hitherto been classed as struma, and will be so styled for many years, are yet really due to a variety of morbid causes. Some occur in the tubercular diathesis, some are the direct consequences of one or other of the exanthems, some are due to inherited syphilitic taint, whilst others appear to be chiefly due to a peculiarly feeble state of the capillary circulation. It is quite possible to group the various strumous disorders in relation to their different causes, though very frequently the result is complicated by the co-existence of several of the influences mentioned. Instead, however, of attempting to disuse the term struma altogether, I would propose to acknowledge that it is, when used alone, destitute of all precision as to the exact pathology of the disorder so designated, and to habitually append to it the adjectives, "tubercular," "heredito-syphilitic," "post-exanthematous," etc., as the case may be.

Hippocrates

BOOK I. OF THE EPIDEMICS

Sec. 1.—Constitution First*

2. Early in the beginning of spring, and through the summer, and towards winter, many of those who had been long gradually declining, took to bed with symptoms of phthisis; in many cases formerly of a doubtful character the disease then became confirmed; in these the constitution inclined to the phthisical. Many, and in fact, the most of them, died, and of those confined to bed, I do not know if a single individual survived for any considerable time; they died more suddenly than is common in such cases. But other diseases, of a protracted character, and attended with fever, were well supposed, and did not prove fatal: of these we will give a description afterwards. Consumption was the most considerable of the diseases which then prevailed, and the only one which proved fatal to many persons. Most of them were affected by these diseases in the following manner: fevers accompanied with rigors, of the continual type, acute, having no complete intermissions, but of the form of the semi-tertians, being milder the one day and the next having an exacerbation, and increasing in violence; constant sweats, but not diffused over the whole body; extremities very cold, and warmed with difficulty; bowels disordered, with bilious, scanty, unmixed, thin, and pungent, and frequent dejections. The urine was thin, colorless, unconcocted, or thick, with a deficient sediment, not settling favorably, but casting down a crude and unseasonable sediment. Sputa small, dense, concocted, but brought up rarely and with difficulty; and in those who encountered the most violent symptoms there was no concoction at all, but they continued throughout spitting crude matters. Their fauces, in most of them, were painful from the first to last, having redness with inflammation; defluxions thin, small, and acrid; they were soon wasted and became worse, having no appetite for any kind of food throughout; no thirst; most persons delirious when near death. So much concerning the phthisical affections.

*The Genuine Works of Hippocrates, translated by Francis Adams, p. 294.

Tuberculosis of the Spine with Tubercles in the Lungs†

"The vertebrae of the spine when contracted into a hump behind from disease, for the most part cannot be remedied, more especially when the gibbosity is above the attachment of the diaphragm to the spine. Certain of those below the diaphagm are carried off by varices in the legs, more especially by such as occur in the vein at the ham; and in those cases where the gibbosities are removed, the varices take place also in the groin; and some have been carried off by a dysentery when it becomes chronic. And when the gibbosity occurs in youth before the body has attained its full growth, in these cases the body does not usually grow along the spine, but the legs and the arms are fully developed, whilst the parts (about the back) are arrested in their development. And in those cases where the gibbosity is above the diaphragm, the ribs do not usually expand properly in width, but forward, and the chest becomes sharppointed and not broad, and they become affected with difficulty of breathing and hoarseness; for the cavities which inspire and expire the breath do not attain their proper capacity. And they are under the necessity of keeping the neck bent forward at the great vertebra, in order that their head may not hang downward; this, therefore, occasions great contraction of the pharynx by its inclination inward; for, even in those who are erect in stature, dyspnoea is induced by this bone inclining inward, until it be restored to its place. From this frame of body, such persons appear to have more prominent necks than persons in good health, and they generally have hard and unconcocted tubercles in the lungs, for the gibbosity and the distension are produced mostly by such tubercles, with which the neighboring nerves communicate. When the gibbosity is below the diaphragm, in some of these cases nephritic diseases and affections of the bladder supervene, but abscesses of a chronic nature, and difficult to cure, occur in the

† The Genuine Works of Hippocrates, translated by Francis Adams, I, New York, Wm. Wood, p. 114.

loins and groins, and neither of these carries off the gibbosity; and in these cases the hips are more emaciated than when the gibbosity is seated higher up; but the whole spine is more elongated in them than in those who have the gibbosity seated higher up, the hair of pubes and chin is of slower growth and less developed, and they are less capable of generation than those who have the gibbosity higher up. When the gibbosity seizes persons. who have already attained their full growth, it usually occasions a crisis of the then existing disease, but in the course of time some of them attack, as in the case of younger persons, to a greater or less degree; but for the most part, all these diseases are less malignant. And yet many have borne the affection well, and have enjoyed good health until old age, more especially those persons whose body is inclined to be plump and fat; and a few of them have lived to beyond sixty years of age, but the most of them are more short-lived. In some cases the curvature of the spine is lateral, that is to say, either to the one side or the other; the most of such cases are connected with tubercles (*abscessts?*) within the spine; and in some, the positions in which they have been accustomed to lie co-operate with the disease. But these will be treated of among the chronic affections of the lungs; for these the most suitable prognostics of what will happen in these cases are given."

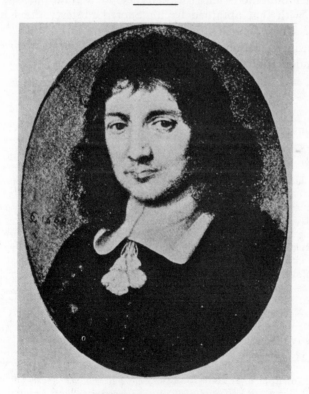

RICHARD WISEMAN (1622-1676)
From a miniature in the possession of His Grace,
the Duke of Rutland

Richard Wiseman

Richard Wiseman was born in 1622, probably at London, and was apprenticed to the Barber-Surgeons' Company in 1637. He began his professional career as a surgeon in the Dutch navy. He served in the English army under Charles I and narrowly escaped capture at Weymouth. After the death of Charles he returned to London, where he was imprisoned with other Royalists and spent several months in the Tower and in Lambeth House, then used as a prison. On being set at liberty he practised for a time in London and then served in the Spanish Navy until 1660. After the Restoration he returned to London and was appointed by King Charles II "Surgeon in Ordinary for the Person." In 1672 Charles appointed him "Our principall Chirurgion and our Sergeant-Chirurgion." He died in 1676 and was buried at St. Paul's in Covent Garden.

Wiseman was a skillful surgeon and occupied as prominent a place in the surgery of his day as did Willis and Sydenham in medicine. His *Chirurgical Treatises* contain an interesting essay on the "King's Evill" which records his attempts to treat this widespread malady. Although he treated the disease both by hygienic methods and with surgery, he admits that his success could not compare with that obtained by his Sacred Majesty the King, who could cure with the Royal Touch.

The following selections are from Wiseman's *Eighth Chirurgical Treatises*, 3rd Ed. (London, 1696), pages 239-246.

A TREATISE OF THE KING'S-EVILL*

THE FOURTH BOOK. CHAP. I

Of the Cure of the EVILL
by the KING's *Touch*

What great difficulty we meet with in the Cure of the KING's *Evill*, the daily experience both of Physicians and Chirurgeons doth shew, I thought it therefore worth my while to spend a whole Treatise upon the Subject, and very particularly to go through the description of it, informing thereby the young Chirurgeon whatever is requisite to the Cure, at least as far as it cometh within the compass of our Art. But when upon trial he shall find the contumaciousness of the Disease, which frequently deluded his best care and industry, he will find reason of acknowledging the goodness of God; who hath dealt so beautifully with this Nation, in giving the Kings of it, at least from *Edward* the Confessor downwards (if not for a longer time), an extraordinary power in the miraculous Cure thereof. This our Chronicles have all along testified, and the personal experience of many thousands now living can witness for his Majesty that now reigneth, and his Royal Father and Grandfather. His

Majesty that now is having exercised that faculty with wonderful success, not only here, but beyond the Seas in *Flanders*, *Holland* and *France* itself. The King of this last pretends to a Gift of the same kind, and hath often the good hap to be alone mentioned in Chirurgical Books, as the sole possessor of it, when the *French* themselves are the Authors: yet even they when they are a little free, will not stick to own the Kings of England as partakers with him in that faculty; witness the Learned Tagaultius, who in his Institutions takes notice of King *Edward's* faculty of doing the same Cure, and the continuance of it in his Successors. *Italy* as well as *France* hath made the like acknowledgments in the Book of *Polydore Virgil*, who reciting the Gift given to Saint *Edward* the Confessor, doth subjoyn these words: *Quod quidem immortale munus quasi haereditario jure ad posteriores Reges manavit: nam Reges Angliae etiam nunc tactu, ac quibusdam hymnis, non sine ceremoniis, prius recitatis, strumosos sanant.* "Which Immortal gift hath been derived as it were by an hereditary right to the latter Kings; for the Kings of *England* even now also do Cure the *Struma* by Touch, &c."

Indeed if Historians of our Nation be diligently compared with the *French*, we shall

* Wiseman, Richard, *Eight Chirurgical Treatises*, III Ed., London, Tooke and Meredith, 1696, p. 239.

find that the *French* Kings had this Gift later than ours. *Dupleix* a most diligent Writer of that History, deriving it no further than *Philip* the first, and *Lewis* the gross; saying, that before their times no man had that power: whereas we on the contrary meet with the general acknowledgments of all our Writers of the same miraculous power in Saint *Edward's* time, which were enough for this Controversie: and not only so, but with strong surmises, that this Miracle was ancienter; it being notorious in the days of *Malmsburiensis*, who lived not long after his Reign, that it was then disputed, whether the Cure of the Evil were a peculiar reward of the King's Holiness, or rather a Hereditary faculty attending the *English* Crown. Which Gift, that it was not taken away upon our departure from the Church of *Rome*, we have not only our daily experience to testifie, but also the confession of Doctor *Harpsfield*, a great Divine of the *Romish* perswasion; who, after he hath in the Ecclesiastical History of *England* described at large the Miracle wrought by the Confessor, doth add, *Quam strumosos sanandi admirabilem dotem in posteros suos Anglorum Reges, ad nostra usque tempora transfudisse & "perpetuasse, merito creditur.* Which admirable faculty of Curing the *Struma*, he "is justly believed to have transmitted to his Posterity, the Kings of *England*, and to have continued it amongst them to those times in which he wrote." And when Bishop *Tooker* would make use this Argument to prove the Truth of our Church, *Smitheus* doth not thereupon go about to deny the Matter of fact; (nay indeed both he and *Cope* acknowledge it) but he rather chuseth first to retort upon him the Protestant argument against Miracles which they will not allow to be the necessary mark of a true Church, because they may also be performed by Infidels. But withal he himself, who is not willing to let go so specious an Argument from his own Church, finds another Solution of the difficulty, attributing it to the great Goodness of God, and the great Grace of Saint *Edward, Quod nec in indigna haerede defecerit*, that the Gift did not fail in an unworthy Successor: Such as he calleth Queen *Elizabeth*, and adds, that she did perform that Cure, *non virtute propria, sed virtute signi crucis;* not by her own vertue, but by vertue of the Sign of the Cross, by whomsoever made, were sufficient to work a Miracle. What would we now say

were he living, and had seen it done by three Generations of Kings without the Sign of the Cross? But it is not my business to enter into Divinity-controversies: all that I pretend to is first, the attestation of the Miracles; and secondly, a direction for such as have not opportunity of receiving the benefit of that stupendious Power. The former of these, one would think, should need no other proof than the great concourse of Strumous persons to *White-hall*, and the success they find in it. I myself have been a frequent Eye-witness of many hundreds of Cures performed by his Majestie's Touch alone, without any assistance of Chirurgery; and those, many of them, such as had tired out the endeavours of able Chirurgeons before they came thither. It were endless to recite what I myself have seen, and what I have received acknowledgments of by Letter, not only from the several parts of this Nation, but also from *Ireland, Scotland, Jersey* and *Garnsey*. It is needless also to remember what Miracles of this nature were performed by the very Bloud of his late Majesty of Blessed memory, after whose decollation by the inhumane Barbarity of the Regicides, the reliques of that were gathered on Chips, and in Hankerchiefs, by the pious Devotes, who could not but think so great a suffering in so honourable and pious a Cause, would be attended by an extraordinary assistance of God, and some more than ordinary Miracle; nor did their Faith deceive them in this point, there being so many so much of vertue, what shall we say of his living Image, the Inheritor of his Cause and Kingdom? whom though it hath pleased God to deliver out of those dangers that overwhelmed his Royal Father: yet it was with so long an exercise of afflictions, that though (God be thanked) he be not now like to increase the catalogue of Martyrs, yet he may well be added to the number of Confessors. This we are sure, the Miracle is not ceased.

But since matter of Fact itself is, in such difficult cases as these, liable to exception; I shall take notice of the Evasions, that obstinate and incredulous Men have used to avoid so great a notoriety of Experience. But since it cannot be denied that many go away cured, some will impute it only to the Journey they take, and the change of Air; others to the effects of imagination; and others to the wearing of Gold.

The first of these is easily confuted by the

hundreds of instances that are to be given of Inhabitants of this City, who certainly could meet with little change of Air, or indeed of exercise, in a Journey to *White-hall*. The second is as readily taken off by the Examples of Infants, who have been frequently healed, though they have not been old enough to imagine any thing of the Majesty, or other secret rays of Divinity, that do attend Kings. or do any other act that way to contribute to the Cure. The third hath more of colour in it, because many that have been touched, have upon loss of their Gold felt returns of their Malady, which upon recovery of that have vanished. But in this case also we have many Evidences of the contrary.

* * *

Chap. III

The History of the Disease with the Diagnosticks and Prognosticks

The *Kings-Evils* is already described in short, but that will not serve the uses of a young Practitioner unless he may have the History of it more fully delivered, which cannot be well done unless we give an account of the Parts themselves which are concerned in it. Now the Parts usually affected are either Glandules, *Parts affected* Muscles, *Viscera* Membranes, Tendons or Bones. I do not remember ever to have seen the Nerves or Brain affected immediately with *Nerves and Brain* any Humour of this kind: or if they have, the Juices of those Parts are rather dissolved, and the Fibres corroded by this Accidity after the likeness of Marrow and Bones, then coagulated into a Tumour; which Corrosion when it happens, the Disease gets another name, and being indeed mortal needs not be insisted upon in this Treatise, it admitting of no other doctrine but that of a Prognostick

So a young Lady having overgrown Tonsils, which were judged Strumous, was cured by me by Extirpation, as you may see in the *Observat* *chap. of Tonsils:* but the same, years after, labouring under great pains of her Head, and being upon the way coming up to *London* for Cure, died suddenly; her Head being opened, her Brain was found corroded, and much wasted with great putrefaction, the inner Table of the Skull carious.

Veins and Arteries The Veins and Arteries do indeed dilate themselves in all congestions of Matter, whether natural or preternatural; but have not any particular Affection in the *Strumae* distinct from what they have in other cases.

Glandules Glandules are a very notorious seat of this Distemper, insomuch that Authors generally have confined it to them as its subject. Here we have a great deal to say, *viz.* that this Part is the most commonly affected when-ever the Patient is Strumous; and if the outward and more visible Glands remain whole, yet generally *Mesentery* speaking the inward ones, those especially of the Mesentery, are obstructed and swell'd. Of these I have seen divers examples, especially in Children, and have passed my Judgment that they have been Strumous, when the outer Signs could not so far justifie my conjecture as to make others of my mind: yet when the Patient hath been dead, the truth hath appeared upon dissection. In one of this sort Dr. *Walter Needham* hath lately been my witness. Nay, whenever the outward Glands do appear swell'd, you may safely conclude the Mesentericks to be so too, they being usually the first Part that is attacqued by this Malady.

Conglobate Nor is the Mesentery alone, but all the conglobated Glandules partake with it: which word *Sylvius* hath appropriated to the reductive Glands that serve the Lymphaeducts. These are frequently liable to this Distemper, their offices being a percolation of the *Serum;* therefore whensoever that is amiss, these must needs suffer. This is outwardly visible in the Neck. on the sides of the *musculus mastoideus* quite *Neck* down to the Clavicle. whence they pass into the *Thorax* down a-long the Spine, and about the Lungs; which themselves also do frequently abound with Strumous coagulations. *Laurentius* adds the *Bronchocele* as a *species* of this Disease.

Groines Axillae Conglomerate more seldom It is as easie to be seen in the Groin. *Axillae.* &c. in both which places they do often appear; but no-where more commonly and frequently than in the Neck. of which every day sheweth examples. Nor are the conglomerate Glandules free of the like malady. under which name *Sylvius* contains all the excretory ones, which I do reckon to be the Salivals bigger and less, the Tonsils, the *Glandulae Lachrymates*, the *Thymus*, the *Pancreas*, the *Mammae*, the Testicles, Prostates, &c.

These are sometimes affected together with the Conglobates, sometimes separably. Many instances may be given thereof, in some we Salivals have found all the conglobate Glandules of the Neck swell'd, and many of them to press hard upon and between the parts of the Salivals; yet they remained found.

The like hath been seen concerning the *Pancreas* and *Thymus*, which have been both surrounded with *Strumae*, yet themselves remained untouched; but very often Ranula the Conglomerates are affected by themselves, of which we have a great example in the *Ranula*, it being but the Tumour of the *Glandula falivalis inferior*, which in a man lieth immediately under the sides of the Tongue. The *Parotis* also which is the external Salival, is very often preternaturally affected; and in the *Pancreas* the learned Dr. *Walter Needham* saith, he hath seen a Strumous Tumour suppurated, which held a pint of matter when the other Glands of the Mesentery remained sound.

Breasts The Breasts are evidently obnoxious to it, as common practice testifies.

In a late private Healing I presented a young Woman with one in the right Breast and 1 near that lying between the 2 Breasts, as large as Pheasants eggs.

Testicles and Prostates The Testicles and Prostates may be liable, but I cannot instance in them; and it may be that we do the less acknowledge their being affected with this Disease, because we are apt in all these cases to suspect another distemper.

Tonsils The over-grown Tonsils are so frequently Strumous, that they need not be insisted on.

The *Glandulae Lachrymales* are often infected, and do according to the variety of their disorders produce several sorts of Tumours about the eye; the most usual of which is a *Lippitudo*, an affection of the ends of the Lachrymal Vessels, which being derived from them do terminate near the *cilia*: so also the *Hordeoli*, &c. nay it is not rare to see the whole ball of the Eye thrust out by the Tumour of these Glandules.

Ophthalmia Fistula Lachrymalis *Ophthalmia* it self is often a consequent of the Disease; so is also the *Fistula Lachrymalis* which often oweth its original to this cause.

Besides all these Glandules which are naturally born with us, there are many more which do arise upon the occasion of this Disease in the several interstices of the Muscles, as I have seen in both Adventitious Glands, Face, Legs Arms, Skin, Muscles, Membranes the arms of one person now under my Cure near the *musculus biceps*. The like happens to others in the Legs and Feet, also the very Fingers and Toes.

In a Child of six years of age I saw them scattering all over the Body, as in the balls of the Cheeks, and upon that part of the *Os zygoma* nearest the external *canthus* of the Eye, higher than the *parotis* reacheth: but whether that were part of the *parotis* or not, the others were certainly adventitious which appeared upon the sides, back, breast, belly, shoulders, arms, and thighs, scattering up and down, some superficial in the skin, others deep.

Viscera The *Viscera* are often found with great *Strumae* growing in them, or from them. Nor are we to wonder at it if *Malpighius's* doctrine be true, who supposeth most of the *Viscera* to be made up of Glandules. In them we frequently find Strumous Swellings as in the Liver, Lungs, Spleen, and sometimes appendants to them. Dr. *Walter Needham* declared in one of his late Lectures of Anatomy at our Hall, that he saw a Strumous Swelling hang at the cone of the Heart that weighed two ounces.

The Tendons are sometimes involved with a great gumminess and collection of Strumous matter, especially the fingers, hands, feet, and toes; yea upon the *musculus mastoideus* it self we find them very distinguishable from glandulous Tumours, and hard to be managed. Elbows, knees, anckles, are very remarkable Seats of this *species* of the Disease.

Bones cariuous from within Bones are as frequently affected as any part of the Body, Glandules only excepted: but there the manner of the Tumour differs; for though the Bone swell, and the outward shell thereof appear hard, yet the inward Juices are all putrid and rotten. This sort of Tumour is sometimes called *Spina ventosa*, how properly let others judge; but it is certain that not only the Bones of the fingers, *carpus, metacarpus, tarsus, metatarsus,* and Toes, are liable to this Evil, but also the Skull itself and the Jaw-bones, and all the other Bones of the body; the venomous nature of which will be seen by those who upon opening some of these Tumours have found the Bone when laid bare at the first appearance found, but when pierced into to be in the heart wholly rotten.

Bones are likewise affected on the outside by any Strumous Tumour that toucheth them,

Bones outwardly carious

whether Membrane or Tendon, &c. which we often experience in opening of them when they lie near such parts; for when we do, we most commonly find the Bone it self bare, if not carious. There is a mixed case of Membranes and Bones which frequently is found Strumous, I mean the *Ozoena,* which requires your utmost diligence; the Bones and Cartilages there soon rotting, leave a blemish to the scandal of the Patient.

Franciscus Sylvius

There has been much confusion between the two Sylviuses, Jacobus and Franciscus. They have been frequently mistaken for each other and there has been similar confusion in regard to their discoveries. Jacobus Sylvius has been credited with the discovery of the aqueduct of Sylvius, the fissure of Sylvius and the ventricle of Sylvius, although recent investigations have established with certainty that these discoveries were made by Franciscus Sylvius.

Franciscus Sylvius was born at Hanau, Germany, in 1614. His family was of French origin and had been driven out of France by the religious persecutions of those days. He was christened François de le Boë, but latinized it into Franciscus Sylvius. His family name originally was Dubois, but had been changed according to the usage of the Languedoc into de le Boë.

Sylvius was described as a youth of remarkable charm and mental ability and after studying at Sedan, Basle, Leyden, and Paris, took his doctor's degree at Basle when twenty-three years of age. He began practice in Hanau, but later removed to Amsterdam, where he rapidly acquired both fame and a large practice. In 1658, he was offered the chair of medicine in the University of Leyden, then one of the first universities in Europe. With characteristic modesty, he hesitated for some time, doubting whether he possessed the necessary knowledge and ability to fill this post, but he finally accepted and immediately achieved great success. Students flocked to him from all over Europe and among his famous pupils were DeGraaf, Stensen, Swammerdam, and van Horne. Sylvius attained distinction in the fields of anatomy, physiology, pathology, and internal medicine. He was one of the earliest teachers to introduce bedside teaching into the medical curriculum. His investigations in pathology led him to a conviction of the rôle played by tubercles in the production of phthisis and he is given credit for this epochal discovery. Sylvius exercised a profound influence upon the medicine of his day. He recognized the importance of Harvey's discovery of the circulation of the blood and attempted to reconstruct medicine on two bases, on the circulation of the blood and on chemistry. He believed that when either acid or alkali predominated in the body, disease resulted, and attempted to explain all morbid processes on the basis of what we should now term acidosis and alkalosis. This chemical conception of disease was accepted by Thomas Willis, who propagated these ideas in England.

Sylvius died in 1672, at the age of fifty-eight, and was buried in St. Peter's Church in Leyden, in a tomb which he had prepared seven years before.

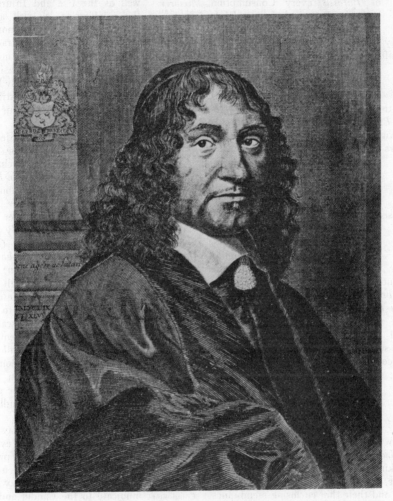

FRANCISCUS DE LE BOË SYLVIUS (1614-1672)
An engraving by T. L. Durant. Frontispiece to *Opera
medica* (Geneva, 1680)

TRACTATUS IV

DE PHTHISI*

How
Phthisis
arises

I. Among the Conditions Causing *Ulcerations* of the *Lungs*, and which is commonly followed by a condition causing *Feebleness of the entire body*, in the first place *Pleuritis* should be mentioned, which is as often either neglected or on the other hand not overcome and leads to Suppuration; for not infrequently Pus collected in the Cavity of the Chest forms an *Empyema*, from whose acrid humor the lungs are frequently attacked and *Phthisis* is produced: concerning which I will not treat.

* Franciscus Deleboe Sylvius, *Opera Medica*, Geneva, de Tournes, 1680, p. 526.

What is commonly meant by the name Phthisis

II. It should be known also that we do not understand by the name of *Phthisis* every Consumption but only that which *follows Ulcer of the Lung*, since this word is commonly employed among Physicians with this significance alone.

Its Symptoms

III. For besides a *wasting away of the Entire Body* other Symptoms are also observed in Phthisis peculiar to it, for instance *Cough* with *secretion of Pus;* to which a *Hectic Fever* is added, with exacerbations apparent one or two hours after taking Food.

The disease can be hereditary

XXXVI. Besides it is known, this disease can be hereditary, transmitted from parents to children; but in whatever this hereditary consists, is also not known.

What is a Vomica to others?

L. So it must be explained briefly, what is meant by *Vomica:* For some understand by Vomica *Blood,* not in the substance of the Lungs, but *visibly poured out* into the *capsular membrane, collected in the same place and then terminating in Pus*. Indeed this I may not venture to deny can happen, although I do not remember ever to have observed such in autopsies, or any thing from which I could satisfactorily deduce and conclude the same.

What to the author?

LI. Therefore, what has been my lot to observe, I may mention and which for me therefore is a *Vomica,* I may clearly communicate I saw many times *Glandulous Tubercles in the Lungs,* which sometimes contained various kinds of pus as a section showed. Therefore, these Tubercles visibly changing into Pus and their thin enclosing membranes I consider to have produced the Vomica, at least *from them* I detected not infrequently phthisis to have taken its origin.

The Vomica the cause of hereditary Phthisis

LII. Indeed, in these Tubercles, if any other things evident to the external senses, I will not fear to define as that hereditary and deadly Disposition in certain families to Phthisis: for these Tubercles are accustomed to increase with age, and visibly proceed to suppuration.

LIII. I can not limit myself, rather on this occasion. I may proceed with my conjectures, which are openly communicated, with the favor of Physicians, dedicated to Truth alone.

The conjectures of the author concerning the Glands small by nature becoming abnormally large

For from these and others, from similar observations, investigations, as well as the Use and Injuries of the neighboring, as well as the distant parts; I came moreover constantly upon various traces of Glands small and almost invisible to the eyes, except occasionally when they were unnaturally larger, and I have seen them present distributed throughout the Viscera and Flesh of our entire Body.

In Plexa Choroideida in the Lung in various parts

LIV. From these Conjectures and Cogitations of mine there have been drawn the conclusions. First *Glands in the Choroid Plexus* are visible only in an abnormal state, sometimes, however, growing to a great size, obviously larger when separated. 2. *Noteworthy Glands only in the Lung* or Tubercula Glandulosa. 3. *Glands manifest in various parts of the body in strumous or scrofulos constitution:* now moreover there are not only enough small ones apparent constantly in the Mesentery and sides of the Neck which grow to great size and hardness, but besides, scattered widely, unknown, they make themselves known by suffering: and besides all Conglobate glands, not so the Conglomerate which we have observed to remain whole and healthy, although the Conglobate glands themselves were for the most part adherent and diseased.

The Division of Glands into Conglobate and Conglomerate

LV. Whence, that I may refer also to this in passing, it is evident, not that I may seem to propose something new and yet useless. but however, that I may communicate to the Candid and honest, a true thing, in itself, indeed, old and very useful, to divide the glands of the human Body primarily and most commonly into *Conglobate* and *Conglomerate*. Which distinction, however, some Scholars revered although ignorant of these things, attack ignorantly and awkwardly and calumiate, demonstrating their ill-will and their fondness for slander.

Phthisis arises from Bloody Sputum

LX. Among the Causes of Ulceration of the Lungs we shall mention secondly, Bloody sputum, either neglected by the Patient or not properly treated by the Physician.

LXIX. And these were the antecedent necessary Causes of the Ulcers in the Lungs leading to Phthisis. Besides these mention of Contagion is made sixthly by Medical Authors, according to which Air

Phthisis from Contagion

expired from the Phthisic was exhaled and inhaled by the mouth and nostrils close by: from whose foetid and Acrid miasma, others especially Relatives were affected, attacked and finally died from the same disease, Phthisis.

Richard Morton

Richard Morton was born in Worcestershire, England, in 1637, the son of Robert Morton, a minister. He studied at Oxford, where he received his

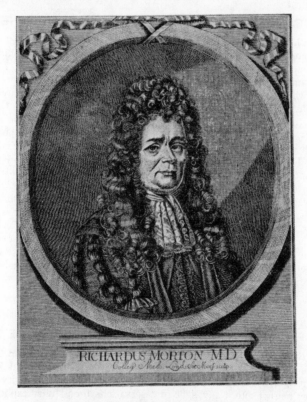

RICHARD MORTON (1637-1698)
From the frontispiece to *Phthisiologia: or a Treatise of Consumptions* (London, 1694)

B.A. degree in 1656. He took orders in the Church and in 1659, after receiving his M.A. degree, became vicar of Kinver in Staffordshire. In 1662 Parliament passed the Act of Uniformity which ordered the expulsion of all clergymen who refused to express approval of the whole of the Book of Common Prayer. Morton would not conform to the requirements of the Act and was ejected from his living. He then began the study of medicine and received his M.D. at Oxford in 1670. Morton settled in London, became a fellow of the College of Physicians and later physician to the King. He died in 1698.

Morton's most important medical work was his *Phthisiologia* first published in London in 1689. In this work he described all the conditions of wasting or consumption that he had observed, without reference to their underlying pathology. He described not only the wasting due to tubercles in the lungs, but the wasting produced by jaundice, gout, and intermittent fevers. His most important contribution was his proof that tubercles in the lungs produced one of the most widespread types of consumption that afflicted the human body. His writings were based upon his own clinical observations with but little reference to the books of others.

CHAP. I

OF THE CAUSES OF AN ORIGINAL CONSUMPTION OF THE LUNGS*

6. An Ill-Air

Sixthly, also a foggy and thick Air, and that which is filled with the Smoak of Coals, does extreamly promote a Consumption by vitiating the Animal Spirits, which are so necessary to the Natural Fermentation of the Blood; and also by stuffing and weakning the Lungs; that serve for Respiration, which are the Seat and Theatre of this Distemper. Seventhly, An Hereditary Disposition from the Parents does very often bring a Consumption of the Lungs, when every Body knows very well, that those who come of Consumptive Parents, are apt to fall into the same Distemper. Eighthly, an ill formation of the Breast, whether it be Natural or Accidental, is another cause of this Disease, I call that

7. An Hereditary Disposition

8. An ill formation of the Breast

Natural, where the Breast is narrow, the Neck long, and the Shoulder-blades stand out like Wings; and that I call Accidental, where there is a crookedness or distortion of the Breast, whereby not only the parts of the Breast and especially the Lungs being once weakned in their Tone, are rendered subject to the Flux of Rheumes; but also the Lungs wanting their necessary expansion, and being streightned, do heap up in themselves, and retain the vitiated *Serum* of the Blood, from whence it comes to pass, that at length they come to have Obstructions. Ninthly, This Disease is also propagated by Infection. For this Distemper (as I have observed by frequent Experience) like a Contagious Fever does infect those that lye with the Sick Person with a certain taint.

9. Infection

CHAP. V

OF THE DIFFERENCES OF AN ORIGINAL CONSUMPTION OF THE LUNGS

Here I could easily make several Divisions of a Consumption of the Lungs, and those such as are confirm'd by daily Experience; but, because they neither afford any light to the forming of a true Notion of this Distemper in general, nor help us to a clearer or more distinct Understanding of the general Prognostick Signs and Indications of Cure, I shall not so much as mention them, at least in this place. But yet there is one Division of a Consumption of the Lungs, which is into an Acute, and a Chronical Consumption, without the knowledge of which, a Physician must needs be very often mistaken, as well in the making of his Prognosticks, as in the dis-

The Division of a Consumption into Acute and Chronical

covery of the Indications of Cure. And therefore, no one ought to think it improper, if I here add with what Brevity I can, my Observations for a fuller explication of it. For as I have seen some taken away by this Distemper within the space of one, or at most of the few Months, so I have observed a great many others, that were far gone in a Consumption, by due care, and by making use of proper means, who have lived, though in a sickly and crazy state, for many Years, as for Example, Mr. *Haither,* who after the Cure of a spitting of Blood, which he had been seized withal when he was a Youth, is

* Morton, Richard, *Phthisiologia: or, a Treatise of Consumptions,* London, Smith and Walford, 1694, p. 64.

yet living in the fiftieth Year of his Age, though in the whole course of this time he has been lean, troubled with a Cough, and often had touches of a Fever, and been freed from several Putrid Fevers by our Art. And thus my dear Father, who himself was a very skilful Physician, though he was troubled with a continual Cough, a difficulty of Breathing, frequent Putrid Fevers, a light degree of Hectical Heat, though continual, did nevertheless by this means spin out his Life, though he continued sickly, from the thirtieth to the sixtieth Year of his Age; and at last did not dye of a Consumption of his Lungs (from which he seemed for the last three Years of his Life to be more free than he had been before), but of that Epidemical, that continued Putrid Fever, which reigned publickly all over *England* in the Year 1658. The same thing I observed in Mrs. *Davison*, a Merchant's Wife in *London*, for the space of fifteen Years, and in a certain Merchant that lived in *Philpot-Lane*, who after several Inflammatory Fevers, that returned often in a Year from every little occasion, at length happened to have such an extraordinary exulceration of his lungs, that he dyed of it, together with a Dropsie, and the other usual Symptoms of a Fatal Consumption of the Lungs, when he was about Sixty Years old. I could likewise give several Histories of this Nature, but at present I study brevity. As for the cause of this difference, to me it seems to proceed from the different disposition of the Blood, and of that Humour, which is supplyed to the Tubercles of the Lungs, and differs according to the various dyscrasy of the Blood. For if the Stuffing of the Lungs, and the Tubercles, which arise from it, by reason of some peculiar dyscrasy of the Blood, have their Original from some malignant or cancrous Humour, or a Humour that is apt to cause a Gangreen, (as I remember it has sometimes happened) the Distemper is not only certainly Mortal, but also quick, and very Acute, and such as carries off the Patient in a few Months, and it may be Weeks.

The cause of this difference

* * *

First, as the Inflammatory Fever, or the Putrid which arises from it, is more or less acute and dangerous, according to the Nature of the Swellings, as they are more or less Malignant, and disposed to an Inflammation, and an Exulceration, so likewise the Consumption from thence grows more or less quick and incurable.

Observation 1. The Nature of the Swelling makes the Fever more or less Acute

Secondly, The frequent taking of Cold, and often committing of Errors in their Diet, Exercise, and Passions of the Mind, &c. do by bringing Inflammatory and Putrid Fevers, that return in the same manner upon the Hectick Heat they had before, bring this Distemper sooner to a fatal end, making that Acute, yea, very Acute, which otherwise would have been in its own Nature Chronical.

Observ. 2. Taking of Cold &c. makes a Consumption more Acute

Thirdly, The Consumption of Young Men, that are in the Flower of their Age, when the heat of the Blood is yet brisk, and therefore more disposed to a Feverish Fermentation, is for the most part Acute. But in Old Men, where the Natural Heat is decayed, it is more Chronical.

Observ. 3. A Consumption more acute in young than in old persons

Fourthly, A Consumption that proceeds from Fevers, especially such as are from an Inflammation of the Lungs, or from the Suppression of Malignant Ulcers, is almost always Acute: But when it depends upon a Scrophulous and Scrobutical disposition, so in a cold and phlegmatick Temper, it is Chronical.

Observ. 4. When— from Acute Distemper, it is Acute

Fifthly, The omission of Bleeding, or taking away too little Blood, or bleeding too late in the Inflammatory Fever of such as have a lingering Consumption, makes that Consumption, which otherwise was in its own Nature slow and lingering, very Acute, and presently Mortal; because the parts of the Lungs that are stufft and harden'd, having heated for some time, do from that grow more apt to be inflamed, to putrefie, and to be exulcerated.

Observ. 5. For want of bleeding in the Inflammatory Fever makes a Consumption to be Acute

Gaspard-Laurent Bayle

Gaspard-Laurent Bayle was a native of Provence, born at Vernet in 1774. He was the son of wealthy parents and in his youth was very carefully instructed in religion and Latin. He decided to become a priest and in 1790 entered a seminary to study for holy orders. On the eve of his ordination as a priest he decided suddenly that he could never be perfect enough to live the life of a priest and instead embraced the profession of law, entering an advocate's office to begin his legal studies. At the age of nineteen he made a brief excursion into politics and was elected a member of the council of his department. Shortly afterwards his parents became alarmed at the turn of political events and sent him to Montpellier where he began the study of medicine. He returned to Paris in 1798, and in 1801 received the degree of doctor of medicine.

Bayle became rapidly a leader of his profession in Paris. In 1807 he was appointed to the Charité and the following year was appointed physician to the imperial household and left for Spain. On his return to Paris he devoted himself to his practice. He rapidly achieved great distinction and reputation, but died in 1816 at the age of forty-two.

Bayle was one of the most distinguished physicians of his generation and stressed the importance of pathological anatomy in the explanation of diseases. His best known work was his *Recherches sur la phthisie pulmonaire* in which he described quite accurately the various types of lesions seen in phthisis and in which he stressed the importance of the tubercles in this disease.

FIRST CHAPTER
ESSENTIAL CHARACTER OF PULMONARY PHTHISIS*

I think I should enter first into certain details of the definition of pulmonary phthisis, which I shall content myself henceforth in calling phthisis. To prevent all equivocation I am calling attention to different diseases of other organs which have also been designated by the name of phthisis and produce consumption. The generic character of phthisis can be deduced from the symptoms of the disease or from its nature and location: that is to say, it can be either artificial or essential. But it appears to me indispensable to write these two characteristics, the artificial which is deduced from the symptoms, is not applicable neither to all degrees nor to all cases of phthisis, the essential characteristic which expresses the nature and the seat of the malady, which agrees with it in its degrees and all forms it may take: but it would be sufficient to cause it to be recognized during life.

* Bayle, G.-L., *Recherches sur la Phthisie Pulmonaire,* Paris, Gabon, 1810, p. 4

Here is, according to the results of my investigations the *essential characteristic* of phthisis. One should call pulmonary phthisis *every lesion of the lung, which left to itself, produces a progressive disintegration of this organ, as the result of which ulceration appears and finally death.* One recognizes ordinarily phthisis with the aid of the following *artificial characteristic,* which is taken from the Nosographie Philosophique of M. Pinel (see the 3 edition, volume 3 p. 588): *cough, difficulty in breathing, emaciation, hectic fever, and sometimes purulent expectoration.* It is seen that it was necessary to unite the two characteristics of which we have spoken. Indeed the cough, the emaciation, the hectic fever, the purulent expectoration are the results of the distintegration of the lung. The existence of these symptoms show that the disintegration is advanced, but the malady is none the less real in its beginning, the period when the essential characteristic is already applicable. Besides, this disease can exist without showing a group of so-called pathognomonic signs (observations 38 and 39). Many writers have already remarked that different individuals succumb to phthisis although they never showed evident signs; also patients have been seen to die in the sage of hectic fever and emaciation, without cough or expectoration, and there have been found in the lungs numerous tubercles, and what is more inconceivable, large ulcerations. The same lesions have been found in other individuals, some of whom do not seem to have had more than an excessive diarrhea and to have died from nothing but inanition, while others have had only vague pains or nervous affections. All however, having marked lesions of the lungs ought to be considered victims of phthisis.

It is because we have not paid enough attention to the essential characteristics of pulmonary phthisis that we have frequently failed to recognize the traces of this disease in opening bodies in which it was not advanced. As the result of this error we have been deprived of the light which pathological anatomy could throw upon the first stages of this affection. This has led the best minds to be prejudiced against the name phthisis. It is necessary to remove the cause of this prejudice: that is the reason which leads us to disclose some truths which appear to us important to establish or rather to recall. Many physicians seem to have confused phthisis with its characteristic signs, and as emaciation and the hectic fever are two of the ordinary symptoms of phthisis, it seems absurd to them to consider an individual as suffering from phthisis, in whom no fever nor emaciation can be discovered. This manner of considering phthisis is just as ridiculous as that of a naturalist, who seeing a young oak tree, would refuse absolutely to give it this name because it did not yet show all its generic and specific characteristics. Moreover the oak which has just grown out of the ground, although it is a very feeble plant is none the less a tree whose trunk will acquire a great deal of strength. It is the same with phthisis: in the beginning it seems scarcely a slight indisposition; in its last stages it strikes down the strongest man, it devours, consumes and reduces to a skeleton those whose plumpness, freshness and health appeared inalterable. Nevertheless it would be unreasonable to refuse to admit that it is always the same disease, and to maintain this opinion and insist that in its earliest stages it did not show all the symptoms which characterize it today.

It is not necessary then to be a slave of methods, and still less of established characteristics to distinguish types of disease; it is this however which has happened in regard to phthisis. Although until now we have not been in agreement regarding the true meaning of the word *pulmonary phthisis*, most of those who employ it mean that progressive Emaciation of the entire body, which is the result of ulceration of the lung. It should be agreed that according to the etymology of the word *phthisis corruption*, *Consumption*, we should only call those phthisics who are very emaciated and who expectorate pus. It is probable that in earlier times, the physicians who designated a malady by this name wished to characterize it by the significant name they gave it. But today our knowledge is too advanced to fail to diagnose phthisis in the first stages of this disease, although frequently there has been no perceptible loss of weight and not the slightest trace of pus in the expectoration. Besides, many phthisics never expectorate pus in any evident manner it is not necessary then to take the term phthisis entirely literally, because in certain cases it would also be as improper as that of chrysanthemum when it is applied to the meadow daisy, which is named *chrysanthemum leucanthemum* which means *yellow flower, white flower*. Following the idea which I have given of pulmonary phthisis, one sees that I should regard as phthisics those individuals who have neither fever nor emaciation, nor purulent expectoration: it suffices that the lungs are affected by a lesion which tends to disintegrate and ulcerate them. One should not regard this lesion as a simple cause of phthisis, but as the first stage of this disease, since phthisis is this legion itself the continuation and subsequent development of which leads to death. It would be hardly reasonable to wish to wait before diagnosing pulmonary phthisis until it had arrived at its last stage which is the time when its pathognomonic symptoms are well marked. Is it not then undebatable that a physician should seek to know a disease from its beginning, through all the stages of its development, and in all its forms, just as the gardener distinguishes the plants which he cultivates through all the stages of their growth, and as an entomologist recognizes an insect in all its metamorphoses?

I know very well that there will always remain some things obscure to the practitioner: but one must not persist in missing, either during life or after death, the signs of a disease which is already apparent, although it does not yet show all the symptoms, all the lesions which it will present in a more advanced stage. If I have given too much emphasis to this discussion, it was indispensable because of what one observes in individuals who have died during the first stages of pulmonary phthisis and have not yet shown any symptoms of this disease. It was also useful to combat some sanctioned prejudices and bring a deceiving term to its proper value. Nothing is more powerful than the influence of language and erroneous terms, confusing definitions and false viewpoints call for in turn error, confusion and the most grave faults, especially in the sciences which, like medicine offer practical applications.

Jean-Antoine Villemin

Jean-Antoine Villemin was born in Prey, a small village in Vosges, in 1827. His father died when he was nine years of age and he was sent by his uncle to the college at Bruyères. He wished at first to become a teacher but was conscripted into the army in 1848 and was later stationed at Strassburg. Here he was advised by the colonel of his regiment to study medicine and began his medical studies at the military hospital of Strassburg. He completed his medical studies in 1853 and the same year was admitted to the school of Val-de-Grâce where he was promoted to the rank of major in the medical corps. He served in the army from 1854 to 1858, and in 1863 was appointed professeur agrégé at the army medical school of Val-de-Grâce where he remained for the rest of his medical career. He became a member of the Academy of Medicine in 1874 and vice-president in 1891. He died in 1892 at the age of sixty-five.

Villemin's great work *Études sur la Tuberculose* was published at Paris in 1868. In this work he demonstrated conclusively that tuberculosis is an infectious disease and can be transferred from a human patient to a rabbit. He also showed that the sputum of tuberculous patients, when inhaled, can give rise to pulmonary tuberculosis and when ingested, to intestinal tuberculosis. Professor Rieux in his eulogy on the occasion of the centenary of Villemin's birth, remarked that the three fundamental advances in the history of tuberculosis were made by three men, "Laënnec, who proclaimed its unity; Villemin, who demonstrated it was due to a virus; R. Koch, who discovered and identified its pathogenic agent."

FOURTH PART
EXPERIMENTAL PROOFS OF THE SPECIFICITY AND
INOCULABILITY OF TUBERCULOSIS
SIXTEENTH STUDY

Tuberculosis is Inoculable

The series of studies which we have just surveyed have demonstrated sufficiently to

*J.-A. Villemin, *Études sur la Tuberculose*, Paris, Baillière, 1868, pp. 528-530, 540-542.

us that tuberculosis does not rise from ordinary causes, that it pursues the course of a general affection, resulting from a morbid agent which infects the entire organism, that it developes and is propagated under conditions common to zymotic diseases, that it has the greatest analogy with syphilis, but especially with glanders, etc., etc., and we have been led to suppose that it ought to be inoculable like the diseases it resembles. The experiments which form the subject of this study have fully confirmed our hypothesis, as one can readily see.

§1.—Inoculation of Man to Rabbit

First series.—March 6, 1865, we took two

sumptive, who had been dead twenty-three hours. On March 30th and April 4th, we repeated the inoculation with a small fragment of tubercle.

June 20th, that is, at the end of three months and fourteen days, there was no appreciable change in the health of the animal, it had grown very much, we sacrificed it and noted the following:

A tablespoonful of serous fluid in the

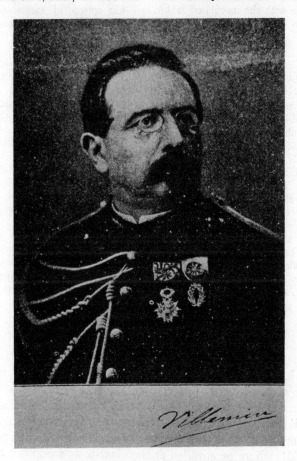

JEAN-ANTOINE VILLEMIN (1827-1892)

rabits about three weeks old, very healthy, still nursing their mother and living with her in a cage raised above the ground and properly sheltered. In one of these rabbits, we introduced into a little subcutaneous wound behind each ear, two small fragments of tubercle and a small amount of purulent liquid from a tuberculous cavity, removed from the lung and the intestine of a con-

peritoneal cavity; tubercular implants along the greater curvature of the stomach, seated in two parallel rows on each side of the midline and formed of very small gray, oblong granulations; many show in the center a small yellow opaque spot. In the intestine, approximately two or three centimeters from the stomach, there is a tubercle the size of the hemp-seed. Other tubercles, small and less noticeable, are disseminated throughout the small intestine.

The lungs are full of large tubercular masses, formed, in an obvious manner, from the agglomeration of numerous granulations; these masses have the size of a large pea: on incising them one sees on cutting, a grey transparent nodule, many small yellowish white points.

The other rabbit, who had shared the same conditions of life with the inoculated rabbit, was then put to death and did not show a single tubercle.

* * *

§3.—Inoculation of the Tubercle from Rabbit to Rabbit

When we had made known our first inoculations, it was objected that when we inoculated with a tubercle taken from a man dead for twenty-four or thirty-six hours, we inoculate by this act a cadaveric material, which bears some relation perhaps, to the effect produced. This question was easy to solve, but it could only be answered later, waiting until we had a perfectly fresh tubercle, as it was necessary to begin by producing it in animals with a tubercle of human origin. The following observations do not lack a certain interest from more than one point of view.

First series.—April 30th we inoculate two young rabits of good stock, with a tubercle taken from the lungs and kidneys of another rabbit, which we had just sacrificed. At the moment of the inoculation the heart of the animal which furnished the tuberculous material, was still beating.

No. 1.—Put to death June 16th, this animal showed the following lesions:

The two lungs contain a considerable number of tubercles still transparent, some very small and the others the size of a hemp-seed.

The spleen, of normal size, contains numerous yellowish tubercles.—Many follicles close to the appendix and the last plaques of the small intestine are tubercular.—The mesenteric glands are swollen and knotted with large tubercles, which are yellowish white and partly softened.

No. 2.—June 30th, exactly two months after the inoculation, the second rabbit of this series was found dead in his pen.

The two lungs are infiltrated with such a quantity of tubercles that there scarcely remains any particles of healthy parenchyma. These tubercles produce irregular confluent masses.—One sees several tubercles on the parietal pleura, especially on the diaphragmatic position.

The liver shows, on its peritoneal surface and inside, a large number of tubercles.— The two kidneys are sown with tubercles, large enough to produce projections on the surface of this organ.—The same is true of the spleen.

René-Théophile-Hyacinthe Laënnec

R.-T.-H. Laënnec was born at Quimper in Brittany, in the year 1781. At the age of eight, he went to live with his uncle Guillaume, a physician at Nantes, and in 1795, at the age of fourteen, began his medical studies with his uncle. His studies were interrupted by the civil wars and, in 1800, he joined the army, serving in the medical corps during his campaign. He went to Paris in 1801, where he enrolled at the Charité as a pupil of Corvisart, then chief of the medical service in that hospital. He also worked with Dupuytren and became a close friend of Bayle. These three men exercisd a profound influence upon the young medical student.

Laënnec received his doctor's degree in 1804 and in 1814 became physician to the Necker Hospital. He made his name immortal by his discovery of the stethoscope in 1816 and by the publication of his *Traité de l'auscultation médiate,* which appeared first in 1819. "Every physician throughout the world, who auscultates any part whatsoever of a human being, is, by this act alone, a disciple of Laënnec." (Letulle)

Laënnec's original stethoscope was a roll of paper, developing later into a rod of wood, and finally a cylinder of wood one foot long. Laënnec's *Traité* was written while its author was in very bad health, as he wrote later, "I know that I risked my life, but the book I am going to publish will be, I hope, useful enough sooner or later to be of more value than the life of a man." Laënnec, who suffered from tuberculosis, died in 1826, soon after the appearance of the second edition of his *Traité*. In this work he laid the foundations of auscul-

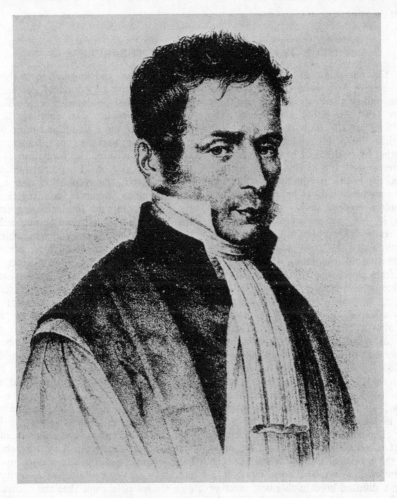

RENÉ-THÉOPHILE-HYACINTHE LAËNNEC (1781-1826)
Lithograph by Formentin, published by Rosselin

tation, describing most of the pathological processes in the lung with which we are today familiar, and introducing most of the terms now employed in auscultation. He also described the condition now known as atrophic cirrhosis of the liver.

The following selection on the physical signs of tubercles is from his *Traité* as are the later selections on mitral stenosis, pneumonia, pleurisy, pneumothorax, emphysema of the lungs and atrophic cirrhosis of the liver, since known as Laënnec's cirrhosis. Laënnec designated the condition "cirrhosis" because the color of the small nodules, which he considered new growths— the terms "cirrhosis" being derived from the Greek, κερρός (russet or yellowish brown). It was learned at a later date that the characteristic pathological lesion is a fibrosis of the liver and the color is not distinctive. The term "cirrhosis," however, has, by universal consent, become too firmly established to be displaced.

SECT. IV. PHYSICAL SIGNS OF TUBERCLES*

With the exception of some very rare cases, tubercles first make their appearance in the summit of the lungs. It is in this place therefore, that we must seek them. The earliest signs usually shew themselves below the clavicle. Small tubercles, separated from one another by portions of healthy lung, cannot be recognized. But at this period of their progress, the health is commonly still good, and the cough too slight to induce the patient to consult a medical man.

Signs of the accumulation of crude or miliary tubercles. When miliary tubercles are accumulated in great numbers in the upper portion of the lungs, the sound resulting from percussion of the clavicles becomes less, and is usually unequal. The right lung being in general the earliest and most severely affected, the defect of resonance is almost always on the right side. This deficiency of sound extends sometimes lower the upper and fore parts of the chest as low as the fourth rib. These, indeed, are the only parts of the chest where the mere accumulation of tubercles can give rise to this phenomenon; if we except the inter-scapular region, in which we sometimes find a deficiency of sound, owing to the great accumulation of tubercles at the roots of the lungs and in the bronchial glands. When the sign just mentioned exists, and even where it is wanting, a diffused bronchophonism, more or less marked, is perceived beneath the clavicle, over the infraspinal fossa of the scapula, and in the axilla. We must, however, disregard this last sign, if it is perceived only about the inner and upper angle of the scapula, on account of the vicinity of the bronchia.

Signs of the softening of the tubercles. When the tubercles begin to soften, the same signs continue; and in addition to these, the cough gives rise to a kind of gurgling, as if the matter that produced it were thick, and agitated *en masse.* The gurgling, however, soon becomes more liquid and more like the mucous rattle; and the cough, transformed to *cavernous,* indicates the formation of a pulmonary excavation. In proportion as this empties itself, the respiration also assumes the cavernous character, and together with the cough, points out the increasing extent of the cavity. The diffused bronchophonism then gives way to pectoriloquism, which is at first imperfect, and frequently interrupted, but gradually becomes more distinct. Sometimes, in proportion as the excavation empties itself, the resonance of the chest, which had been obscure, becomes clearer; and I have known physicians deceived by this circumstance, as to imagine that their patient was improving. Most frequently, however, even after the formation of a considerable excavation, the sound does not become louder, because there is developed at the same time around it, a great number of crude tubercles. It is also at this time, when the tuberculous matter begins to soften, that we sometimes perceive on percussion, a gurgling, or a jar, like that yielded by a cracked pot, and accompanied by a peculiar resonance indicative of the presence of a cavity. This sign always points out that the excavation is very near the surface of the lung; and is never observed except in lean subjects, the walls of whose chest are thin, and the ribs more than usually moveable. When a superficial excavation has some of its walls thin, soft, and not adhering to the costal pleura, the phenomenon which I have termed the auricular *puff, simple* or *veiled,* frequently accompanies the cavernous respiration and cough, as well as the pectoriloquism. In this case, every word is followed by a puff like that used in blowing out a candle, and which

---

* Laënnec, R.-T.-H., *A Treatise on the Diseases of the Chest and on Mediate Auscultation,* translated by John Forbes, M.D., New York, Samuel Wood & Sons, 1830, p. 339.

would be mistaken for a puff in reality, if the sense of touch did not rectify that of hearing. By making the patient speak in monosyllables, we ascertain that the puff immediately succeeds, rather than accompanies the voice.

Signs of the complete discharge of the tuberculous matter. When a tuberculous excavation is completely empty, this state is clearly indicated by the cavernous respiration and cough. In most cases the cavernous rattle is no longer heard; and if it sometimes takes place, owing to a secretion going on from the walls of the cavity, it is only temporarily, and frequently disappears for several hours, after the patient has expectorated. At this period, and often long before this pectoriloquism becomes quite perfect. I have in a former part of this volume described pectoriloquism, the most important of those signs which point out a pulmonary excavation. On account of its great value, however, I think it proper to enlarge a little more on it, in this place. I formerly stated that pectoriloquism may be *perfect, imperfect* or *doubtful,* that it may be suspended for some time, and in certain cases even disappear entirely. When pectoriloquism is doubtful and exists only in the interscapular region, below the axilla, or towards the junction of the clavicle and sternum, we must lay no stress on it. Indeed we may extend the same restriction to the whole of the upper parts of the chest as low as the upper rib, when the phenomenon is very doubtful, and as perceptible on one side as the other. This restriction is founded on the circumstance of there being more bronchial tubes of a certain diameter in the top of the lungs than elsewhere. These are sometimes very superficial; and when this is the case they frequently give rise to the phenomenon in question; which is, in point of fact, only bronchophonism. When we explore the space between the clavicle and upper edge of the trapezius muscle, we must be very careful to keep the stethoscope perpendicular; because if we give it the slightest direction towards the neck, we hear the natural resonance of the voice in the larynx and trachea, and will be very apt to confound this with pectoriloquism, if not much accustomed to the practice of auscultation. But when this doubtful pectoriloquism is observed below the third or fourth rib, or on one side only, it affords at least a strong presumption of the existence of an excavation; and if at the same time, it does not exist in the points above mentioned, the presumption may be considered as amounting to certainty; we have only to think that the cavity is situated deep within the pulmonary substance, or that it is still, in a great measure, filled with tuberculous matter imperfectly softened. In whatever part of the chest it may be, when the resonance of the voice is much stronger than on the opposite side, and particularly if it is so intense as to seem louder and nearer the ear of the observer, then the natural voice heard without the stethoscope, we may consider the sign quite as certain as if the voice traversed the tube of the instrument; and in such a case we say the pectoriloquism is *imperfect* and not doubtful. Between the most *perfect* pectoriloquism and that which is completely *doubtful,* there are many degrees which can only be learned by habit, and which it would be as difficult as it would be superfluous to describe. In one degree, for example, the voice seems to enter a short way into the extremity of the tube, but does not traverse it completely. Pectoriloquism is more distinct according as the voice of the individual is more sharp; and as women and children are the subjects in which this character is most strikingly marked, we must be particularly on our guard, in them, not to confound with pectoriloquism the doubtful bronchophonism which exists naturally in some points of the chest. In men, on the other hand, who have a very deep voice, pectoriloquism is frequently imperfect, and sometimes doubtful, even when there exists in the lungs excavations of the sort best calculated for producing it.

PLAGUE

The selection of passages referring to plague presents certain difficulties, since many different kinds of epidemics have been described by this term. The famous plague of Athens described by Thucydides was possibly not bubonic plague and there is much doubt whether the pestilence of Rome during the reign of Marcus Aurelius was this disease. The account of Rufus of Ephesus, by contrast, is an unmistakable description of bubonic plague, the earliest

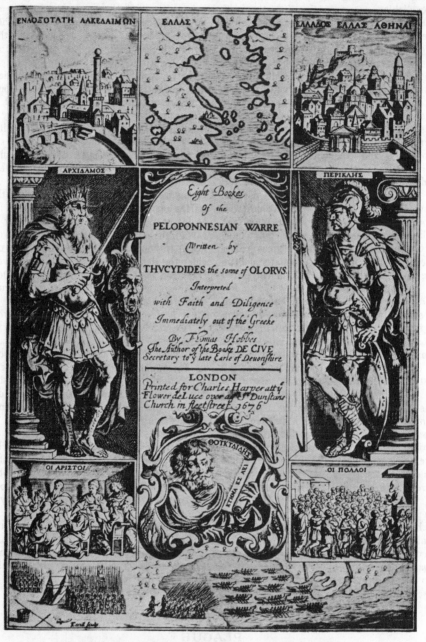

Frontispiece of Thucydides' *History of the Peloponnesian War*, translated by Thomas Hobbes (London, 1676)

account in medical literature. Piazza's account, while brief, is also unmistakable and points out the extreme contagiousness of the malady. One of the most famous of all accounts is that of Guy de Chauliac, the great French surgeon, called by many of his admirers "the father of surgery." Guy de Chauliac describes with great vividness the ravages of the "great mortality" at Avignon and gives an account of his own illness and recovery from the plague. Knutsson's book on the plague was widely read for several centuries and the accounts of Boccaccio and of Defoe are two of the most vivid in literature, although neither writer was an eye-witness of the scenes he describes with such fidelity. Kircher's account is noteworthy for his insistence that the disease is due to small animalcules and for the fact that it records the employment, for the first time, of the microscope in the study of disease. Paré's treatise, whether purloined from other sources or not, is clothed in the picturesque verbiage of one of the most interesting characters in the history of medicine. The literature on plague is enormous, and those interested in this subject should consult the writings of Dr. Arnold C. Klebs.

The Plague of Thucydides

Thucydides, the great historian, was born in Athens, probably in 471 B.C. The facts of his life are few, but his place in literature was assured by his *History of the Peloponnesian War,* one of the greatest historical works ever written. Thucydides was a witness of many of the events related in this history and was unquestionably acquainted with the great men of his time, although it is striking that he makes no reference to the poets Aeschylus, Sophocles, Euripides, and Aristophanes, the sculptor Pheidias, the philosophers Anaxagoras and Socrates, nor to Hippocrates. He was an eyewitness of the plague which he describes and also suffered himself from it.

The "plague of Thucydides" has been a subject of dispute for centuries. It has been identified as meningitis, measles, yellow fever, scarlet fever, typhus fever, typhoid fever, smallpox, and even as ergot poisoning. Wilhelm Ebstein in his monograph *Die Pest des Thukydides* discusses the plague at great length, but draws the conclusion only that it was some kind of a very contagious infectious epidemic. Francis Adams, the learned translator of Hippocrates and great authority on Greek medicine says however, "To my mind, then, there can be no doubt that the pestilence which prevailed during the Peloponnesian war partook of the nature of the glandular plague. What has tended to create doubts on this subject, in the minds of many learned men, is the omission of any distinct mention of buboes in the graphic description of it given by Thucydides."

The translation which follows is by Thomas Hobbes (1588-1679), the well-known English philosopher. Although he is described in this work as the author of the book *De Cive,* he is best known by his *Leviathan.*

Year II. The second invasion of Attica, by the Lacedaemonians

In the very beginning of Summer the *Peloponnesians* and their Confederates, with two thirds of their Forces, as before invaded *Attica,* under the Conduct of *Archidamus* the son of *Zeuxidamus,* King of *Lacedaemon,* and after they had encamped themselves, wasted the Country about them.*

* *Eight Bookes of the Peloponnesian Warre written by Thucydides the sonne of Olorus,* Interpreted with Faith and Diligence Immediately out of the Greeke by Thomas Hobbes, the Author of the Booke *De Cive,* Secretary to ye late Earle of Devonshire, London, Clark, 1676, p. 72.

The plague at *Athens*

They had not been many days in *Attica* when the Plague first began among the *Athenians*, said also to have seised formerly on divers other parts, as about *Lemnos,* and elsewhere; but so great a Plague and mortality of men, was never remembered to have happened in any place before. For at first, neither were the Physicians able to cure it, through ignorance of what it was, but died fastest themselves, as being the men that most approached the sick, nor any other Art of man availed whatsoever. All supplications to the *Gods,* and enquiries of *Oracles,* and whatsoever other means they used of that kind,

It began in *Æthiopia* proved all unprofitable, insomuch as subdued with the greatness of the evil, they gave them all over. It began (by report) first, in that part of *Æthiopia* that lieth upon *Ægypt,* and thence fell down into *Ægypt,* and *Africk,* and into the greatest part of the Territories of the *of Persia* *King. It invaded *Athens* on a sudden, and touched first upon those that dwelt in *Piraeus;* insomuch as they reported that the *Peloponnesians* had cast poison into their Wells, for Springs there were

The *Peloponnesians* supposed to have poisoned their wells not any in that place. But afterwards it came up into the high City, and then they died a great deal faster. Now let every man, Physician or other, concerning the ground of this Sickness, whence it sprung, and what causes he thinks able to produce so great an alteration, speak according to his own knowledge, for my own part, I will deliver but the manner of it, and lay open onely such things as one may take

The Author sick of this disease his Mark by, to discover the same if it come again, having been both sick of it my self, and seen others sick of same. This year by confession of all men, was of all other, for other Diseases most free and healthful. If any

The description of the Disease man were sick before, his Disease turned to this; if not, yet suddenly, without any apparent cause preceding, and being in perfect health, they were taken first with an extream ach in their Heads, redness and inflammation of the Eyes;

Ach of the head. Redness of the eyes. Sore throat. Unsavoury breath and then inwardly their Throats and Tongues grew presently bloody, and their Breath noisom and unsavoury. Upon this followed a sneezing and hoarseness, and not long after, the pain, together

with a mighty Cough came down into the Brest: and when once it was settled in the *stomach, it caused Vomit, and with great torment came up all manner of bilious purgation, that Physicians ever named. Most

Vomitings. *Καρδια here taken for the stomach. Hyckyexe of them had also the Hickeyexe. which brought with it a strong Convulsion and in some ceased quickly, but in others was long before it gave over. Their bodies outwardly to the touch, were neither very hot nor pale, but reddish livid, and beflowred with little Pimples and Whelks; but so burned inwardly, as not to endure the lightest clothes or linnen

Extreme heat of their bodies. Livid pustules nen garment to be upon them, nor any thing but meer nakedness; but rather most willingly to have cast themselves into the cold water. And many of them that were not looked to, possessed with insatiate thirst, ran unto the Wells, and to drink much or little

Insatiate thirst. Want of sleep was indifferent, being still from ease, and power to sleep, as far as ever. As long as the Disease was at the height, their bodies wasted not, but resisted the torment beyond all expectation, insomuch, as the most of them either died of their inward burn-

After 7, or 9 days, death ing, in nine or seven days, whilest they had yet strength, or if they had escaped that, then the disease falling down into their Bellies, and causing there great exculcerations and immoderate looseness, they died many of them afterwards through weakness. For the disease

Disease in the Belly. Looseness (which took first the head) began above and came down, and passed through the whole body; and he that overcame the worst of it was yet marked with the loss of his extream parts;

Loss of the parts where the Disease brake out for breaking out both at their privy members, and at their fingers and toes, many with the loss of these escaped. There were also some that lost their eyes, and many that presently upon their recovery, were taken

Oblivion of all things their done before sickness with such an oblivion of all things whatsoever, as they neither knew themselves, nor their acquaintance. For this was a kind of Sickness which far surmounted all expression of words, and both exceeded humane nature, in the cruelty wherewith it handled each one, and appeared also otherwise to be none of those diseases that are bred amongst us, and that especially by this. For all, both Birds and Beasts, that use to feed on humane Flesh, though many men lay abroad unburied, either came not, at them, or tasting perished. An argument whereof as touching the Birds, is the manifest defect of such Fowl, which were not then seen, neither about the Carcasses, or any where else: But by the Dogs, because they are familiar with men, this effect was seen much clearer. So that this Disease (to pass over many strange particulars of the accidents that some had differently from others) was in general such as I have shown, and for other usual Sicknesses, at that time no man was troubled with any. Now they died some for want of attendance, and some again with all the care and Physick that could be used. Nor was there any to say, certain Medicine, that applied must have helped them; for if it did good to one, it did harm to another; nor any difference of body, for strength or weakness that was able to resist it; but it carried all away, what Physick soever was administered. But the greatest misery of all was, the dejection of mind, in such as found themselves beginning to be sick (for they grew presently desperate, and gave themselves over without making any resistance) as also their dying thus like Sheep, infected by mutual Visitation, for the greatest Mortality proceeded that way. For if men forbore to visit them, for fear; then they died forlorn, whereby many Families became empty, for want of such as should take care of them. If they forbore not, then they died themselves, and principally the honestest men. For out of shame they would not spare themselves, but went in unto their Friends, especially after it was come to this pass, that even their Domesticks, wearied with the lamentations of them that died, and overcome with the greatness of the calamity, were no longer moved therewith. But those that were recovered, had much compassion both on them that died, and on them that lay sick, as having both known the misery themselves, and now no more subject to the danger. For this disease never took any man the second time, so as to be mortal. And these men were both by others counted happy, and they also themselves, through excess of present joy, conceived a

Birds and Beasts perished that fed on Carkasses

Want of attendance

Dejection of mind

No man sick of it mortally the second time

kind of light hope never to die of any other Sickness hereafter. Besides the present affliction, the reception of the Countrey people and of their substance into the City, oppressed both them, and much more the people themselves that so came in. For having no houses, but dwelling at that time of the Year in stifling Booths, the Mortality was now without all form; and dying men lay tumbling one upon another in the Streets, and men half dead about every Conduit through desire of Water. The temples also where they dwelt in Tents, were all full of the dead that died within them; for oppressed with the violence of the Calamity, and not knowing what to do, men grew careless both of holy and prophane things alike. And the Laws which they formerly used touching Funerals, were all new broken; every one burying where he could find room. And many for want of things necessary, after so many deaths before, were forced to become impudent in the Funerals of their Friends. For when one had made a Funeral *Pile, another getting before him, would throw on his dead and give it fire. And when one was in burning, another would come, and having cast thereon him whom he carried, go his way again. And the great licentiousness, which also in other kinds was used in the City, began at first from this disease. For that which a man before would dissemble, and not acknowledge to be done for voluptuousness, he durst now do freely, seeing before his eyes such quick revolution, of the rich dying, and men worth nothing inheriting their Estates; in so much as they justified a speedy fruition of their goods, even for their pleasure, as men that thought they held their lives but by the day. As for pains, no man was forward in any action of honour to take any, because they thought it uncertain whether they should die or not, before they atchieved it. But what any man knew to be delightful, and to be profitable to pleasure, that was made both profitable and honourable. Neither the fear of the Gods, nor Laws of men, awed any man. Not the former, because they concluded it was alike to worship or not worship, from seeing that alike they all

Men died in the Streets

Disorder in their Funerals

A Pile of Wood, which when they had laid the Corps on it, they fired, and afterwards buried the bones

Licentiousness of life justified

Neglect of Religion and Law

perished: nor the latter, because no man expected that lives would last, till he received punishment of his crimes by judgment. But they thought there was now over their heads, some far greater judgment decreed against them; before which fell, they thought to enjoy some little part of their lives. Such was the misery into which the *Athenians* being fallen, were much oppressed; having not onely their men killed by the Disease within, but the Enemy also laying waste their Fields and Villages without. In this sickness also, (as it was not unlikely they would) they called to mind this Verse, said also of the elder fort to have been uttered of old:

Predictions called to mind

A Dorick War shall fall,
And a great *Plague withall.

*Λοιμὸς.

Now were men at variance about the word, some saying it was not Λοιμὸς, (i. *the Plague*) that was by the Ancients, mentioned in that Verse, but Λιμὸς, (i. *Famine.*) But upon the present occasion the word Λοιμὸς deservedly obtained. For as men suffered, so they made the Verse to say. And I think, if after this, there shall ever come another *Dorick War,* and with it a Famine, they are like to recite the Verse accordingly. There was also reported by such as knew, a certain answer given by the Oracle to the *Lacedaemonians,* when they enquired whether they should make this War, or not, *That if they warred with all their Power, they should have the Victory, and that the *God himself would take their parts:* and thtreupon they thought the present misery to be a fulfilling of that Prophecie. The *Peloponnesians* were no sooner entered *Attica,* but the sickness presently began, and never came into *Peloponnesus,* to speak of, but regained principally in in *Athens,* and in such other places afterwards as were most populous. And thus much of this Disease.

An ambiguous Prophecie expounded by the event

*Apollo, *to whom the Heathen attributed the immission of all epidemick or ordinary Diseases*

Rufus of Ephesus

SECT. XXXVI.—ON THE PLAGUE, FROM THE WORKS OF RUFFUS*

In the plague there is everything which is **dreadful, and nothing of this kind is wanting** as in other diseases. For there are delirium, vomitings of bile, distension of the hypochondrium, pains, much sweatings, cold of the extremities, bilious diarrhoeas, which are thin and flatulent; the urine watery, thin, bilious, black, having bad sediments, and the substances floating on it most unfavorable; trickling of blood from the nose, heat in the chest, tongue parched, thirst, restlessness, insomnolency, strong convulsions, and many other things which are unfavorable. Should a person foresee that the plague is coming, by attending to the badness of the season, and the unhealthy occupations of the inhabitants, and from observing other animals perishing; when one observes these things, let him also observe this—what is the character of the present season, and what that of the whole year, for you will be able thereby to find out the best regimen; such,

for example, as if the temperature of the season ought to have been dry, but has become humid; in that case, it will be necessary, by a drying diet, to consume the superabundant moisture. Care also must be had of the belly, and when there is phlegm in the stomach it must be evacuated by emetics. And when a fulness of blood prevails, a vein should be opened. Purgings also by urine, and otherwise by the whole body, are proper. But, if the patient is affected with ardent fever, and has a fiery heat about the breast, it will not be improper to apply cold things to the breast, and to give cold drink, not in small quantities, for it only makes the flame burn more; but in full draughts, so as to extinguish it. But if an ardent fever prevails within, and the extremities are cold, and the skin cold, the hypochondrium distended, and the stomach sends the matters which have been melted, some upwards, and others downwards; if watchfulness, delirium, and roughness of the tongue, are present; in these cases, calefacient remedies are wanted to diffuse the heat all over the body, and every

* The Seven Books of Paulus Aegineta, translated by Francis Adams, London, Sydenham Society, 1844, I, 277.

other means ought to be tried, in order to determine the heat from the internal to the external parts. The following propoma may be used; of aloes, two parts; of ammoniac perfume, two parts; of myrrh, one part; pound these in fragrant wine, and give every day to the quantity of half a cyathus (z,v.) I never knew a person, says Ruffus, who did not recover from the plague after this draught So says Ruffus: but Galen says, concerning pestilential putrefactions, that to drink Armenian bole, and, in like manner, the theriac from vipers, is of great service; and that, in the plague which prevailed in Rome, all died who were not benefited by either of these things.

Michele di Piazza

The following early account of the plague was written by a Franciscan monk, Michele di Piazza in his History of Sicily—Michaelis Platiensis, *Historia Sicula ab anno 1337 ad annum 1361.* He describes cases of plague brought into the port of Messina by Venetian galleys in October, 1347.*

Which on account of infection of the breath among them mingled together talking, so one infected the other, since all were seen as if racked with pain, and in a measure, severely shaken; from the pain of which, by shaking and infection of the health, pustules appear on the thigh or arm in the manner of lenticulae, which thus infected and penetrated the body, wherefore, they violently spit forth blood; thus they shall spit for three days, incessantly without any cure for the dreaded disease they depart from life; and not only whoever talks to them dies, but indeed whoever should acquire, touch or seize anything belonging to them.

Guy de Chauliac

Guy de Chauliac, the most famous surgeon of the Middle Ages, was born in the hamlet of Chauliac near Auvergne, France, about 1300. He received his early education at Montpellier, where he obtained the degree of Master in Medicine, then proceeded to Bologna, and later studied in Paris. Like most of the learned men of that time, Guy de Chauliac took orders in the Church, and practised for a time at Lyons, where he was also a Canon of the Chapter of St. Just. Later he went to Avignon where he was physician successively to Popes Clement VI, Innocent VI, and Urban V. Guy de Chauliac was in Avignon during the epidemic of plague in 1348 and, unlike many of the other physicians, did not flee, but remained to treat the patients. He contracted the disease but recovered. His *Surgery* which he completed in 1363 was, he says, "ad solatium senectutis, ad solum mentis exercitium" (for the solace of old age, solely for the exercise of his mind). Guy de Chauliac died in Lyons in 1368

Guy de Chauliac's *Surgery* was the authoritative text in surgery until the eighteenth century. Sixteen editions appeared in Latin, forty-three in French, five in Italian, four in Dutch, several in German, five in Spanish, and one in English. The work is essentially a compilation rather than an account of his own surgical experience. However, his account of the plague, "the great mortality," is that of an eyewitness. He discusses the prevalence of the disease

* Kindness of F. H. Garrison.

throughout Asia and Europe, describes the havoc it wrought at Avignon, and differentiates the pneumonic type from the bubonic type.

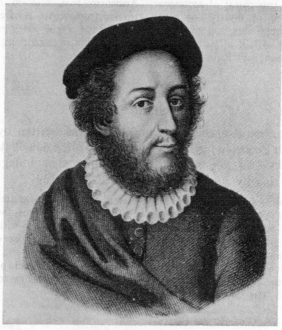

Courtesy of the Surgeon General's Library

GUY DE CHAULIAC (1300(?)-1368)

FIFTH CHAPTER*
OF THE APOSTEMS OF THE CHEST

This we have seen manifestly in the great mortality & the like of which one has not heard, which appeared in Avignon, the year of our Lord 1348, in the sixth year of the pontificate of Clement sixth, in whose service I, undeserving, was at that time, by his grace.

And it may not displease you if I recount it, on account of its wonders & because of its violence which happened again and again.

The said mortality commenced with us in the month of January & lasted the space of seven months.

It was of two kinds: the first lasted two months, with continued fever & expectoration of blood. And they died of it in three days. The second was, all the rest of the time, also with continued fever & apostems & carbuncles on the external parts, principally in the armpits & groin: & they died of it in five days. And was of such great contagiousness, (especially that which had expectoration of blood) that not only in visiting but also in looking at it, one person took it from another: so that the people died without servants & were interred without Priests.

The father did not visit his son, nor the son his father.

Charity was dead & hope destroyed.

I call it great because it spread out through all the world or very little was spared.

For it commenced in the Orient & so

*La Grande Chirurgie de M. Guy de Chauliac, Médecin très fameux de l'Université de Montpelier composée l'an de grâce 1363, Restituée par M. Laurens Joubert, Tournon, Michel, 1619, p. 172.

throwing its arrows against the world passed through our country towards the Occident.

And it was so great that it scarcely left behind one quarter of the population.

And I say it was such the like of which one has not heard: for we read of that of the city of Cranon & of Palestine, & of others in the book of the Epidemics, which were of the time of Hippocrates: & of that which came to the subjects of the Romans, at the time of Galen, in the book on good humor: & of that of the city of Rome at the time of Gregory.

It was not like these. For these did not infest but one region, ours the entire world: the one curable in some, the other in none.

So it was useless & shameful for the physicians, since they did not dare visit the sick for fear of being infected: & when they visited them, they did not make them well, & gained nothing: for all the sick died, except a few at the end, who escaped it with mature buboes.

Many were in doubt as to the cause of this great mortality.

In some quarters it was believed the Jews had poisoned the people & thus killed them.

In some other quarters, that it was the poor cripples & they chased them away.

And others that it was the nobles: & so they were afraid to go among the people.

Finally they went so far that they placed guards at the cities & villages: & did not permit anyone to enter who was not well known. And if they found powders or ointments on anyone, fearing that these were poisons, they made them swallow them.

But whatever the people said, the truth is, that the cause of this mortality was two-fold: the one an agent, universal: the other the patient, particular.

The universal agent was, the disposition of a certain conjunction of the greatest, of three superior bodies Saturn, Jupiter & Mars: which had proceeded it in 1345. The twenty fourth day of the month of March, at the fourteenth degree of Aquarius. For the greatest conjunctions (as I have said in the book I have written on Astrology) signify wonderful, violent & terrible things: as changing of reigns, coming or prophets, & great mortalities.

And they are arranged according to the nature of the signs, & the aspects of those to which they belong. It is not necessary to be astonished, if this great conjunction signifies a marvelous & terrible mortality, for it was not solely the greatest but the very great. And because it was a human sign, it caused distress to human nature: & since it was a sixth sign, it signified a long duration.

For it commenced in the Orient, a little after the conjunction: & lasted through the year fifty in the Occident. It impressed such a form on the air, & on other elements, and as the diamond cuts the iron so it produced great harsh & poisonous humors: & collecting them within, it produced apostems; from which continued fevers arose & expectoration of blood at the beginning, so that the said variety was powerful & tormented nature.

Then when it was calmed nature was not so troubled & cast it out as it was able, principally in the arm-pits, & in the groins: & caused buboes & other apostems: in such a way that these external apostems were the result of internal apostems.

* * *

The carbuncles were cupped, scarified & cauterized. And I, to avoid infamy, not daring to absent myself, with continual fear, I treated myself as much as I could, using the said remedies.

Nevertheless, toward the end of the mortality, I fell into a continued fever, with an apostem on the groin, and sick nearly six weeks, & was in such great danger that all my companions believed that I would die, but the apostem becoming mature, & treated as I have said, I escaped by the will of God. And after the year sixty & the eighth of the Pontificate of Pope Innocent sixth, in coming back from Germany & the Northern regions, the mortality returned to us. And commenced at the feast of St. Michael with swellings, fevers, carbuncles & boils, increasing little by little: & sometimes returning towards the middle of the year sixty one.

Then it raged furiously, until the following three months, so that in many places it did not leave behind more than half of the people. It differed from the preceding, in that in the first more of the populace died: & in this one there were more of the rich & nobles, & many infants & few women. During the same I concocted & composed a theriacal electuary like that of Master Arnold of Villanova & of the doctors of Montpellier and of Paris.

Boccaccio's Account of the Plague

Giovanni Boccaccio (1313-1375), the Italian author, wrote a description of the plague at Florence, which is universally recognized as a masterpiece of epic vividness. It appears as an introduction to the stories in his *Decameron*, which first appeared in 1353, and earned for its author the title of "Father of Italian Prose." Boccaccio's description of the plague of Florence was based largely upon hearsay and his own imagination, since in 1348 he was living in Naples and could not have been an eyewitness of the harrowing scenes he describes. The first printed edition of the *Decameron* appeared in 1469, and the number of printed editions that have appeared far exceed one hundred. The first complete English translation appeared in 1620.

INTRODUCTION
TO THE LADIES

As often, most gracious ladies, as, taking thought in myself, I mind me how very pitiful you are all by nature, so often do I recognize that this present work will, to your thinking, have a grievous and a weariful beginning, inasmuch as the dolorous remembrance of the late pestiferous mortality, which it beareth on its forefront, is universally irksome to all who saw or otherwise knew it. But I would not therefore have this affright you from reading further, as if in the reading you were still to fare among sighs and tears. Let this grisly beginning be none other to you than is to wayfarers a rugged and steep mountain, beyond which is situate a most fair and delightful plain, which latter cometh so much the pleasanter to them as the greater was the hardship of the ascent and the descent; for, like as dolor occupieth the extreme of gladness, even so are miseries determined by imminent joyance. This brief annoy (I say brief, inasmuch as it is contained in a few pages) is straightway succeeded by the pleasance and delight which I have already promised you and which, belike, were it not foresaid, might not be looked for from such a beginning. And in truth, could I fairly have availed to bring you to my desire otherwise, than by so rugged a path as this will be, I had gladly done it; but being in a manner constrained thereto, for that, without this reminiscence of our past miseries, it might not be shown what was the occasion of the coming about of the things that will hereafter be read, I have brought myself to write them.

I say, then, that the years [of the era] of the fruitful incarnation of the Son of God had attained to the number of one thousand three hundred and forty-eight, when into the notable city of Florence, fair over every other of Italy, there came the death dealing pestilence, which, through the operation of the heavenly bodies or of our own iniquitous dealings, being sent down upon mankind for our correction by the just wrath of God, had some years before appeared in the parts of the East and after having bereft these later of an innumerable number of inhabitants, extending without cease from one place to another, and now unhappily spread toward the West. And thereagainst no wisdom availing nor human foresight (whereby the city was purged of many impurities by officers deputed to that end and it was forbidden unto any sick person to enter therein and many were the counsels given for the preservation of health) not yet humble supplications, not once but many times both in ordered processions and on otherwise made unto God by devout persons—about the coming of Spring of the aforesaid year, it began in horrible and miraculous wise to show forth its dolorous effects, yet not as it had done in the East, where, if any bled at the nose, it was a manifest sign of inevitable death; nay, but in men and women alike there appeared at the beginning of the malady, certain swellings, either on the groin or under the armpits, whereof some waxed of the bigness of a common apple, others like unto an egg, some more and more less, and these the vulgar named plague-boils. From these two parts the aforesaid death-bearing plague-boils proceeded, in brief space, to appear and come indifferently in every part of the body; wherefrom, after awhile, the fashion of the contagion began to change into black or livid blotches, which showed themselves in many (first on the arms and on the thighs and (after spread to) every other part of the person, in some large and sparse and in others small and thick-sown, and like as the plague-boils had been first (and yet were) a very certain token of coming death, even so were these for every one to whom they came.

To the cure of these maladies nor counsel of physicians nor virtue of any medicine appeared to avail or profit aught; on the contrary,—whether it was that the nature of the infection suffered it not or that the ignorance of the physicians (of whom, over and above the men of art, the number, both men and women, who had never had any teaching of medicine, was become exceeding great) availed not to know whence it arose and consequently took not due measures thereagainst,—not only did few recover thereof, but well nigh died within the third day from the appearance of the aforesaid signs, this sooner and that later, and for the most part without fever or other accident. And this pestilence was the more virulent for that, by communication with those who were sick thereof, if gat hold upon the sound, no otherwise than fire upon things dry or greasy, whereas they are brought very near thereunto. Nay, the mischief was yet greater; for that not only did converse and consortion with the sick give to the sound infection or cause of common death, but the mere touching of the clothes or of whatsoever other thing had been touched or used of the sick appeared of itself to communicate the malady to the toucher. A marvelous thing to hear is that which I have to tell and one which had it not been seen of many men's eyes and of my own, I had scarce dared credit, much less set down in writing, though I had heard it from one worthy of belief. I say, then, that of such efficience was the nature of the pestilence in question in communicating itself from one to another, that not only did it pass from man to man, but this, which is much more, it many times visibly did;—to wit, a thing, which had pertained to a man sick or dead of the aforesaid sickness, being touched by an animal foreign to the human species, not only infected this later with the plague; but in a very brief space

of time killed it. Of this mine own eyes (as hath a little before been said), had one day, among others, experience on this wise; to wit, that the rags of a poor man who had died of the plague, being cast out into the public way, two hogs came up to them and having first, after their wont, rooted amain among them with their snoots, took them in their mouths and tossed them about their jaws, then, in a little while, after turning round and round, they both, as if they had taken poison, fell down dead upon the rags with which they had in an ill hour intermeddled.

* * *

The condition of the common people (and belike in great part, of the middle class also) was yet more pitible to behold, for that these, for the most part retained by hope or poverty in their houses and abiding in their own quarters, sickened by the thousands daily and being altogether untended and unsuccored died well nigh all without recourse. Many breathed their last in the open street, whilst other many, for all they died in their houses, made it known to the neighbors that they were dead rather by the stench of their rotting bodies than otherwise; and of these and others who died all about the whole city was full. For the most part one same usance was observed by the neighbors, moved more by fear lest the corruption of the dead bodies should imperil themselves than by any charity they had for the departed; to wit, that either with their own hands or with the aid of certain bearers, whereas they might have any, they brought the bodies of those who had died forth of their houses and laid them before their doors, where especially in the morning, those who went about might see corpses without number; then they fetched biers and some, in default thereof, they laid upon some board or other. Nor was it only one bier that carried two or three corpses, nor did this happen but once, nay, many might have been counted which contained husband and wife, two or three brothers, father and son or the like. And an infinite number of times it befell that, two priests going with one cross for some one, three or four biers, borne by bearers, ranged themselves behind the latter, and whereas the priests thought to have but one dead man to bury, they had six or eight, and whiles more. Nor therefore, were the dead honored with aught of tears or candles or funeral train; nay, the thing was come to such a pass that folk recked no more of men that died than nowadays they would of goats; whereby it very manifestly appeared that that which the natural course of things had not availed, by dint of small and infrequent harms, to teach the wise to endure with patience, the very greatness of their ills had brought even the simple to expect and make no account of. The consecrated ground sufficing not to the burial of the vast multitude of corpses aforesaid, which daily and well nigh hourly came carried in crowds to every church—especially if it were sought to give each his own place, according to ancient usance,—there were made throughout the churchyards, after every other part was full, vast trenches, wherein those who came after were laid by the hundred and being heaped up therein by layers, as goods are stored aboard ship, were covered with a little earth, till such time as they reached the top of the trench.

Moreover,—not to go longer searching out and recalling every particular of our past miseries, as they befell throughout the city,— I say that, whilst so sinister a time prevailed in the latter, on no wise therefore was the surrounding country spared, wherein, (letting be the castles, which in their littleness were like unto the city,) throughout the scattered villages and in the fields, the poor and miserable husbandmen and their families, without succor of physicians or aid of servitor, died, not like men, but well nigh like beasts, by the ways or in their tillages or about the houses, indifferently by day and night. By reason whereof, growing lax like the townfolk in their manners and customs, they recked not of anything or business of theirs; nay, all, as if they looked for death that very day, studied with all their wit, not to help to maturity the future produce of their cattle and their fields and the fruits of their own past toils, but to consume those which were ready to hand. Thus it came to pass that the oxen, the asses, the sheep, the goats, the swine, the fowls, nay the very dogs, so faithful to mankind, being driven forth of their own houses, went straying at their pleasure about the fields, where the very corn was abandoned, without being cut, much less gathered in; and many, well nigh like reasonable creatures, after grazing all day, returned at night, glutted, to their houses, without the constraint of any herdsman.

To leave the country and return to the city, what more can be said save that such and so great was the cruelty of heaven (and in part, peradventure, that of men) that, between March and the following July, what with the virulence of that pestiferous sickness, and the number of sick folk ill tended or forsaken in their need, through the fearfulness of those who were whole, it is believed for certain that upward of an hundred thousand human beings perished within the walls of the city of Florence, which, peradventure, before the advent of that death-dealing calamity, had not been accounted to hold so many. Alas, how many great palaces, how many goodly houses, how many noble mansions once full of families, of lords and of ladies, abode empty even to the meanest servant. How many memorable families, how many ample heritages, how many famous fortunes were seen to remain without lawful heir. How many valiant men, how many fair ladies, how many sprightly youths, whom, not others only but Galen, Hippocrates or Easculapius themselves, would have judged most hale, breakfasted in the morning with their kinsfolk, comrades and friends and that same night supped with their ancestors in the other world.

Bengt Knutsson

One of the most interesting mediaeval treatises on the plague is "A litil boke the whiche traytied and reherced many gode thinges necessaries for the ... Pestilence ... made by the ... Bisshop of Arusiens," published in London about 1485. A beautiful facsimile of this treatise was published in London about 1485. A beautiful facsimile of this treatise was published by the University of Manchester Press in 1910, with an introduction by Guthrie Vine, M.A.

The author of this work is said to be Bengt Knutsson, (Benedict Kanuti), who became bishop of Arosia (Västeros), near Stockholm, in 1461. Knutsson was a man of good birth, travelled far and wide and had studied medicine at Montpellier, then the foremost medical school in Europe. No further details of his life have been preserved. The author of this treatise on the plague according to Sudhoff was Johannes Jacobi, professor in Montpellier and physician to the

First page of "a litil boke" by the "Bisshop of Arusiens," Bengt Knutsson, published in London about 1485. Reproduced from the facsimile edition published by the University of Manchester Press in 1910.

Pope. Jacobi's treatise was written before 1380, probably in 1373. Jacobi died in 1384.

The following extract is from the facsimile edition mentioned above.

THE LITIL BOKE OF THE BISSHOP OF ARUSIENS

Here begynneth a litil boke the whiche traytied and reherced many gode thinges necessaries for the infirmite & grete sekenesse called Pestilence and whiche often times enfecteth us made by the most expert Doctour in phisike Bisshop of Arusiens in the realme of Denmark etc.

At the reverence & Worschip of the blessed Trinite & of the glorious Virgyn saynt Marye & the conservation of the comyn Wele of alle cristen people, as Wel for them that ben hole as for remedie of them that been seke. I the Bisshop of Arusiens in the wyalme of Denmark doctour of Phisique Wille Write by the moost experte and famous doctours auctorised in Phisike somme thynges of the infirmitie of pestilence Whiche dayly enfecteth, & sone suffreth be to departe oute of this lyfe First I Will Write the tokenes of this infirmite

The second the causes Whereof yt cometh

The thirde remedies for the same

The fourth comfort for the herte & the principal membres of the Body

The V When it schall be season to be lett Blode

First I sayde the tokenes of this infirmite Vii thynges ought to be noted in the same. The first is Whan in a sommers daye the Weder often times chaungeth, as in the morning the Wedyr appereth to rayne, after Ward it apperith cloudy & atte last Wyndy in the south

The seconde token is Whan in sommer the dayes apperith al derke & like to rayne & yet hit rayneth not. And if many dayes so continue it is to drede of grete Pestilence

The thirde tokyn is Whan grete multitude of flyes ben Upon the eerthe thenne it is signe the ayer is venemous and enfect

The fourth token is, Whan the sternes semen afte times to falle: then hit is token that the ayer is enfecte With moche venemous vapours

The V token is Whan a blasyng sterne is see in the element, thenne it sholde fortune some after to be grete manslaughter in batayle

The Vi token is, Whanne there is grete lyghtnynge and thundre namely oute of the southe

The Vii token is Whan grete Wyndes passen out of the south they be Foule & Unclene therfore Whan these tokens appere

it is drede grete pestilence but god of His mercy Wille remeve it

These thinges folowyng be the causes of pestilence

The Pestilence cometh of thre thinges, somtime it cometh fro the rote bynethe, Other While fro the rote above, so that We may fele sensibly howe the chaunge of the ayer appereth Unto Us. And somtyme it cometh of bothe to gider as Wele fro the rote above as fro the rote bynethe. As We sce a sege or prevy next to a chambre or of any other particuler thyng Whiche corrupteth the ayer in his substance & qualite Whiche is a thinge may happe every daye. And ther of cometh the ague of Pestylence. And aboute the same many phisicions be deceyved: not supposyng this axes to be a Pestilence. Sometime it cometh of dede cereyn or corrupcion of standing Waters in diches or sloughs & other corrupt places & these things somtyme be Universall & somtime particular: Fro the rote above it fortuneth the causes of the bodyes above in the ayer by Whome the spyryte of lyfe ys corrupte in a man or in a beste. In like Wyse as Avycenne sayth in his fourthe boke, by the Forme of thayer above the Bodyes benethe lightly be infecte. For thynpssyons above corrupteth the ayer, and soo the spirytes of a man ben corrupte. This infirmite cometh also from the rote above & bynethe. Whanne of thynpssions above the ayer is corrupt and of the putrefaccion or rotyn careyn of the Vyle places bynethe an infirmite is caused in a man. And suche an infirmite sometime is an axes, sometimes a postume or a swellying and that ys in many thinges.

Also the ayer inspired sometime is venemous and corrupt, hurtyng the herte that nature many Wayes ys greved, so that he perceyveth not hys harme. For the Uryne appereth fayer and sheweth gode dygestion, yet neverthelesse the paycent ys lyke to dye.

Athanasius Kircher

Now* when they (the corpuscula) are warmed in such clothes, so it is just as if resin and pitch were attacked by fire, for this poison is drawn through the breath and through the sweat pores of the body, from which later such fearful symptoms and effects result, as for example harmful absesses, tumors, boils and bumps, carbuncles and buboes of various forms, spots and eruptions, which project from the skin and seem sown throughout the body, like

The effects and symptoms of the plague

* Kircher, Athanasius, *Natürliche und Medicinalische Durchgründung der laidigen ansteckenden Sucht und so genanten Pestilentz*, Augsburg, Brandan, 1680, p. 39

hempseed. Then there comes to the patient loss of the senses and unconsciousness, weakness and vomiting, hiccoughing or coryza with fever, then when the foulness without ignites and spoils the humors of the heart, it drives them out by way of the arteries, either into a Humor or an abscess under the arm-pits, from the heart, or in the brain, or in the liver, and when the brain is still strong and powerful, it drives the poison away from it

In which parts of the body the plague causes buboes

and it breaks out in sore by the ears, which is called apostem, by the doctors parotides or ear afscess. If however the brain has already been weakened by the poison, is no longer strong enough by itself to drive out the poison, so the poison remains in the brain and its coverings or also in the the brain, called meninges. From this then little vessels between the two coverings of arises unconsciousness, phrenesis, and as soon as the inflammation attacks the first part of the brain, the patient begins to have phantasies and talk wildly, if it however begins to penetrate more deeply, then according to the view of the Arabian Physicians, the patient loses all judgment and understanding, and when it finally penetrates into the innermost part of the brain, all memory of things is taken away from the patient. I have spoken of the brain in accordance with the teachings of the Arabians and Avicenna, I know quite well that Galen discusses the matter somewhat differently, and has a different opinion regarding the vessels of the brain.

From this, then, it is clear that the harmful ear tumors and abscesses come from the poisoned brain when however the pestilential poison is driven by the heart into the liver, it is in turn driven by the liver to the secret places and the private parts of the human body, where the pestilential buboes and obscesses develope, which immediately spoil such weak and ignoble members with a harmful inflammation. The carbuncle however arises, when on all parts of the body

What the causes of the effects are

from the heart and appears like black, yellow, pale or reddish and fiery small pox which looks from within outwards black, and likewise soon becomes full of pus. When however the small pox eruption is pale red, so it is a sign that bile is mixed with blood; if it is black, that is a sign of black bile and melancholy humors; finally when the eruption is pale and whitish, it shows that there is trouble with the phlegm, and these signs are generally seen in the midst of the inflammation. When this is all past and the patient has lost his strength, and can not more fight against this illness, then it happens that these spots are pustules spread to the surface of the skin, meanwhile this poison rages within, conquers the entire body and overwhelms him and finally brings about death.

The other signs, which this evil guest brings are severe headache, with wakefulness and disturbed slumber and commonly loss of speech and delirium, anxiety and pain about the heart, heat within the breast, distaste for all food, then follows often vomiting, fainting, straining of the heart, great thirst, heat and burning of the throat, sticking and lividity of the tongue, foul breath, frequent stools and severe nose bleed. But now we will consider all these changes.

* * *

The pestilential vapor from the dead bodies of those dead of the plague increase the plague and scatter it further

Strangely enough, the power of this contagion is spread through the bodies of those who have died of the plague. For often the breath of life and the inward heat are driven out, and foulness remains, and exercises its power and might in all the inner and outer parts of the body, and continues in this, that is in a putrid carcase and in this foulness are the true seeds of the past hidden. These are partly activated within and partly without in the foul air, and the poisonous corpuscula are thrown off, become more poisonous and the contagion is spread still further.

Nathaniel Hodges

Nathaniel Hodges was born in Kensington, September 13, 1629. After studying at Westminster School, he obtained a scholarship at Trinity College, Cambridge, but later migrated to Oxford, where he was appointed by the parliamentary visitors a student of Christ Church. There he obtained the degrees of B.A. (1641), M.A. (1654), and M.D. (1659). He became a member of the College of Physicians in 1659.

When the plague raged in London in 1665 he did not flee as did so many of his colleagues, but attended all who sought his aid. He arose early each morning and soon afterwards entered his consulting room, where there was a large crowd of patients waiting. For three hours he examined them, prescribed for them, and when he had seen all, he had his breakfast. In spite of his constant exposure he escaped the disease and, in rcognition of his service to the citizens, he received a stipend from the city authorities.

In 1671 Hodges wrote an account of the plague, which was published in 1672 as 'Λοιμλογἰα' "sive Pestis nuperae apud Populum Londinensem grassantis Narratio Historica." In this work he mentions the behaviour of vermin during the plague epidemic and describes what is believed to be a case of acute pericarditis. He was elected a Fellow to the Royal College of Physicians in 1672, and in 1683 delivered the Harveian oration. Later his practice declined. Becoming poor, he was imprisoned in Ludgate Prison for debt, dying there in 1688.

SECTION I

Of the Rise and Progress of the Late Plague*

The Plague which we are now to give an Account of, discovered the Beginnings of its future Cruelties, about the Close of the Year 1664; for at that Season two or three Persons died suddenly in one Family at Westminster, attended with like Symptoms, that manifestly declared their Origin: Hereupon some timerous Neighbours, under Apprehensions of a Contagion, removed into the City of *London,* who unfortunately carried along with them the pestilential Taint; whereby that Disease, which was before in its Infancy, in a Family or two, suddenly got Strength, and spread Abroad its fatal Poisons; and meerly for Want of confining the Persons first seized with it, the whole City was in a little Time irrecoverably infected. Not unlike what happened the Year following, when a small Spark, from an unknown Cause, for Want of timely Care, increased to such a Flame, that neither the Tears of the People, nor the Profusion of their *Thames,* could extinguish; and which laid Wast the greatest Part of the City in three Days Time: and therefore as happens

to be no great Difference between these two grievous Calamities, this Mention of them together may not be improper; and the more especially, because by a like irresistable Fate from a Fever and a Conflagration, both the Inhabitants and their Houses were reduc'd to Ashes.

* * *

SECTION II

Of the Cause of a Pestilence, and a Contagion

And for what concerns that Pestilence now under Enquiry, this we have as to its Origin, from the most irrefrigable Authority, that it first came into this Island by Contagion, and was imported to us from *Holland,* in Packs of Merchandice; and if any one pleases to trace it further, he may be satisfied by common Fame, it came thither from *Turkey* in Bails of Cotton or Silk, which is a strange Preserver of the pestilential Steams. For that Part of the World is seldom free from such Infections, altho' it is sometimes more severe than others, according to the Disposition of Seasons and Temperature of Air in those Regions: But if any would yet more intimately be acquainted with its Origin, it concerns him to know all the Changes the Air in these Climates is subject to, and its various Properties of Dryness, Moisture, Heat, Cold, etc.

* * *

*Nath. Hodges, M.D., *Loimologia: or an Historical Account of the Plague in London, in 1665,* London, E. Bell and J. Osborn, 1720, pp. 1, 30, 41, 64, 106.

For further Illustration hereof it may be observed, that the nitrous Spirit which circulates through the subterraneous Caverns may, instead of Obtaining a further Purification, take along with it corrupt and poysonous Vapours from arsenical or other Minerals; and loaded therewith, break out into the open Air: And this we have confirmed from common Observation in the Western Climes of *Africa,* that lye under the *Equator,* wherein the very Showers seem to be endued with a Stiptick or Caustick Power, so as to taint the Cloaths and Skin of the Travellers, and burn, as it were, upon them pestilential Characters. From which Disposition it cannot be a Wonder to any, that the Plague should reign after Earthquakes; because a poysonous Spirit at such Times break out into the Air; as also that Nitre thus loaded with an impure Mixture, and sometimes too that which is deadly, should of it self, like the Occursion of an Acid, force out its Way wherever there is Room, and leave behind in its Passage many Marks of Malignity; so that subterraneous Animals, such as Moles, Mice, Serpents, Conies, Foxes, etc. as conscious of approaching Mischief, leave their Burrows, and lie open in the Air; which is also a certain Sign of a Pestilence at Hand: Hence also a sudden Death of Fish; and a Departure of the Birds of the Air, to secure their Safety in that which is more wholesome.

* * *

As for that opinion of the famous *Kircher,*

about animated Worms, I must confess I never could come at any such Discovery with the Help of the best Glasses, nor ever found the same discovered by any other; but perhaps in our cloudy Island we are not so sharp-sighted as in the serene Air of *Italy;* and with the Submission to so great a Name, it seems to me very disconsonant to Reason, that such a pestilential *Seminium,* which is both of a nitrous and poisonous Nature, should produce a living Creature.

* * *

SECTION V

Of the Manifest Signs of the Late Pestilence

But how vehemnently the Heart may beat on this Occasion, appears very manifest from a remarkable Instance; I was sent for to a Youth of about fourteen Years of Age, who had continued free of the Infection, after his Mother and the rest of the Family had been visited by it, when all on a sudden he was seized with such a Palpitation at Heart, That I and several others could hear it at some considerable Distance, and it continued so to do till he died, which was soon after; many Medicines being given without any manner of Success: But in so extraordinary a Case as this, I am apt to conjecture it rather owing to a Pestilential Carbuncle seizing the Heart it self, than from the Vellication and *Stimulus* only of pungent Particles passing through it.

* * *

Ambroise Paré
OF THE PLAGUE*
THE TWENTY-SECOND BOOK

Chap. I
The Description of the Plague

What the Plague is   The Plague is a cruel and contagious diseas, which everiewhere, like a common diseas invadeing Man and Beast, kill's verie manie, being attended, and as it were associated with a continual fever, botches, carbuncles, spots, nauseousness, vomitings, and other

* *The Workes of that famous Chirurgion Ambrose Parey,* translated by Tho. Johnson, London, Cotes, 1644, p. 535.

Sect. 3. aphor   such malign accidents. This diseas is not so pernicious or hurtful, by anie elementairie qualitie, as from a certain poisonous and venenate malignite, the force whereof exceed's the condition of common putrefaction. Yet I will not denie, but that it is more hurtful in certain bodies, times and regions, as also manie other diseases, of which *Hippocrates* makes mention. But from hence wee can onely collect, that the force and malignite of the plague may bee encreased, or diminished, according to the condition of the elementarie qualities concurring with it; but not the whole nature and essence thereof to depend thereon.

This pestiferous poison prin- How it comes to kill cipally assail's the vital spirit, the store-hous and original whereof is the heart, so that if the vital spirit proov stronger, it drive's it far from the heart; but if weaker, it beeing overcom and weakned, by the hostile assault, flie's back into the fortress of the heart, by the like contagion infecting the heart, and so the whole bodie, beeing spread into it by the passages of the arteries.

Hence it is, pestilent fevers are sometime simple and solitarie; other-whiles associated with a troop of other affects, as botches, carbuncles, blanes and spots, of one or more colors.

It is probable such effects have The original buboes, carbuncles, &c. in the plague their original from the expulsive facultie, whether strong or weak, provoked by the malignite of the rageing matter: yet assuredly divers symptoms and changes arise, according to the constitution of the bodie of the patient, and condition of the humor in which the virulencie of the plague is chiefly inherent, and lastly, in the nature of the efficient caus.

I thought good, by this description, to express the nature of the plague, at this my first entrance into this matter; for wee can scarce comprehend it in a proper definition. For although the force thereof bee definite, and certain in nature, yet it is not altogether certain and manifest in mens mindes, becaus it never happen's after one sort: so that in so great varietie, it is verie difficult to set down anie thing general and certain.

* * *

CHAP. V

WHAT SIGNS IN THE AIR AND EARTH
PROGNOSTICATE A PLAGUE

Wee may know a Plague to bee at hand and hang over us, if at anie time the air and seasons of the year swarv from their natural constitution, after those waies I have mentioned before; if frequent and long continuing Meteors, or sulphureous Why abortions are frequently in a pestilent season Thunders infect the air; if fruits, seeds and puls bee worm-eaten: If Birds forsake their nests, eggs or young, without anie manifest caus; if wee perceiv women com-

monly to abort, by continual breathing in the vaporous air, being corrupted and hurtful both to the Embryon and original of life, and by which it beeing suffocated, is presently cast forth and expelled. Yet notwithstanding those airie impressions do not solely corrupt the air, but there may bee also others raised by the Sun from the filthie exhaltations and poisonous vapors of the earth and waters, or of dead carkasses, which by their unnatural mixture, easily corrupt the air, subject to alteration, as which is thin and moist, from whence divers Epidemial diseases, and such as everie-where seiz upon the common sort, according to the several kindes of corruptions, such as that famous *Catarrh* with difficultie of breathing, A *Catarrh* with difficultie of breathing killing maniac which in the year 1510 went almost over all the world, and raged over all the Cities and Towns of France, with great heaviness of the head (whereupon the French named it *Cuculla*) with a straightness of the heart and lungs, and a cough, a continual fever, and sometimes raveing.

This, although it seized upon manie more then it killed, yet becaus they commonly died who were either let blood, or purged, it shewed it self pestilent by that violent and peculiar and unheard of kinde of malignitie.

Such also was the English The English Sweating sickness *Sweating-Sickness,* or *Sweating-fever* which unusual, with a great deal of terror invaded all the lower parts of Germanie, and the Low-Countries, from the year 1525 unto the year 1530, and that chiefly in Autumn.

As soon as the pestilent diseas entered into anie Citie, suddenly two or three hundred fell sick on one day, then it departed thence to som other place. The people strucken with it languishing, fell down in a swound, and lying in their beds, sweat continually, haveing a fever, a frequent, quick and unequal puls; neither did they leav sweating, till the disease let them, which was in one or two daies at the most, yet free'd of it, they languished long after, they all had a beating, or palpitation of the heart, which held som two or three years, and others all their life after.

At the first beginning it killed manie, before the force of it was known: but afterwards verie few, when it was found out by practice and use, that those who furthered and continued their sweats, and strengthened

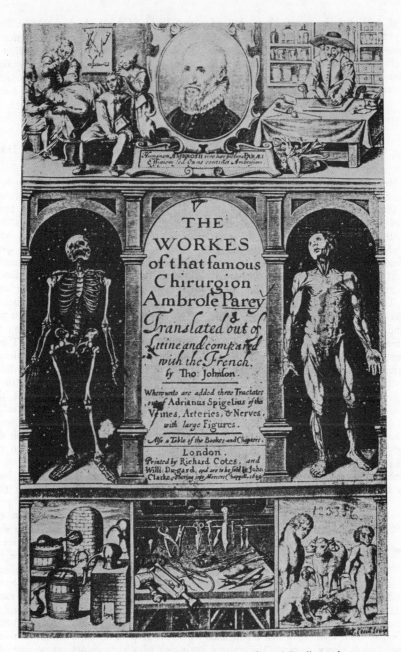

Frontispiece of Thomas Johnson's translation of Paré's works,
published in London, 1644

themselves with cordials, were all restored. but at certain times many other popular diseases sprung up, as putrid fever, fluxes, bloodie-fluxes, catarrhs, coughs, phrenzies, squinnances, plurisies, inflammations of the lungs, inflammations of the eies, apoplexies, lithargies, small pocks and meazles, scabs, carbuncles, and malign pustles. Wherefore the Plague is not alwaies, nor everie-

The Plague is not the definite name of one disease

where of one and the same kinde, but of divers; which is the caus that divers names are imposed upon it, according to the varietie of the effects it bring's and symptoms which accompanie it, and kindes of putrefaction, and hidden qualities of the air.

What signs in the earth foretell a plague — They affirm, when the Plague is at hand, that Mushroms grow in greater abundance out of the earth, and upon the surface thereof manie kindes of poisonous *insecta* creep in great numbers, as Spiders, Caterpillars, Butter-flies, Grass-hoppers, Beetles, Hornets, Wasps, Flies, Scorpions, Snails Locusts, Toads, Worms and such things as are the off-spring of putrefaction. And also wilde beasts tired with the vaporous malignite of their dens and caves in the earth, forsake them; and Moles, Toads, Vipers, Snakes, Lizards, Asps and Crocodiles are seen to flie away, and remoov their habitations in great troops. For these, as also som other creatures, have a manifest power by the gift of God, and the instinct of Nature, to presage changes of weather, as rains, showrs, and fair weather; and seasons of the year, as the Spring, Summer, Autumn, Winter, which they testifie by their singing, chirping, crying, flying, playing, and beating with their wings, and such like signs: so also they have a perception of a Plague at hand. And Moreover, the carkasses of som of them which took less heed of themselvs, suffocated by the pestiferous poison of the ill air contained in the earth, may bee everie-where found, not onely in their dens, but also in the plain fields.

How pestilent vapors may kill plants and trees — These vapors corrupted not by a simple putrefaction, but an occult malignitie, are drawn out of the bowels of the earth into the air, by the force of the Sun and Stars, and thence condensed into clouds, which by their falling upon corn, trees and grass, infect and corrupt all things which the earth produceth, and also kill's those creatures which feed them; yet brute beasts sooner then men, as which stoop and hold their heads down towards the ground (the maintainer and breeder of this poison) that they may get their food from thence. Therefore, at such time, skilful husband-man, taught by long experience, never drive their Cattel or Sheep to pasture, before that the Sun, by the force of his beams, hath wasted and dissipated into air this pestiferous dew hanging and abideing upon boughs

and leavs of trees, herbs, corn and fruits.

But on the contrarie, that pestilence which proceed's from som malign qualitie from above, by reason of evil and certain conjunction of the Stars, is more hurtful to men and birds, as those who are nearer to heaven.

* * *

CHAP. XIII

OF THE SIGNS OF SUCH AS ARE INFECTED WITH THE PLAGUE

Whence certain signs of the Plague may be taken — Wee must not stay so long before wee pronounce one to have the Plague, until there bee pain and a tumor under his arm-holes, or in his groin, or spots (vulgarly called *Tokens*) appear over all the bodie, or carbuncles arise: for manie die through the venenate malignitie, before these signs appear. Wherefore the chiefest and truest signs of this diseas are to bee taken from the heart, beeing the mansion of life, which chiefly and first of all is wont to bee assailed by the force of the poison. Therefore they that are infected with the Pestilence, are vexed with often swoundings and fainting; their puls is feebler and slower then other, but sometimes more frequent, but that is specially in the night-season; they feel prickings over all their bodie, as if it were the pricking of needles; but their nostrils do itch especially by occasion of the malign vapor's riseing upwards from the lower and inner, into the upper parts, their breast burneth, their heart beateth with pain under the left dug, difficultie of takeing breath, ptissick, cough, pain of the heart, and such an elation or puffing up of the *Hypocandria,* or sides of the bellie, distended with the abundance of vapors raised by the force of the feverish heat, that the patient will in a manner seem to have the Tympanie. They are molested with a desire to vomit, and oftentimes with much and painful vomiting, wherein green and black matter is seen, and alwaies of divers colors, answering in proportion to the excrements of the lower parts, the stomach being drawn into a consent with the heart, by reason of the vicinitie and communion of the vessels; oftentimes blood alone, and that pure, is excluded and cast up in vomiting and is not onely cast up by vomiting out of the stomach, but also verie often out of the nostrils, fundament; and

The cause of vomiting in such as have the plague

in women, out of the womb; the inward parts are often burned and the outward parts are stiff with cold, the whole heat of the patient beeing drawn violently inward, after the manner of a Cupping-glass, by the strong burning of the inner parts; then the eie-lids wax blew, as it were through som contusion, all the whole face hath a horrid aspect, and as it were the color of lead, the eies are burning red, and as it were swoln, or puffed up with blood, or anie other humor, shed tears; and to conclude, the whole habit of the bodie is somwhat changed, and turned yellow.

Their looks are sud-denly changed

Manie have a burning fever, which doth shew itself by the patient's ulcerated jaws, unquenchable thirst, driness and blackness of the tongue, and it causseth such a phrensie by inflameing the brain, that the patients, running naked out of their beds seek to throw themselves out of windows into the pits and rivers that are at hand. In som the joints of the boddie are so weakned, that they cannot go nor stand; from the beginning they are as it were buried in a long swound and deep sleep, by reason that the fever sendeth up to the brain the gross vapors from the crude and cold humors, as it were from green wood newly kindled to make a fire.

Why some that are taken with the plague are sleepie

Such sleeping doth hold him especially while the matter of the sore or carbuncle is drawn together, and beginneth to com to suppuration. Oftentimes when they are awaked out of sleep, there do spots and marks appear dispersed over the skin, with a stinking sweat. But if those vapors bee sharp that are stirred up unto the head, in stead of sleep they caus great wakeing, and alwaies there is much diversitie of accidents in the urine of those that are infected with the Plague by reason of the divers tempera-ture and condition of bodies; neither is the urine at all times, and in all men of the same consistence and color: For sometimes they are like unto the urine of those that are found and in health, that is to say, laud-able in color and substance, becaus that when the heart is affected by the venemous air, that entreth in unto it, the spirits are more greatly grieved and molested then the humors: but those, *i.e.* the spirits, are infected and corrupted when these do begin to corrupt.

Why their urines are like those that are found

But Urines onely shew the dispositions of the humors or parts in which they are made, collected together, and through which they pass.

This reason seemeth truer to mee then theirs which say, that nature terrified with the malignities of the poison avoid's contention, and doth not resist or labor to digest the matter that causseth the diseas.

Manie have their appetites so overthrown, that they can abstain from meat for the space of three daies together.

And to conclude, the varietie of accidents it almost infinite, which appear and spring up in this kinde of diseas, by reason of the diversitie of the poison, and condition of the bodies and grieved parts: but they do not all appear in each man; but som in one, and som in another.

Daniel Defoe

The following observations on the plague are from Daniel Defoe's *A Journal of the Plague Year, being Observations or Memorials of the most remarkable Occurrences as well publick as private, which happened in Lon-don during the Last Great Visitation in 1665.* Daniel Defoe was born in 1661 and was therefore only four years old in the Plague year, 1665. Daniel Defoe's two great literary masterpieces were *Robinson Crusoe* published in 1719, and his *Journal of the Plague Year* which appeared in 1722. The latter work pre-sents such a striking picture of the plague that Dr. Richard Mead was led into the error of quoting from it as from the narrative of an eye-witness. One of the most interesting paragraphs in this *Journal* refers to the destruction of dogs, cats, and particularly mice and rats "especially the latter" because these animals probably spread the infection.

I cannot undertake to give any other than a Summary* of such Passages as these, because it was not possible to come at the Particulars, where sometimes the whole Families, where such Things happen'd were carry'd off by the Distemper: But there were innummerable Cases of this Kind, which presented to the eye, and the Ear; even in passing along the streets, as I have hinted the Plague rag'd at the Easter-most Part of the Town; how for a long Time the People of those parts had flattered themselves that they should escape; and how they were surprized, when it came upon them as it did; for indeed, it came upon them like an armed Man, when it did come. I say, this brings me back to the three poor Men, who wandered from *Wapping,* not knowing whether to go, or

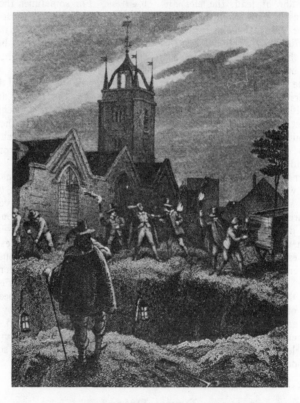

BURYING OF THE DEAD IN THE GREAT PIT

A drawing by George Cruikshank from Defoe's *Journal of the Plague Year,* edition of 1876

above, nor is it easy to give any Story of this, or that Family, which there was not divers parrallel Stories to be met with of the same Kind.

But as I am now talking of the Time when

what to do, and who I mention'd before; one a Biscuit-Baker, one a Sail-maker, and the other a Joiner; all of *Wapping,* or thereabouts.

The Sleepiness and Security of that Part, as I have observ'd, was such, that they not only did not shift for themselves as others did; but they boasted of being safe, and of Safety being with them; and many People fled out of the City, and out of the infected Suburbs, to *Wapping, Ratcliff, Lime-house, Poplar,* and such Places, as to Places of Se-

*From *The History of the Great Plague in London in the Year 1665. Containing, Observations and Memorials of the most remarkable Occurrences, both Public and Private, that happened during that dreadful Period.* By a Citizen, who lived the whole Time in LONDON, London, F. and J. Noble, 1754, p. 139, 224.

curity; and it is not at all unlikely, that their doing this help'd to bring the Plague that way faster, than it might otherwise have come. For tho' I am much for Peoples flying away and emptying such a Town at this, upon the first Appearance of a like Visitation, and that all People that have any possible Retreat, should make use of it in Time, and begone; yet, I must say, when all that will fly are gone, those that are left and must stand it, should stand stock still where they are, and not shift from one End of the Town, or one Part of the Town to the other; for that is the Bane and Mischief of the whole, and they carry the Plague from House to House in their very Clothes.

Wherefore, were we ordered to kill all the Dogs and Cats: But because as they were domestick Animals and are apt to run from House to House, and from Street to Street, so are they capable of carrying the Effluvia or Infectious Steams of the Bodies infected, even in their Furrs and Hair; and therefore, it was that in the beginning of the Infection, an Order was published by the Lord Mayor, and by the Magistrates, according to the Advice of the Physicians, that all the Dogs and Cats should be immediately killed, and an Officer was appointed for the Execution.

It is incredible, if their Account is to be depended upon, what a prodigious Number of these Creatures were destroy'd: I think they talk'd of forty thousand Dogs, and five times as many Cats, few Houses being without a Cat, and some having several, and sometimes five or six in a House. All possible Endeavours were us'd also to destroy the Mice and Rats, especially the latter, by laying Rats-Bane, and other Poisons for them, and a prodigious Multitude of them were also destroy'd.

* * *

The Manner of its coming first to *Londen,* proves this also, (viz.) by Goods brought over from *Holland,* and brought thither from the Levant; the first breaking of it out in a House in *Long-Acre,* where those Goods were carried, and first opened; its spreading from that House to other Houses, by the visible unwary conversing with those who were sick, and the infecting the Parish Officers who were employed about the Persons dead, *and the like;* these are known Authorities for this great Foundation Point, that it went on, and proceeded from Person to Person, and from House to House, and no otherwise; In the first House that was infected there died four Persons, a Neighbour hearing the Mistress of the first House was sick, went to visit her, and went Home and gave the Distemper to her Family, and died, and all her Household. A Minister call'd to pray with the first sick Person in the second House, was said to sicken immediately, and die with several more in his House: Then the Physicians began to consider, for they did not at first dream of a general Contagion. But the Physicians being sent to inspect the Bodies, they assur'd the People that it was neither more or less than *the Plague* with all its terrifying Particulars, and that it threaten'd an universal Infection, so many People having already convers'd with the Sick or Distemper'd and having, as might be suppos'd, received infection from them, that it would be impossible to put a stop to it.

Here the Opinion of the Physicians agreed with my Observations afterwards, namely, that the Danger was spreading insensibly; for the Sick cou'd infect none but those that came within reach of the sick Person; but that one Man, who may have really receiv'd the Infection, and knows it not, but goes Abroad, and about as a sound Person, may give the Plague to a thousand People, and they to greater Numbers in Proportion, and neither the Person giving the Infection, or the Persons receiving it, know anything of it, and Perhaps not feel the Effects of it for several days after.

For Example, Many Persons in the Time of this Visitation never perceiv'd that they were infected, till they found to their unspeakable Surprize, the Tokens come out upon them, after which they seldom liv'd six Hours; for those Spots they call'd the Tokens were really gangreen Spots, or mortified Flesh in small Knobs as broad as a little silver Peny, and hard as a piece of Callus or Horn; so that when the Disease was come up to that length, there was nothing could follow but certain Death, and yet, *as I said,* they knew nothing of their being Infected, nor found themselves so much as out of Order, till those mortal Marks were upon them: But every Body must allow, that they were infected in a high Degree before, and must have been so some time; and consequently their Breath, their Sweat, their very Cloaths were contagious for many Days before.

MALARIA

The following references to malaria from the early history of Greece and Rome were written by laymen with one exception—that of Hippocrates. Aristophanes, the poet and dramatist (450-380 B.C.), was a contemporary of Hippocrates, his *Plutus* is a remarkable satire on the disciples of Æsculapius and the cures in the temple, and his *Wasps* contains an unquestioned reference to malaria.

Marcus Terentius Varro (116-27 B.C.) is best remembered for his treatise on agriculture which contains the shrewd guess that certain diseases are due to invisible living creatures. Aulus Cornelius Celsus, who lived during the reign of Tiberius, was a member of the noble patrician family Cornelius and was the first of the great encyclopedists. He wrote a series of books on agriculture, military science, oratory, jurisprudence, philosophy, and medicine. The book on medicine, which alone has survived, was written between 25 and 35 A.D. This work, ignored by contemporaries, and unknown to the medieval physicians, was discovered in manuscript by Pope Nicholas V and was *the first medical book printed after the discovery of printing*. Since this first edition, printed in Florence in 1478, innumerable editions have appeared. Celsus' book on medicine was highly prized not only for its learning but because of his chaste Latin style. Celsus was one of the great masters of Latin prose. Pliny the Elder (23-79 A.D.), author of the famous *Natural History*, mentions malaria several times in this work. Pliny, according to his nephew, was always studying "except when he was actually in his bath" and "deemed all time wasted that was not employed in study." Pliny, as is well known, perished during the great eruption of Vesuvius which overwhelmed Pompeii and Herculaneum. Martial (43-104 A.D.) the epigrammatist, satirist and scourger of the morals of Rome, is today the chief source of our information regarding the sexual perversions and pornography of the Romans.

Hippocrates
SECTION III*

12. Fevers are,—the continual, some of which hold during the day and have a remission at night, and others hold during the night and have a remission during the day,[3] semi-tertians, tertians, quartans, quintans, septans, nonans. The most acute, strongest, most dangerous, and fatal diseases, occur in the continual fever. The least dangerous of all, and the mildest and most protracted, is the quartan, for it is not only such from itself, but it also carries off other great diseases.[4]

In what is called the semi-tertian, other acute diseases are apt to occur, and it is the most fatal of all others, and moreover phthisical persons, and those labouring under other protracted diseases, are apt to be at-

* Hippocrates: *Epidemics*—Book I. *The Genuine Works of Hippocrates* translated by Francis Adams, LL.D., London, Sydenham Society, 1859, Vol. I, p. 368.

[3] Having already stated in this work, as well as in the *Commentary on Paulus Aegineta*, Book II, 27, my opinion respecting the nature of the continual fevers, I need not enlarge on the subject in this place. Whoever wishes for more information may find much to interest him in the *Commentary of Galen*. Respecting the septans and nonans, he remarks, that, although conversant with fevers from his youth, he had never met with any cases of these.

[4] Galen, in illustration, states that epilepsy is sometimes carried off by an attack of quartan fever.

tacked by it.[1] The nocturnal fever is not very fatal, but protracted; the diurnal is still more protracted, and in some cases passes into phthisis. The septan is protracted, but not fatal; the nonan more protracted, and not fatal. The true tertian comes quickly to a crisis, and is not fatal; but the quintan is the worst of all, for it proves fatal when it precedes an attack of phthisis, and when it supervenes on persons who are already consumptive.[2] There are peculiar modes, and constitutions, and paroxysms, in every one of these fevers; for example,—the continual, in some cases at the very commencement, grows, as it were, and attains its full strength, and rises to its most dangerous pitch, but it is diminished about and at the crisis; in others it begins gentle and suppressed, but gains ground and is exacerbated every day, and bursts forth with its heat about and at the crisis; While in others, again, it commences mildly, increases, and is exacerbated until it reach its acme, and then remits until at and about the crisis.[3] These varieties occur in every fever, and in every disease. From these observations one must regulate the regimen accordingly. There are many other important symptoms allied to these, part of which have been already noticed, and part will be described afterwards, from a consideration of which one may judge, and decide in each case, whether the disease be acute, and whether it will end in death or recovery; or whether it will be protracted, and will end in death or recovery; and in what cases food is to be given, and in what not; and when and to what amount, and what particular kind of food is to be administered.

12. Those diseases which have their paroxysms on even days have their crises on even days; and those which have their paroxysms on uneven days have their crises on uneven days. The first period of those which have the crisis on even days, is the 4th, 6th, 8th, 10th, 14th, 20th, 40th, 60th, 80th, 100th; and the first period of those which have their crises on uneven days, is the 1st, 3d, 5th, 7th, 9th, 11th, 17th, 20th, 21st, 27th, 31st. It should be known, that if the crisis take place on any other day than on those described, it indicated that there will be a relapse, which may prove fatal. But one ought to pay attention, and know in these seasons what crises will lead to recovery and what to death, or to changes for the better or the worse. Irregular fevers, quartans, quintans, septans, and nonans should be studied, in order to find out in what periods their crises take place.

Aristophanes

THE WASPS[1]

But He, when the monstrous form he saw,
    no bribe he took and no fear he felt,
For you he fought, and for you he fights:
    and then last year with adventurous hand
He grappled beside with the Spectral Shapes,

[1] The semitertian was always looked upon as a very formidable form of fever. See *Paulus Aegineta*, Book II, 34. Galen gives a prolix, but not a very distinct account of it.

[2] Galen, in his *Commentary*, states that he had often seen persons in consumption attacked with tertian and quotidian intermittents, but admits that he had no more experience of quintans than he had of septans and nonans. Avicenna, however, is not so sceptical as to the occurrence of these rare forms of intermittents. Indeed he says, he had often met with quintans, and that a truthworthy physician of great experience had assured him that he had met with nonans. (iii, 1, 3, 67.) Rhazes also would appear to acknowledge the occurrence of all these varieties of intermittent fever. (Contin., XXX, 10, 1, 409.)

[3] The text is much improved in Littré's edition, so that the meaning is pretty intelligible without any commentary. Galen states in explanation, that the three varieties of fever are thus marked and distinguished from one another: in the first, the fever attains its height at the commencement, and gradually diminishes until the crisis; in the second, it begins mild, and gradually reaches its height at the crisis; in the third, the fever begins mild, gradually attains its height, and then gradually subsides until the crisis.

[1] *Aristophanes* with the English translation of Benjamin Bickley Rogers, M.A., D.Litt., barrister-at-law, London, William Heinemann, New York, G. P. Putnam's Sons, 1924, Vol. I, p. 507.

the Agues and Fevers that plagued our land;[*]
That loved in the darkdome hours of night
        to throttle fathers, and grandsires choke,
That laid them down on their restless beds,
        and against your quiet and peaceable folk
Kept welding together proofs and writs
        and oath against oath, till many a man
Spring up, distracted with wild affright,
        and off in haste to the Polemarch ran.[f]

Marcus Terentius Varro

CHAPTER XII[*]

THE SITE OF THE FARM HOUSE

You must be careful to place the farm-house at the base of a well-wooded mountain —the best situation—where there are wide pastures, and see that it face the healthiest winds which blow in the district. The farmhouse which faces the equinoctial East has the best aspect, for it has shade in summer, and in winter gets sunshine. If you should be obliged to build close to a river, you must be careful not to build your farmhouse to face it, for in winter it will become exceedingly cold, and in summer unwholesome. Note also if there be any swampy ground, both for the reasons given above, and because certain minute animals, invisible to the eye, breed there, and, borne by the air, reach the inside of the body by way of the mouth and nose, and cause diseases which are difficulty to be rid of.[1] Said Fundanius: What shall I do to escape malaria, if I am left an estate of such a kind? Why, said Agrius, even I can answer that question. You must sell it for as many pence as you can get, or if you can't sell it you must quit it.

Scrofa went on: You must not allow your farmhouse to face a quarter from which an unwholesome wind commonly blows, nor must you place it in a basin surrounded by hills, but its situation should rather be lofty than low. Such a place being wind-swept, if any evil thing should be carried thither, it is easily blown away. Morover, as it gets the sun all day long, it is healthier, for any small insects which breed or are carried there are either blown away or quickly perish from drought.

Sudden rainstorms and rivers in flood are dangerous to those who have their dwellings on lowly ground or in hollows; there is danger also from sudden bands of robbers who can more easily surprise them. For both these reasons high ground is the safer.

Aulus Cornelius Celsus

CHAPTER III

Of the several kinds of fevers.[3]

THESE are the rules to be observed by such as are in health, that are only apprehensive of the cause. We next proceed to the cure of fevers, which is a kind of disease, that affects the whole body, and is the most common of all. Of these one is a quotidian, another a tertian, and a third a quartan. Some-

---

[*] He refers to the attack on the Sophists made the year before in the *Clouds*. "As agues and fevers," says the Scholiast, "harm men's bodies, so do these men the City."

[f] *i.e.* for help: Aris. Pol. *Ath.* 58.

[*] *Varro on Farming*, translated by Lloyd Storr-Best, London, G. Bell and Sons, Ltd., 1912, pp. 38-40.

[1] *Difficilis Morbos.* Columella, i, 5, 6, speaks of marshes breeding *infestis aculeis armata animalia*, i.e., mosquitoes. Schneider's comment on this passage is amusing. "Am I to believe that

Varro attributed lingering diseases to these small gnats? Never did any doctor ancient or modern make such an assertion." Varro, however, though he may appear to speak of malarial microbes, does not connect them with "small gnats" as their carrier.

[3] Celsus, A. Cornelius. *Of medicine in eight books.* Translated with notes critical and explanatory, by James Greive, London, Wilson and Durham, 1756, p. 114.

times some fevers also return after a longer period, but that seldom occurs. With regard to the former they are both diseases in *themselves,* and a cure for *others.*

But quartan fevers are more simple. They begin commonly with a shuddering; then a heat breaks out; after the paroxysm is over, the patient is well for two days. So that it returns upon the fourth day.

Of tertians again there are two kinds. One of them both beginning and ending like the quartan; with this difference only, that there is one day's intermission, and it returns upon the third. The other kind is much more fatal, which indeed returns upon the third day, but of forty-eight hours thirty-six are occupied by the fit (and sometimes either less or more) nor does it entirely cease in the remission; but is only mitigated. This kind most physicians call semitertian.

But quotidians are various, and different in their appearances. For some of them begin with a heat, others with a coldness, others with a shuddering. I call that a coldness, when the extremities of the limbs are chilled; a shuddering, when the whole body trembles. Again, some end, so as to be followed by an interval quite free from indisposition; others so, as that tho' the fever somewhat abates, yet some relicks remain, till another paroxysm come on; and others often remit little or nothing, but continue as they begun. Some again are attended with a very vehement heat, others more tolerable: some are equal every day, others unequal, and alternately milder one day and more severe another: some return at the same time the following day, others either later or sooner: some by the fit and the intermission take up a day and a night, some less, others more: some, when they go off, cause a sweat, others do not; and in some leaves the patient well, in others it only renders the body weaker: sometimes also one fit comes on each day, sometimes two or more. Whence it frequently happens, that every day there are several both paroxysms and remissions; yet so as that each of them answers to some preceding one. Sometimes too the fits are so irregular, that neither their durations nor intermissions can be observed. Nor is it true, which is alledged by some, that no fever is irregular, unless it arises from a vomica, or an inflammation, or an ulcer. For the cure would always be easier, if this were fact. For what is occasioned by the evident causes, may also proceed from the occult. Nor do those dispute about things but words, who allege, that when feverish paroxysms come on in different manners in the same distemper, these are not irregular returns of the fever, but new and different fevers successively arising. Which however would have no relation to the method of cure, tho' it were true. The intervals also are sometimes pretty long, at other times scarce perceptible.

Pliny the Elder
BOOK XXX
REMEDIES DERIVED FROM LIVING CREATURES*

CHAP. 30—REMEDIES FOR FEVERS

In the treatment of quartan fevers, clinical medicine is, so to say, pretty nearly powerless; for which reason we shall insert a considerable number of remedies recommended by professors of the magic art, and, first of all, those prescribed to be worn as amulets: the dust, for instance, in which a hawk has bathed itself, tied up in a linen cloth, with a red string, and attached to the body; the longest tooth of a black dog; or the wasp known by the name of "pseudosphex,[32] which is always to be seen flying alone, caught with the left hand and attached beneath the patient's chin. Some use for this purpose the first wasp that a person sees in the current year. Other amulets are, a viper's head, severed from the body and wrapped in a linen cloth; a viper's heart, removed from the reptile while still alive; the muzzle[33] of

* *The Natural History of Pliny.* Translated with copious notes and illustrations by the late John Bostock, M.D., F.R.S., and H. T. Riley, Esq., B.A., late scholar of Clare Hall, Cambridge. London, Henry G. Bohn, York Street, Covent Garden, 1856, Vol. v, p. 453, 354. Vol. iv, p. 260.

[32] "Bastard-wasp."
[33] "Rostellum." Holland renders it "The little prettie snout's end of a mouse."

a mouse and the tips of its ears, wrapped in red cloth, the animal being set at liberty after they are removed; the right eye plucked from a living lizard, and enclosed with the head, separated from the body, in goat's skin; the scarabaeus also that forms pellets[34] and rolls them along.

It is on account of this kind of scarabaeus that the people of a great part of Egypt worship those insects as divinities; an usage for which Apion gives a curious reason, asserting as he does, by way of justifying the rites of his nation, that the insect in its operations pictures the revolution of the sun. There is also another kind of scarabaeus, which the magicians recommend to be worn as an amulet—the one that has small horns[36] thrown backwards; it must be taken up, when used for this purpose, with the left hand. A third kind also, known by the name of "fullo,"[37] and covered with white spots, they recommend to be cut asunder and attached to either arm, the other kinds being worn upon the left arm. Other amulets recommended by them, are, the heart of a snake taken from the living animal with the left hand; or four joints of a scorpion's tail, together with the sting, attached to the body in a piece of black cloth; due care being taken that the patient does not see the scorpion, which is set at liberty after the operation, or the person who has attached the amulet, for the space of three days: after the recurrence, too, of the third paroxysm, he must bury the whole in the ground. Some enclose a caterpillar in a piece of linen with a thread passed three times around it, and tie as many knots, repeating at each knot why it is that the patient performs that operation. A slug is sometimes wrapped in a piece of skin, or the heads of four slugs, cut from the body with a reed: a millepede is rolled up in wool: the

small grubs that produce the gadfly,[38] are used before the wings of the insect are developed: or any other kind of hairy grub is employed that is found adhering to prickly shrubs. Some persons attach to the body four of these grubs, enclosed in an empty walnut shell, or else some of the snails that are found without a shell.

In other cases, again, it is the practice to enclose a spotted lizard in a little box, and to place it beneath the pillow of the patient, taking care to set it at liberty when the fever abates. It is recommended also, that the patient should swallow the heart of a sea-diver, removed from the bird without the aid of iron, it being first dried and then bruised and taken in warm water. The heart of a swallow is also recommended, with honey: and there are persons who say that, just before the paroxysms come on, the patient should take one drachm of swallow's dung in three cyathi of goats' milk or ewes' milk, or of raisin wine: others, again, are of opinion that the birds themselves should be taken, whole. The nation's of Parthia, as a remedy for quartan fevers, take the skin of the asp, in doses of one-sixth of a denarius, with an equal quantity of pepper. The philosopher Chrysippus has left a statement to the effect, that the phryganion,[39] worn as an amulet, is a remedy for quartan fevers; but what kind of animal this is he has nowhere informed us, nor have I been able to meet with any one who knows. Still, however, I felt myself bound to notice a remedy that was mentioned by an author of such high repute, in case any other person should happen to be more successful in his researches. To eat the flesh of a crow, and to use nitre in the form of a liniment, is considered highly efficacious for the treatment of chronic diseases.

In cases of tertian fever—so true it is that suffering takes delight in prolonging hope by trying every remedy—it may be worth while to make trial whether the web of the spider called "lycos"[40] is of any use, applied, with the insect itself, to the temples and forehead in a compress covered with resin and wax; or the insect itself, attached to the body in a

---

[34] Of cowdung. It was supposed that there was no female scarabaeus, and that the male insect formed these balls for the reproduction of its species. It figures very largely in the Egyptian mythology and philosophy as the emblem of the creative and generative power. It has been suggested that its Coptic name *"skalouka"* is a compound word, signifying—"The ox-insect that collects dirt into a round mass." See B. XI, c. 34.

[36] Probably the "lucanus" mentioned in B XI, c. 34; supposed to be the same as the stag-beetle.

[37] The "fuller," apparently. This name may possibly be derived, however, from the Greek φυλλὸν, a "leaf."

[38] See B. XI, c. 38.

[39] Some suppose that this was an insect that lived among dry wood, and derive the name from the Greek φρυγανὸν. Queslon is of opinion that it is the salamander.

[40] The "Wolf" spider. See c. 17 of this book.

reed, a form in which it is said to be highly beneficial for other fevers. Trial may be made also of a green lizard, enclosed alive in a vessel just large enough to receive it, and worn as an amulet; a method, it is said, by which recurrent fevers are often dispelled.

BOOK XXVIII

REMEDIES DERIVED FROM LIVING CREATURES*

Chap. 66.—Remedies for Fevers

Deer's flesh, as already[86] stated, is a febrifuge. Periodical and recurrent fevers are cured, if we are to believe what the magicians tell us, by wearing the right eye of a wolf, salted, and attached as an amulet. There is one kind of fever generally known as "amphemerine;"[87] it is to be cured, they say, by the patient taking three drops of blood from an ass's ear, and swallowing them in two semisextarii of water. For quartan fever, the magicians recommend cats' dung to be attached to the body, with the toe of a horned owl, and, that the fever may not be recurrent, not to be removed until the seventh paroxysm is past. Who,[88] pray, could have ever made such a discovery as this? And what, too, can be the meaning of this combination? Why, of all things in the world, was the toe of a horned owl made choice of?

Other adepts in this art, who are more moderate in their suggestions, recommend for quartan fever, the salted liver of a cat that has been killed while the moon was on the wane, to be taken in wine just before the paroxysms come on. The magicians recommend, too, that the toes of the patient should be rubbed with the ashes of burnt cow-dung, diluted with a dog's urine, and that a hare's heart should be attached to the hands; they prescribe, also, hare's rennet, to be taken in drink just before the paroxysms come on. New goats' milk cheese is also given with honey, the whey being carefully extracted first.

BOOK XX

REMEDIES DERIVED FROM THE GARDEN PLANTS

Chap. 55.—Wild Pennyroyal: Seventeen Remedies

For all the purposes already mentioned, wild pennyroyal[83] has exactly the same properties, but in a still higher degree. It bears a strong resemblance to wild marjoram,[84] and has a smaller leaf than the cultivated kind: by some persons it is known as "dictammos."[85] When browsed upon by sheep and goats, it makes them bleat, for which reason, some of the Greeks, changing a single letter in its name, have called it "blechon,"[86] (instead of "glechon.")

This plant is naturally so heating as to blister the parts of the body to which it is applied. For a cough which results from a chill, it is a good plan for the patient to rub himself with it before taking the bath; it is similarly employed, too, in shivering fits, just before the attacks come on, and for convulsions and gripings of the stomach. It is also remarkably good for the gout.

---

* *The Natural History of Pliny.* Translated. with copious notes and illustrations by the late John Bostock, M.D., F.R.S., and H. T. Riley, Esq., B.A., late scholar of Clare Hall, Cambridge. London, Henry G. Bohn, York Street, Covent Garden, 1856, Vol. v, 354.

[86] In B. VIII. c. 50. Because the animal itself was supposed to be free from fever.

[87] Or "quotidian," daily fever.

[88] A rather singular episode in his narrative. It looks like a gloss.

[83] It differs in no respect whatever from the cultivated kind, except that the leaves of the latter are somewhat larger.

[84] Of origanum.

[85] Whence our name "dittany."

[86] The "bleating plant"; from βληχάομαι, "to bleat." Dioscorides, B. II, c. 36, says the same of cultivated pennyroyal.

Martial

II XL*

Tis a false report that Tongilius is being consumed by a semi-tertian fever. I know the tricks of the man; he is hungry and thirsty.

LV LXXX

You declaim in a fever, Maron; if you don't know that this is frenzy, you are not sane, friend Maron. You declaim when you are ill, you declaim in a semi-tertain; if otherwise you can't perspire, there is some reason in it. "Yet it is a great thing." You are wrong; when fever burns up your vitals 'tis a great thing to hold your tongue, Maron.

*Martial: *Epigrams*, translated by Walter C. A. Ker, M.A. (New York, G. P. Putnam, 1920.

X LXXVII

Nothing more scandalous, Maximus, was ever done by Carus than his dying of fever, and it too committed an outrage. The cruel fatal fever should have been at least a quartan! That malady should have been reserved for its own doctor.

(Carus was a specialist in quartan fever)

XII XC

For his old friend, ill of a severe and burning semi-tertian fever, Maro—and aloud—made a vow that, if the sick man were not sent down to the Stygian shades, there should die a victim welcome to mighty Jone. The doctors begin to guarantee a certain recovery. Maro now makes vows not to pay his vow.

Sir Robert Tabor

The popularity of quinine in the treatment of malaria was largely due to the publicity given it by Robert Tabor or Talbor or Talbot. Robert Tabor was born probably in 1642, the son of John Tabor, Registrar to the Bishop of Ely. While still a youth Tabor was apprenticed to an apothecary at Cambridge and became interested in giving powdered cinchona bark to patients suffering from ague. He was admitted as asizar at St. Johns College, Cambridge, in 1663 but did not take his degree and presently went to Essex, where there was much malaria, to study the effect of the bark on patients. He then returned to London, set up his sign and wrote a book describing his marvelous results in treating the ague.

Tabor's powders became so famous that in spite of opposition he was appointed Physician-in-Ordinary to Charles II, with a salary of 100 pounds a year and was knighted at Whitehall. As he was not a member of the College and liable to prosecution for practicing without a license, the King gave orders that he was not to be molested. He successfully treated the King for an attack of tertian malaria and then went to France to treat the Dauphin who was suffering from the ague. The French physicians were quite naturally hostile to the intruder and asked him pointedly "what is fever." Tabor replied "I do not know; you gentlemen may explain the nature of fever; but I can cure it which you cannot." The Dauphin recovered and the King in gratitude created Tabor a Chevalier, gave him a yearly pension of one hundred pounds and bought the secret of his remedy for two thousand pounds. Further he granted to Tabor a monopoly of the remedy for ten years and forbade the French physicians its use. The remedy proved to be an infusion of cinchona bark in "good claret wine."

Tabor died in 1681, was buried in Holy Trinity Church, Cambridge and a monument was erected in the church describing him as *Febrium malleus*. Thus as

Sir Humphry Rolleston remarks, "Tabor had a short, but financially successful life." His amazing career has been described in a most interesting fashion by Sir Humphrey Rolleston and by Dr. George Dock in the *Annals of Medical History*.

QUINQUINA*

Quinquina, or *Kinakina,* is the bark of an *Indian Tree,* of the bigness of a *Cherry*-Tree, whose leaves much resemble the leaves of a young Oak, and bareth a fruit not unlike to an Acorn, the figure thereof given by *Johnstonus* may be seen at the end of the *History of Trees* written by *Mantissa*.

It is hardly as yet thirty years since this Drug become known in Europe: Since that time many Authors have wrote of it, as *Johnstonus, James Chifflet, Denis Touquet,* in his *Royal Garden of Plants; Roland Sturmius, Melipus, Conigius, Gaudentius, Brunatius, Wolfangus, Hoeferus, Willis, Rolfincius,* a Physitian of *Leyden* that hath added to *Scroderus, M. de Muva,* in his *Pharmaceutick Dictionary,* the Author of the Treatise of the *Cure of Feavers, &c.* And last of all Mr. *Lemery* in the fourth Edition of his *Course of Chymistry:* several other curious Remarks are to be found in our *Journals of Medicine* upon the same subject.

These Authors do not all agree upon the Etimology of its name, nor upon the place from whence it is brought; for some affirm that it comes from *China,* and therefore many have called it *Cortex sineasis,* and to distinguish it from that Root which is called *China* or *Kina,* they have named it *Quinquina,* or (which is that same thing) *Kinakina:* others again who are more in numbers, maintain that it is brought from *Peru,* where the Feavor or Ague is called *Quina,* whence comes the name *Quinquina;* That the Natives of that Countrey call it *Gannateride;* that because of its extraction it ought to be called in *Latin, Cortex Peruviana,* and in the vulgar Language the Bark of *Peru,* and that the name of *Jesuits Powder* by which it commonly goes, was given it, because the *Jesuits* were the first that brought it from *America,* of which *Peru* is a part. However the matter be, they begin now to call it in *Latin, Cortex febrilis;* and the *Spaniards* name it, *Palo de Culenturas,* i.e. *Feaverwood.*

*Talbor, Sir Robert, *The English Remedy or Talbor's Wonderful Secret,* London, Wallis, 1682, p. 1.

The reason why it was thought to come from *China,* was because much of it was brought from *Portugal,* but that makes nothing against the common opinion, because it is known that the *Portugueze* have Commerce with both *Indies.*

Some Authors make two kinds of *Quinquina,* one which they say is wild and of little value, and another which they think is cultivated, and therefore say that it is the better of the two; but to make a true estimate of their quality, it were fit one should be upon the place where they grow.

It is certain nevertheless that the goodness of it may be known by some marks which experience hath discovered; for the best hath always its upper rind or skin cut transversally or crossways with pretty deep streaks or lines, and long-ways with very superficial ones when it is fresh, and now the most part of the little squares or interslices of its skin, are of a sliver white colour; it is otherways of a clear reddish colour, compact, very bitter, and gives to the boxes wherein it is kept a sweet and pleasant smell.

But it is to be observed that that smell is much weaker and less aromatick than the scent of *Cassia Cariophilata,* which by cheats is Sold for *Quinquina,* mingling it with the bark of *Cherry*-Tree, which for some days before they have steept in Water wherein *Aloes* hath been dissolved; and this is a very culpable sophistication, seeing these kinds of barks have nothing of the virtue of *Quinquina.*

There is besides this, another way of cheating the Publick as to the matter of the *Jesuits Powder,* for there are some *Droguists* that infuse it entire, and having by that means extracted the first *Tincture* out of it, for their own advantage, sell it afterward at the same rate as if it had not lost his chief virtue.

Hitherto the price of *Quinquina* or *Jesuits Powder,* hath been very various and uncertain. When it was only in the hands of the *Jesuits,* it was sold at *Rome* and *Paris* for *Eight* or *Nine* Shillings *Sterling* the *Dose,* which consisted only of *Two Drachms;* but as soon as *Droguists* began to Trade in it, it began to fall in Price, so that *Three* or *Four* Years ago, the best might have been had for about *Forty* Shillings the Pound weight; but no sooner began the *English* Remedy to be in vogue, but men began every where to make Experiments with the Bark of *Peru*, which much enhansed the value of it: yet that was not all which raised it to the highest price; for Sir *Robert Talbot* observing that *Febrifuges* were prepar'd which came very near his own, and fearing least some body at length might discover it, resolved to buy up all the *Quinquina*, that he could find in *Paris*, and the other chief Towns of *France*, and of *England* also. The execution of this Design making some noise, several *Physitians*, *Chirurgeons* and *Apothecaries*, thought it concerned them, to make all hast to provide themselves, and some that they might not be wanting in Precaution, caused a considerable quantity of the Bark to be brought from *Roan* and *Bourdeaux*, so that Mr. *Andry* and Mr. *Vilain*, the two most famous *Droguists* in *Paris*, having Sold all they had at the Rate of about *Fifteen* Pound the pound-weight; and not being able to procure any more from any place, for above a Fortnight there was not a bit to be had at any *Droguist's* shop in *Paris*, nevertheless some small quantity came at length, but it was held up so dear, that it was like to have gone off at the rate of an *Hundred* Crowns the pound-weight: since that time the Merchants having imported much from *Spain* and *Portugal*, and the English Remedy having lost the Advantages of the *Mode;* the price of that Commodity hath fallen daily, in so much that at present it does not yield above *Four* or *Five* Pound the pound-weight; and I make no doubt, but that in a short time a Fleet from the *West-Indies* will make it much cheaper.

Amongst the Authors whom I have named, there are some who endeavoring to explain the properties of *Quinquina* or the *Jesuits Powder*, according to the principles of the ancient Medicine, think it enough to say that it is hot and dry in the beginning of the *Second Degree:* and some others of the number of those who have introduced bad Principles into the *New-Philosophy*, think to mend the matter by saying, That Quinquina *as an* Alkali *stops the motion of the acid which occasions the Feaver:* but that is to illustrate one obscurity by others that are far more obscure.

That we may give the World somewhat more satisfactory as to that point, we must in the first place, (with *Willis*,) take our measures from *Experience*, and allow with him, That all things which are actually bitter, have great virtue in sifting preternatural fermentations; and upon that account it was that the Root of *Gentian* was heretofore in so great reputation for curing of *Quartan Agues;* and that the Flowers of the lesser *Cantaury*, the Root of *Contrayerva* and *Serpentaria*, the leaves of *Wormwood* and *Chervil, Scammony*, and many other bitter *Drogues*, are really *Febrifuges*, though in virtue far inferior to the *Jesuits Powder.*

Having laid down this from undoubted Truth, we must now enquire into the *Natural Causes* which produce Bitterness in mixt bodies: now supposing (as it is reasonable we should) that the true Elements of Bodies are acid, liquid, fiery, etherean, and terrestrial corpuscles; it will be a very easie matter to discover those *Causes:* for seeing all bitter things penetrate the Tongue, in such a manner that they leave therin a sense of their action for a long time after, and that of all the elements none are so proper as acids to produce that effect, we must conclude that they are predominant in mixts which have that tast; but also since being mingled with many liquid corpuscles, they produce only sharp and corroding liquors, as the spirits of *Salt, Vitriol, Alum,* &c. that being joyned to fiery corpuscles, they make only *Causticks*, as *corrosive sublimat;* the spirit of *Nitre, cauteres*, &c. and that being in intimate conjunction with *Sulphurous* and *Oily* Particles, they only produce sweet mixts, as *Honey, Sugar,* &c. It follows that none but terrestrial corpuscles mingled with them in a proportionable quantity, can produce a bitter tast, and in effect the more of *Earth* there is in *Salt*, the bitterer it is, and on the contrary, the more it is refined and depurated, the less bitter it is: thus *Sea Salt* dissolved in a moist *Air*, and afterward filtrated through brown paper, has no other tast than of an acid spirit, though before that dissolution and filtration it was considerably bitter.

Now since among the Elements that I have named, the acid is heaviest, and by consequence the coldest; and that though the terrestrial be not so heavy as it, nor yet as the liquid, yet it is more ponderous than the fiery and ethereal, we may say that it is temperat; I mean, of a quality equally distant from the two extreams, and that so, being with the acid predominant in a mixt body, the mixt must certainly be cooling, or at least proper to preserve the just temperature of our body.

But because there are no bitter things made up solely of acid and terrestrial corpuscles, and that there are some wherein either the fiery, the ethereal or liquid particles are likewise in a considrabl quantity; so there are some more or less bitter, and even more or less cooling and temperate; but if we mind the dryness of *Quinquina*, and yet how unapt it is to take fire, it will not be hard to conclude, That the three Elements which I have named last, enter but in a very small quantity into the composition thereof, and that by consequence amongst all bitter mixts none can be of a more temperate quality than it.

From the Principle which I have not laid down concerning the nature of *Quinquina*, all the other properties thereof may be deduced; for seeing its predominant parts are the acids, whose property is to coagulate the more substantial liquors, such as *Blood, Milk, &c.* and the terrestrial which by absorbing the humidity and unctuosity that relaxes the solid parts, does bind and strengthen them of necessity it must be stiptick and astringent, and it is in effect in these two qualities principally, that the rarity and wonderfulness of its operation does conflict, as I have made appear in former observations.

Albert Freeman Africanus King

Albert Freeman Africanus King was born in Oxfordshire, England in 1841. His father, Dr. Edward K. King, was much interested in the colonization of Africa, an interest which led him to christen one of his sons "Africanus." A. F. A. King attended school in Bichester near Oxford and when ten years of age came with his parents to America. The King family lived first at Alexandria, Virginia, and later purchased a plantation near Warrenton, Virginia.

A. F. A. King began the study of medicine in the National Medical College of Washington where he graduated at the age of twenty. He began practice in Haymarket, Virginia, and upon the breaking out of the Civil War attended the Confederate soldiers after the battle of Bull Run. Dr. King subsequently attended the University of Pennsylvania, where he obtained the degree of M.D. in 1865. He came to Washington to practice and was present at Ford's Theatre the night Abraham Lincoln was assassinated. Dr. King was seated in the orchestra near the president's box and after the fatal shot was fired, climbed into the box, gave the wounded president first aid and helped carry him across the street to the house where he died.

Dr. King was for many years professor of obstetrics in George Washington University and in the University of Vermont. The latter institution conferred upon him the degree of LL.D. in 1904. Dr. King died in 1914 at the age of seventy-five.

Dr. King was widely known as the author of a *Manual of Obstetrics* which first appeared in 1882 and passed through eleven editions. Posterity, however, will probably remember him best for a paper read before the Philosophical Society of Washington on February 10, 1882, and published in the *Popular Science Monthly* for September 1883. In this paper he gives nineteen reasons for believing that malaria is transmitted by the mosquito. This paper attracted attention far and wide and had a profound influence upon the thought of men studying tropical diseases.

INSECTS AND DISEASE—MOSQUITOES AND MALARIA*

By Professor A. F. A. KING, M.D.

The animalculae, or insect, origin of disease is not a new idea. It was suggested by Linnaeus, by Kircher, and by Nyander, but gained little ground. It received a new impetus after the publications of Ehrenberg on the Influsoria. Later, it received attention in Bradley's work on "The Plague of Mar-

(London *Medical Times and Gazette,* January 12, 1878, p. 69; September 7, 1878, p. 275; December 28, 1878, p. 731; June 4, 1881, p. 615).

Still later, M. le Dr. Ch. Finlay has hypothetically considered the mosquito an agent of transmission of yellow fever ("El mos-

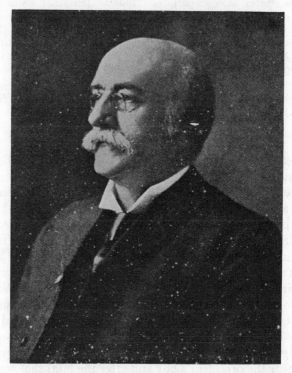

ALBERT FREEMAN AFRICANUS KING (1841-1914)

seilles," in Dr. Drake's books on "Epidemic Cholera" and on "The Topography and Diseases of the Mississippi Valley," as well as in Sir Henry Holland's "Medical Notes," and other works.

More recently the researches of Dr. Patrick Manson in China, Dr. Bancroft in Australia, Dr. J. R. Lewis in India, and Dr. Sonsino in Egypt, have tended to show that the mosquito "acts as the intermediary host of *Filiria sanfuinis hominis,*" and is thus indirectly instrumental in the production of Chyluria, elephantiasis, lymphscrotum, etc.

* Popular Science Monthly, New York, Sept., 1883.

quito hipoteticamente considerado como agente de transmission de la fiebre amarilla," Havana, 1881; and "Pathogonia de la fiebre amarilla," 1882). These papers were communicated to l'Academie royale des sciences medicales, physiques et naturalles at the dates mentioned. A review of them, by Dr. A. Corre, appears in the *Archives de med. Navale,* tome XXXIX, pp. 67-70, 1883, Paris. (See also "Lancet," 1878, I, p. 69.)

Viewed in the light of our modern "germ theory" of disease, the punctures of proboscidian insects, like those of Pasteur's needles, deserve consideration, as probable means by which bacteria and other germs may be inoculated into human bodies, so as to infect the blood and give rise to special fevers. It has long been demonstrated that "malignant pustule" is produced in man by the bite of a fly (*British Medical Journal,* January 24, 1863, p. 239). Dr. Budd, in the article just quoted, refers to the greater frequency of this disease in hot, dry summers where insect life is active and teeming; and this, he thinks, would go far to explain the greater frequency of the malignant pustule in Burgundy than in England and the north of France, as also its greater frequency in Siberia and Lapland, where insects of the mosquito tribe are the great pest of the traveler. In Lapland the popular belief was long ago universal that the disease was caused by a peculiar insect which suddenly descended from the air, and as suddenly disappeared. In the London *Times* (1860) it is reported that four hundred persons lost their lives in the south of Russia and in the province of Kiev from the sting of a "venomous fly" imported from Asia, the same fly having made its appearance there on another occasion, sixty or seventy years before. Virchow, who has made malignant pustule a special study says: "Most probably, insects with piercing proboscces effect the inoculation, such as gadflies (Bremse); but flies which make no wound may also implant the poison on the skin by their soiled wings and feet." The bites of these same flies may be generally harmless; they have no venomous power of their own, but only poison from sources of infection to man and animals.

* * *

I now propose to present a series of facts—some of the best known and most generally established facts—with regard to the so-called "malarial poison" and to show how they may be explicable by the supposition that the mosquito is the real source of disease, rather than the inhalation or cutaneous absorption of a marsh-vapor. These facts are briefly, as follows:*

1. Malaria affects, by preference, low and moist localities—in fact, swamps, fens, jungles, marshes, etc. This statement no one will dispute. Conformably with it we find the mosquito does the same. The female lays her

* Most of them are quoted from a paper read by Dr. John T. Metcalfe. U. S. Sanitary Commission, 1862; see also, Flints' *Practice,* p. 826, edition of 1867.

eggs, to the number of two hundred and fifty or three hundred, in a boat-shaped mass, on the surface of any natural or artificial receptacle for fresh water. Early in the spring the larvae are found in the bottoms of pools and ditches, feeding upon decaying matter (hence the works on entomology state that they are of great benefit in *clearing swamps of miasms* (?). These larvae are the so-called "wrigglers," or "wigglers," to be found in great numbers in any stagnant pool of water during summer. They change into pupae, and, in a few days more, the pupa-skin is cast, and floating on this latter, like a raft, the insect finally takes flight, a full-developed gnat. Many thousands perish by drowning, or are devoured by fish while extricating themselves from their pupa-cases. As the eggs develop into perfect insects in three or four weeks, many broods are hatched during the warm season, which accounts for their increasing numbers during the later summer and autumnal months. Some species deposit their eggs in soft mud or in dry sand, but all require moisture in the larval state.

2. Malaria is hardly ever developed at a lower temperature than 60° Fahr. A temperature of 60° F. is necessary for the development of the mosquito.

3. "The evolution or active agency of malaria is checked by a temperature of 32° F." The mosquito is killed or paralyzed, so that its active agency is checked, by a temperature of 32°.

4. Malaria "is most abundant and most virulent as we approach the equator and the sea-coast." The swarms of mosquitoes (as well as of sand-flies, ants, and other insect-plagues) that infest many equatorial regions are well known; and, with regard to sea-coasts, the accumulation of mosquitoes is both a fact and easily susceptible of explanation. Under the influence of gentle land-breezes the mosquito is wafted towards the ocean, but, in the absence of strong winds that would carry it out to sea, the water will form a barrier to its farther progress seaward, for it is not a marine insect. Mosquitoes, therefore, accumulate on sea-coasts—notably at some of our familiar summer resorts, Cape May, Atlantic City, etc.

5. Malaria "has an affinity for dense foliage, which has the power of accumulating it when lying in the course of winds blowing from malarious localities."

6. "Forests or even woods have the power of obstructing or preventing its transmission under these circumstances."

These last two propositions, embodying, first, the "accumulation," and second, the "obstruction," of malaria by forests and trees, may be considered together. That a wind coming from a marsh (from, in fact, a mosquito nursery), and bearing a colony of mosquitoes, should be screened or sifted of its insect burden by passing through the foliage of a forest, or a belt of trees, is certainly far more comprehensible than the conception of a malarial vapor being screened by virtue of its "affinity for foliage." And though, in the case of a single belt of trees, even the mosquital filter may *appear* imperfect, the insect, should it have been carried far, is probably anxious to settle, and may so vary its course by steering as to take the first opportunity of clinging to anything that may come in its way; and, having settled, we may readily conceive its shifting round to the leeward side of a leaf or branch, and there holding on until the wind sufficiently subsides to allow of safer flight. Thus mosquitoes, like malaria, may both accumulate in, and be obstructed by forests and trees.

The conduct, or rather the mechanical properties, of the mosquito, when carried by the wind, can hardly be better described than in the following verbatim quotation from Sir Francis Day, in his description of malaria. He says: "Malaria may be carried by the winds to places where it was not generated; it is obstructed by and hangs in the foliage of trees, or in mosquito-curtains; it subsides into low places, and may be blown over a hill, and, may be very virulent on the side opposite to that on which it was formed. In like manner it may be taken up the side of a hill, and, as a lull takes place in the atmosphere, consequent upon its weight it rolls down, and may thus envelop its base with a deadly belt of fever, for there, hanging in the leaves of the trees, it gradually sinks through them to the earth beneath, in which situations it is most dangerous to pass the night." (Sir Francis Day's work, p. 87).

7. "By atmospheric currents it (malaria) "is capable of being transported to considerable distances, probably as far as five miles." So, certainly, is the mosquito.

8. "It (malaria) may be developed in previously healthy places by turning up of the soil, as in making excavations for the foundations of houses, tracks for railroads, and beds for canals." Here two things are confounded, viz; 1. Turning up of the soil, as by plowing or digging; and, 2. Making excavations. Which of these two is the more fruitful in producing malaria is not stated, nor is the *modus operandi* of either suggested. In Hong-Kong, an island consisting of little more than bare and barren rocks of weather-beaten granite, and whose soil contains but two percent of organic matter, malarial disease was formerly unknown, and only became prevalent, as it is at present, after *excavations* had been made in digging granite for building purposes. So, again, tanks and pools of water—cess-pools, mill-ponds, reservoirs, and bilge-water on shipboard—appear to be especially productive of malaria. In Ceylon, the tanks of Candelay and Minery—the one twenty miles in circumference, the other twelve—have been considered the cause of malaria in that region (see Davy on "Disease of the Army," p. 51, etc.). It is easy to comprehend how such pools, tanks and excavations containing water may constitute mosquito nurseries, where the female may deposit her eggs and propagate, which would probably have been prevented in the absence of such water accumulations. How simply digging up the soil may contribute to the formation of malaria, or to the development of mosquitoes, *without excavations* I am not able to explain.

* * *

10. "In proportion as countries, previously malarious, are cleared up and thickly settled, periodical fevers disappear." Here, too, we may remark that in such countries the land is cultivated, and its swamps and pools drained, so that the mosquito can not so readily find a place suitable to deposit her eggs. And, as the forests and underbrush disappear before the implements of the agriculturist, colonies of mosquitoes, wafted from a distance by winds, are not "obstructed" and "accumulated" by foliage, nor can the insect so readily escape, as before, the numerous fly-catching birds that feed upon it. Even here, however, artificial pools, tanks, and excavations containing water, may constitute mosquito nurseries from which many millions may be developed in a single summer.

11. Malaria usually keeps near the surface

of the earth; it is said to "hug the ground" or "love the ground." When blown by the wind, however, or drifting up ravines, it has been known to rise several thousand feet. Dr. Russell, in his address before the New York Public Health Association, April 13, 1876, stated that, "under ordinary circumstances, a certain altitude affords immunity from malaria, although low elevations of 200 or 300 feet above a miasmatic tract are often more dangerous than the flat lands, the poison seeming to float upward and become intensified." This, he says, has long been noticeable on the heights of Bergen Hill, West Hoboken, and Weehawken, which overlook the Jersey flats. In accordance with the malarial vapor theory, these facts are completely mysterious. The mosquito, on the other hand, is known to hover near the ground (or water) from which it springs, and, being wafted by winds, can readily be understood to be "obstructed" and "accumulated" by forests on the brows of hills, etc.

12. Malaria is most dangerous when the sun is down, and it seems almost inert during the day. Of this there is no doubt, and the various hypotheses on the marsh-vapor theory, that have been alleged in explanation of it, are almost as numerous as they are unsatisfactory. With regard to the mosquito, however, it is well known that it remains, for the most part, during the day, harbored in woods, weeds, or low underbrush, and comes out after sunset and at night to indulge its blood-sucking proclivities.

13. The danger of exposure after sunset is greatly increased by the person exposed sleeping in the night air. Again have the hypotheses based on the marsh-vapor theory been altogether insusceptible of explaining this circumstance satisfactorily. With regard to mosquital inoculation, however, it is undoubtedly true that, while awake, the person exposed will move about, or brush away the insect, while he will submit to be bitten during sleep.

14. In malarial districts, the use of fire, both in-doors, and to those who sleep out, affords a comparative security against malarial disease. Explanations on the marsh-vapor theory are numerous, various and unsatisfactory. With regard to the mosquito, however, it is well known to be attracted by lamps, and fires, into which it heedlessly flies at the cost of life. In countries where these insects are extremely numerous, lamps are extinguished by the accumulation of their dead bodies. Every fire, therefore, whether in-doors or out, is a sort of mosquito hades. In some tropical countries, despite heat of climate, fires are kept up all night in every apartment as a preventive against fevers; and experience has demonstrated that they are more effective when placed between the open window (or door) and the body of the person to be protected. In this way it is easy to comprehend how every mosquito will fly directly into the light and the fire before reaching the thus protected sleeper.

15. "The air of cities in some way renders the poison innocuous, for, though a malarial disease may be raging outside, it does not penetrate far into the interior."

In conformity with this statement, we may easily conceive that mosquitoes, while invading cities during their nocturnal pilgrimages, will be so far arrested by walls and houses, as well as attracted by the lights in the windows and streets of the suburbs, as that many of them will in this way be prevented from penetrating far "into the interior." Even a single row of houses, on one side of the road, with its contiguous fences, lamps, and closely-knit hedge-rows, may so far completely obstruct the onward flight of mosquitoes coming from some neighboring swamp as to prevent their crossing the street. The curious instances in which people living on the other side escape, as on the high-road between Chatham and Feversham (see Macculloch on "Malaria," p. 121) and in Civita Vecchia (see Johnson on "Tropical Climates," p. 315) are quite as susceptible of possible explanation by the mosquito theory as by the marsh-vapor conception, for that the infected air from the marshes does not cross the street is inconceivable.

16. Malarial diseases are most prevalent toward the latter part of summer and in autumn.

It has been already explained in what manner—and the fact is a common observation—mosquitoes are more numerous also during the later summer and autumn months.

17. Malaria is arrested, not only by trees, walls, etc., but also by canvas curtains, gauze veils, and mosquito-nets.

Sir Francis Day (p. 87) tells us that travelers besides being warned against night and morning temperature, should be instructed at night to employ mosquito-curtains "through which malaria can seldom or never pass."

Dr. Macculloch (pp. 137, 138) says that, by surrounding the head with a gauze veil or conopeum, the action of malaria is prevented, and that thus it is possible even to sleep in the most pernicious parts of Italy without hazard or fever. The prophylactic efficacy of fine cloth or gauze at night is further attested by Dr. Johnson ("Tropical Climates," pp. 316, 317) as quoted on p. 318 of LaRoche's well-known work. (See also p. 416 of Dr. Johnson's work, and p. 15 of Dr. W. J. Evans on "Endemic Fevers of West Indies," 1837.) Dr. Oldham ("What is Malaria?" p. 172)

tells us that the Jeevas of the Punjaub, employed in fishing and catching wild-fowl, spend the whole night in the midst of malaria"; but they are wrapped from "head to foot" in a peculiar costume that completely envelopes them, and which they always put on at sunset, and, moreover, a smoldering fire is kept up in the boat.

It is almost needless to add that, while these nets, curtains, etc., can hardly be conceived to intercept marsh-air, they certainly can and do intercept and protect from mosquitoes.

Sir Ronald Ross

Ronald Ross, one of the greatest of modern sanitarians and of investigators in tropical medicine, was born in Almora, India, in 1857. His father was Major Ross of the Indian Army who subsequently became General Sir Campbell Ross and had a distinguished career in the British army. Ronald was the eldest of ten children and at the age of eight was sent to England to begin his education. At the age of seventeen young Ross began the study of medicine, not because of any predilection but at the express wish of his father who wished him to enter the Indian Medical Service. In 1874 he entered St. Bartholomew's Hospital in London as a student of medicine. In 1881 he passed his examinations "without distinction," received a commission as Surgeon in the Indian Medical Service, and sailed for India.

Ross early in his career in India became interested in mosquitoes. While stationed at Bangalore they nearly devoured him in his bungalow, until he discovered they were breeding in a tub outside his window and got rid of them by simply upsetting the tub. "When I told the Adjutant of this miracle," Ross says, "and pointed out that the Mess House could be rid of mosquitoes in the same way (they were breeding in the garden tubs, the tins under the dining-table and even the flower vases) much to my surprise he was very scornful and refused to allow men to deal with them for, he said, it would be upsetting the order of nature, and as mosquitoes were created for some purpose it was our duty to bear with them! I argued in vain that the same thesis would apply to bugs and fleas, and that according to him it was our duty to go about in a verminous condition! I did not know then that this type of fool is very common indeed."

In India, Ross was often much depressed by the incompetence, inefficiency, mental lethargy and often hostility he encountered among his ranking superiors in the army, and was several times on the point of resigning from the army. Despite all handicaps he persisted in his studies on the mosquito and, in 1897, discovered malarial parasites in the stomach of an anopheles mosquito and thereby proved the rôle of the mosquito in the transmission of malaria. In 1899 Ross retired from the Indian Medical Service and was appointed lecturer on tropical medicine at the University of Liverpool. In 1902 Ross received the Nobel Prize in medicine and in 1911 the order of knighthood was conferred upon him. In 1926 the Ross Institute, an institution for medical research named in his honor, was dedicated. His death in 1932 was mourned by the entire world.

No modern scientist has shown the remarkable versatility of Ross, indeed such examples are rare in history. Besides his remarkable scientific researches, Ross was a first rate mathematician who contributed important articles to mathematical journals, a talented musician who composed chamber music,

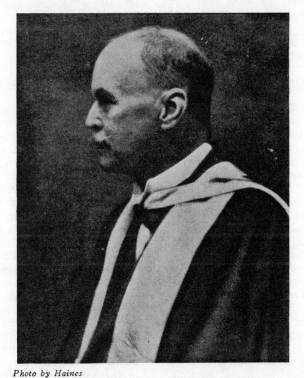

Photo by Haines

SIR RONALD ROSS (1857-1932)
From *Ronald Ross* by R. L. Mégroz (Allen & Unwin, London.)

a novelist who wrote stories which belong to real literature, a playwright whose dramas have received great praise from dramatic critics and a poet whose poem *In Exile* moved John Masefield, the Poet Laureate of England to write, "it is by far the most splendid poem of modern times. It is magnificent." It should also be mentioned that Ross invented a system of shorthand and devised a method of phonetic spelling in which some of his poems were written.

The discovery of Ross marks the beginning of scientific attempts to stamp out malaria. As Manson wrote, "Ross had hammered out the key; others might take the trouble to open the door."

The life story of this remarkable man has been told in a most interesting and fascinating way by R. L. Mégroz in his *Ronald Ross: Discoverer and Creator.*

PIGMENTED CELLS IN MOSQUITOES*

By Surgeon-Major Ronald Ross, I.M.S.

In the *British Medical Journal* of December 18th, 1897, you did me the honor to publish an article by me on this subject, together with notes by Surgeon-Major Smyth, Dr. Manson, Mr. Bland Sutton, and Dr. Thin, on the original preparations. My sincere thanks are due to these gentlemen for the interest they have taken in the matter, and for the courtesy of their remarks, and I hope that the existence of the cells as attested by them may now be considered as established. As to the nature of the cells, however, doubt still remains, and I should therefore like to give two more instances in which they have been found, both having an important bearing on this point.

It will be remembered that the pigmented cells were not found in a large number of brindled and grey mosquitoes, unfed or fed on healthy or crescent-bearing blood, but were seen for the first time in two large "dapple-winged" insects (Cases I and II) of a rare species, fed on crescent blood. Since then (September 1897) I have observed them in two more insects. Case III: Some scores of small dapple-winged mosquitoes, unfed or fed on healthy blood, had been examined without finding the cells. At last two of this species were persuaded to feed on a patient with crescents. One of them was killed the next day; no pigmented cells could be found. The second was killed forty-eight hours after feeding; numerous pigmented cells were present. They were all small, much smaller than epithelial cells, ovoid, about 7µ in the major axis, and each contained about 20 granules of typical pigment which were often arranged circumferentially, just as in the malaria parasite. No more insects of this species fed on malarial blood have since been examined. Case IV.—A hundred or more grey or "barred-back" mosquitoes (wings, legs, belly plain: back of abdomen transversely striated) unfed, or fed on healthy or crescent blood have been dissected without finding the pigment cells. At last one was observed feeding on a patient whose blood that morning had been seen to contain

numerous mild tertian parasites. I judged for many reasons that it had been feeding occasionally on the same man for several days. It was killed three days afterwards, when it must have been quite a week old (after hatching from pupa). Its stomach contained a large number of pigmented cells of all sizes, from 8 µ to 25 µ. They were very defined and distinct, especially the larger ones, and contained each from 10 to 20 granules of typical pigment. Some of the largest cells appeared to have a uniform structure without vacuoles, but with a central nucleus (?)

I thought I observed a few similar bodies without any pigment. Besides these cells, the stomach cavity contained numbers of swarm spores, never before seen in any Secunderabad mosquito, but found in the mosquitoes of the malarious Sigur ghat. In May a number of these swarm spores had been given to a person who volunteered to drink them, and he had been attacked with fever five days afterwards.[1] I could trace no connection between the pigmented cells and the clusters of swarm spores; that is, I could find no pigment in the latter; though it would have been difficult to do so even if it had been present, owing to the numbers of struggling flagellulae. Since then I have examined no more grey mosquitoes fed on tertian blood; and indeed, have not been in a position to continue researches on malaria; but I have dissected thirty horse flies (tabanus), parasitic on tame pigeons, whose blood contained halteridium (Labbe). Though halteridium was found in the blood in the insects' stomach cavity, the stomach walls never contained pigmented cells; yet the histology of tabanus is closely like that of culex. It is interesting to note that in the four instances in which the cells have been found, their size is in proportion to the length of time between the feeding and death of the insects—namely, 7 µ after two days, 17 µ after four days, 19 µ after five days,. and 25 µ after about a week.

[1] No parasites found. Vide *Proceedings* of South Indian Branch, British Medical Association, 1897.

* *Brit. M. J.*, 1898, I, 550.

I must correct an error due to the unfortunate use of formalin as a preservative in the two specimens sent to England. Pigment appears to have been found, not only in the pigmented cells, but also in the ordinary, stomach cells, and elsewhere; and Dr. Thin draws the natural inference from this that the former are an altered form of the latter, induced by the absorption of malarial pigment from the stomach cavity. The effect is due to formalin, which not only blackens the green and yellow granules and globules always found in the tissues of culex, but converts traces of haemoglobin in the stomach cavity into a multitude of minute acicular crystals very like pigment, and even has the same effect on the pigment of the pigmented cells. I know this to be the case from specimens in my possession, one of which now appears to contain pigment everywhere. I can say with confidence, and after special and repeated search for it, that when the specimens were fresh pigment was to be found nowhere else in them except in the pigmented cells; nor, except in the pigmented cells, have I ever found pigment in the stomach walls of mosquitoes fed on malarial blood.

So long as the cells had been found only in two individuals (the only two properly examined) of a rare species of mosquito, it was quite possible to suppose them some kind of physiological cell, either pigment-producing or pigment-absorbing; the new facts show them to be too exceptional for this. If they be normal pigment-producing cells, they should be found in most individuals of a species in one of which they have been observed. But Cases III and IV show that they may occur in a single individual out of many scores of the same species examined, while, except in these four instances, I have never observed them in allied diptera (pulex, tabanus, musca) nor even in allied species of culex. If, as Dr. Thin believes, they be ordinary epithelial stomach cells which have taken up the pigment of dead malarial parasites from the stomach cavity, they should, if found in one individual of a species fed on malarial blood, be found also in others of the same species similarly fed; but Case IV, in which they were observed in an insect fed on tertian blood, but not at all in many insects of the same species fed on crescent blood, is in direct opposition to this postulate—unless we can venture to assume that the stomach cells of this species are capable of taking up tertian pigment to the exclusion of crescent pigment. But there are now many reasons against Dr. Thin's theory. Thus, in Case III, the cells were much too small to be epithelial cells. Again, the pigmented cells are not like phagocytes in one important particular—they all contain roughly the same amount of pigment and an arrangement of it, which, as Dr. Manson says, forcibly recalls the arrangement of pigment in the malaria parasite. Phagocytes contain varying amounts of pigment, from one granule to several large clumps of it, according to the quantity they have been able to seize (compare phagocytes with parasites in malarial blood for example). Still further, if the pigment in the cells is due merely to phagocytosis, how comes it that they do not contain other granules from the stomach cavity besides, such as the yellow detritus of ingested blood corpuscles? Lastly, it remains to be proved that the stomach cells of culex are capable of taking up solid particles from the cavity. I have never seen any evidence of such, either in culex or in other families of diptera. Yet the stomach of the larva and imago contains multitudes of coloured vegetable and haemoglobinous particles which could easily be detected if contained in the interior of the cells of the stomach wall. I have never observed such a phenomenon. Why, then, should these cells absorb matter so exceptional in the ingesta as malarial pigment, and reject the numerous other granules which are much more commonly presented to them? The cells of the stomach are not scavengers like the phagocytes of the blood; what object can they possibly have in taking up the pigment of dead parasites, which otherwise will be naturally evacuated by the bowel? Or, are we to suppose that this dead pigment has the power of forcibly entering the cells? In short, I doubt whether this hypothesis will bear careful scrutiny.

Hence, the facts already collected, especially the new ones, make it difficult, if not impossible, to believe that the pigmented cells can be any kind of normal physiological cells, whether pigment-producing or pigment-absorbing cells. It would seem then that they must be some kind of pathological cells. What kind—whether new growths, or parasites peculiar to the mosquito, or a developmental form of the parasites of malaria in the mosquito—I cannot say. If not the last of these, it will always remain a curious coincidence that they should contain pigment so closely like malaria pigment, and that they should as yet have been found only in insects fed on malarial blood.

ON SOME PECULIAR PIGMENTED CELLS FOUND IN TWO MOSQUITOES FED ON MALARIAL BLOOD*

By Surgeon-Major RONALD ROSS, I.M.S.
(With Note by Surgeon-Major SMYTH, M.D., I.S.M.

For the last two years I have been endeavoring to cultivate the parasite of malaria in the mosquito. The method adopted has been to feed mosquitoes, bred in bottles from the larva, on patients having crescents in the blood, and then to examine their tissues for parasites similar to the haemamoeba in man. The study is a difficult one, as there is no *a priori* indication of what the derived parasite will be like precisely, nor in what particular species of insect the experiment will be successful, while the investigation requires a thorough knowledge of the minute anatomy of the mosquito. Hitherto the species employed have been mostly brindled and grey varieties of the insect; but though I have been able to find no fewer than six new parasites of the mosquito, namely a nematode, a fungus, a gregarine, a sarco-sporidium (?), a coccidium (?), and certain swarm spores in the stomach, besides one or two doubtfully parasitic forms, I have not yet succeeded in tracing any parasite to the ingestion of malarial blood, nor in observing special protozoa in the evacuations due to such ingestion. Lately, however, on abandoning the brindled and grey mosquitoes and commencing similar work on a new brown species, of which I have as yet obtained very few individuals, I succeeded in finding in two of them certain remarkable and suspicious cells containing pigment identical in appearance to that of the parasite of malaria. As these cells appear to me to be very worthy of attention, while the peculiar species of mosquito seems most unfortunately to be so rare in this place that it may be a long time before I can procure any more for further study, I think it would be advisable to place on record a brief description both of the cells and of the mosquitoes.

The latter are a large brown species, biting well in the daytime, and incidentally found to be capable of harbouring the filaria sanguinis hominis. The back of the thorax and abdomen is a light fawn colour; the lower surface of

* *Brit. M. J.*, 1897, II, 1786.

the same, and the terminal segment of the body a dark chocolate brown. The wings are light brown to white, and have four dark spots on the anterior nervure. The haustellum and tarsi are brindled dark and light brown. The eggs—at least, when not fully developed—are shaped curiously like ancient boats with raised stern and prow, and have lines radiating from the concave border like banks of oars—so far as I have seen, a unique shape for mosquitoes' eggs. The species appears to belong to a family distinct from the ordinary brindled and grey insects; but there is an allied species here, only more slender, whiter, and much less voracious. My observations on the characteristics of these mosquitoes were not very careful, as when I first obtained them I did not anticipate any difficulty in procuring more.

On August 16th eight of them were fed on a patient whose blood contained fair to few crescents (and also filaria). Unfortunately four were killed at once for the study of flagellate bodies (flagellulae cysts). Of the remainder two were examined on the 18th and 20th respectively, without anything being noted. The seventh insect was also killed on the 20th, four days after having been fed. On turning to the stomach with an oil-immersion lens I was struck at once by the appearance of some cells which seemed to be slightly more substantial than the cells of the mosquito's stomach usually are. There were a dozen of them lying among (or within?) the cells of the upper half of the organ, and though somewhat more solid than these, still very delicate and colourless. They were round, or oval, 12 μ to 16 μ in diameter when not compressed (that is, considerably larger than the largest haemamoeba in man); the outside sharp but very fine; the contents full of stationary vacuoles; and no sign of apparent nucleus, contractile vesicle or amoeboid or intracellular movement. So far it would have been impossible for any but a person very familiar with the insect's anatomy to have distinguished them from the neighbouring cells; but what now arrested attention was the fact that each of these bodies contained a few granules of black pigment absolutely identical in appearance with the well-known and characteristic pigment of the parasite of malaria (large quartans and crescent-derived spheres).

The granules were more scanty in comparison to the size of the cell than in the haemamoeba, and numbered from 10 to 20 in each. They were not dispersed throughout the cells, but were collected in groups, or arranged in lines transversely or peripherally, or in a small circle round the centre (just as in some forms of the haemamoeba). They were black or dark brown, and not refractive on change of focus. In some cases they showed rapid oscillation within a small range, but did not change their position. Owing to their blackness, so different from the bluish, yellow, and green granules and *debris* found in and about the neighbouring cells, they arrested the eye at once; and it must clearly be understood that I have not confounded them with normal objects. In short (except perhaps that rods were shorter or absent) these granules of pigment were indistinguishable from those of the haemamoeba.

The eighth and last mosquito was killed next day, five days after having been fed. The stomach contained precisely the same cells, 21 in all, again toward the oesophageal end of the organ. In this case, however, they were distinctly larger and more substantial than in the seventh mosquito, and had a decidedly thicker outline. The size (along the major axis) appeared now sometimes to reach nearly 20 μ, on a rough computation made without a micrometer. There thus appeared to be a marked increase in bulk and definition between these cells of the fourth and fifth days, suggesting that they had grown in the interval.

Both specimens were irrigated with 40 per cent. formalin, and sealed. The result of the formalin was, as anticipated, that the bodies became slightly more visible than before, as compared with the stomach cells.

In spite of all attempts, I have not yet succeeded in obtaining any more of the species of mosquito referred to. Thinking, however, that I may have overlooked these delicate cells in former dissections, I have again examined a large number of brindled and grey mosquitoes, fed on malarial blood. Their stomachs certainly contained no such cells. Next I caught by hand a number of the more slender and white, but allied, species already referred to (I have failed in finding their grubs also), and examined them. Some had not been fed at all, and others had fed themselves on (presumably) healthy blood, two, three, or four days previously. The results were again negative. I may add that I have not yet succeeded in getting this species fed on malarial blood.

To sum up: The cells appear to be very exceptional: they have as yet been found only in a single species of mosquito fed on malarial blood: they seem to grow between the fourth and fifth day: and they contain the characteristic pigment of the parasite of malaria. It would, of course, be absurd to attempt final conclusions as yet; but I think we may venture to draw some cautious inferences on these observations. First, as to the nature of the cells. Judging from the facts that the elementary cells of allied species of mosquitoes are always alike, or very similar, and that I have never observed such bodies in previous or subsequent dissections of mosquitoes (I suppose I must have examined quite a thousand more or less carefully by this time), we may reasonably conjecture that these are no normal physiological cells—in other words, that they are parasites; and this view is fortified by the comparative substantiality of the bodies, by the appearance of growth between the fourth and fifth days, and, most notably, by their possession of pigment, a substance in my experience certainly quite foreign to the physiological cells of the mosquito. Secondly, as to the connection of these presumable parasites with the parasite of malaria: they have been found in two consecutive insects fed on malarial blood (owing to their delicacy, and to my attention not having yet been attracted by them, I may have overlooked them in the fifth and sixth mosquitoes), a fact which may encourage us to believe that they may exist in a large percentage of similar insects similarly fed; and as they have not been found in an allied species fed on presumably healthy blood, we may hazard a conjecture that their presence in the original species was due to the ingestion of malarial blood. These considerations, taken together with the remarkable fact that the cells contain pigment just like that of the haemamoeba (a characteristic product which is, I believe, unknown in any other protozoa except some allied haematozoa) seem to open the question of their being indeed the form of the haemamoeba we are in search of—namely, the alternative form in the mosquito of the parasite of malaria in man.

On the other hand, the parasitic nature of the cells cannot finally be accepted until certain facts as to structure, sporulation, and so on, have been demonstrated. Even if this be done, it remains to be seen whether the bodies are not parasites common in the particular species of mosquito referred to, and quite independent of the ingestion of malarial blood and of the haemamoeba in man. I must, however, confess to feeling personally that the presence of pigment, so distinctive of the haemamoeba, renders this last supposition rather unlikely.

In conclusion I may note that the pigment in the cells may be derived from the hemo-globin in the insect's stomach, in the walls of which the cells are situated. With reference to their being found as yet only in one species of mosquito, it may be remembered that Manson originally conjectured that each species of haemamoeba might require a special species of mosquito for development extraneous to man, just as filaria embryos do.

The two specimens containing the cells described above will be forwarded to Dr. Manson. Former specimens of microscopic objects sent to England by me have perished *en route,* and lest these should experience a similar fate, I have thought it well to have an independent note on the subject on record. With this object I append a description of the cells furnished by Surgeon-Major Smyth, who has very kindly examined the specimens. I should add that his measurements, made with a micrometer, are more exact than mine.

YELLOW FEVER
Mathew Carey

Mathew Carey, the son of a Dublin baker, was born in 1760. In 1783, after suffering imprisonment because of his editorship of the *Volunteers Journal,* he emigrated to America and settled in Philadelphia where he founded the *Pennsylvania Herald.* He wrote several articles or tracts on various political topics and in 1820, founded a medical journal with Dr. Nathaniel Chapman as editor. This journal which was published by Carey, was first called the *Philadelphia Journal of the Medical and Physical Sciences,* which was renamed in 1824 the *American Journal of Medical Sciences.* Carey, although not a physician, wrote one of the best accounts of the epidemic of yellow fever which prevailed in Philadelphia in the year 1793. Mathew Carey died in Philadelphia in 1839.

*   *   *

The malignant fever, which has committed such ravages in Philadelphia, made its appearance here, about the end of July. Dr. Hodge's child, probably the first victim, was taken ill on the 26th or 27th of July, and died on the 6th or 7th of August. A Mr. Moore,* in Mr. Denny's lodging house, in Water street, was seized on Friday, the 2nd of August, and died on Sunday, the fourth. Mrs. Parkinson, who lodged in the same house, caught the disorder, on the 3d of August, and died on the 7th.

On the origin of the disorder, there prevails a very great diversity of opinion. Dr. Hutchinson maintained that it was not imported, and stated, in a letter which he wrote on the subject to Captain Falconer, the health officer of the port of Philadelphia, that "the general opinion was, that the disorder originated from some damaged coffee, or other putrified vegetable and animal matters." To

* This man had been walking along the wharves, where the coffee lay, and at which the *Sans Culottes* was moored, in the morning; and on his return home, was so extremely ill, as to be obliged to be to bed, from which he never rose again.

Mathew Carey, *A Short Account of the Malignant Fever, lately prevalent in Philadelphia,* Philadelphia, Printed by the Author, 1793, ɪɪ, Ed., pp. 16-19, 21-23, 30-37.

this opinion, though he did not give it absolutely as his own, he seemed strongly to incline; and mentioned, that at a wharf, a little above Arch-street, there was not only a quantity of damaged coffee*, extremely offensive, but also some putrid animal and vegetable substances. The doctor rested his opinion, that the disorder was not imported, on two circumstances, which prove to be mistaken, viz., that no foreigners or sailors were infected on the 27th of August, the time of writing, and that it had not been found in lodging houses. This opinion was so far from being just, that the second place in which it is known to have made its appearance, was a lodging house, and some of the earliest patients were French lads.

Dr. Rush is of the same opinion with Dr. Hutchinson, and says he has in his possession sufficient documents to prove that the disorder is not an imported one, but of native growth. As he has not yet communicated his proofs to the public, it is impossible to decide on them.

That it is an imported disorder, is the opinion of almost all the inhabitants of Philadelphia. However, there is much diversity of sentiment, as to the time and manner of its introduction. I shall state some of the various reports current, and let the reader judge for himself.

Some assert, that it was brought by *Il Constante*, capt. Fiscovisch, which arrived here from Ragusa, after having touched at Martinico, about the beginning of May. This is very unlikely, as the lower part of the city, where she lay, was free until the disorder spread there from the upper part.

Another opinion is, that it was introduced by the *Mary*, captain Rush, which arrived here on the 7th of August, with some of the French emigrants from the cape. But the existence of the disorder previous to her arrival, sets aside this opinion at once.

Others again say that a vessel from Tobago, which arrived here in July, lost nearly all her hands with a malignant fever. In the river, she shipped fresh hands, many of whom died. From her they believe the disorder spread. With respect to this report, I cannot aver any thing.

Another opinion is, that the privateer *Sans*

---

* The stench of the coffee was so excessively offensive, that the people in the neighborhood could hardly bear to remain in the back part of their houses.

Culottes Marseillois, with her prize, the *Flora*, which arrived here the 22nd of July, introduced the fever. The privateer was in a foul, dirty condition—her hold very small—and perhaps as ill calculated for the accommodation of the great number of people that were on board, as any vessel that ever crossed the ocean. All her filth was emptied at a wharf between Arch and Race street. A dead body, covered with canvass, lay on board the *Flora*, for some time, and was seen by mr. Lemaigre and other gentlemen*.

* * *

The first official notice taken of the disorder, was on the 22d of August, on which day, the mayor of Philadelphia, Matthew Clarkson, esq. wrote to the city commissioners, and after acquainting them with the state of the city, gave them the most peremptory orders, to have the streets properly cleansed and purified by the scavengers, and all the filth immediately hauled away. These orders were repeated on the 27th, and similar ones given to the clerks of the market. The 29th the governor of the state, in his address to the legislature, acquainted them, that a contagious disorder existed in the city; and that he had taken every proper measure to ascertain the origin, nature and extent of it. He likewise assured them that the health officer and physician of the port, would take every precaution to allay and remove the public inquietude.

The 26th of the same month, the college of physicians had a meeting, at which they took into consideration the nature of the disorder, and the means of prevention and of cure. They published an address to the citizens, signed by the president and secretary, recommending to avoid all unnecessary intercourse with the infected; to place marks on the doors or windows where they were; to pay great attention to cleanliness and airing the rooms of the sick; to provide a large and airy hospital in the neighbourhood of the city for their reception; to put a stop to the tolling of the bells; to bury those

---

* Mr. Vanuxem has published a lengthy statement to prove that the disorder was not brought here by either of these vessels. Dr. Currie and Dr. Cathrall, who have taken great pains to elucidate the subject, assert there were sundry sick people on board, in opposition to mr. Vanuxem's declaration. To their respective publications I beg leave to refer the reader.

who died of the disorder in carriages and as privately as possible; to keep the streets and wharves clean; to avoid all fatigue of body and mind, and standing or sitting in the sun, or in the open air; to accommodate the dress to the weather, and to exceed rather in warm than in cool clothing; and to avoid intemperance, but to use fermented liquors, such as wine, beer, and cider, with moderation. They likewise declared their opinion, that fires in the streets were very dangerous, if not ineffectual means of stopping the progress of the fever, and that they placed more dependence on the burning of gunpowder. The benefits of vinegar and camphor, they added, were confined chiefly to infected rooms; and they could not be too often used on handkerchiefs, or in smelling bottles, by persons who attended the sick.

In consequence of this address, the bells were immediately stopped from tolling. This was a very expedient measure; as they had before been kept pretty constantly going the whole day, so as to terrify those in health, and drive the sick, as far as the influence of imagination could produce that effect, to their graves. An idea had gone abroad, that the burning of fires in the streets, would have a tendency to purify the air, and arrest the progress of the disorder. The people had, therefore, almost every night large fires lighted at the corners of the streets. The 29th, the mayor published a proclamation, forbidding this practice. As a substitute, many had recourse to the firing of guns, which they imagined was a certain preventative of the disorder. This was carried so far, and attended with such danger, that it was forbidden by the mayor's order, of the 4th of September.

* * *

While affairs were in this deplorable state, and people at the lowest ebb of despair, we cannot be astonished at the frightful scenes that were acted, which seemed to indicate a total dissolution of the bonds of society in the nearest and dearest connexions. Who, without horror, can reflect on a husband deserting his wife, united to him perhaps for twenty years, in the last agony—a wife unfeelingly abandoning her husband on his death bed—parents forsaking their only children—children flying from their parents, and resigning them to chance, often without an enquiry after their health or safety—masters hurrying off their faithful servants to Bush-

hill, even on suspicion of the fever, and that at a time, when, like Tartarus, it was open to every visitant, but never returned any—servants abandoning tender and humane masters, who only wanted a little care to restore them to health and usefulness—who, I say, can even now think of these things without horror? Yet such were daily exhibited in every quarter of our city.

These desertions produced scenes of distress and misery, of which few parallels are to be met with, and which nothing could palliate, but the extraordinary public panic, and the great law of self preservation, the dominion of which extends over the whole animated world. Many men of affluent fortunes, who have given employment and sustenance to hundreds every day in the year, have been abandoned to the care of a negro, after their wives, children, friends, clerks, and servants, had fled away, and left them to their fate. In many cases, no money could procure proper attendance. With the poor, the case was, as might be expected, infinitely worse than with the rich. Many of these have perished, without a human being to hand them a drink of water, to administer medicines, or to perform any charitable office for them. Various instances have occurred, of dead bodies found lying in the streets, of persons who had no house or habitation, and could procure no shelter.

A woman, whose husband had just died of the fever, was seized with the pains of labour, and had nobody to assist her, as the women in the neighbourhood were afraid to go into the house. She lay for a considerable time in a degree of anguish that will not bear description. At length, she struggled to reach the window, and cried out for assistance. Two men, passing by, went up stairs; but they came at too late a stage. She was striving with death—and actually in a few minutes expired in their arms.

A woman, whose husband and two children lay dead in the room with her, was in the same situation, without a midwife, or any other person to aid her. Her cries at the window brought up one of the carters employed by the committee for the relief of the sick. With his assistance, she was delivered of a child, which died in a few minutes, as did the mother, who was utterly exhausted by her labour, by the disorder, and by the dreadful spectacle before her. And thus lay in one room, no less than five dead bodies, an entire family, carried off in an hour or two. Many instances have occurred, of respectable women, who, in their lying-in, have been obliged to depend on servant women for assistance—and some have had none but their husbands. Some of the midwives were dead—and others had left the city.

A servant girl, belonging to a family in this city, in which the fever had prevailed, was apprehensive of danger, and resolved to remove to a relation's house, in the country. She was, however, taken sick on the road, and returned to town, where she could find no person to receive her. One of the guardians of the poor provided a cart, and took her to the alms house, into which she was refused admittance. She was brought back, and the guardian offered five dollars to procure her a single night's lodging, but in vain. And in fine, after every effort made to provide her shelter, she absolutely expired in the cart.

To relate all the frightful cases of this nature that occurred, would fill a volume. Let these few suffice. But I must observe, that most of them happened in the first stage of the public panic. Afterwards, when the citizens recovered a little from their fright, they became rare.

Great as was the calamity of Philadelphia,

it was magnified in the most extraordinary manner. The hundred tongues of rumour were never more successfully employed, than on this melancholy occasion. The terror of the inhabitants of all the neighbouring states was excited by letters from Philadelphia, distributed by every mail, many of which told tales of woe, whereof hardly a single circumstance was true, but which were every where received with implicit faith. The distresses of the city, and the fatality of the disorder, were exaggerated as it were to see how far credulity could be carried. The plague of London was, according to rumour, hardly more fatal than our yellow fever. Our citizens died so fast, that there was hardly enough of people to bury them. Ten, or fifteen, *or more* were said to be cast into one hole together, like so many dead beasts.* One man, who could find his feeling easy enough, to be facetious on the subject, acquainted his correspondent, that the only business carrying on, was *grave digging,* or rather *pit digging*†

And at a time when the deaths did not exceed from forty to fifty daily, many men had the modesty to write, and others, throughout the continent, the credulity to believe, that we buried from one hundred to one hundred and fifty.*

* The following extract appeared in a Norfolk paper about the middle of September:

Extract of a letter from Philadelphia, to a gentleman in Norfolk, Sept. 9.

"Half the inhabitants of this city have already fled "to different parts, on account of the pestilential disorder "that prevails here. The few citizens who remained in "this place, die in abundance, so *fast that they drag them* "*away, like dead beasts, and put ten, or fifteen, or more in a hole* "*together. All the stores are shut up.* I am afraid this city "will be ruined: for nobody will come near it hereafter. "I am this day removing my family from this fatal "place."

†*From a New York paper of October 2,*
Extract of a letter from a gentleman in Philadelphia, dated Sept. 23.

"The papers must have amply informed you of the "melancholy situation of this city for five or six weeks "past. Grave-digging has been the only business carrying "on; and indeed I may say of late, pit-digging, where "people are interred indiscriminately in three tiers of "coffins. From the most accurate observations I can make "upon matters, I think I speak within bounds, when "I say, eighteen hundred persons have perished (I do not "say all of the yellow fever) since its first appearance."

From the Maryland Journal, of Sept. 27th.
Extract of a letter from Philadelphia, dated Sept. 20th.

"The disorder seems to be much the same in this "place, as when I last wrote you; about 1500 have fal- "len victims to it. Last Sunday, Monday, and Tuesday, "there were not less than 350 died with this fever disor-

Thousands were swept off in three or four weeks.* And the nature and danger of the disorder, were as much misrepresented, as the number of the dead. It was said, in defiance of every day's experience, to be as inevitable by all exposed to the contagion, as the stroke of fate.

AN ACCOUNT
of the
BILIOUS REMITTING YELLOW FEVER
as it
APPEARED IN PHILADELPHIA,
IN THE YEAR. 1793
By Benjamin Rush, M.D.*

* * *

The weather, for the first two or three weeks in August, was temperate and pleasant. The cholera morbus and remitting fevers were now common. The latter were attended with some inflammatory action in the pulse, and a determination to the breast. Several dysenteries appeared at this time, both in the city and in its neighbourhood. During the latter part of July, and the beginning of this month a number of the distressed inhabitants of St. Domingo, who had escaped the desolation of fire and sword, arrived in the city. Soon after their arrival, the influenza made its appearance, and spread rapidly among our citizens. The scarlatina still kept up a feeble existence among children. The above diseases were universal, but they were not attended with much mortality. They prevailed in different parts of the city, and each appeared occasionally to be the ruling epidemic. The weather continued to be warm and dry. There was a heavy rain on the twenty-fifth of the month, which was remembered by the citizens of Philadelphia, as the last that fell for many weeks afterwards.

There was something in the heat and drought of the summer months which was uncommon, in their influence upon the human body. Labourers every where gave out (to use the country phrase) in harvest, and

---

"der!!! As I informed you before, this is the most dis-
"tressed place I ever beheld. Whole families go in the dis-
"order, in the course of twelve hours. For your own
"sakes, use all possible means to keep it out of Balti-
"more."

Extract of a letter from Philadelphia, of the same date:

"The malignant fever which prevails here, is still in-
"creasing. Report says, that above one hundred have
"been buried per day for some time past. It is now
"thought to be more infectious than ever. I think you
"ought to be very careful with respect to admitting
"persons from Philadelphia into your town."

* From a Chestertown paper, of Sept. 10.

Extract of a letter from a respectable young mechanic, in Philadelphia, to his friend in this town, dated the 5th inst.

"It is now a very mortal time in this city. The yellow
"fever hath killed *some thousands* of the inhabitants.
"Eight thousand mechanics, besides other people, have
"left the town. Every master in the city, of our branch
"of business, is gone." The *"some thousands"* that were
killed at that time did not amount to three hundred.
The *authentic* information in this letter, was circulated
in every state in the union, by the news papers.

* Rush, Benjamin, *Medical Inquiries and Observations,* Philadelphia, Benj. and Thos. Kite, 1818, Vol. III, pp. 40-44, 80-81, 84-85.

frequently too when the mercury in Fahrenheit's thermometer was under 84°. It was ascribed by the country people to the calmness of the weather, which left the sweat produced by heat and labour to dry slowly upon the body.

The crops of grain and grass were impaired by the drought. The summer fruits were as plentiful as usual, particularly the melons, which were of an excellent quality. The influence of the weather upon the autumnal fruits, and upon vegetation in general shall be mentioned hereafter.

I now enter upon a detail of some solitary cases of the epidemic, which soon afterwards spread distress through our city, and terror throughout the United States.

On the 5th of August, I was requested by Dr. Hodge to visit his child. I found it ill with a fever of a bilious kind, which terminated (with a yellow skin) in death on the 7th of the same month.

On the 6th of August, I was called to Mrs. Bradford, the wife of Mr. Thomas Bradford. She had all the symptoms of a bilious remittent, but they were so acute as to require two bleedings, and several successive doses of physic. The last purge she took was a dose of calomel, which operated plentifully. For several days after her recovery, her eyes and face were of a yellow colour.

On the same day, I was called to the son of Mrs. M'Nair, who had been seized violently with all the usual symptoms of a bilious fever. I purged him plentifully with salts and cream of tartar, and took ten or twelve ounces of blood from his arm. His symptoms appeared to yield to these remedies; but on the 10th of the month an haemorrhage from the nose came on, and on the morning of the 12th he died.

On the 7th of this month I was called to visit Richard Palmer, a son of Mrs. Palmer, in Chestnut-street. He had been indisposed for several days with a sick stomach, and vomiting after eating. He now complained of a fever and head-ach. I gave him the usual remedies for the bilious fever, and he recovered in a few days. On the 15th day of the same month I was sent for to visit his brother William, who was seized with all the symptoms of the same disease. On the 5th day his head-ach became extremely acute, and his pulse fell to sixty strokes in a minute. I suspected congestion to have taken

place in the brain, and ordered him to lose eight ounces of blood. His pulse became more frequently, and less tense after bleeding, and he recovered a day or two afterwards.

On the 14th day of this month I was sent for to visit Mrs. Leaming, the wife of Mr Thomas Leaming. I suspected at first that she had the influenza, but in a day or two her fever put on bilious symptoms. She was affected with an uncommon disposition to fait. Her pulse was languid, but *tense.* I took a few ounces of blood from her, and purged her with salts and calomel. I afterwards gave her a small dose of laudanum which disagreed with her. In my note book I find I have recorded that "she was worse for it." I was led to make this remark by its being so very uncommon for a person, who had been properly bled and purged, to take laudanum in a common bilious fever without being benefited by it. She recovered, however, slowly, and was yellow for many days afterwards.

On the morning of the 18th of this month I was requested to visit Peter Aston, in Vine-street, in consultation with Dr. Say. I found him on the third day of a most acute bilious fever. His eyes were inflamed, and his face flushed with a deep red colour. His pulse seemed to forbid evacuations. We prescribed the strongest cordials, but to no purpose. We found him, at 6 o'clock in the evening, sitting upon the side of his bed, perfectly sensible, but without a pulse, with cold clammy hands, and his face of a yellowish colour. He died a few hours after we left him.

None of the cases which I have mentioned excited the least apprehension of the existence of a malignant or yellow fever in our city; for I had frequently seen sporadic cases in which the common bilious fever of Philadelphia had put on symptoms of great malignity, and terminated fatally in a few days, and now and then with a yellow colour on the skin, before or immediately after death.

On the 19th of this month I was requested to visit the wife of Mr. Peter LeMaigre, in Water-street, between Arch and Race-streets, in consultation with Dr. Foulke and Dr. Hodge. I found her in the last stage of a highly bilious fever. She vomited constantly, and complained of great heat and burning in her stomach. The most powerful cordials and tonics were prescribed, but to no purpose.

She died on the evening of the next day.

Upon coming out of Mrs. LeMaigre's room I remarked to Dr. Foulke and Dr. Hodge, that I had seen an unusual number of bilious fevers, accompanied with symptoms of uncommon malignity, and that I suspected all was not right in our city. Dr. Hodge immediately replied, that a fever of a most malignant kind had carried off four or five persons within sight of Mr. LeMaigre's door, and that one of them had died in twelve hours after the attack of the disease. This information satisfied me that my apprehensions were well founded. The origin of this fever was discovered to me at the same time, from the account which Dr. Foulke gave me of a quantity of damaged coffee which had been thrown upon Mr. Ball's wharf, and in the adjoining dock, on the 24th of July, nearly in a line with Mr. LeMaigre's house, and which had putrified there to the great annoyance of the whole neighbourhood.

After this consultation I was soon able to trace all the cases of fever which I have mentioned to this course. Dr. Hodge lived a few doors above Mr. LeMaigre's which his child had been exposed to the exhalation from the coffee for several days. Mrs. Bradford had spent an afternoon in a house directly opposite to the wharf and dock on which the putrid coffee had emitted its noxious effluvia, a few days before the sickness, and had been much incommoded by it. Her sister, Mrs. Leaming, had visited her during her illness at her house, which was about two hundred yards from the infected wharf. Young Mr. M'Nair and Mrs. Palmer's two sons had spent whole days in a counting house near where the coffee was exposed, and each of them had complained of having been made sick by its offensive smell, and Mr. Aston had frequently been in Water-street near the source of the exhalation.

This discovery of the malignity, extent, and origin of a fever which I knew to be attended with great danger and mortality, gave me great pain. I did not hesitate to name it the *bilious remitting yellow fever*. I had once seen it epidemic in Philadelphia, in the year 1762. Its symptoms were among the first impressions which diseases made upon my mind. I had recorded some of these symptoms as well as its mortality. I shall here introduce a short account of it, from a note book which I kept during my apprenticeship.

"In the year 1762, in the months of August, September, October, November and December, the bilious yellow fever prevailed in Philadelphia, after a *very hot summer*, and spread like a plague, carrying off daily, for some time, upwards of twenty persons.

"The patients were generally seized with rigours, which were succeeded with a violent fever, and pains in the head and back. The pulse was full, and sometimes irregular. The eyes were inflamed, and had a yellowish cast, and a vomiting almost always attended.

"The 3d, 5th, and 7th days were mostly critical, and the disease generally terminated on one of them, in life or death.

"An eruption on the 3d or 7th day over the body proved salutary.

"An excessive heat and burning about the region of the liver, with cold extremities, portended death to be at hand."

* * *

From the accounts of the yellow fever which had been published by many writers, I was led to believe that the negroes in our city would escape it. In consequence of this belief, I published the following extract in the *American Daily Advertiser*, from Dr. Lining's *History of the Yellow Fever*, as it had four times appeared in Charleston, in South Carolina.

"There is something very singular (says the doctor) in the constitution of the negroes, which renders them not liable to this fever; for though many of them were as much exposed as the nurses to the infection, yet I never knew of one instance of this fever among them, though they are equally subject with the white people to the bilious fever."*

A day or two after this publication the following letter from the mayor of the city, to Mr. Claypoole, the printer of the *Mail*, appeared in his paper.

"Sir,

"It is with peculiar satisfaction that I communicate to the public, through your paper, that the African Society, touched with the distresses which arise from the present dangerous disorder, have voluntarily undertaken to furnish nurses to attend the afflicted; and that, by applying to Absalom Jones and

* *Essays and Observations, Physical and Literary*, Vol. XI, p. 409.

William Gray, both members of that society, they may be supplied.

MATTH. CLARKSON
Mayor.

September 6th 1793.

It was not long after these worthy Africans undertook the execution of their humane offer of services to the sick before I was convinced I had been mistaken. They took the disease in common with the white people, and many of them died with it. I think I observed the greatest number of them to sicken after the mornings and evenings became cool. A large number of them were my patients. The disease was lighter in them than in white people. I met with no case of haemorrhage in a black patient.

The tobacconists and persons who used tobacco did not escape the disease. I observed snuff-takers to be more devoted to their boxes than usual, during the prevalence of the fever.

* * *

The disease. which was first confined to Water-street, soon spread through the whole city. After the 15th of September, the atmosphere of every street in the city was charged with miasmata; and there were few citizens in apparent good health, who did not exhibit one or more of the following marks of their presence in their bodies.

1. A yellowness in the eyes, and sallow colour upon their skin.
2. A preternatural quickness in the pulse.
I found but two exceptions to this remark, out of a great number of persons whose pulses I examined. In one of them, it discovered several preternatural intermissions in the course of a minute. This quickness of pulse occurred in the negroes, as well as in the white people. I met with it in a woman who had had the yellow fever in 1762. In two women, and in one man above 70 the pulse beat upwards of 90 strokes in a minute. This preternatural state of the pulse during the prevalence of a pestilential fever, in persons in health, is taken notice of by Riverius.*

3. Frequent and copious discharges by the skin of yellow sweats. In some persons, these sweats sometimes had an offensive smell, resembling that of the washings of a gun.
4. A scanty discharge of high coloured or turbid urine.
5. A deficiency of appetite, or a greater degree of it than was natural.
6. Costiveness.
7. Wakefulness.
8. Head-ach.
9. A preternatural dilatation of the pupils. This was universal. I was much struck in observing the pupil in one of the eyes of a young man who called upon me for advice, to be of an oblong figure. Whether it was natural, or the effect of the miasmata acting on his brain, I could not determine.

* "Pulsus sanorum pulsibus similes admodum periculosi." *De Febre Peatilenti*, p. 114.

Josiah C. Knott

Dr. Josiah C. Knott deserves to be remembered for his work on yellow fever, and also because as an obstetrician, he presided at the birth of William C. Gorgas, whose name became one of the best known in the field of yellow fever research. Some writers have described him as having a clear idea that yellow fever was transmitted by the mosquito, but Dr. Robert Wilson has advanced good reasons for believing that Knott had no essential knowledge of the role of the intermediate host.

Josiah Knott was born in Columbia, South Carolina, on March 31, 1804, the son of Abraham Knott, a native of Connecticut, who in early life settled in South Carolina. Josiah, after graduating from South Carolina College in 1824, studied medicine in the University of Pennsylvania, taking the degree of M.D. in 1827 and remaining two years longer as demonstrator of anatomy for Dr. Physick. In 1830 he returned to Columbia and began the practice of medicine. In 1835 he went to Paris for further study, and on his return to America settled in Mobile, Alabama, where he rapidly rose to the head of his profession and enjoyed a large and lucrative practice. In 1840 he made observations upon the mosquito as conveyor of yellow fever and published his conclusions in the following extract.

At the close of the Civil War he came first to Baltimore, and then he moved to New York, where he practiced for several years, returning, however, to Mobile in 1872. Dr. Knott died on March 31, 1873.

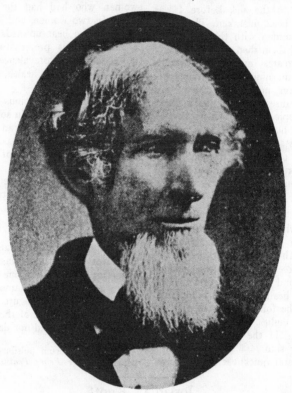

JOSIAH C. KNOTT, (1804-1873)
From *American Journal of Obstetrics* (1913, LXVII, 958)

Dr. Knott had eight children, four of whom died during an epidemic of yellow fever in 1853, while two sons died during service in the Confederate Army.

YELLOW FEVER CONTRASTED WITH BILOUS FEVER—REASONS FOR BELIEVING IT A DISEASE SUI GENERIS—ITS MODE OF PROPAGATION—REMOTE CAUSE—PROBABLE. INSECT OR ANIMALCULAR ORIGIN, &c. By JOSIAH C. KNOTT, M.D., Mobile, Alabama*

In the April number, 1845, of the *American Journal* I published an essay on the Pathology of Yellow Fever as presented to our notice in Mobile. I now purpose to give the results of my observations on the peculiar habits, or what may be called the Natural

The New Orleans Medical and Surgical Journal, 1848, IV, 563, 565, 568, 588, 592.

History of this disease, and my reasons for supposing its specific cause to exist in some form of Insect Life. Malaria, which, according to the received doctrine of the day, is a gaseous or molecular emanation from the earth's surface, is, in my opinion, wholly inadequate to the explanation of the mode of propagation of this disease, and I am therefore induced to offer a different solution which is strongly supported by the phenomena attending it. The whole doctrine of Malaria is but an hypothesis, and if we can substitute another for it which is better sustained by reason and analogies, and which conflicts with no known law of nature, it is the part of sound philosophy to give it a preference, until a less objectionable one can be found.

There is no novelty in the doctrine of Insect or Animalcular origin of diseases. Many of the older writers, amongst whom are conspicuous Linnaeus, Kircher and Nyander, have promulgated such an opinion, and it has been vaguely presented from time to time to the notice of the profession, but it is only since the publication of Ehrenberg's great work on Infusoria (1838) that its bearings can be fully appreciated. The medical periodicals of late years have made occasional allusions to the subject. Dr. Wood, of Philadelphia, Dr. Watson, of London, and others make honorable mention of it, but the most elaborate and ingenious article I have met with is that in Sir Henry Holland's *Medical Notes: On the Hypothesis of Insect Life as a Cause of Disease.*

* * *

The first Epidemic I witnessed was that of 1837, which was announced by a single case on the 10th of September. Four more cases occurred about the 20th, and it is remarkable that all these cases occurred at points so remote from the shipping and so distant from each other as to preclude the idea of recent importation, or propagation by contagion. They seemed to arise, each from an independent focus. The next cases did not appear until about the 10th of October, or some twenty days after the last mentioned cases, when it commenced spreading rapidly in all directions as an Epidemic, and carried off about 350 persons before it was arrested by a "killing frost." There was nothing in the character of the weather to account for the slow progress during the first thirty days, and it assumed the Epidemic character a few days after a very heavy southern gale which caused the water of the river to overflow the low parts of the town on its margin.

The next Epidemic occurred in 1839, and commenced during the first days of August, where it should have been the least expected, viz: on the corner of Government and Hamilton streets, half a mile from the shipping, in a clean, well ventilated and fashionable part of the town. For a short time the disease spread slowly around this focus, but at length it burst forth in every direction with extraordinary violence, ravaging not only the town, but the environs for several miles. This was one of those great Epidemics, in which the disease, shaking off complications, assumes its true and undisguised character, and usurping the field, swallows up every thing else in the shape of Fever. Number of deaths, 480. Almost all the seaports on the Gulf were visited by Yellow Fever this season in severe form. There was nothing peculiar in the weather, but on the contrary it had been pleasant, temperate and showery. There was no imaginable cause why the dormant germ of Yellow Fever should have been aroused to such extraordinary an activity at so many distant points at the same time.

In 1842 we again see the disease, commencing the 29th of August, in Spanish Alley, a very filthy place near the docks, where it would naturally be expected. From this point it spread with surprising deliberation in a north westerly direction—travelling slowly from house to house, and taking more than a month to reach and extend along Dauphin street, which runs the whole length of the town, dividing it into two equal parts. Its course and progress could be traced step by step, and its ravages were confined to one half of the town, leaving the other almost untouched. Had frost kept off a few weeks longer, there is every reason to believe it would have continued its course and marched over the other half of the town. Another Epidemic appeared in 1843, commencing about the 19th of August in the opposite or northern extreme of the town, and pursuing a course the reverse of the preceding year, viz: south east—taking about the same length of time to extend itself over the northern, that it had over the southern half in 1842—leaving the southern part almost untouched. Number of deaths 240, and checked by a severe frost.

* * *

The Insect theory is perhaps as applicable to Periodic as Yellow Fever. We can well understand how Insects wafted by the winds (as happens with mosquitoes, flying ants, many of the Aphides, etc.,) should haul up on the first tree. house or other object in their course, offering a resting place; but no one can imagine how a gas or emanation, entangled or not with aqueous vapor, while sweeping along on the wings of the wind, could be caught in this way; and we, on the contrary, often see fogs and clouds swept by winds *through the forest.* Another insuperable difficulty, too, is found in the fact that the dews are deposited as heavily on the one side as on the other of the protecting woods. I have very strongly impressed on my memory an instance of this kind: at my father's summer residence in South Carolina, our house stood upon a hill which gradually declined for half a mile till it terminated in the lowlands of the plantation; a row of trees, which were so scattered as but imperfectly to obstruct the view of the fields below, stood about midway between the latter and the residence; though the fact was inexplicable, this imperfect barrier did protect us, and our family lived there for fourteen summers, with uninterrupted health. The trees presented scarcely any impediment to the force of the winds, and I *never saw heavier dews than those on the rich grass plot around the house.* After my father's death, the old residence fell into the hands of my brother-in-law, and the protecting row of trees having been cut down, it has become so subject to marsh fevers, that he has been compelled to abandon it.

If these emanations are attracted by and attached to trees, how do they get loose again and come down to attack persons in *lower stories?*

They should remain on the trees until again evaporated by the morning's sun—these miasms must have some power per se of migrating, and clustering in trees, else these facts could not exist. It should be borne in mind, too, that the very writers who thus run their Malaria up trees, are those who tell us that its specific gravity is so great that it lies on the ground!

* * *

Those gentlemen who contend for the absolute non-transmissibility of Yellow Fever would do well to weight these and all the facts of similar import before they rudely condemn others of equal honesty and ability, holding opposite opinions. The argument is utterly inconclusive, though a thousand instances be proven that vessels or steamboats

with Yellow Fever on board have gone to distant ports, or ascended the Alabama and Mississippi Rivers without spreading the disease. Half a dozen well authenticated facts to the contrary are amply sufficient to overthrow it. Yellow Fever, like many other diseases, cannot be propagated in certain localities where the local circumstances are uncongenial to it. You cannot carry it to the interior towns on the Alabama River because some local condition is wanting; still it would seem that the germ of the disease lurks about steamboats, as in those seasons when Yellow Fever prevails in Mobile, it appears almost invariably in the old boats lying up and repairing on the Bay or Rivers within ten or fifteen miles of the town. Small Pox is known to be one of the most contagious of all diseases, and yet it has not extended in our city for the last twelve years, though vessels are bringing in cases every winter, and occasional sporadic cases are occurring which cannot be accounted for. How often too do we see solitary cases of Scarlet Fever occurring in families without contaminating other children, and we have already mentioned the fact that this disease cannot be propagated in the Antilles.

Can any one of the anti-contagionists explain why these contagious diseases are not communicable at one time, and so deadly at another? or why the Asiatic Cholera should suddenly assume an Epidemic form and encircle the globe?

In conclusion (on this point) I would remark, that admitting my suggestions to be true, they do not afford any ground for the vexatious and ruinous quarantine laws which have been enacted against Yellow Fever. A vessel *with Yellow Fever on board* should not be allowed to lie near a town, but here the restrictions should cease. If Yellow Fever is transportable by vessels at all, the instances are so rare, as not to justify very rigid quarantine regulations. Commerce is one of the *great necessities* of society, and law-makers should take into consideration the injuries as well as the benefits of their acts.

As, according to the theory we are discussing, the Natural History of Yellow Fever is closely allied to the Natural History of Insects, it is proper that I should say a few words more on the latter. The Infusoria, or Microscopic animalcules particularly demand a passing notice, as few of our readers have access to original sources on this curious subject. It has, I think, been pretty clearly shown that the propagation of Yellow Fever cannot be explained by the Malarial theory, and it must remain with the reader to determine whether the chain of anologies offered, render the Insect theory more probable.

Carlos Finlay

Carlos Finlay, who first proved that yellow fever was transmitted by the bite of a mosquito, was born in Camagüey, Cuba, in 1833. Although typically Cuban in sentiment and feeling, there was not a drop of Spanish blood in his veins, his father being a native of Scotland and his mother a French woman.

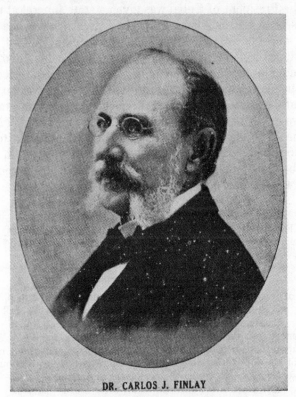

DR. CARLOS J. FINLAY

CARLOS J. FINLAY (1833-1915)
Courtesy of Surgeon General's Library

Finlay's early education was obtained in Havre and Rouen, and his medical education in the Jefferson Medical College of Philadelphia where he graduated in 1855. While in Philadelphia, he was greatly influenced by Dr. John K. Mitchell, one of the early champions of the microbic origin of disease, and also formed a lasting friendship with Weir Mitchell, the son of John K. Mitchell.

After his return to Cuba, Finlay became a general practitioner in Havana. After many years of study Finlay became convinced that yellow fever was transmitted by the bite of a mosquito then known as the *Culex fasciata,* but now called *Stegomyia calopus*. This theory Finlay advocated at a meeting of the International Sanitary Conference held at Washington in 1881. In the article which follows Finlay elaborates this theory and supports it with a series of experimental inoculations in which he describes the production of yellow fever by the bite of infected mosquitoes. He assisted the work of the yellow fever commission of the United States Army in Cuba in many ways and supplied them with the first mosquitoes used in their experiments.

Finlay was elected an honorary member of the Philadelphia College of Physicians, in 1908 was decorated with the Legion of Honor by the French government, and in 1911 the Paris Academy of Medicine elected him a corresponding member. Carlos Finlay died in 1915 at the age of eighty-two and, by decree of the President of Cuba, was given a state funeral at public expense.

Finlay was possessed of a keen mentality, great persistence and a remarkable geniality and charm of manner. He was convinced that the stegomyia mosquito produced yellow fever and "would discuss his favorite topic with any chance acquaintance, and at length. At the slightest encouragement he would bring out his records and his mosquitoes—for he was so wedded to the hypothesis that he always kept a small menagarie of the stegomyia in his office, and always had a large supply of dry eggs on hand." (Marie Gorgas) Finlay was one of the first friends Gorgas made when the latter was ordered to Havana. Gorgas described him as "a most lovable man in character and personality," but in spite of his arguments in favor of the mosquito theory, Gorgas adds "I remained unconvinced."

YELLOW FEVER:

ITS TRANSMISSION BY MEANS OF THE CULEX MOSQUITO*

By CHARLES FINLAY, M.D.

Member of the Academy of Medical, Natural, and Physical Sciences of Havana, and of the Sociedad de Estudios Clinicos

In the month of May, of last year, when the yellow fever epidemic was commencing at Vera Cruz, Dr. Carmona, of Mexico, inoculated six prisoners with the dried residue of yellow fever urine. In two of the six, the local symptoms of the inoculation were immediately followed by those of fatal yellow fever, and, a few days later, both died *on the same day* (Carmona, *Leçons sur l'étiologie et la prophylaxie de la fièvre jaune*, p. 265). This unfortunate result agrees with the views that I have entertained since 1881, viz., that whereas the disease is not spontaneously transmissible by infection through the air nor by contact, it can be communicated by inoculation. In searching for a natural agent capable of fulfilling this condition, I was led to fix upon the Culex mosquito as the most likely one. Before submitting, however, the

experimental results which, so far, appear to confirm my theory, it will be necessary to describe the habits and peculiarities of this insect.

Most books on natural history inform us that only the *female* mosquito stings human beings and animals for the purpose of sucking their blood, the *males* feeding only on sweet juices or nutrient liquids. The fecundated females, in cold climates, hibernate during winter, in a state of apparent death, in dark corners, in cellars, etc., to revive with the return of warm weather, when they will lay eggs and propagate their species. I was unable, however, to ascertain from previous writers whether gnats, in general, suck blood more than once, how long they live after their first bite, and many other particulars essential for my investigation. I was, therefore, obliged to undertake a systematic study of the species generally found in Havana.

*Am. J. M. Sc., 1886. xcii. 395.

to which alone the following remarks must be understood to apply, leaving future inquiries to determine whether the same may be true of others that are known to exist in the interior of the island and in foreign countries.

Two species of mosquitoes are commonly observed in Havana. One, the Culex cubensis (La Sagra), *zancudo,* or long-legged mosquito, is from five to six mm. in length, of a yellowish or fawn color, with long, thin legs, and no noticeable spots upon its body or legs. This species is nocturnal, coming out exclusively at night and retiring before daybreak; they are often found in the morning, in a state of torpor, gorged with blood, inside of mosquito nets. I have never succeeded in getting these *zancudos* to sting a second time after they had once become filled; but as they can be kept alive, by feeding with sugar, over a period of forty days, it is unlikely that they should not bite more than once when in a state of freedom. The female of this species lays its eggs pretty much in the same manner as the European gnat, described by Reaumur, forming a boatlike aggregate of eggs, where over one hundred are closely packed together, standing upright, side by side, the tiny raft being left floating upon the water.

The other species is the Culex mosquito (Robineau Desvoidy), lately described, I am told, as "Culex fasciatus." There are several varieties, principally distinguishable by their dimensions and shades of color; some being small and nearly black, while others are stronger, almost as large as the nocturnal species, and of a brown or steel color; the general characteristics being the same in the two or three varieties that I have observed.

The body of the C. mosquito is dark colored, the ventral surface coated with a thick skin and marked with gray or white rings; on each side of the abdomen is a double row of white dots, between which stretches a transparent membrane through which the blood can be seen when the insect is full. The most striking feature consists in five white rings on its hind legs, corresponding to the tarsal and metatarsal articulations. Others less apparent are on the fore and middle legs; white spots are visible on the sides of the thorax and front of the head, while the corselet presents a combination of white lines in the figure of a two-stringed lyre. The wings, when closed, do not cover the end of the body.

The *males* are known by their bushy antennae and long palps lying close to the proboscis, and curved near the point; whereas the *females* have delicate antennae and short palps drawn up close to the root of the proboscis.

The female of this species lays its eggs in in a different manner from the *zancudo,* not in a boat-like aggregate but singly, having previously deposited a viscous substance through which they lie scattered in irregular groups, either upon the liquid surface or upon the sides of the vessel, close to the water's edge.

* * *

My first inoculation by means of mosquitoes were performed under the following circumstances: A group of twenty unacclimated soldiers, who were quartered on the heights of the Cabanas, on the other side of the bay, were picked out for my observations, and were only allowed to cross the bay in batches of four or five on the days they were sent to my office, where I tried their blood for hematimetric purposes. Five of the group were inoculated by me at different dates between the 29th of June and the end of August, 1881. The first three were followed, at the end of five or fourteen days' incubation, by an attack of fever of several days' duration, diagnosticated by the attending physicians at the military hospital as "regular yellow fever" in the first case, and "abortive yellow fever" in the two others. The fourth inoculated soldier suffered only from continued headache, and, on the fifteenth day after the inoculation, came to my office with slight fever (temperature 100.7°F., pulse 100), but was not laid up. The fifth did not return to my office. I was informed that he had felt poorly a few days after the inoculation, but was not laid up. I have been able to trace the history of these five cases until the beginning of last year. None of them had been reported, up to that date, as subsequently attacked with yellow fever. Of the remaining fifteen soldiers of the group, upon whom the inoculation *was not performed,* none were attacked with yellow fever during the period of my observation, June 28 to September, 1881.

Case I.—On the 30th of June, 1881, one of the soldiers of the above group (F.B.), twenty-two years of age, three months in Havana, having had previously some attacks of intermittent fever, was inoculated by means of a mosquito which had bitten, two days before (June 28th), a patient in the fourth day of yellow fever and who died thirty-six hours later.

July 14. The inoculated soldier was taken sick and went to the Military Hospital, where I was only able to see him on the 16th (third day of his illness). I found him with a slight fever, slight yellowish tinge of conjunctivae, pains of invasion almost disappeared; the urine gave distinct evidence of albumen with heat and with nitric acid, not having presented any in the morning. The clinical report of the attending physician, together with my own observation, gave the following result.

1st day, July 14. Invasion preceded by a few days of discomfort.

2nd day. Morning: Temp. 101.8°F.; pulse 92; resp. 28; face and eyes injected; intense headache; slight epigastralgia; pains in the spine; tongue coated; no vomiting or other remarkable symptoms. Treatment: Ipecacuanha four grammes in four doses; cream of tartar lemonade; absolute diet. Evening: Temp. 100.4°F.; pulse 88; resp. 26; headache less intense. Night: Intense thirst; urine scanty.

3d day. Morning: Temp. 99.6°F.; pulse 72; resp. 34; skin pale; slight yellowness of conjunctivae; congested gums; epigastralgia; no nausea; no albumen in the urine. Evening: Albumen detected in the urine. Night: Same condition; insomnia. Treatment: One gramme of sulphate of quinine in ten doses; cream of tartar lemonade; mustard plasters to the extremities.

4th day. Morning: Temp. 98.9°F.; pulse 72; resp. 34; no headache; some appetite; gums gave a little blood on compression; urine treated by heat and nitric acid, gives a more abundant precipitate of albumen. Evening: Normal temperature and pulse.

5th day. Temp. 98.9°F.; pulse 78; respiration normal; slight jaundice; urine contains albumen.

6th day. Convalescent; urine not examined; broth allowed.

7th day. Continues well.

12th day. Cured.

The distinct evidence of albumen in the urine, notwithstanding the mildness of the fever and general symptoms, leaves no doubt regarding the diagnosis, which was unhesitatingly reported as "regular yellow fever."

* * *

Case IV.—A Spaniard (J.B.) employed as a servingman to my friend Dr. Delgado, twenty-five years of age, nine months in Havana, having never been ill since his arrival, was inoculated on the 22nd of June, 1883, by two mosquitoes, which had both bitten, two days before, a fatal case of yellow fever in the sixth day of his illness.

July 9th (seventeen days after the double inoculation), J.B. was taken ill with symptoms of yellow fever. The following morning an emetic was administered, followed by a dose of castor oil; no other medicine being given in the course of the illness, and absolute diet maintained until the sixth day, only water being allowed.

2nd day. Morning: Temp. 101.3°F.; pulse 80; face flushed; pains in the loins. Evening: Temp. 101.8°F.

3d day. Morning: Temp. 101.4°F.; pulse 70; no albumen in the urine. Evening: Temp. 101.8°F.; face less flushed; straw color of the conjunctivae; intense thirst, anorexia.

4th day. Morning: Temp. 99.5°F.; pulse 68; no albumen. Evening: Temp. 101.3°F. pulse 70.

5th day. Morning: Temp. 100.4°F.; pulse 68; no albumen; conjunctivae yellowish; gums do not bleed on pressure.

6th day. Morning: Temp. 101.4°F.; pulse 72. Midday: Temp. 103.1°F.; pulse 52; appetite returning; rapid convalescence.

The general type of the fever, with remission on the fourth day, and defervescence on the seventh, bears a strong resemblance to some forms of natural yellow fever that I have observed. The patient has since remained protected.

The following case is remarkable from the circumstance that most of the conditions were fulfilled that can well be secured in the vicinity of Havana, in order to avoid the chances of independent infection from other sources besides the inoculation. The place selected for the experiment was the same country residence or "Quinta" rented by the Jesuit Fathers since 1872, near the "Quemados de Marianao," to which Dr. Stanford E. Chaille has alluded in his remarkable report as President of the Yellow Fever Commission which visited Havana in 1879 (*An-*

nual Report of the National Board of Health, Washington, 1880, p. 276). In the course of eleven years (1872-1883), the only case of yellow fever developed among the many liable subjects who had spent their summer vacations at this place, during their stay, occurred in 1880 in a young priest who had been going backward and forward to Havanna during the previous fortnight, and who was attacked with the disease during his last visit to the city, where he remained and died. It is more than likely that he had contracted the infection in town, and not at the "Quinta."

Toward the end of June, 1883, several priests and a servant, all unacclimated and having arrived from Spain the previous autumn, happened to be staying at this country-place, and I availed myself of their willingness to submit to my inoculation experiments.

Case V.—P. U., one of the unacclimated priests, a young man of spare habit, having gone to the "Quinta" toward the end of June, 1883, did not again visit the city nor the neighboring town of Marianao until the following September. On the 15th of July a first unsuccessful attempt was made with a mosquito contaminated from a case in the seventh day of yellow fever; a full month was then allowed to elapse before a second attempt on the same person.

August 18, 1883, P. U. was inoculated with a mosquito which had bitten on the 13th and 16th two separate cases of yellow fever, each in the sixth day of their illness. On the 26th of August, eight days after inoculation, P. U. was taken ill about 8 A.M. with headache, pains in the loins, and fever (temp. 100.7°F.). I saw him at 4 P.M. and from that time followed the case, keeping accurate notes of the symptoms.

1st day. 4 P.M., felt very poorly, complained of headache and pains in the loins and calves; face flushed and covered with perspiration; eyes injected; was sent to bed, and after a while presented: Temp. 102.2°F.; pulse 100, dicrotic. Treatment: Castor oil with lime juice. Night: Temp. 102.3°F.; pulse 104; vomited five or six times through the night and had several passages; thirst; eyes injected.

2d day. Morning: Temp. 101.3°F.; pulse 88; resp. 20; eyes injected without yellow tinge; urine natural in appearance. Evening: Temp. 101.4°F.; pulse 90; resp. 30: somewhat drowsy; urine less copious than usual, acid reaction, not affected by boiling. Treat-

ment: Hyposulphite of soda; boiled orange-ade for common drink.

3d day. Morning: Temp. 101.8°F., pulse 80; resp. 27; urine contains no albumen; restless night, insomnia; tongue white; thirst; face less flushed. Evening: Temp. 101.8°F.; pulse 84; resp. 26; subicteric tinge of conjunctivae. Same treatment.

4th day. Morning: Temp. 100.4°F.; pulse 60; resp. 27; subicteric tinge more marked; the pains have ceased; urine scanty, contains biliverdine, but no albumen; the gums bled on pressure. Treatment: Chlorade of potash. Evening: Temp. 101.4°F.; pulse 80; restlessness; urine scanty, no albumen; thirst; anorexia.

5th day. Morning. Temp. 101.1°F.; pulse 76; resp. 29. Evening: Temp. 101.8°F.; pulse 83. Night: During a thunderstorm became very nervous; ten hours without passing urine; urine presents traces of albumen. Treatment: Morphia syrup.

6th day. Morning: Temp. 101.8°F.; pulse 72; urine not altered by ebullition; quiet night; expectorated some bloody sputa. Broth allowed. Evening: Temp. 100.7°F.; pulse 75.

7th day. Morning. Temp. 99.6°F.; pulse 62; resp. 20; subicteric tint of conjunctivae; some bloody sputa; gums bleed on pressure; urine scanty, no albumen. Evening: Temp. 98.9°F. pulse 57.

8th day. Morning: Temp. 98.7°F.; pulse 58; subicteric tint of conjunctivae.

* * *

From the evidence adduced in the preceding pages, I conclude that while yellow fever is incapable of propagation by its own unaided efforts, it may be artificially communicated by inoculation, and only becomes epidemic when such inoculations can be verified by some external natural agent, such as the mosquito.

The history and etiology of yellow fever exclude from our consideration, as possible agents of transmission, other blood-sucking insects, such as fleas, etc., the habits and geographical distribution of which in no wise agree with the course of that disease: whereas, a careful study of the habits and natural history of the mosquito shows a remarkable agreement with the circumstances that favor or impede the transmission of yellow fever. So far as my information goes, this disease appears incapable of propagation wherever tropical mosquitoes do not or are not likely to exist, ceasing to be epidemic at the same limits of temperature and altitude which are incompatible with the functional activity of those insects; while, on the other hand, it spreads readily wherever they abound. From these considerations, taken in connection with my successful attempts in producing experimental yellow fever by means of the mosquito's sting, it is to be inferred that these insects are the habitual agents of its transmission. It cannot be denied, however, that other such agents may and probably do occasionally occur, but not being endowed with the same facilities for rapid and extensive operation, their influence becomes insignificant as compared with the action of the Cuban culex.

Walter Reed

Walter Reed was born in Gloucester County, Virginia, in 1851. He was a bright lad and entered the University of Virginia at the age of sixteen by special dispensation as he was under the required age. After a year's course he

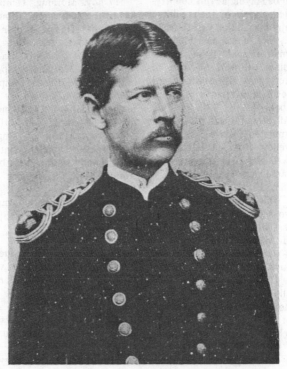

WALTER REED (1851-1902)
Courtesy of Surgeon General's Library

inquired of the faculty whether he would be allowed the degree of doctor of medicine if he could pass the necessary examinations. The faculty agreed to his request, thinking it an utter impossibility. Reed then began his medical studies and worked so hard that he passed the examinations and received his degree nine months later in 1869, at the early age of eighteen, standing third in his class. A few months after his graduation Reed went to New York City, entered the Bellevue Hospital Medical College and received the degree of

M.D. one year later. In 1875, he received a commission as First Lieutenant in the Medical Corps of the United States Army.

Reed spent thirteen years in various army posts mostly on the frontier and in 1890 was ordered to Baltimore where he worked in pathology and bacteriology under Dr. William H. Welch at the Johns Hopkins Hospital. In 1893, he was appointed curator of the Army Medical Museum and professor of bacteriology in the Army Medical School in Washington. During the next few years, he published important papers on typhoid fever and malaria. In 1900 yellow fever appeared among the American troops stationed in Havana and the government appointed a commission to study the disease. Reed was appointed chairman, the other members of the commission being Dr. James Carroll, Dr. Jesse W. Lazear, and Dr. Aristide Agramonte.

When the Yellow Fever Commission went to Havana, they received the hearty cooperation of Colonel Gorgas and of Dr. Carlos Finlay. The latter, who believed that yellow fever was due to the Stegomyia mosquito, was ready on all occasions and at all places to discuss his favorite theory and by many was regarded as a harmless crank. Gorgas had been unsuccessful in his attempts to stamp out the disease but believed it was due to filth and was not convinced by the reasoning of his friend Dr. Finlay. Reed was much impressed by Finlay's ideas and, although he regarded the mosquito hypothesis as an unproved theory, he determined to test out thoroughly this interesting possibility and was supplied with Stegomyia mosquitoes by Finlay. The commission began its experiments in August and by December had proved that yellow fever was transmitted by the bite of the Stegomyia mosquito and was not carried by fomites. This work cost the life of Dr. Lazear, and left Dr. Carroll with a serious heart affection to which he later succumbed.

Walter Reed died in 1902 from acute appendicitis and is buried in Arlington. Over his tomb is a tablet with the simple inscription: "He gave to man control over that dreadful scourge—Yellow Fever."

The story of the work of the Yellow Fever Commission has been told in a fascinating way by Dr. Howard A. Kelly in his *Walter Reed and Yellow Fever*, published in 1906.

ORIGINAL ARTICLES

THE ETIOLOGY OF YELLOW FEVER*
A Preliminary Note[1]

By WALTER REED, M.D., Surgeon, U.S.A.,

and

JAMES CARROLL, M.D., A. AGRAMONTE, M.D., JESSE W. LAZEAR, M.D.[2]
Acting Assistant Surgeons, U.S.A.

The writers, constituting a board of medical officers, convened "for the purpose of pursuing scientific investigations with reference to the acute infectious diseases prevalent on the Island of Cuba," arrived at our station, Columbia Barracks, Quemados, Cuba, on June 25 of the present year, and pro-

* *Med. Rec.*, 1900, VI, 790, 791-793, 796.
[1] Read at the Meeting of the American Public Health Association, held in Indianapolis, Ind., October 22-26, 1900.

[2] Died of yellow fever at Camp Columbia, Cuba, September 25, 1900.

ceeded under written instructions from the Surgeon-General of the Army, to "give special attention to questions relating to the etiology and prevention of yellow fever."

Two of its members (Agramonte and Lazear) were stationed on the Island of Cuba, the former in Havana, and the latter at Columbia Barracks, and were already pursuing investigations relating to the etiology of this disease.

Fortunately for the purposes of this board, an epidemic of yellow fever was prevailing in the adjacent town of Quemados, Cuba, at the time of our arrival, thus furnishing us an opportunity for clinical observations and for bacteriologic and pathologic work. The results already obtained, we believe, warrant the publication, at this time, of a Preliminary Note. A more detailed account of our observations will be submitted to Surgeon General Sternberg in a future report.

The first part of this Preliminary Note will deal with the results of blood-cultures during life and of cultures taken from yellow-fever cadavers; reserving for the second part a consideration of the mosquito as instrumental in the propagation of yellow fever; with observations based on the biting of nonimmune human beings by mosquitoes which had fed on patients sick with yellow fever, at various intervals prior to the biting.

In prosecuting the first part of our work, we isolated a variety of bacteria, but of this we do not purpose to speak at present. It will suffice for our purpose if we state the results as regards the finding of *Bacillus icteroides*, leaving the mention of other bacteria to our detailed report.

The cases studied during the Quemados epidemic had been diagnosed by a board of physicians, selected largely by reason of their familiarity with yellow fever. This board consisted of Drs. Nicolo Silverio, Manual Herera, Eduardo Angles, and Acting Assistant Surgeon Roger P. Ames, and Jesse W. Lazear, U. S. Army.

Those studied in Havana were patients in Las Animas Hospital, and had been diagnosed as such by a board of distinguished practitioners of that city.

An examination of Table 1 will show the character of the attacks. The milder cases studied, few in number, were attended by jaundice and albumin in the urine.

* * *

II

The Mosquito as the Host of the Parasite of Yellow Fever

Having failed to isolate B. icteroides, either from the blood during life, or from the blood and organs of cadavers, two courses of procedure in our further investigations appeared to be deserving of attention, viz., first, a careful study of the intestinal flora in yellow fever in comparison with the bacteria that we might isolate from the intestinal canal of healthy individuals, in this vicinity, or of those sick with other diseases; or, secondly, to give our attention to the theory of the propagation of yellow fever by means of the mosquito—a theory first advanced and ingeniously discussed by Dr. Carlos J. Finlay, of Havana, in 1881 (*Anales de la Real Academia,* vol. XVIII, 1881, pp 147-169).

We were influenced to take up the second line of investigation by reason of the well-known facts connected with the epidemiology of this disease, and, of course, by the brilliant work of Ross and the Italian observers, in connection with the theory of the propagation of malaria by the mosquito.

We were also very much impressed by the valuable observations made at Orwood and Taylor, Miss. during the year 1898, by Surgeon Henry R. Carter, U. S. Marine Hospital Service (*A note on the interval between infecting and secondary cases of yellow fever, etc.,* Reprint from *New Orleans Medical Journal,* May 1890). We do not believe that sufficient importance has been accorded these painstaking and valuable data. We observe that the members of the yellow fever commission of the Liverpool School of Tropical Medicine, Drs. Durham and Meyers, to whom we had the pleasure of submitting Carter's observations, have been equally impressed by their importance (*British Medical Journal,* September 8, 1900, pp. 656-7).

The circumstances under which Carter worked were favorable for recording with considerable accuracy the interval between the time of arrival of infecting cases in isolated farmhouses and the occurrence of secondary cases in these houses. According to Carter, "the period from the first (infecting) case to the first group of cases infected at these houses, is generally from two to three weeks."

The houses having now become infected,

susceptible individuals thereafter visiting the houses for a few hours, fall sick with the disease in the usual period of incubation, 1 to 7 days.

Other observations made by us since our arrival confirmed Carter's conclusions, thus pointing as it seemed to us the presence of an intermediate host, such as the mosquito, which having taken the parasite into its stomach, soon after the entrance of the patient into the noninfected house, was able after a certain interval to reconvey the infecting agent to other individuals, thereby converting a noninfected house into an "infected" house. This interval would appear to be from 9 to 16 days (allowing for the period of incubation), which agrees fairly closely with the time required for the passage of the malarial parasite from the stomach of the mosquito to its salivary glands.

In view of the foregoing observations we concluded to test the theory of Finlay on human beings. According to this author's observation of numerous inoculations in 90 individuals, the application of one or two contaminated mosquitoes is not dangerous, but followed in about 18% by an attack of what he considers to be very benign yellow fever at most.

We here desire to express our sincere thanks to Dr. Finlay, who accorded us a most courteous interview and has gladly placed at our disposal his several publications relating to yellow fever, during the past 19 years; and also for ova of the variety of mosquito with which he had made his several inoculations. An important observation to be here recorded is that, according to Finlay's statement, 30 days prior to our visit, these ova had been deposited by a female just at the edge of the water in a small basin, whose contents had been allowed to slightly evaporate; so that these ova were at the time of our visit entirely above contact with the water. Notwithstanding this long interval after deposition, they were promptly converted into the larval stage, after a short period, by raising the level of the water in the basin.

With the mosquitoes thus obtained we have been able to conduct our experiments. Specimens of this mosquito forwarded to Mr. L. A. Howard, Entomologist, Department of Agriculture, Washington, D.C., were kindly identified as *Culex fasciatus,* Fabr.

* * *

Case 3.—Dr. Jesse W. Lazear, Acting Assistant-Surgeon, U. S. Army, a member of this board, was bitten on August 16, 1900 (Case 3, Table III) by a mosquito (Culex fasciatus) which 10 days previous had been contaminated by biting a very mild case of yellow-fever (fifth day). No appreciable disturbance of health followed this inoculation.

On *September 13, 1900 (forenoon)*, Dr. Lazear, while on a visit to Las Animas Hospital, and while collecting blood from yellow-fever patients for study, was bitten by a Culex mosquito (variety undetermined). As Dr. Lazear had been previously bitten by a contaminated insect without after-effects, he deliberately allowed this particular mosquito, which had settled on the back of his hand, to remain until it had satisfied its hunger.

On the evening of September 18, 5 days after the bite, Dr. Lazear complained of feeling "out of sorts," and had a chill at 8 P.M.

On September 19, 12 o'clock noon, his temperature was 102.4°, pulse 112; his eyes were injected and his face suffused; at 3 P.M. temperature was 103.4°, pulse 104; 6 P.M. temperature was 103.8° and pulse 106; albumin appeared in the urine. Jaundice appeared on the third day. The subsequent history of this case was one of progressive and fatal yellow fever, the death of our much-lamented colleague having occurred on the evening of September 25, 1900.

As Dr. Lazear was bitten by a mosquito while present in the wards of a yellow fever hospital, one must, at least, admit the possibility of this insect's contamination by a previous bite of a yellow-fever patient. This case of accidental infection therefore cannot fail to be of interest taken in connection with Cases 10 and 11.

For ourselves, we have been profoundly impressed with the mode of infection and with the results that followed the bite of the mosquito in these three cases. Our results would appear to throw new light on Carter's observations in Mississippi, as to the period required between the introduction of the first (infecting) case and the occurrence of secondary cases of yellow fever.

Since we here, for the first time, record a case in which a typical attack of yellow fever has followed the bite of an infected mosquito, within the usual period of incubation of the disease, and in which other sources of infection can be excluded, we feel confident that the publication of these observations must excite renewed interest in the mosquito-theory of the propagation of yellow fever, as first proposed by Finlay.

From the first part of our study of yellow fever, we draw the following conclusions:

1. The blood taken during life from the general venous circulation, on various days of the disease, in 18 cases of yellow fever, successively studied, has given negative results as regards the presence of B. icteroides.

2. Cultures taken from the blood and organs of 11 yellow-fever cadavers have also proved negative as regards the presence of this bacillus.

3. *Bacillus icteroides (Sanarelli) stands in no causative relation to yellow fever, but when present, should be considered as a secondary invader in this disease.*

From the second part of our study of yellow fever, we draw the following conclusion:

The mosquito serves as the intermediate host for the parasite of yellow fever, and it is highly probable that the disease is only propagated through the bite of this insect.

TETANUS
Hippocrates

The master of a large ship mashed the index finger of his right hand with the anchor. Seven days later a somewhat foul discharge appeared; then trouble with his tongue—he complained he could not speak properly. The presence of tetanus was diagnosed, his jaws became pressed together, his teeth were locked, then symptoms appeared in his neck: on the third day opisthotonos appeared with sweating. Six days after the diagnosis was made he died.*

Aretaeus
CHAPTER VI†

TETANUS, in all its varieties, is a spasm of an exceedingly painful nature, very swift to prove fatal, but neither easy to be removed. They are affections of the muscles and tendons about the jaws; but the illness is communicated to the whole frame, for all parts are affected sympathetically with the primary organs. There are three forms of the convulsions, namely in a straight line, backwards and forwards. Tetanus is in a direct line, when the person labouring under the distension is stretched out straight and inflexible. The contractions forwards and backwards have their appellation from the tension and the place; for that backwards we call Opisthotonos; and that variety we call Emprosthotonos in which the patient is bent forwards by the anterior nerves. For the Greek word τόνος is applied both to a nerve, and to signify tension.

The causes of these complaints are many; for some are apt to supervene on the wound of a membrane, or of muscles, or of punctured nerves, when, for the most part, the patients die; for, "spasm from a wound is fatal." And women also suffer from this spasm after abortion; and, in this case, they seldom recover. Others are attacked with the spasm owing to a severe blow in the neck. Severe cold also sometime proves a cause; for this reason, winter of all the seasons most especially engenders these affections; next to it, spring and autumn, but least of all summer, unless when preceded by a wound, or when any strange diseases prevail epidemically. Women are more disposed to tetanus than men, because they are of a cold temperament; but they more readily recover, because they are of a humid. With respect to the different ages, children are frequently affected, but do not often die, because the affection is familiar and akin to them;

---

* Beck, Theodor. *Hippokrates Erkenntnisse,* Jena, Diederichs, 1907, p. 132.

† *The Extant Works of Aretaeus, the Cappadocian,* edited and translated by Francis Adams, LL.D., London, Sydenham Society, 1856, p. 253.

striplings are less liable to suffer, but more readily die; adults least of all, whereas old men are most subject to the disease and most apt to die; the cause of this is the frigidity and dryness of old age, and the nature of the death. But if the cold be along with humidity, these spasmodic diseases are more innocent, and attended with less danger.

In all these varieties, then, to speak generally, there is a pain and tension of the tendons and spine, and of the muscles connected with the jaws and cheek; for they fasten the lower jaw to the upper, so that it could not easily be separated even with levers or a wedge. But if one, by forcibly separating the teeth, pour in some liquid the patients do not drink it but squirt it out, or retain it in the mouth, or it regurgitates by the nostrils; for the isthmus faucium is strongly compressed, and the tonsils being hard and tense, do not coalesce so as to propel that which is swallowed. The face is ruddy and mixed colours, the eyes almost immovable, or are rolled about with difficulty; strong feeling of suffocation; respiration bad, distension of the arms and legs; subsultus of the muscles; the countenance variously distorted; the cheeks and lips tremulous; the jaw quivering, and the teeth rattling, and in certain rare cases even the ears are thus affected. I myself have beheld this and wondered! The urine is retained, so as to induce strong dysuria, or passes spontaneously from contraction of the bladder. These symptoms occur in each variety of the spasms.

But there are peculiarities in each; in Tetanus there is tension in a straight line of the whole body, which is unbent and inflexible; the legs and arms are straight.

Opisthotonos bends the patient backward, like a bow, so that the reflected head is lodged between the shoulder-blades; the throat protrudes; the jaw sometimes gapes, but in some rare cases it is fixed in the upper one; respiration stertorous; the belly and chest prominent, and in these there is usually incontinence of urine; the abdomen stretched, and resonant if tapped; the arms strongly bent back in a state of extension; the legs and thighs are bent together, for the legs are bent in the opposite direction to the hams.

But if they are bent forwards, they are protuberant at the back, the loins being extruded in a line with the back, the whole of the spine being straight; the vertex prone, the head inclining towards the chest; the lower jow fixed upon the breast bone; the hands clasped together, the lower extremities extended; pains intense; the voice altogether dolorous; they groan, making deep moaning. Should the mischief then seize the chest and the respiratory organs, it readily frees the patient from life; a blessing this, to himself, as being a deliverance from pains, distortion, and deformity; and a contingency less than usual to be lamented by the spectators, were he a son or a father. But should the powers of life still stand out, the respiration, although bad, being still prolonged, the patient is not only bent up into an arch but rolled together like a ball, so that the head rests upon the knees, while the legs and back are bent forwards, so as to convey the impression of the articulation of the knee being dislocated backwards.

An inhuman calamity! an unseemly sight! a spectacle painful even to the beholder! an incurable malady! owing to the distortion, not to be recognized by the dearest friends; and hence the prayer of the spectators, which formerly would have been reckoned not pious, now becomes good, that the patient may depart from life, as being a deliverance from the pains and unseemly evils attendant on it. But neither can the physician, though present and looking on, furnish any assistance, as regards life, relief from pain or from deformity. For if he should wish to straighten the limbs, he can only do so by cutting and breaking those of a living man. With them, then, who are overpowered by this disease, he can merely sympathise. This is the great misfortune of the physician.

DIPHTHERIA

Diphtheria was known to the ancient Hebrews and is mentioned in the Babylonian Talmud. Aretaeus described it as the *ulcera Syriaca* and noted that some patients when they drank returned the fluid by their nostrils—the first record, apparently, of paralysis of the soft palate. Baillou described the disease quite clearly and noted the characteristic membrane. Tulp saw the disease in Amsterdam, and Fothergill's description remains a classic although he confused it with scarlet fever. Huxham's account is interesting, like all contributions from his pen, and Bard's description of the epidemic in New York is an early classic in American medical literature. Francis Home described diphtheria in his *Principia Medicinae,* first published in 1758, and in his *Enquiry into the Nature, Cause and Cure of Croup,* which appeared in Edinburgh in 1765. His *Enquiry* has been described as the first systematic study of diphtheria. The work of Bretonneau, a model of careful clinical observation, of meticulous precision in pathological study, and lucid and cogent reasoning, was however, the outstanding one in the whole history of diphtheria. Bretonneau pointed out the contagiousness of the disease, the important role of the diphtheritic membrane, and the specificity of the disease, and differentiated it from scarlatinal angina and from spasmodic croup. He practised with success tracheotomy in diphtheria and demonstrated the great value of this procedure.

Aretaeus

CHAPTER IX

ON ULCERATIONS ABOUT THE TONSILS*

Ulcers occur on the tonsils; some, indeed, of an ordinary nature, mild and innocuous; but others of an unusual kind, pestilential and fatal. Such as are clean, small, superficial, without inflammation and without pain, are mild; but such as are broad, hollow, foul, and covered with a white, livid, or black concretion, are pestilential. Aphtha is the name given to those ulcers. But if the concretion has depth it is an Eschar and is so called: but around the eschar there is formed a great redness, inflammation, and pain of the veins, as in carbuncle; and small pustules form, at first few in number, but others coming out, they coalesce, and a broad ulcer is produced. And if the disease spread outwardly to the mouth, and reach the columella (*uvula*) and divide it asunder, and if it extend to the tongue, the gums, and the alveoli, the teeth also become loosened and black; and the inflammation seizes the neck; and these die within a few days from the inflammation, fever, foetid smell, and want of food. But, if it spread to the thorax by the windpipe, it occasions death by suffocation

* *The Extant Works of Aretaeus, the Cappadocian,* Edited and translated by Francis Adams, LL.D., London Sydenham Society, 1856, p. 253.

within the space of a day. For the lungs and heart can neither endure such smells, nor ulcerations, nor ichorous discharges, but coughs and dyspnoea supervene.

The cause of the mischief in the tonsils is the swallowing of the cold, rough, hot, acid and astringent substances; for these parts minister to the chest as to the purposes of voice and respiration; and to the belly for the conveyance of food; and to the stomach for deglutition. But if this affection occur in the internal parts, namely, the belly, the stomach, or the chest, as ascent of the mischief by eructions takes place to the isthmus faucium, the tonsils, and the parts there; wherefore children, until puberty, especially suffer, for children in particular have large and cold respiration; for there is most heat in them; moreover, they are intemperate in regard to food, having a longing for varied food and cold drink; and they bawl loud both in anger and in sport; and these diseases are familiar to girls until they have their menstrual purgation. The land of Egypt especially engenders it, the air thereof being dry for respiration, and the food diversified, consisting of roots, herbs of many kinds, acrid seeds, and thick drink; namely, the water of the Nile, and the sort of ale prepared from barley. Syria also, and more especially Coelosyria, engenders these diseases, and hence they have been named Egyptian and Syrian ulcers.

The manner of death is most piteous; pain sharp and hot as from carbuncle;[1] respiration bad, for their breath smells strongly of putrefaction, as they constantly inhale the same again into their chest; they are in so loathsome a state that they cannot endure the smell of themselves; countenance pale or livid; fever acute, thirst as if from fire, and

[1] The term in the original, ἄνθραξ, may either signify "a live coal," or the disease of "Carbuncle." See Paulus Aegineta, iv, 25. It is somewhat doubtful to which of these significations our author applies it here; indeed, the former would be the more emphatic.

yet they do not desire drink for fear of the pains it would occasion; for they become sick if it compress the tonsils, or if it return by the nostrils; and if they lie down they rise up again as not being able to endure the recumbent position, and if they rise up, they are forced in their distress to lie down again; they mostly walk about erect, for in their inability to obtain relief they flee from rest, as if wishing to dispel one pain by another. Inspiration large, as desiring cold air for the purpose of refrigeration, but expiration small, for the ulceration, as if produced by burning, is inflamed by the heat of the respiration. Hoarseness, loss of speech supervene; and these symptoms hurry on from bad to worse, until suddenly falling to the ground they expire.

Guillaume de Baillou

Guillaume de Baillou or Ballonius was born in Paris in 1538, the son of a famous mathematician and architect. He studied medicine in Paris, where he graduated in 1570. He practiced medicine for forty-six years in Paris and became dean of the medical faculty in 1580. When Henry of Navarre became King of France and Paris opened the gates of the city to welcome him, Baillou was chosen to present the keys of the city to the new king. Baillou died in 1616 at the age of seventy-eight.

Baillou was a pupil of Fernel and had a great veneration for his master. He was a skillful physician, a brilliant teacher, and a masterful writer and speaker. He insisted upon the study of patients, of nature, and of disease pictures, and was a vehement champion of the methods of Hippocrates. He was intensely interested in the relationship between climate, temperature, and diseases, and his observations in these matters pointed out a method of study later pursued with great success by Sydenham.

Baillou was the first modern epidemiologist and has left us striking descriptions of the plague, of diphtheria, or rheumatic fever, and of whooping cough. Baillou's reference to adhesive pericarditis is mentioned by Morgagni as one of the earliest descriptions of this disease. The following selection describes an epidemic of diphtheria in Paris during the year 1576. In discussing a similar epidemic in 1578, Baillou suggests the value of tracheotomy. "I have often asked myself," he writes, "if, in angina, after all else has failed, it would not be advisable to make an opening in the larynx. Certainly the operation is not without danger; but if it were carried out by a skilled operator who knew how to avoid the recurrent nerves, perhaps it might be without danger and would give certainly some chance of recovery." In another passage in his *Epidemiorum et Ephemeridum* he describes a young man who "was attacked during the night by an angina which threatened to suffocate him. He opened his throat with the aid of a sword: he lost much blood but recovered. In an urgent case would it not be possible to attempt a similar operation?" Baillou, although suggesting tracheotomy, does not seem to have performed it himself. This operation, although mentioned by Asclepi-

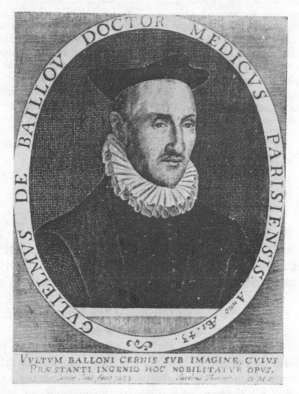

GUILLAUME DE BAILLOU (1538-1616)
Etching by Jasper Isac from Baillou's De morbis mulierum ac virginum liber Paris 1643

ades of Bithynia (B.C. 124) and by Avenzoar (1140), was first used extensively by Marco Aurelio Severino in 1610 and later popularized by Bretonneau. None of Baillou's writings were published during his lifetime.

CONSTITUTIO HIEMALIS*
ANNI DOMINI 1576

A Spaniard, Nicolaea Honorata, Nicolaus Dubuisson, the granddaughter of the wife of Gilbert all died from an almost identical illness. This was the despair of all the physicians. However I should venture to affirm they did not understand the disease. The

greatest difficulty was in breathing, respiration was continuously rapid & shallow until death. They seemed to breathe as if dried up. Neither cough nor sputum. They were not able to hold their breath for a moment. They breathed thus with their bodies erect frequently & in small breaths. The fever was not great, nor should it have made such breathing necessary. The physicians accused

* Ballonius, Gulielmus, *Epidemiorum et Ephemeridum libri duo. Opera omnia*, Venice, Jeremia, 1734, p. 130.

the lungs; others thought it to be a catarrh, others an inflammation or burning of the lungs, though it was not likely since the fever had not been at all marked. Neither venesection nor purging was of avail. Nicolaea Honorata had suffered from a mild fever, & had eaten well began to breathe superficially & frequently. Respiration ceased until she died. We referred it to a disease in the lower abdomen not to the lungs. The others were against me. I opened the body, I found the right kidney purulent. Therefore it is probable the dry breathing came from the malignant vapor. However it is unbelievable that the symptoms from which she suffered arose entirely from poisonous vapors. The history of Joannes Tassina proves this. And also we present other theories. After daily fever or other affections, different in the skin, different in the joints, different remnants of poison were deposited in other parts. Thus some were spotted with horrible scabies, others had pains of the joints, others hemicrania, others certain species of catalepsy, aphonia and apoplexy sometimes appeared: examples of this we have considered in the first book of our Consilia and given its reason. It was however, if after a marked obstruction of the upper parts that we find it was of such innate strength, that it produced pain & such suffering that a difficulty in breathing followed.

Now the manner in which the affection of the lower parts causes shallow & rapid respiration, I have explained at length in volume two of our Consilia. Besides the lungs of the girl were sound. A very small part adhered to the ribs, but it was not badly diseased. Nicholas Dubuisson died with the same symptoms. Moreover this resulted from a poisonous vapor. Now he had passed regularly a purulent secretion by the urethra since the age of fifteen or nineteen. It was from the kidneys. Excretion was not normal. A colicky pain commenced. Then difficulty in breathing without coughing and some similar symptoms. Death. It should be asked whether this dyspnoea could be the result of the colicky pains or the noxious vapors. We sectioned him and looked for the expected findings: In the Spaniard & the granddaughter of Gilbert nothing of this sort was

observed in the kidneys. Furthermore we were in doubt about this affection whether we could properly call it dry or bloody orthopnoes. Furthermore it has some affinity with a certain affection which Hippocrates calls dry orthopnoes.

* * *

ANNOTATIONS

7. The difficulty was in breathing. Moreover the cause of this was not in the lung itself, rather in the region of the liver or spleen. Since from the beginning of the fever either or continuous or intermittent nausea, dyspnoea, dry cough, anxiety, prostration, suppression and a kind of nightmare was produced: thus if the matter was moved it was affected inwardly by any kind of fever, it could cause this difficulty in breathing which we could neither lay to the suffocating catarrh nor to a disease of the lungs. . . . There was dyspnoea, a marked harsh rustling was heard. This was due to the harsh juice, or to the malignant breathing produced in the lung. Or this was a sign of rubeola appearing. Or if this dyscrasia lie not in the lungs in such a manner as when in danger of measles or that the difficulty in breathing arose from this? Perhaps it is not entirely dissimilar. Another boy 7 years old died of the same disease. Nothing was found of the origin of the illness & the cause of the difficult breathing. At this time there raged a cough, commonly called Quinta, of which a little later. And since at intervals the cause of the Quinta cough was fleeting, the same certain cause produced it. This difficulty in breathing persisted until death. The son of Doctor le Noir died from this difficulty in breathing, hence he had this dog-like raucity and a little swelling of the pharynx. The right part of the lung was partly diseased. Gervais Honoré my father-in-law died in the same manner almost suffocated. The surgeon said he sectioned the body of the boy with this difficult breathing, & with the disease (as I said) of unknown cause; sluggish resisting phlegm, was found which covered the trachea like a membrane and the entry & exit of air to the exterior was not free: thus sudden suffocation.

Nicholas Tulp

Nicholaas or Nicholas Tulp was born in 1593 in Amsterdam, the son of Peter Dirks, a prominent merchant of this city. In early life he was known as Claes Pieter or Nicholaus Petreus, but later adopted the name of Tulp, or Tulpius—a tulip. He spent his entire life in Amsterdam and was elected

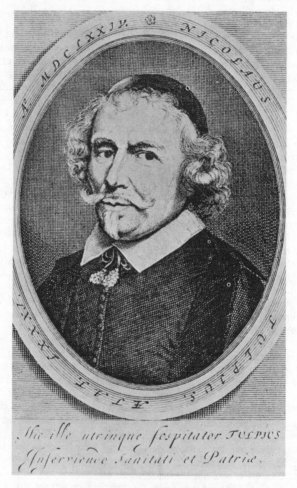

NICHOLAS TULP (1593-1674)
Engraving by L. Visscher. The frontispiece to *Observationes medicae* (Leyden, 1716)

Mayor four times. He died at eighty-one after leading a most active life both in medical practice and in the services of the city.

Tulp's personal appearance has been immortalized in Rembrandt's celebrated picture "The Anatomy Lesson," which depicted Tulp dissecting before a group of surgeons. This has resulted perhaps in making Tulpius an artistic rather than a scientific figure. "We gaze with such interest at Nicholas

Tulp's tassels and his exquisite lace collar that we forget the ileo-cecal valve is still known as Tulp's valve" (Robinson).

Tulp's best known work was his *Observationes Medicae* called by Haller "a golden work," which first appeared in 1641. This work contains many medical items of great interest, and from it we learn that Tulp was intensely interested in pathological anatomy and checked up his diagnoses by post-mortem dissections. This work describes and pictures the ileo-cecal valve, an orang-outang, a two-headed monster with three arms and three legs, kidney stones, and a tapeworm. It also contains an account of what was probably diphtheria, a description of a bronchial cast which is pictured on page 516, and one of the earliest European descriptions of beriberi.

Tulp is also said to have cured Rembrandt, by suggestion, of a mental disease which caused the famous painter to believe that his bones were turning into jelly.

CHAPTER II

ANGINA INTERNA*

The types of angina are various, but none is more pernicious than that which produces either a dislocation of the vertebra within; or an inflammation of the muscles on the inside of the larynx. A deep swelling of which, if indeed it should compress the narrow top of the treachea; & pressing upon its cord (which are the nearest instruments of speech) not only the voice itself is suppressed; but moreover the passage of air is shut off, or rather of life itself. Which without air he does not last a single day. And in like manner Hippocrates, not without reason says in his book III of prognostics "a hidden angina is fatal either the first or second day."

A sailor of large frame was attacked in the dead of night, by a severe constriction of the pharynx; immediately he drew his breath with such difficulty that fever was produced & inflammation of the throat, forthwith he fell into heavy sighing, disturbed breathing then death itself. In this extremity by which he was carried away, everything was attempted; for the necessity was more urgent & more necessary as he was strangled by the obstruction of air, so that of aid were the prompt withdrawal of blood from both arms; or cutting a swelling or cupping glasses, gargles, clysters, cataplasms, and other things applied with sufficient celerity.

Nor would their wholesome remedies aid this angina, without any swelling visible in

the mouth or a very slight one: therefore if anything is to be hoped for, if one is not provided with the remedies generally used in the past which can destroy rapidly the swelling. With too rapid a dissolving of these, moreover blood is frequently produced, but not so much from the part affected as from the entire body. It is evident through the trunk of the jugular vein, whose blood more plentifully drawn towards the place by itself easily suffocates the man by choking. Such now is the example of this unfortunate man we have discussed.

But the nature of this disturbed breathing does not remain hidden very long to anyone, that is the abnormal breathing was strikingly evident in this patient. Nothing was better known to Hippocrates than to designate the certain hopelessness of this disease, both with Πνεῦμα ἀμαυρόν or, hidden, or with Πνεῦμα Θολερόν troubled breathing.

For as it is called obscure breathing it is near to extinction: Disturbed because it comes from the mixture either of vapors or humors very harsh and dark; so that the true nature of the air is lost, which consists in the ethereal excellence and invisible exhalation; the heart is not exhilarated further; much less easily it digests the inspired air; much less it separates poorly the soot but is seen to be spread by this strong force & to come forth, like some smoke stirred up by a violent wind storm or from damp and dark hovel or from smouldering coal.

Indeed the heart becomes faint with such

* Tulp, Nicholas, *Observationes Medicae*, Leyden, du Vivie, 1716, p. 93.

breathing & thus the vital heart becomes faint: so that the vapor retained or the air falsely mixed either oppress or kill a man. See what Hippocrates says so clearly in book 1 of prognostics. "In acute feeble sweats around the head, bad: but especially with black urine and disturbed breathing."

As he says if indeed the man be so weak: that the sweats do not disturbe save in the head & besides the urine appears blackish either from the extinction of inward heat or from the black bile most freely mixed: it is dangerous. The patient does not die if the before mentioned defects of bad breath are to be seen particularly, the breathing has become disturbed & health itself indeed save such a man. For the breathing becomes disturbed only in the extreme struggle, in which now it is content to impede the breath, which can cause death itself, it excites by its violent force whatever in the body is movable.

And mixed with the clear spirits, either harsh or blackish, either black bile or with blood of whatever kind, it makes this very disturbed: besides this the thick unequal spirit excites this noisy trouble by aggitating the air: which in the dying moreover is confused with stertor, well known by physicians.

From which neverless indeed it is well to distinguish this breathing; observe with care the noise either of a man suffering from apoplexy; or of an ox dying at a butcher's hand. If you will examine their chests after death, you will see the treachea filled everywhere with foamy blood: as it were the true refuse of the disturbed breathing, which without doubt, also the poet knew, when he wrote:

Behold now the bull smoking under the heavy plow
He falls & vomits blood mixed with foam by mouth

John Fothergill

John Fothergill was born in Wensleydale, Yorkshire, in 1712, the son of John Fothergill, a prosperous farmer. The Fothergills were Quakers and for generations had worked and suffered for their faith. Young John Fothergill was apprenticed at the age of sixteen to an eminent Friend apothecary, Benjamin Bartlett, and at the age of twenty entered the University of Edinburgh, for the study of medicine, since as a Dissenter the universities of his own country were closed to him. At Edinburgh he was a most diligent student and took his doctor's degree in 1736.

After receiving his degree Fothergill enrolled in St. Thomas' Hospital in London, for a course in medical practice under Edward Wilmot, the son-in-law of Dr. Mead. He spent two years studying at St. Thomas' Hospital and in 1740 began practice in London. While at St. Thomas' Hospital his kindness to poor patients won him their regard and the poor now sought him out. This practice brought him little pecuniary return, but gradually increased his reputation, so that he remarked in later years "I climbed on the backs of the poor to the pockets of the rich."

In 1748 he published a monograph *An Account of the Sore Throat attended with Ulcers,* which contains a striking account of both diphtheria and scarlatinal angina but fails to differentiate between the two conditions. This book was widely read, several editions were soon published, and Fothergill almost immediately found himself famous and much sought after by patients. At thirty-six years of age he had one of the largest practices in London and for thirty years led a most busy life. Few physicians have worked so hard. He commonly worked sixteen or seventeen hours daily and often went for twenty hours without sleep. Benjamin Franklin writing him in 1764 asked "By the way, when do you intend to live?"

Fothergill was proposed in 1774, by Lord North, as one of the Royal physicians. Fothergill, however, declined the appointment, either through modesty, or because of his Quaker faith. Fothergill, as a prominent Quaker,

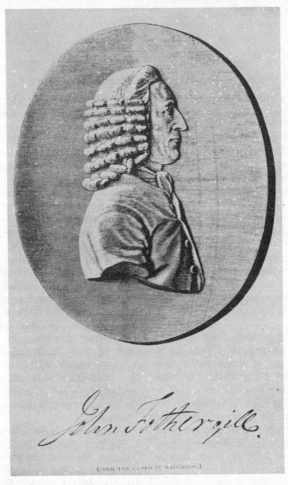

(FROM THE CAMEO BY WEDGWOOD.)

JOHN FOTHERGILL (1712-1780)
From the frontispiece to *A Sketch of the Life of John Fothergill* by James Hack Tuke (London, n.d.) From the cameo by Wedgewood

had many friends in America, particularly in Philadelphia, and worked hard to prevent the rupture between England and the American Colonies. After the American Revolution he aided some young Americans who came to London for their medical education, and gave a large sum of money to the Pennsylvania Hospital at Philadelphia. He died in 1780 at the age of sixty-eight years.

Fothergill was not only a great physician, but a great humanitarian and philanthropist. He was very active in prison reform, in the improvement of medical education, and in the abolition of slavery, and was throughout his life a strict and consistent Quaker. While his description of epidemic sore-throat is his best known work, his account of *tic douloureux*, is the first clear description of this affection and his paper on angina pectoris contains the first record of sclerosis of the coronary arteries in this disease—an observation confirmed later by Jenner and Parry.

PART II

Of the Sore Throat attended with Ulcers;
As it has appeared in This City and Parts adjacent*

ACCORDING to the Information I have received from several eminent Persons of the Faculty, it was in the Year 1739, that a Disease was first taken notice of, which was thought to be the *Morbus strangulatorius,* already described, and which differed in no essential Circumstance, as far as I can learn, from the Distemper which is the Subject of this Treatise.

The sudden Death of two Children in a Family of Distinction, and of some others near the same Part of the Town, whose Complaints had chiefly been of a sore Throat, seem to have occasioned this Suspicion: But as very few Cases of the like Nature occurred after these, or if they happened, passed unobserved, little mention was made of it during several Years.

It began however to shew itself again in 1742, but not in so general a Way as to render it the Subject of much public Discourse; for tho' such of the Faculty, as were in the most extensive Practice, met with it now-and-then, in the City especially, it remained unknown to the greater Part of the Practitioners, till within these two or three Years, in which Time its Appearance hath been more frequent, both in Town, and in the Villages adjacent.

* * *

In this Country, as well as in those where the *Angina maligna* was first taken notice of, Children and young People are more exposed to it than Adults: A greater Number of Girls have it than Boys; more Women than Men; and the infirm of either Sex are more liable to have the Disease, and to suffer from it,

than the healthy and vigorous: I have seen but few Adults of this Constitution affected by it, and not one who died of it.

When it breaks out in a Family, all the Children are commonly affected with it, if the healthy are not kept apart from the sick; and such Adults as are frequently with them, and receive their Breath near at hand, seldom escape some Degree of the same Disease.

It generally comes on with such a Giddiness of the Head, as commonly precedes Fainting, and a Chilness or Shivering like that of an Ague-Fit: This is soon followed by great Heat; and these interchangeably succeed each other during some Hours, till at length the Heat becomes constant and intense. The Patient then complains of an acute Pain in the Head, of Heat and Soreness, rather than Pain, in the Throat, Stiffness of the Neck, commonly of great Sickness, with Vomiting, or Purging, or both (b). The Face soon after looks red and swelled, the Eyes inflamed and watry, as in the Measles; with Restlessness, Anxiety, and Faintness.

This Disease frequently seizes the Patient in the fore Part of the Day: As Night approaches, the Heat and Restlessness increase, and continue till towards Morning; when after a short disturbed Slumber (the only Repose they often have during several Nights), a sweat breaks out; which mitigates

(b) The Vomiting and Purging were but seldom observed to accompany this Disease, at its first Appearance amongst us, as I have been informed by some Physicians of Eminence, who saw it early; but it is generally agreed, that these Symptoms almost constantly attended, in the manner here described, during the Years 1747 and 1748, the Time in which these Observations were collected: And I have since found, that the abovementioned Symptoms have not so regularly appeared as at that time.

*An Account of the Sore Throat Attended with Ulcers, by John Fothergill, London, Davis, 1754, IV Ed., pp. 28, 31, 47.

the Heat and Restlessness, and gives the Disease sometimes the Appearance of an Intermittent.

If the Mouth and Throat be examined soon after the first Attack, the *Uvula* and *Tonsils* appear swelled; and these Parts, together with the *Velum Pendulum Palati*, the Cheeks on each Side near the Entrance into the *Fauces,* and as much of them, and the *Pharynx* behind, as can be seen, appear of a florid red Colour. This Colour is commonly most observable on the posterior Edge of the Palate, in the Angles above the *Tonsils,* and upon the *Tonsils* themselves. Instead of this Redness a broad Spot or Patch, of an irregular Figure, and of a pale white Colour, is sometimes to be seen, surrounded with a florid Red; which Whiteness commonly appears like that of the Gums immediately after having been pressed with the Finger, or as if Matter ready to be discharged was contained underneath.

Generally on the second Day of the Disease, the Face, Neck, Breast, and Hands to the Fingers Ends, are become of a deep erysipelatous Colour, with a sensible Tumefaction; the Fingers are frequently tinged in so remarkable a manner, that, from seeing them only, it has not been difficult to guess at the Disease.

A great Number of small Pimples, of a Colour distinguishably more intense than that which surrounds them, appear on the Arms, and other Parts. They are larger, and more prominent in those Subjects, and in those Parts of the same Subject, where the Redness is least intense; which is generally on the Arms, the Breast, and lower Extremities (a).

As the Skin acquires this Colour, the Sickness commonly goes off, the Vomiting and Purging cease of themselves, and rarely continue after the first Day.

The Appearance in the *Fauces* continues to be the same; except that the white Places become more Ash-coloured; and it is now discoverable, that what at first might have been taken for the superficial Covering of a suppurated Tumour, is really a Slough, concealing an Ulcer of the same Dimensions.

(a) The Redness and Eruption have not accompanied this disease so regularly, during the latter Part of this Winter, as they did in the preceding Seasons: In some Cases they did not appear at all, in others not till the third or fourth Day; and, as I have heard, in some not till the fifth, and even later.

All the Parts of the *Fauces* above-mentioned are liable to these Ulcerations; but they generally are first discernible in the Angles above the *Tonsils,* or on the *Tonsils* themselves; though they are often to be seen in the Arch formed by the *Uvula* and one of the *Tonsils;* and also on the *Pharynx* behind, on the Inside of the Cheeks, and the Base of the Tongue, which they cover in the manner of a thick Fur. Instead of these Sloughs, where the Disorder is mild, a superficial Ulcer, of an irregular Figure, appears in one or more of these Parts, scarce to be distinguished from the sound, but by the Inequality of Surface it occasions.

* * *

The *Uvula* and *Tonsils* are sometimes so much swelled, as to leave but a very narrow Entrance into the Gullet, and this Entrance frequently surrounded with Ulcers or Sloughs; yet the Patients often swallow with less Difficulty and Pain than might be expected under such Circumstances (e).

They frequently complain, soon after they are taken ill, of an offensive putrid Smell, affecting their Throats and Nostrils, which oft occasions Sickness before any Ulcerations appear.

In those who have this Disease in a severe manner, the Inside of the Nostrils, as high up as can be seen, frequently appears of a deep red, or almost livid Colour: After a Day or two, a thin corrosive *Sanies,* or with it a white putrid Matter of a thicker Consistence, flows from them, which is so acrid, as to excoriate the Part it lies upon any considerable time. This is most observable in Children, or in young and very tender Subjects, whose Lips likewise are frequently of the Colour above-mentioned, and covered on the Inside with Vesicles containing a thin *Ichor,* which excoriates the Angles of their Mouths, and the Cheeks where it touches them.

It is probable, that Part of the same acrid Matter passes with the Nourishment into the Stomach; especially in Children; and it is perhaps owing to this Cause in part, that they suffer much more from the Distemper than Adults; this corrosive Fluid without Doubt producing the same Effects on the

(e) I have seen many Cases, where these Glands were so inlarged, as to force back thro' the Nostrils most Part of what was attempted to be swallowed.

Stomach and Bowels, as it does when applied to the much less sensible Skin of the Face; *i.e.*, it excoriates the Parts it touches; which in fact seems to be the Case: For, if they get over this Stage of the Disease, a Purging sometimes succeeds, attended with the Symptoms of Ulcerations in Bowels; and after enduring great Pain and Misery, perhaps some Weeks, they at length die emaciated: I have been informed, that some Children have had the Parts about the *Anus* excoriated (f); the *Sanies* retaining its Virulency thro' the whole Tract of the Intestines.

* * *

A copious Flux of pituitous Matter to the Glands, and other Parts about the *Fauces*, seemed to be the Cause of sudden Death, in a Girl about 12 Years old. She was seized

(f) Some Adults, who have had the Disease in a violent Degree, have suffered very much from the same cause: Emollient mucilaginous Liquids taken plentifully, and also applied externally, by way of Fomentation, to the Part affected, frequently give speedy Relief.

in the common Way, with Shivering, Headach, Sickness, Vomiting, and Purging. The Discharges abated in a few Hours, and were succeeded by great Heat, Redness of the Skin, and a sore Throat; the *Uvula, Tonsils,* and contiguous Parts, were red, and so swelled in eight or ten Hours, as to touch each other, and seemed to close the Entrance into the *Pharynx.* She breathed without much Difficulty, swallowed with less Pain than could be imagined, and spit up large Quantities of Phlegm. About six in the Evening she was seized with a Difficulty of breathing, as if strangled: Those about her raised her up, thinking she was in a Fit; she recovered herself a little, but expired upon being again laid down in Bed, in somewhat less than 24 Hours from the first Attack. A larger Quantity of viscid Phlegm, with which, after she was dead, her Mouth appeared to be filled, together with the tumefied *Uvula, Tonsils,* and *Velum Palati,* had perhaps jointly closed the *Rima Glottidis,* and put a Stop to Respiration.

John Huxham

John Huxham was born at Totness in the County of Devon, in 1692. He went to school at a private academy in Exeter and, in 1715, proceeded to the University of Leyden to study medicine. He was attracted to Leyden by the fame of the great Boerhaave, whose lifelong influence upon him contributed greatly to his later success. His financial resources, however, were inadequate for the three years of study at Leyden, so he went presently to Rheims, where he received the degree of Doctor of Medicine. Upon his return to England, he settled first at Totness, but presently moved to Plymouth, where he lived with a Mr. Colker, one of the most influential Dissenters of that city. In Plymouth he affected great gravity and dignity of manner, wearing striking clothes —a scarlet coat with ruffles at the sleeves and a cocked hat. He carried a gold-headed cane and in warm weather was always attended by his servant, who carried his gloves. "He would," it was said, "go to Chapel, order his servants to call him out in haste, when he was not really wanted, get upon his horse and ride furiously out of one gate of the town and in at the other."

In spite of these expedients, his progress at Plymouth was very slow and he had much time for study, the fruit of which appeared in his later writings. His *Essay on Fevers,* which appeared in 1739, brought him great fame and a European reputation. He was consulted in the illness of the Queen of Portugal, who was suffering from a fever, and, upon her recovery, the King of Portugal had his treatise translated into the Portuguese language and sent him a richly bound copy as a token of his gratitude.

In 1757 he wrote a dissertation *On the malignant, ulcerous sore throat,* which contains an excellent account of diphtheria, but fails to distinguish diphtheria from the angina of scarlet fever. His *Method for preserving the Health of Seamen in Long Cruises and Voyages,* recommends the use of fresh vegetables and fruit juices as a preventive of scurvy. His account of diphtheria follows and his methods of preventing scurvy appears later in his book.

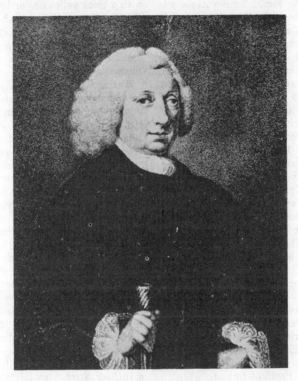

JOHN HUXHAM (1692-1768)
Portrait by T. Rennell, engraved by J. Jenkins

Huxham also wrote a classical account of Devonshire colic and made observations upon antimony which were rewarded with the Copley Medal. He was elected a Fellow of the Royal Society in 1739, and after accumulating a considerable fortune, died in 1768 at the age of seventy-six.

A DISSERTATION
ON THE
MALIGNANT ULCEROUS SORE-THROAT*

The attack of this Disease was very different in different Persons.—Sometimes a Rigor, with some Fulness and Soreness of the Troat, and painful Stiffness of the Neck, were the very first Symptoms complained of. —Sometimes alternate Chills and Heats, with some Degree of Head-ach, Giddiness, or Drowsiness, ushered in the Distemper.—It

* Huxham, John, *An Essay on Fevers, to which is now added a Dissertation on the Malignant, Ulcerous Sore-Throat,* III Ed., London, Hinton, 1757, p. 276.

seized others with much more feverish symptoms, great Pain of the Head, Back, and Limbs, a vast Oppression of the Praecordia, and continual Sighing.—Some grown Persons, on the contrary, moved about for a Day, or two, neither sick or well, as it were, but under Uneasiness and Anxiety till they were obliged to lie for it. Thus various was the Disease at the *onset*. But it commonly began with Chills and Heats, Load and Pain of the Head, Soreness of Throat and Hoarseness, some cough, Sickness at Stomach, frequent Vomiting and Purging, in Children especially, which were sometimes very severe, though a contrary State was more common to the Adults.—There was in all a very great Dejection of Spirits, very sudden weakness, great Heaviness on the Breast, and Faintness, from the very Begining.—The Pulse in general was quick, small and fluttering, though sometimes heavy and undose.—The Urine commonly pale, thin and crude, however, in many grown Persons in small Quantities, and high-colored, or like turbid Whey. —The Eyes were heavy, reddish and as it were weeping.—The Countenance very often full, flushed and bloated, though sometimes pale and sunk.

How slight soever the Disorder might appear in the Day-time, at Night the Symptoms became greatly aggravated, and the feverish Habit very much encreased, nay, sometimes a Delirium came on the very first Night; and this Exacerbation constantly returned in the Evening through the whole Course of the Disease.—Indeed, when it was considerably on the Decline, I have been often pretty much surprized to find my Patient had passed the whole Night in a Phrenzy, whom I had left tolerably cool and sedate in the Day.

Some few Hours after the Seizure, and sometimes cotemporary with it, a Swelling and Soreness of the Throat was perceived, and the Tonsils became very tumid and inflamed, and many times the parotid and maxillary Glands swelled very much, and very suddenly, even at the very Beginning; sometimes so much as even to threaten Strangulation. The Fauces also very soon appeared of a high florid Red, or rather of a bright Crimson Colour, very shining and glossy; and most commonly on the *Uvula, Tonsils, Velum Palatinum,* and back Part of the *Pharynx,* several whitish, or Ash-coloured Spots appeared scattered up and down, which

oftentimes encreased very fast, and soon covered one, or both the Tonsils, Uvula, &c: these in Event proved the *Sloughs* of superficial Ulcerts (which sometimes however eat very deep into the Parts). The Tongue at this Time, though only white and moist at the Top, was very foul at the Root, and covered with a thick yellowish, or brown Coat.—The Breath also now began to be very nauseous, which offensive Smell encreased hourly, and in some became at length intolerable, and that too sometimes even to the Patients themselves.

The second, or third Day, every Symptom became much more aggravated, and the Fever much more considerable, and those, that had struggled with it tolerably well for thirty or forty Hours, were forced to submit—The Restlessness and Anxiety greatly encreased, as well as the Difficulty in Swallowing.—The Head was very giddy, pained, and loaded; there was generally more or less of a Delirium, sometimes a Pervigilium and perpetual Phrenzy, though others lay very stupid, but often starting and muttering to themselves.—The Skin was very hot, dry and rough; there was very rarely any Disposition to sweat. The Urine pale, thin, crude, often yellowish, and turbid. Sometimes a Vomiting was urgent, and sometimes a very great Loosness, in Children particularly. The Sloughs were now much enlarged, and of a darker Colour, and the surrounding Parts tended much more to a livid Hue.—The Breathing became much more difficult, with a Kind of a *rattling Stertor,* as if the Patient was actually strangling, the Voice being exceeding hoarse and hollow, exactly resembling that from *venereal Ulcers in the Fauces;* this Noise in Speaking and Breathing was so peculiar; that any Person in the least conversant with the Disease might easily know it by this odd Noise; from whence indeed the *Spanish Physicians* gave it the Name of *Garotillo,* expressing the Noise such make as are strangling with a Rope.—I never observed in one of them the shrill, barking Noise, that we frequently hear in inflammatory Squinzies. The Breath of all the Diseased was very nauseous, of some insufferably foetid, especially in the Advance of the Distemper to a Crisis; and many about the fourth or fifth Day spit off a vast Quantity of stinking, purulent Mucus, tinged sometimes with Blood, and sometimes the Matter was quite livid, and of an abominable Smell.

The Nostrils likewise in many were greatly inflamed and excoriated, continually dripping down a most sharp *Ichor*, or *fanious Matter*, so excessively acrid, that it not only corroded the Lips, Cheeks, and Hands of the Children, that laboured under the Disease, but even the Fingers and Arms of the very Nurses, that attended them: As this Ulceration of the Nostrils came on, it commonly caused an almost incessant Sneezing in the Children, but few Adults were affected with it, at least to any considerable Degree. It was surprising what Quantities of Matter some Children discharged this Way, which they would often rub on their Face, Hands and Arms, and blister them all over.—A sudden Stoppage of this Rheum from the Mouth and Nostrils actually choaked several Children; and some swallowed such Quantities of it, as occasioned Excoriations of the Intestines, violent Gripings, Dysentery, &c; nay, even Excoriations of the Anus and Buttocks.—Not only the Nostrils, Fauces, &c. were greatly affected by this extreamly sharp Matter, but the Wind-pipe itself was sometimes much corroded by it, and Pieces of its internal Membrane were spit up, with much Blood and Corruption, and the Patients lingered on for a considerable Time, and at length died tabid; tho' there were more frequent Instances of its falling more suddenly and violently on the Lungs, and killing in a peripneumonic Manner.

Francis Home

Francis Home was born, probably at Edinburgh in 1719. He was apprenticed to a practitioner named Rattray and later served as a regimental surgeon from 1742 to 1748 in Flanders, during the War of the Austrian Succession. While in Flanders, he continued, during lulls in the campaign, his medical studies at the University of Leyden. After the war, he resumed his medical studies at the University of Edinburgh where he received the degree of Doctor of Medicine in 1750. He was later President of the Royal College of Physicians of Edinburgh and an early member of the Royal Medical Society of Edinburgh. In 1768 Home was appointed Professor of Materia Medica at the University of Edinburgh and in 1773 taught the Institutes of Medicine but never became professor of that subject. Later, becoming interested in the scientific study of agriculture, he was appointed the first Professor of Agriculture in the University of Edinburgh. He died in 1813.

Home's *Principia Medicinae,* which first appeared in 1758, was widely used in Great Britain and on the Continent and went through several editions. In this work he described diphtheria quite accurately and clearly and later wrote a more extended treatise, *An Enquiry into the Nature, Cause and Cure of Croup,* Edinburgh, 1765. Several authorities give Home priority for the first, clear, systematic study of diphtheria. Home was also the first observer to point out that yeast fermented the sugar in diabetic urine.

COROLLARY I*

It seems easy, in general, to distinguish the Croup from all other diseases hitherto described. A peculiar sharp shrill voice, not easily described; a remarkable freedom from all complaints, when in imminent danger, so that they will eat a minute before they expire; a quick laborious breathing; a frequent pulse, sometimes strong at first, but always soft and weak toward the end; scarce any

* Home, Francis: *An Inquiry into the Nature, Cause and Cure of the Croup,* Edinburgh, Kincaid and Bell, 1765, pp. 32, 51, 59.

difficulty of deglutition, or remarkable inflammation in the *fauces;* a dull pain, often, and sometimes an external swelling in the upper part of the *trachea;* senses quite distinct to the last; and all the symptoms most rapid in their progress, characterize sufficiently this disease. I have not mentioned a cough, as that symptom is sometimes absent; and when it attends the Croup, it is not of

dangerous. But we have seen, that the lungs are totally free from any inflammation, and are not the seat of the disease. The *Catarrhus suffocativus* of *Etmuller* seems, likewise, to have been a peripneumony. And, as he describes no peculiarity in the voice; as the symptoms seem to have been, apparently, severer; and as it returned, at stated and regular periods, we must consider them as

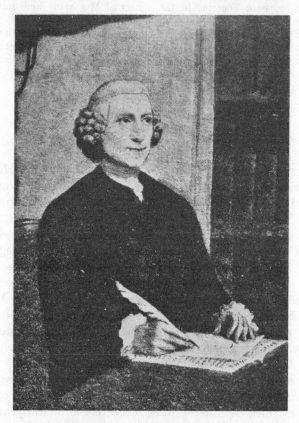

Francis Home (1719-1813)
From Comrie's *History of Scottish Medicine*

the common kind, but more short and stiffled, and less convulsive, with little or no expectoration.

The other symptoms, that often attend it, such as a red swelled face, oedematous feet, drought, urine sometimes with, and, at other times, without a sediment, reachings, &c. are not so constant as the former; and therefore, are not so characteristical.

Those not conversant in this disease, often mistake peripneumoniacal complaints, and severe colds, for it; and, as they frequently cure these, they are apt to look on it as not so

different diseases, tho' similar in many points.

As this disease has different vulgar names, for I am told, that on the west coast, they call it the *Chock,* or *Stuffing,* a technical one becomes absolutely necessary. A name is best given from the apparent symptoms, which are always conspicuous, while the cause is generally hidden, and often doubtful. The leading symptoms here, are, the shrill voice, and difficult breathing. It, therefore, may properly be called *Suffocatio stridula.*

COROL. II. As it appears peculiar to a certain age, and local, in a great measure, as to its situation, so it seems to attend certain seasons of the year. All the preceding cases showed themselves during the course of the winter, from the month of *October* to the month of *March*, except one in *August*, which was probably owing to the antecedent small-pox; for long catarrhs from the small pox, measles, or chin-cough, are strong predisponent causes to this disease. The moist and cold weather in winter, seems to have great power in producing this disease.

COROL III. Very different have been the opinions, with regard to the seat of the *Suffocatio stridula*. Some placing it in the *glottis* and its muscles; some in the coats of the *trachea;* while others have fixt its seat in the lungs themselves. None of all these opinions appear to be true. The *glottis* is never found contracted or inflamed; the lungs are quite sound; and the coats of the *trachea* seem to suffer only by second hand.

The seat of this distemper appears to be the cavity of the wind-pipe. The place first, and most particularly, affected, is the upper part of the *trachea,* about an inch below the *glottis;* for in that part they complain of a dull pain; the external swelling has been observed there; and the morbid membrane we have found stretching from that place downwards. The back part of the *trachea,* where there are no cartilages, seems, from the inspection of those that die of this disease, to be its first and principal seat, as this morbid membrane is often found there, when it is in no other part.

* * *

COROL. VII. This disease appears, in general, to be a very dangerous one, and the more so, as it is silent in its progress, and gives no visible alarm, till death is near at hand. The first stage of this distemper, often, passes unobserved; and, before we see it, is beyond all remedy. As it happens, frequently, to young children, who are unable to speak or describe their feelings, we have double reason to be afraid.

If we be not called till the third or fourth day; if the breathing appears much affected, the pulse quick and weak, the face red, great anxiety, and frequent tossing, the danger is great and pressing. But if we see the patient the first or second day of the attack; if the breathing is not very bad; the pulse, though frequent, strong, and firm; and more especially, if the voice is only altered, in its stronger exertions of crying or coughing, but more natural in its common state, we may entertain hopes of a recovery. The first sign commonly of safety, is the cough becoming stronger and less dry, with that peculiar sound which attends moistened lungs; for this shows that the membrane is not formed, or is already dissolved, and that the inflammatory state is abated.

The case seems very desperate, when the membrane is once forced, and the lungs filled with matter. In the latter case, the patient is soon suffocated, as effectually, tho' more slowly, as if he was immersed over the head in it.

It appears, from the preceding cases, that the membrane, alone, is sufficient to kill, as there was but little matter found in the lungs of some of them.

* * *

To effectuate a solution of the morbid membrane, after it is once completely formed and consolidated, seems to me impossible by any internal or external medicine that I know. To effectuate its expulsion appears equally impossible. We have, then, no method remaining to save the patient's life, but that of extraction. That cannot be done thro' the *glottis.* When the case is desperate, may we not try *bronchotomy?* I can see no weighty objection to that operation, as the membrane can be so easily got at, and is very loose. Many a more hazardous operation is daily performed. I would propose, however, that it should be first tried on a dead subject, that we may proceed with all manner of caution and assistance. But something ought to be tried in this dangerous situation.

We have now brought our Inquiry to a conclusion. The facts, we hope, will appear curious, exact, and sufficiently numerous for our purpose; the method such as is used in mathematics and natural philosophy, for discovering unknown truths; and the conclusions new, surprising, and naturally arising from the facts. If we have not brought this Inquiry to that degree of perfection, in every point, that we could have wished, we have the satisfaction, at least, to think, that, so far as we go, our discoveries are certain, as they are built on the foundation of Nature. Shunning, with all imaginable care, fruitless and deceitful speculations, however entertaining, we have constantly kept our facts and experiments in view, as the only road to the improvement of medicine, and the good of mankind.

ANGINA MALIGNA*

1. Malignant angina, or the strangling disease, or the pestilential affection of the throat is accompanied by acute fever and ulcers destroying these parts. Ulcer of the Egyptians, or of the Syrians, was the name selected by Araeteus, who described it accurately. After this it was either a hidden disease, or was overlooked by physicians until at the beginning of the seventeenth century it showed itself in Spain and Italy with the most dreadful symptoms and demanded the attention of physicians.

2. Those of tender age are attacked more violently and more severely than adults, girls than boys, infirm than vigorous, leucophlegmatic than sanguine. It appears especially in autumn and at the beginning of spring, before warm weather.

3. The immediate cause of this disease is a miasma sui generis, which is communicated to the body from the air or from bodies previously affected. The frequent transmission of the disease to those near by, or to a whole family, by the breath or by the bloody matter ejected from the mouth, proves it a contagious disease.

4. The virus introduced in the body spreads in the entire mass of humors, but especially in the throat, and the fluids secreted from the glands there, by their innate acerbity tend to putrefaction and sharpness. This is clearly apparent from the symptoms, the remedies and from dissection of the bodies.

5. It makes its appearance with a chill, then burning and intense heat; dizziness; headache; immobility of the neck; an annoying sensation in the throat; nausea, and vomiting; diarrhea; inflamed and watery eyes; face tumid and suffused with redness; restlessness; anxiety; fainting; alienation of the mind; rapid and often weak pulse, slow, active and hard; blood florid, lax and dissolute in the beginning, sometimes inflamed; urine at first crude and serous, later as if stained with bile; tongue moist and frequently covered with mucus; swallowing not very painful or obstructed; unpleasant odor in the throat; breath ill-smelling and putrid;

*Home, Francis, *Principia Medicinae*, III Edition, Amsterdam, DeTournes, 1766, p. 114.

uvula, tonsils and pharynx swollen and shiny red, followed afterwards by white spots near the tonsils, a foul ulcer and covered everywhere by foul blood; redness and excoriations of the nostrils; face, neck, chest and arms, even to the fingers, swollen, glistening scarlet in color, and often erysipelatous; the hands here and there covered with pustules; the parotid glands swollen and painful; neck edematous; voice raw and suffocated; hemorrhages from the uterus, anus or nostrils; gangrene of the esophagus down to the stomach, and of the trachea extending to the lungs. The disease by night often is worse; and by morning, a small sweat appearing, is improved.

6. The malignant angina knows neither critical days nor a regular crisis. It terminates favorably or unfavorably between the second and seventh days. When the disease tends to heal the heat diminishes, the color of the skin disappears, the cuticle desquamates, expectoration increases, the pulse slows, the swelling of the neck subsides and the ulcers heal.

7. The vomiting and diarrhoea arise from the caustic foul discharge descending into the stomach and intestine; and probably from the rapid inflammation of these parts as well as of the skin. From the same putrid discharge, a very foul odor. The swelling of the nasal tissues and the pustules partly from the morbific material carried to these parts. Hemorrhages, from the bad blood and vessels eroded by the discharge.

8. Malignant angina is distinguished from inflammatory angina, by vomiting and diarrhoea; erysipelatous swelling, foul ulcers of the throat, and covered with a white crust; rough voice; light delirium quickly supervening; no certain crisis, and increase of symptoms after evacuations. It attacks here strong men, there most frequently infants and the debilitated. From aphtha, because here it only covers the throat, there white crusts occupy the mouth as well.

9. The nature of this disease is most exceedingly tricky. The disease is always more dangerous in infants than in adults, because they do not have power to expel the corruption and are subject to less help. An ery-

sipelatous swelling is usually a bad omen. When the eyes shine, hope is present; at the time they become dull, death is near. The greater the debility and weakness, the graver the illness; the less, that much better. White ulcers are best, ashen worse, livid and black the worst. Diarrhea, rigor, weak and small pulse, edematous or cadaverous body are bad omens. Scattered or livid exanthemata; blood, especially flowing from the nose, indicate that death approaches.

10. Regarding the treatment of this disease, (1) Stomach and glands of the throat evacuate with a mild emetic, (2) Strong cardiac drugs and milder diaphoretics, refresh with wine and a restoring and antiseptic diet, (3) Treat the swelling of the external parts with tepid heat by which diarrhea is best presented, (4) Antiseptic medicines, especially Peruvian bark, and mineral and vegetable acids, provided that they do not cause diarrhea, (5) Blistering plasters applied to the neck.

Venesection, purgation, and antiphlogistic medicines, experience shows often injure. Venesection is, however, indicated in phethoric individuals and in adults, if labored respiration appears early.

11. At the beginning of the disease it is well to gargle the affected parts, with medicaments gently repelling and resolvent, such as infusion of red roses with vinegar or red dry wine. Gargles of detergents, such as honey, tincture of myrrh, Egyptian honey, and lime water. Repeated gargling separates best, the white crust adhering to the ulcer, which should never be removed with impurity; for inflammation and pain is produced, and often hemorrhage follows. To the hemorrhage astringents and styptics are applied.

Samuel Bard

Samuel Bard, one of the conspicuous figures in American medicine during the Revolution, was born in Philadelphia in 1742. His grandfather, Peter Bard, was a Huguenot who was exiled from France following the revocation of the Edict of Nantes and settled near Philadelphia. His father Dr. John Bard, was practicing medicine in Philadelphia at the time of his son's birth but four years later removed to New York where he became prominent in medical and literary circles. The son showed no precocious talent as a child but was a quick and industrious student. His mother's instruction to the teacher of her two boys was, "If Peter does not know his lesson, excuse him: if Sam does not, punish him, for he can learn at will." Samuel Bard after completing his academic studies at Columbia College decided to study medicine, and accordingly, at the age of nineteen, set sail for Europe in 1761 with Edinburgh as his objective.

At this period England was at war with France and the first letter Dr. John Bard received from his son stated that the latter had been captured by the French and was in prison at Bayonne Castle. Through the assistance of Benjamin Franklin who was at that time in London, young Bard was released from prison and after being detained in France for five months was allowed to proceed to London. In London, Bard became acquainted with Fothergill, John Hunter, and Mackenzie, and then in 1762 went to Edinburgh to begin his medical studies. Edinburgh was then at the height of her fame as a medical center and young Bard came under the influence of the two Monros, Cullen, Hope, Ferguson, and Gregory. He took his degree in 1765 and after a five years' stay abroad returned to America.

In New York, Samuel Bard formed a partnership with his father and as the father had been at great expense for his son's education, the latter for three years refused to take any of the income their partnership earned. The year after his return to New York he was active in the formation of a medical school at King's College and at the age of twenty-six became Professor of the Practice of Physics in this school. During the Revolution he was consulted by Washington for the latter's illness. In 1791, when King's College became Columbia College, Bard was appointed Dean of the Medical Faculty. In 1813 Columbia College

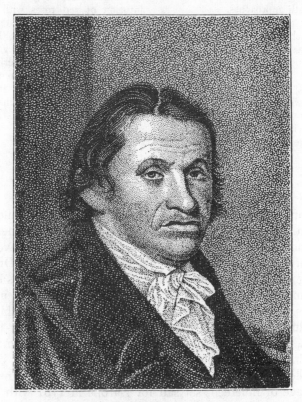

SAMUEL BARD (1742-1821)
Drawing by McCleland. Etching by W. Main. From *American Medical Biography* by James Thacher (Boston, 1828)

was separated from the medical school and Bard became President of the College of Physicians and Surgeons, a position he held until his death in 1821.

Samuel Bard was a man of tremendous energy and industry. He was conservative in his therapy and constantly warned his students against too great enthusiasm for every innovation. "New names," he said, "are always deceiving, new theories are mostly false or useless and new remedies for a time are dangerous." His most noteworthy contribution to medicine was his description of diphtheria in his treatise on *Angina Suffocativa*, which was published in 1771.

An
Enquiry
into the
Nature, Cause, and Cure,
of the
Angina Suffocativa, &c.*

"As a faithful and accurate history of diseases, their various
"symptoms and method of cure, is the most effectual way of
"promoting the art of healing; Physicians should describe, with
"the utmost care, the diseases they would treat of; and the good
"and bad effects of any method or medicines they have used in
"them. But in a more particular manner is this necessary, when
"any new and uncommon distemper occurs, of which the peculiar
"pathognomonic and diagnostic signs should be carefully laid down,
"and a particular account given of what evacuations, regimen,
"and medicines were useful or hurtful in it.

Huxham *on Fevers*, p. 267."

From a conviction of the truth and importance of these observations, and in obedience to the precept of so great a Man as Huxham, I have determined to attempt the history of a disease, which has lately appeared among the children of this city; and which, both as an uncommon and highly dangerous distemper, well deserves an attentive consideration. In delivering it therefore, I shall first carefully enumerate the symptoms with which it was attended, and describe the appearances which occurred on inspecting the bodies of such as died of it; then enquire into its nature and cause; and lastly lay down the method of cure which has been found to be most successful in its treatment.

In general, this disease was confined to children under ten years old, though some few grown persons, particularly women, (while it prevailed) had symptoms in some respects resembling it. Most of those who had it were observed to droop for several days before they were confined. And the first symptoms, in most instances, were a slightly inflammed and watry eye, a bloated and livid countenance, with a few red eruptions here and there upon the face, and in one case a small ulcer in the nose, whence oosed an ichor so sharp as to inflame and erode the upper lip. At the same time, or very soon after, such as could speak, complained of an uneasy sensation in the throat, but without any great soreness or pain. Upon examining it, the tonsils *or almonds,* appeared

* Bard, Samuel, *An Enquiry into the Nature, Cause, and Cure, of the Angina Suffocative, or Sore Throat Distemper, as it is commonly called by the Inhabitants of this City and Colony,* New York, Inslee and Carr, 1771.

swelled and slightly inflamed, with a few white specks upon them, which, in some, increased so as 'to cover them all over with one general slough, and in a few the swelling was so great, as almost to close up the passage of the throat; but this, altho' a frequent symptom, did not invariably attend the disease; and some had all the other symptoms without it. The breath was either no ways offensive, or had only that kind of smell which is occasioned by worms; and the swallowing was very little, if at all, impeded.

These symptoms, with a slight fever, at night, continued in some for five or six days, without alarming their friends; in others a difficulty of breathing came on within twenty-four hours, especially in the time of sleep, and was often suddenly encreased to so great a degree as to threaten immediate suffocation. In general, however, it came on later, increased more gradually, and was not constant, but the patient would now and then enjoy an interval of an hour or two, in which he breathed with ease, and then again a laborious breathing would ensue, during which he seemed incapable of filling his lungs, as if the air was drawn through a too narrow passage.

This stage of the disease was attended with a very great and sudden prostration of strength; a very remarkable hollow dry cough; and a peculiar change in the tone of the voice; not easily described, but so singular, that a person who had once heard it, could almost certainly know the disease again by hearing the patient cough or speak. In some the voice was almost entirely lost, and would continue very weak and low for several weeks after recovery. A constant fever attended this disease, but it was much more remarkable in the night than in the day time; and in some there was a remarkable remission towards morning. The pulse at the wrist was in general quick, soft and fluttering, thought not very low, and it was remarkable that at the same time the pulsations of the heart were rather strong and smart than feeble. The heat was not very great, and the skin was commonly moist.

These symptoms continued for one, two, or three days. By that time it was usual for them to be greatly increased in such as died; and the patients, though commonly somewhat comatous from the beginning, now became much more so; yet even when the disorder was at the worst, they retained their senses, and would give distinct answers, when spoken to; although on being left to themselves, they lay for the most part in a lethargic situation, only raising up now and then to receive their drink. Great restlessness and jactation came on towards the end of the disease, the sick perpetually tossing from one side of the bed to the other, but they were still so far comatous as to appear to be asleep, immediately upon changing their situation or posture. An universal languor and dejection were observed in their countenances; the swelling of the face subsided; a profuse sweat broke out about the head, neck and breast, particularly when asleep; a purging in several came on; the difficulty of breathing increased, so as to be frequently almost entirely obstructed, and the patient died apparently from the suffocation. This commonly happened before the end of the fourth or fifth day; in several within thirty-six hours from the time the difficulty of breathing first came on. One child, however, lived under these circumstances to the eighth day; and the day before he died, his breath and what he coughed up, was somewhat offensive; but this was the only instance in which I could discover any thing like a disagreeable smell, either from the breath or expectoration.

Out of fifteen cases attended with this remarkable suffocation in breathing, seven died; five of them before the fifth day, the other two about the eighth. Of those who recovered, the disease was carried off, in one, by a plentiful salivation, which began on the sixth day; in most of the others, by an expectoration of a viscid mucus.

I have had an opportunity of examining the nature and seat of this disease, from dissection, in three instances. One was a child of three years old. Her first complaint was an uneasiness in her throat. Upon examining it, the tonsils appeared swelled and inflamed, with large white sloughs upon them, the edges of which were remarkably more red than the other parts of the throat. She had no great soreness in her throat and could swallow with little or no difficulty. She complained of a pain under her left breast; her pulse was quick, soft and fluttering. The heat of her body was not very great, and her skin was moist; her face was swelled, she had a considerable prostration of strength, with a very great difficulty of breathing, a very remarkable hollow cough, and a peculiar change in the tone of her voice. The next day her difficulty of breathing was increased, and she drew her breath in the manner before described, as if the air was forced through too narrow a passage, so that she seemed incapable of filling her lungs: She was exceedingly restless, tossing perpetually from side to side, was sensible, and when asked a question, would give a pertinent answer, but otherways she appeared dull and comatous. All these symptoms continued, or rather increased, until the third night, on which she had five or six loose stools, and died early in the morning.

Upon examining the body, which was done on the afternoon of the day she died, all the back parts of the throat, and the root of the tongue were found interspersed with sloughs, which still retained their whitish colour. Upon removing them, the parts underneath appeared rather pale than inflamed. No putrid smell could be perceived from them, nor was the corpse in the least offensive. The Œsophagus, or *gullet,* appeared as in a sound state. The epiglottis, *which covers the wind-pipe,* was a little inflamed, on its external surface, and on the inner side, together with the whole larynx, was covered with the same tough white sloughs, as the glands of the throat. The whole trachea quite down to its division in the lungs, was lined with an inspissated mucus, in form of a membrane, remarkably tough and firm; which, when it came into the lungs, seemed to grow thin and disappear. It was so tough as to require no inconsiderable force to tear it, and came out whole from the trachea which it left with much ease; and resembled more than any thing, both in thickness and appearance, a sheath of thin shammoy leather. The inner membrane of the trachea was slightly inflamed; the lungs too appeared inflamed, as in peripneumonic cases; particularly the right lobe, on which there were many large livid spots, though neither rotten or offensive; and the left lobe had small black spots on it, resembling those marks left under the skin by gun powder. Upon cutting into any of the larger spots, which appeared on the right lobe, a bloody sanies issued from them without frothing, whereas upon cutting those parts which appeared sound, a whitish froth, but slightly tinged with blood, followed the knife.

The second dissection I attended, was of a child about seven years old, who had had all the symptoms with which this disease is commonly attended, except that in this case the glands of the throat, and upper parts of the windpipe, were found entirely free from any complaint, and the disease seemed to be confined to the trachea only, which was lined with this tough mucus, inspissated so as to resemble a membrane: We could trace it into the larger divisions of the trachea, and it was evident that the smallest branches were obstructed by it, for it was very observable, that upon opening the brest the lungs did not colapse as much as is usual, but remained distended, and felt remarkably firm and heavy, as if they were stuffed with the same mucus.

The last was a child of about three years old, who died in thirty-six hours after the difficult breathing first came on; yet even in this case, I discovered and shewed to several by-standers, the inspissated mucus which lined the trachea, and which was so remarkable as to be evident to all who saw it, that it must have been the cause of the child's death.

Pierre Bretonneau

Pierre-Fidèle Bretonneau was born at St. Georges-sur-Cher, France, in 1778. His father and uncle were surgeons and his family for nine generations had produced fifteen physicians, surgeons, or apothecaries. Bretonneau was not a precocious child, did not learn to read until he was nine years of age, and was not taught Latin although his father inspired him with an interest for natural history and medicines.

Bretonneau was sent to Paris at the age of seventeen to study medicine and entered the Ecole de Santé where he had as fellow students Dupuytren, Bayle, and Récamier. Because of ill health he was forced to abandon his studies and return home. In 1799 he returned to Paris, but failing to pass his examinations for the doctorate, he was forced to content himself with the title of "officier de santé" and then returned to Chenonceaux where he began to practice.

He rapidly acquired a reputation as a skillful practitioner and was invited to go to Tours as chief physician to the hospital. To fill this post it was necessary to qualify as a doctor of medicine so Bretonneau returned to Paris, passed the necessary examinations, and received his degree in 1814. Meanwhile he had rapidly acquired a knowledge of Latin and became a very proficient Latin scholar.

Bretonneau became chief physician to the hospital at Tours and held this position for twenty-three years. He was very active during these years, dividing his time between his clinical rounds which began at 6:00 A.M., the autopsy room where he correlated his clinical experiences with the necropsy findings, and the instruction of pupils. He was a great favorite with his students, two of whom, Velpeau and Trousseau, later achieved great fame in Paris and spread the doctrines of their old teacher.

In 1819 an epidemic of sore throat appeared in Tours which Bretonneau studied with scrupulous care. The epidemic was attended by a high mortality and in a short time he had carried out sixty autopsies. In 1821 he read a paper before the Academy of Medicine in Paris showing that croup, malignant angina, and scorbutic gangrene of the gums were all the same malady for which he proposed the name "diphtheritis." His communication was received with approval and he was later elected a corresponding member of the Academy

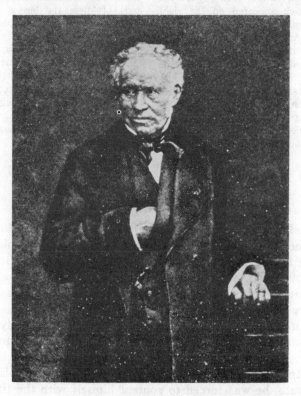

PIERRE BRETONNEAU (1778-1862)
A portrait by Moreau of Tours

Boisseau immediately attacked the term on the ground that it must mean "inflammation of a skin" and that consequently the expression "diphtheritic inflammation" was tautologous. Bretonneau, however, was a better Greek scholar than his critic and immediately pointed out that the termination "itis" did not mean inflammation but was a feminine adjective used as a noun, so "diphtheritis" merely meant the pellicular disease.

Bretonneau's work on typhoid fever, which was written between 1821 and 1827, was based upon autopsies on 120 persons dying from this disease, in all of whom he demonstrated the characteristic ulcers on the Peyer's patches. He pointed out the difference between typhoid ulcers and tuberculous ulcers, and described both intestinal hemorrhage and perforation. He called typhoid fever "dothienenteritis," (from δοθίην a pustule, and ἔυτερον the intestine) and maintained that the eruption on the intestinal mucosa was specific and went through its various stages like the eruption of smallpox.

Bretonneau's third great contribution to medicine was his insistence upon the specificity of infectious diseases, a doctrine which foreshadowed the germ theory of disease.

In 1841 Bretonneau, as the result of opposition from local practitioners resigned his position at the hospital and devoted himself to his practice and his garden. He died in 1862.

"The individuality of M. Bretonneau," says Velpeau, "was exceedingly original, and his everyday life in no way resembled that of others. He worked and slept at all hours, and was indifferent to heat and cold, and his regimen was altogether irregular. He ate and drank when he liked, at night as well as in the daytime, and quite regardless of domestic arrangements. Sometimes he would, without losing his balance, fall asleep whilst riding on horseback, and in the midst of a conversation, or he would drop off while sitting at the bedside of a patient or in the midst of a sentence. As soon as he was awake he resumed the thread of his conversation and his companions were sometimes not even aware that he had thus been absent. Everything he did was spontaneous, and he never troubled himself or others about the future, but when struck by an idea he took it up, and nothing afterwards could draw him away from it. If called to a patient he would tell his servant to ask if it was a case of sore throat or fever; and if it was neither to say that his master was not at home. Again, when returning from the hospital he went into his garden, he immediately forgot all about his patients and thought of nothing but legumes, scions, grafts, saps, and stocks. . . ."

A remarkably intimate picture of Bretonneau is revealed in his letters especially to Trousseau and to Velpeau which have been collected and published by Paul Triaire *Bretonneau et ses correspondants* (Paris, 1892). From these letters we learn that as early as 1818 he pointed out to his students the characteristic lesions of typhoid fever which were the result of a specific transmissible agent. A clear insight into the character of Bretonneau appears in his letters to Trousseau when the physician of Tours writes that the greatest intrinsic value of a man is "neither what he has, what he knows, nor his talents, it is his character." "Profits are perhaps legitimate for business men, for men of affairs; but I am convinced that they degrade the character of a physician."

The following selection is from Bretonneau's *Traité de la diphthérie*, while the later article on typhoid fever is from the pen of his devoted pupil Trousseau, who sets forth clearly the doctrine of his old chief.

TREATISE ON DIPHTHERIA

First Communications upon the Diphtheric Inflammation, or Pellicular Inflammation of the Mouth, of the Larynx, and the Air Passages*

1. The communication which I have the honor of submitting to the judgment of the Academy, is based on a collection of observations upon special inflammations of the mucous membranes. All of the work tends to prove that many of the inflammatory

* P. Bretonneau, *Des inflammations spéciales du tissu muqueux, et en particular de la diphthérite, ou inflammation pelliculaire*, Paris, Crevot, 1826.

lesions of the mucous membranes, have been confused, also that the variations of the same affection have often been mistaken for different diseases.

2. The inflammations of the mucous membranes show just as varied characteristics as cutaneous inflammations, whose classification has tested the talent of the nosographers. The exudation which accompanies them presents itself some marked differences, sometimes it is a thin fluid, sometimes it consists of mucus variously changed; it is sometimes a coating, which has the whiteness and consistency of caseous material. At other times it is a membraneous substance closely adherent, or indeed, a membraneous film, simply attached. The degree of thickness, hardness, the force of cohesion, color, the elevation of the tissue effected, the indefinite or limited margins of the inflammation furnish a host of other differences, which I will not attempt to describe. I will add only, that certain very frequent combinations of those different pictures, co-exist too constantly with the symptoms of certain diseases for one not to see here, the relationship of cause and effect.

3. Far from entering into these distinctions and insisting upon the difference of the inflammatory processes of the mucous membranes, I undertake now to prove the evidence of facts that scorbutic gangrene of the gums, croup and malignant angina are nothing but a single and identical type of inflammation. These facts which are assembled from numerous researches of pathological anatomy, have been noted and collected, during the course of an epidemic, which raged in Tours from 1818 until 1820, and they have been collected either in the town, with a population of twenty-odd thousand, or at the hospital, where the number of patients varied from one hundred and twenty to four hundred. They are also based upon evidence which has been produced in our day, or observed since the earliest antiquity, and when we compare the ideas of our moderns with those which have been transmitted by the ancients, we can explain the certain anomalies and disagreement.

4. It will be a difficult enterprise, especially, for a physician, to prove that the croup is nothing else than the last stage of malignant angina, that malignant or gangrenous angina is not gangrenous, that there are no relationships between the abscess and

between the mortification, as superficial as one supposes it, and the changes that follow this disease.

In a very different position it remains to me to carry out a more delicate task. I have not only to demonstrate the nature and identity of these diseases, I ought still to show that the ancients recognized its identity and moreover, they have retraced the observations they had under their eye with great fidelity; that, in a word, they have painted them so that they can be seen without the aid of pathological anatomy, they are such that the illusion of perspective, which must necessarily be found in their pictures, has become to the modern, a source of great errors; errors all the more dangerous because they have been solemnly consecrated by the assent of so many men who are justly celebrated.

But truth to surmount these obstacles only has to show itself. The moment when chance showed it to me, I thought that before making it known, it was my duty to draw attention anew to the observations of facts, to see them, to re-see them, in all of their aspects.

5. Sixty autopsies have been made in the course of the epidemic. If the examination of the viscera, which during life showed no signs of disease, has been occasionally neglected, at least, the state of digestive tract and the air passages have been studied with great care.

6. I am led to carry my researches upon the bodies of those who have shown particularly the characteristic symptoms of croup, or those of malignant angina, either where there was no attempt to arrest the progress of the disease, or when it has been vainly combatted by active and opposing medications. I have been able to follow, in a large number of subjects, the varied modifications of the disease until its perfect cure obtained under the influence of special, general, or local treatment. One hundred and thirty soldiers and twenty individuals, of every age, have shown diverse variations pellicular chronic, or scorbutic gangrene, limited to the mouth, or extending to the larynx and not differing in the latter case from gangrenous angina.

7. In order not to exceed the limits which I have thought advisable to confine myself, I will limit myself in this first part to an examination of each of these affections and to the

discussion of their general characteristics.

In a second communication, historical evidence will be succinctly analyzed and I will show that the results of this comparison do not differ in any respect from those which direct observation has given me; I will add also all I have been able to discern regarding the contagion of the pellicular inflammation, a question which is very important and difficult to solve. The second division of this communication closes with some therapeutic considerations, the principal facts of which will be summarized in the general view of the epidemic which raged in Tours.

TYPHUS FEVER

Typhus fever was apparently first described by Jerome Cardan, although the credit is usually assigned to Fracastor. The clinical description of the latter is unquestionably superior, as Cardan's account seems to have been written for the purpose of ridiculing the methods of diagnosis and treatment employed by rival physicians. Bravo's account of "tabardillo" in Mexico is one of the earliest contributions to medical science from the New World. Tobias Cober wrote a graphic description of the "Hungarian Disease" which raged in the army of the Archduke Rudolf and also noted the abundance of lice in the quarters of the soldiers. Willis' description of the epidemic in the army of the Earl of Essex is referred to by some authors as an epidemic of typhoid fever, but I have followed Murchison in identifying the *febris pestilens* of Willis with typhus fever, and in considering his *febris putrida* as typhoid fever. Lind's contribution to the subject of typhus fever was his demonstration that it could be carried by bedding. It was Gerhard, a young American physician, however, who demonstrated by pathological studies the difference between typhus and typhoid fever. Nicolle only a few years ago discovered what had escaped observation for four centuries—that typhus fever may be transmitted by the body louse. This important discovery has solved some of the problems that perplexed Cardan, Fracastor, and Willis, and would make clear to Lind the necessity of disinfecting the patient's bedding. It explains the mystery of the famous "Black Assizes" in England where the judges after trying prisoners brought up from jail, sickened and died of "jail fever."

Typhoid fever, long confused with other febrile diseases, was first proved to be a disease *sui generis* by Bretonneau. This remarkable man, because of his characteristic caution and utter disregard for the plaudits of the world and questions of priority, wrote nothing on this subject and we know of his discoveries in typhoid fever only through the writings of his pupils. The oft-repeated statement that Roederer and Wagler in their treatise on the *morbus mucosus* described in detail the typical anatomical lesions of typhoid fever, I, like Murchison, have been unable to confirm. Most of their autopsy reports contain extended accounts of intestinal parasites and ulcers in the colon, and usually dismiss the small intestines in a few words.

Jerome Cardan

Jerome Cardan, Italian mathematician, physician, and astrologer, was one of the most important and interesting persons associated with the renaissance of science in Europe. He was born at Pavia in 1501, the illegitimate son of

Fazio Cardano, an eminent physician, jurist, and mathematician. Jerome Cardan became a student in the University of Pavia at the age of nineteen and later removed to Padua, where he was made doctor of medicine at the age of twenty-five.

Cardan then settled in Sacco, a small town near Padua, where he practised his profession, gambled, spent his money freely, and found time to compose three medical treatises on plague, syphilis, and sputum. After three years he went to Milan and sought membership in the College of Physicians but his petition was denied because of his illegitimate birth. For several years he led a wandering life, most unhappy and unsuccessful, and finally returned destitute to Milan, and was lodged with his wife and son in the city poorhouse. He secured, however, the appointment of physician to the Augustinian Friars and succeeded in curing their prior of a skin disease which had baffled the skill of the most distinguished physicians in Milan.

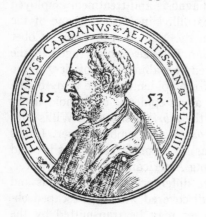

AVTHORIS CARMEN.

*Non me terra teget, cœlo sed raptus in alto
Illustris utiam docta per ora uirûm:
Quicquid uenturis spectabit Phœbus in annis,
Cardanot noscet, nomen & usq; meum.*

JEROME CARDAN (1501-1576)
In his forty-ninth year. Woodcut from *De subtilitate libri* XXI (Basle, 1611)

In 1535 Cardan, who had already written works on geometry, arithmetic, geography, and architecture, determined to write a medical work which might increase his medical reputation. In fifteen days he wrote two books with the title *De malo recentiorum medicorum mendendi usu* (The Bad Practice of Healing among Modern Doctors), a title not especially propitiating or likely to better his standing among his fellow-practitioners. This book was finally published in Venice in 1536. It had a large sale, but received the most violent criticism and condemnation from the doctors in Milan. The book harmed him in almost every respect and as Cardan said, "Where I had looked for honor, I reaped nothing but shame." The book, however, was very clever and contains one of the earliest accounts of typhus fever, which he called *morbus pulicaris* or flea-like disease because the spots resembled flea-bites. This description was published ten years before the more familiar account of Fracastorius.

In 1539, the cure of the child of a Milanese senator brought him renown and from this year his fortune changed. In 1543, he became professor of medicine in Pavia and won fame throughout Europe, from his works on algebra and astrology. He was offered the post of physician to Pope Paul III and to the King of Denmark, but he declined both offers. In 1552, he was called to Edinburgh as the medical adviser of Archbishop Hamilton of St. Andrews. He remained in Scotland for nearly three months and left his patient much improved.

Cardan upon his return to Milan continued to prosper, but in 1562 was suddenly banished by a decree of the senate, the charges not being named. The following year he was called to the University of Bologna, where he soon became a popular teacher and he had the freedom of the city conferred upon him. In 1570, however, Cardan, then a man of almost seventy, was suddenly cast into prison upon the accusation of impiety. He was finally liberated, but prohibited from lecturing or publishing books. Pope Pius V then granted Cardan a pension, so he removed to Rome where he lived until his death in 1576.

Cardan's most interesting career has been told with great charm and interest by Henry Morley whose *Life of Girolamo Cardano of Milan, Physician* (London, 1854), is one of the classics of medical biography. W. G. Waters' *Jerome Cardan* (London, 1898) is also a most interesting and valuable biographical study. Boerhaave's judgment of Cardan was "Sapientior nemo, ubi sapit; dementior nullus, ubi errat." (No one was wiser, when he was wise; nobody was more foolish, when he erred.)

CHAPTER XXXVI*

IN THAT THEY BELIEVE THE MORBUS PULICARIS TO BE MEASLES

The thirty-sixth fatal error is, in that disease, which produces in the body, marks like the bites of fleas. For they seek to call this by the name of measles, we shall call it from its resemblance pulicaris: & although Rhazes says in chapter 8 that blacciae do not have elevations on the skin: & are red in the superficial part of the skin & therefore, this disease is to be regarded as different, moreover he says partly by the authority of Gregory that blacciae is an arid & dry smallpox from which it appears that there is authority on both sides, but there is a difference, because in variola it terminates in pointing & with health, in blacciae, however, neither but it resembles a hot fire, from which it is obvious that the morbus pulicaris, which never is elevated above the skin, cannot have been called blacciae by Rhazes, but that blacciae is measles.

Therefore, they consider the morbus pulicaris to be measles, therefore its treatment necessarily is the same. For the morbus pulicaris is called by the Venetians petechiae, the Milanese also, from this mark. Since the doctors are held fast by this error, an infinite multitude of patients have perished. For they should begin the treatment with nothing of that used in measles, nevertheless

they persist, esteeming that old saying of Hippocrates, making everything secondary to reason, but not resulting from it, nor is it derived from reason: which is obvious from their holding fast to this principle. Hippocrates would by no means wish to persist in these things which work against reason, such as these: for morbus pulicaris is regarded only by a few as not being measles.

Measles are elevated above the skin, from their own nature healing they affect all men, just as small-pox, as Averroës says, is seen on different years, most rarely, & most rarely attacks a man more than once, seldom has mild symptoms, except in boys, and is seen in certain adolescents, is not associated with bubonic plague.

Morbus pulicaris is wholly without elevations, and only spots on the skin are present, in its nature deadly, neither attacking half of the human race: it rages at certain times not during single years, in a vigorous manner, frequently moreover malignant it attacks the same person twice or thrice and four times with the most severe symptoms, infecting all ages even to extreme old age, with the familiar buboes of the plague and rarely these are lacking.

Indeed there may have been some old woman, who clung steadfastly to her opinion, who did not distinguish them, whose treatment in opposite diseases did not pro-

* Cardan, Jerome, *De malo recentiorum medicorum medendi usu*, Venice, Scotus, 1536, p. 44.

duce different results, they obstinately drank concoctions to the point of bursting, as is wont to be done in small-pox & measles: in morbus pulicaris the spots may be the only sign, nothing is excreted from them, this on the other hand is not the sign of measles alone, for it contains some noxious material, which therefore should be expelled.

Now also you should consider me to have separated blacciae from measles, and especially, as one who has been able to escape from the bad accounts which have been written.

Therefore in this disease, when it is pestilential & not only epidemic, it has been preferable to administer the treatment which is necessary for plague, applying with this purpose only, whatever may increase in the thinned blood, soothing in nature so the skin, which is the sole refuge to such, it produces sweating the true crisis of this disease. Also do not fail with adjuvants, nor let up with restraints, give aid to the heart and few treated from the beginning will be in peril. Moreover it is clear from this that those who desire water, with no other remedy, should have as much of this drink as healthful, if other things agree.

Hieronymus Fracastorius

DE MORBIS CONTAGIOSIS

Cap. 6. Concerning a Fever which They Call Lenticular or Punctate or Petechial*

And there are other fevers, which are, so to say, mid-way between true pestilences & diseases not pestilential, from which many indeed perish, many however recover; & for that reason many think them of a pestilential nature; however, they are usually called malignant rather than pestilent: such were those which in the years 1505 & 1528 first appeared in Italy, not formerly known to our generation, although in certain neighboring regions, as in Cyprus, & in neighboring Islands, it was known to our ancestors: it was called "lenticulae" or "puncticulae," it produced lenticular spots or spots like the bites of fleas: indeed by changing the letters, they say petechia; with which we now have to earnestly occupy ourselves, & now also they are seen close together, generally numerous, particularly also by nature spreading: for it is seen in those who go from Italy to other countries, where the same fevers were not present, from which moreover they perished as if they had carried the infection with them, which happened to the most excellent & learned gentleman Andrea Naugerio ambassador of the most Serene Venetian Republic to Francis King of France in the year of grace, 1529.

For, from this illness he died in that country, in which indeed not by name any illness of this kind was known, a man of such learning & ingenuity, and no greater loss to letters

has happened for many years. For that man was not only versed by nature in the best learning, but in many and great things; in managing affairs for the advantage and well being of his country. For it was a most difficult time for the affairs of state, all Europe everywhere was at war. . . . But now we shall return to the lenticular or petechial fever.

This fever, therefore, is contagious, but not rapidly, nor by fomites & from the distance, but only by the handling of the sick: before the onset, moreover all pestilential fevers are still good & mild, then besides it commences slowly, so that the sick hardly wish to have a doctor, & also most of the physicians are at first deceived, expecting resolution of the disease a little later, and not contriving anything against it: indeed soon the signs of a malignant fever are revealed: for although the heat seems mild for the nature of this fever, however inside the commotion takes possession, & now weakness in the whole body and lassitude, fatigued by nature: decubitus appears on the back, the head becomes heavy, senses are drowsy & the mind for the most part, after the fourth or seventh days, not clear, the eyes redden, many words are spoken, the urine at first pale and very much excreted also enough, soon afterwards red & cloudy, like the urine granatorum: pulse slow & small as we say: the excrementa corrupt, foetid: about the fourth and seventh day red spots on the arms, back & breast, &

*Hieronymus Fracastorius Veronensis *Opera Omnia*, Venice, 1584, p. 77-78.

often they break out red like the bites of fleas, often large, resemble freckles, from which the name was given: thirst either little or none, the tongue grows filthy, somnolence comes to some, wakefulness to others, sometimes in one day by turns: this condition in some until the seventh, others until the fourteenth, others beyond that: the urine in some was suppressed, which was a very bad sign: women were not commonly affected, old people most uncommonly, almost none of the Jews perished, but many youth and boys, & indeed the nobles who on the contrary escaped true pestilences, which attacked mainly the common people, these fevers were now seen to spread mostly among the nobles. Certain signs precede dying, just as recovery: it is bad if the patient immediately feels himself deficient in strength, if by the taking of a mild medicine were followed by an intense purging of the abdomen, if improvement does not follow the crisis, for we have seen in them three pints of blood burst forth from the nose, and shortly afterwards die: moreover it is bad if the urine be suppressed, if the spots disappear, if they scarcely erupt, if they are livid and intensely purplish red: wherefore if either all or many are afflicted with such signs, death most certainly follows, escape indeed, if opposite things appear to either all or many.

Francisco Bravo

Francisco Bravo, a physician of the sixteenth century was born at Osuma, Spain. He studied medicine in his native city and later went to Mexico, where he practiced.

His best known work, *Opera medicinalia in quibus quam plurima extant scitu medico necessaria in IV libros digesta quae pagina versa continentur, etc.*, was published in the city of Mexico, in 1570, and was one of the earliest medical publications in the New World.

*If indeed, we are conscious of our skill, by which things become known first to the senses, we investigate: and proceeding from those things perceptible to the hand we are moved to a consideration of the internal appearances of diseases: which principle therefore, is used by us, for without it, we would not now have the slightest knowledge of disease. The method therefore, and the manner of invasion is as follows: a fairly intense fever frequently attacks those affected by this malady, which lasts many days without any intermission; with the greatest fullness and distension of the veins, with the most intense severe lassitude of the entire body, and with pains, especially in the head, in which they suffer the most severe heaviness and pain, and most frequently with dizziness or symptoms of coma and delirium, with extreme redness of the face, with the mouth swollen and of a red color, with a large, forceful, fast and hard pulse, with uneasiness of the heart, with inexplicable thirst, and much dryness and harshness of the tongue, and blackness produced by the humors, and heaviness in the temples, and most intense heat of the entire body: so that they seem to be consumed: and it comes from these above mentioned troubles, and difficulty in breathing: in this disease all these vexing accidents happen, so that on the first day, or the second, or the third, or the fifth, or the seventh, and so on the other days, there break out on the entire skin of the body, spots (pustulae) similar to flea-bites, at first red or livid, or showing a black color when the intensity and severity of the complications are most severe.

* Bravo, Francisco, *Opera Medicinalia,* City of Mexico, 1570. Citation from *Historia bibliográfica de la medicina española* de Don Antonio Hernandez Morejon, Madrid, 1843, III, 166.

Tobias Cober

Tobias Cober, born at Görlitz, studied at the University of Helmstadt where he gained distinction through his Latin comedy "Hospitia" and was crowned poet laureate in 1594. In 1595 he entered the imperial army of Rudolf II, Archduke of Austria, and took part in the campaign against the Turks in Hungary. While serving in the army he collected the material for his most important work, *Observationum medicarum castrensium Hungaricarum decades tres* (Three Decades of Medical Observations in Hungarian Camps),

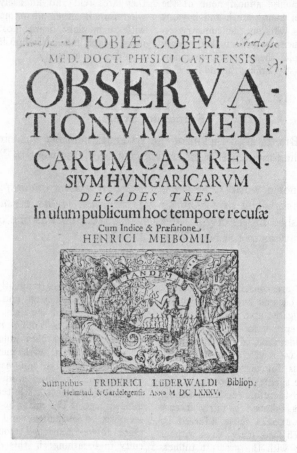

Frontispiece of Cober's *Observationum Medicarum*
Helmstad 1685

first published at Frankfurt in 1606. In this work he describes the notorious Hungarian disease, obviously typhus fever, and notes the prevalence of lice in the infected army camps. Cober describes with harrowing and graphic detail the ravages of disease in the army camps as well as the bestiality and cruelty of the soldiers. He states that the presence of petechiae is necessary for the diagnosis of the Hungarian disease, describes the weakness, mental confusion and fever accompanying the disease but believed it was due largely to eating poorly cooked meat and drinking bad water. He frequently calls the Hungarian disease: the Pannonian languor (Pannonia being the ancient Roman name of a province which included Hungary). After serving for seven years as an army surgeon, he became a physician in Hungary where he died in 1625. His name is often written Kober and in some biographical sketches he is described as Thomas Kober.

OBSERVATIO UNGARICA*

Before we study the Pannonian languor we should first once and for all, place a clear definition of it before our eyes. Therefore the Pannonian languor is a disposition to disease from six things contrary to nature, either from moving about, or from injurious exercise & abuse, disposing a man at first to indifferent health then by neglect of himself gradually causing death. Now among the authors who have described in their writings the terrible languor of the Pannonian pestilence, not the least is Thomas Jordan, who, in the treatise Phenomenon of the plague Chapter 19, while working as an army doctor in an unfortunate expedition during the year 1566, described indeed briefly, yet learnedly, the fury of this deadly disease. Also, among those who have attacked the subject quite happily in the idiom of their country, the least was not Coradinus, whose work, I think, a Doctor departing for the army should consult. But above all, I advise consulting the most learned and on all counts the perfect work of the eminent Doctor Octavianus Roberta Tridentinus on Petechial Diseases, for Petechiae are to be regarded, almost as if by law, a concurrent symptom of the Pannonian languor. Among the Hungarians I saw no other composition on this grave pestilence although I have carefully inquired of the chief of Lower Hungary.

Yet the inhabitants consider it their own particular Pannonian plague, calling it Tschemmerle in their language and think it can be promptly eradicated by violent, almost excoriating massage of the limbs with garlic, and peppery vinegar. By employing this method done to cause healing, a few are injured by the Pannonian plague, fewer still are forced to take to their beds and an extremely small number perish. And indeed I should allow three very acid things, pepper

certainly, garlic and vinegar with a strong odor, which should be stronger from long rubbing and putrid fogs can always be removed from the brain in this distemper. However I have found that these severe treatments in people other than the Hungarians, more often harm than help.

When among many others the generous Lord Stardnitzsky, a noble Pole, leader of the Cossack horsemen, in the year 1599 made intemperate use of massage while he lived upon various edibles, aromatic seasonings & wine. He fell into an acute, dangerous fever shortly after massage, and was so extremely ill that he did not regain his health for a long time. The same may be said of the others, more than a thousand, so I asserted before all that this harsh treatment is as injurious to strangers & less hardy persons as the Hungarian disease itself.

I firmly maintain also that the Pannonian languor arrived as a stranger in the countries of Europe except Hungary, together with other peculiar, indeed heterogenous diseases. And I assert this, that the virus spreads first only in the Pannonian air, heavy itself & dense with the soot of pines, then to the lungs, accustomed to a purer air and to the brain inflamed with poisonous spirits which is the center and seat of the Hungarian disease, and can produce this languor itself. The languor is not of itself a disease. In the beginning, the usual movements of the body are certainly not confused, but gradually disturbances of function appear.

* * *

And I say especially to those of us who understand, and are familiar with the Hungarian languor in the camps, that it, no less than the English sweating sickness & the French disease has lost much of its former severity. Yet at first (and not of the year 1566 when a violent plague like a madness spread everywhere) but from the years 1593 to 96 contagion with atrocious carnage raged everywhere. For they are accustomed

* Cober, Tobias, *Observationum Medicarum Castrensium Hungaricarum decades tres*, Helmstad & Gardelegen, Lüderwald, 1685, pp. 30, 32, 48.

to these bestial ragings of diseases so that continued violence cannot tame nor soften it: moreover because of wars and an unusual series of them lasting beyond ten years, this disease certainly became familiar to the soldiers, I should have added. And if a few of the recruits especially in the first year usually were immune by avoiding the air breathed out from this plague, and by no means in particularly good health, and suffering too many injuries they became quite ill, more often languid, then they soon evaded the fates. Now the gluttony & intemperance of the soldiers, who follow the Hungarians continually is more dangerous to us than any Turk, since very many trade harm for Hungarian delicacies. For among the delights are the flesh of beef, with most crass juices and not living far from sluggish rivers, the flesh of haughty fish boiled just so, which are taken often from the overflowing lakes of Istina, or from the muddy banks of the Danube itself: we say nothing of the seasonal fruits and with the dregs of the wines. No member is affected by all these things at first than the stomach itself, & by which the orifice of the stomach under the sternum is exhausted and torn, who may not perceive.

* * *

And these words concerning the Pannonian languor excited by the eating of meat, badly prepared, should be sufficient, so we take up next the same malady brought on by drinking the marshy Hungarian water.

* * *

There is something peculiar to camps and seen almost nowhere else, since nowhere is a greater collection of bile heaped up in a most sudden display of anger. Many causes may be given for this, no one perhaps really knows, but we can study the causes in turn. For to tell the truth, during the first years the military discipline imparts a harshness to both mind and body, which I think gradually causes a congestion of bile and chyme. I should myself certainly think it would increase when the soldier had been fighting continually with the army all day and night in so many different places. I detested with my whole soul, the madness of this unaccustomed existence, so little congenial to my profession. I was irritated myself at this, since the heat of this ebullient material bore with it a mixture of predisposing factors to

disease, but on reflection, I controlled myself for the sake of the men and also because I feared, and not in vain or without reason, diseases most certain to follow.

When before this, many of our sick with the same ghosts of the furies, were seized with the most severe diseases, and I heard them struggling, I dared scarcely hope they would survive without harm. In addition, monstrous and inhuman barbarities spread through the camp, almost daily many were carried off to the gallows, decapitated, affixed on piles, stabbed with hooks, everywhere one saw the flash of lances and swords, the ears by day were assailed with the sounds of torment. The nostrils were poisoned by fetor and filth, the taste was exposed to all the ills of frequent changes of diet, in quantity most abundant, then scarce, then mediocre, variable. Touch, the most expert index of the whole body, of all the senses, was seen to endure the miseries. One would think they had suffered not so much from laying down on the hard ground, deserted, exposed to rains, extreme lasting cold as well, as from little beasts by day and by night, not only minute but troublesome, which gather on the hands and wait ready for action. Among these are fleas, called Goltzschen. the vilest of the insects and most annoying with their bites, who especially at night in summer, attack all parts of the body. They bore through with their murderous stings, disfiguring often many faces with reddish swellings. How dangerous, although invisible the bites of these vipers may be, no one unless expert would have believed. I know this, for certain, that from their cries and imprecations the enraged soldiers curse this pest usually above everything else. Added to these are pediculi, most loathsome and so nauseous that they are scarcely worthy of a name, who contribute to the accumulation of bile by their continuous crawling about and sucking. Indeed in vain, especially in the first years, you will flee from the stabs of these pests, for with right, they celebrate as if citizens of the camps. Moreover the warmth, softness and thickness of the air is so great, that if you expose the water from washed linen, especially when stagnant, to the drying action of the sun, you will see it all full of worms. Therefore you could not, hope to prevent these future collections and assemblages in the future or even if they were easily generated from the body itself. I thought at first it was possible to avoid these pests by always dressing with fresh linen, but this I have proved, of itself attracts many of them much less destroying them. And so this production of lice by the Egyptian magicians, in olden times considered impossible, I achieved in these places with all possible ease, and this I have known from experience can cause a great deal of bile to collect.

Thomas Willis

CHAP. XIV

Of Pestilential and Malignant Feavers in specie, and of others Epidemical†

After having unfolded the Nature of the Plague, by the order of our Tract, we ought to proceed to the Diseases, which seem to be nearest like its Nature; which chiefly are Feavers, called Pestilent and Malignant; for tis commonly noted, that Feavers sometimes reign popularly, which for the vehemency of symptoms, the great slaughter of the sick, and the great force of contagion, scarce give place to the Pestilence, which however, because they imitate the type of Putrid Feavers, and do not so certainly kill the sick as the Plague, or so certainly infect others, they deserve the name not of the Plague, but by a more minute appellation of a Pestilential Feaver: Besides these, there are Feavers of another kind, the perniciousness and Contagion of which appear more remiss, yet, because they are infectious, beyond the force of Putrid Feavers, and seem to contain in themselves in a manner, the Τὸ Θεῖον or hand of God of Hippocrates, are yet by a more soft appellation, called Malignant Feavers.

Those Feavers differ both from the Pest, and from one another according to the degree, and vehemency of contagion and deadlyness; as the Plague is a Disease highly contagious, and deadly to human kind; tis the Pestilent Feaver, which commonly spreads with a lesser diffusion of its infection, and frequency of burials. When the infection is only suspected, and the Crisis happens beyond the event of vulgar Feavers, only not to be trusted or less safe, tis esteemed for a Malignant Feaver. They are yet more fully described thus.

When the Feaver commonly spreads abroad, which for the variety of symptoms, puts on the likeness of the Putrid Feaver so called, to wit, when there are present, Thirst, Burning, Weariness, Anxiety, roughness of the Tongue, Watchings, Phrensie, Vomiting, want of Appetite, Syncopy, Swooning, Heartpains and a concourse of other most terrible accidents if there happen besides, spots either like the little Flea-bites, or broad ones like black and blew strokes, and livid, we esteem this disease of an evil Nature.

* * *

The pestilent Feaver of late years, hath more rarely spread in these Regions, than the Plague itself: of the only one of this kind, which fell under our observation, I will give you a brief description. In the year 1643, when in the coming on of the Spring, the Earl of *Essex* besieged *Reading*, being held for the King, in both Armies there began a Disease to arise very Epidemical; however, they persisting in that work, till the besieged were forced to a surrender, this Disease grew so grievous, that in a short time after, either side left off, and from that time, for many months, fought not with the Enemy, but with the Disease; as if there had not been leisure to turn aside to another kind of Death, this deadly disease increasing, they being already overthrown by Fate, and as it were falling down before this one Death. *Essexe's* Camp moving to the *Thames,* pitched in the places adjacent, where he shortly lost a great part of his men: But the King returned to *Oxford,* where at first, the Souldiers being disposed in the open Fields, then afterwards among the Towns and Villages suffered not much less: For his Foot, (which it chiefly invaded) being pact together in close houses, when they had filled all things with filthiness, and unwholsom nastiness, and stinking odors (that

† Willis, Thomas, *Practice of physick,* London, Basset, 1684, p. 131.

the very air seemed to be infected) they fell sick by Troops and as it were by Squadrons. At length the Feaver now more than a Camp Feaver invaded the unarmed and peacable Troops, to wit, the entertainers of the Souldiers, and generally all others, yet at first (the Disease being yet but lightly inflicted) tho beset with a heavy and long languishment, however, many escaped. About the Summer Solstice this Feaver began also to increase with the worse provision of Symptoms, and to lay hold on the Husbandmen, and others inhabiting the Country. Then afterwards, spread through our City and all the Country round, for at least Ten miles about. In the mean time they who dwelt far from us, in other Countries remained free from hurt, being as it were without the sphere of the Contagion. But here this Disease became so Epidemical that a great part of the people was killed by it; and as soon as it had entered an house, it run through the same, that there was scarce one left well to administer to the sick, strangers, or such as were sent for to help the sick, were presently taken with the Disease, that at length for fear of the Contagion, those who were sick of this Feaver, were avoided by those who were well, almost as much, as if they had been sick of the Plague.

Nor indeed did there a less mortality, or slaughter of men, accompany this Disease: because Cachectic, and Pthisical old men, or otherways unhealthful, were killed by it; also not a few of Children, young men, and those of a more mature and robust age. I remember in some Villages, that almost all the old men dyed this year, that there were scarce any left, who were able to defend the manners and priviledges of the Parish, by the more anciently received Traditions.

When this Feaver first began, it was something like the figure of a putrid Synochus; but it was harder to be cured and when it seemed to be helped by a sweat or looseness, presently it was wont to be renewed again: but for the most part, after the deflagration of the Blood, continued for six or seven days, this remitting, and instead of a Crisis the adust matter being translated to the Brain, the sick for a long time keeping their Beds with raging somtimes, but more often with a stupefaction, with great weakness, and somtimes with Convulsive motions, scarcely escaped at last. About the middle of the Summer, besides the Contagion and frequent burials, this Disease betrayed its malignity, and pestilential force in open signs, *viz.* By the eruption of the Whelks and Spots: because about this time in many there appeared without any great burning of the Feaver, an unequal, weak and very much disordered pulse; also without a manifest expense of Spirits, their strength presently became languishing, and very much dejected: In others, sick after the same manner, appeared little Blisters or Measles, now small and red, now broad and livid: in many Buboes (as in the Plague) about the glandulas: of these some died silently and unforeseen, without any great strugling of the Spirits, or Feaverish burning excited in the Blood: in the mean time others, by and by becoming furibundous, whilst they lived suffered most horrid distractions of the animal Spirits. Those about to escape from this Disease, without any laudible Crisis, (unless they were the sooner freed by a sweat provoked by Art) the Brain, and nervous stock becoming distempered, at length, with a benummedness of the senses, trembling, vertigo, debility of the members, and Convulsive motions, did not grow well, but of a long time after. During the Dog-days, this Disease being still infectious, began to be handled not as a Feaver, but as a lesser Plague, and to be overcome only by Poyson-resisting Remedies, letting of Blood was believed to be fatal to this: Vomits and Purges, sometimes tho not often, were made use of, but the chiefest means of Cure, were accounted to be produced by Alexiteriums, and timely sweat. For this end, besides the prescripts of Physicians, to be had at the Apothecaries, some Emperical Remedies deserved no small praise; then first of all, the pouder of the Countess of *Kent*, began to be of great esteem in this Country; also of no less note was another prouder, of the colour of Ashes, which a certain Courtier staying by chance in this City, gave to many with good success; and to others approving of the use of it, he sold it at a great price; the sick were wont having taken half a dram of this, in any Liquor, to fall into a most plentiful sweat, and so to be freed from the virulency of the Disease. That Diaphoretick (whose preparation I afterwards learnt from the Cousen German of the Author) was only the pouder of Toads, purged thoroughly with Salt, and then washed in the best Wine, and lightly calcined in an earthern Pot. The Autumn coming on, this Disease by degrees remitted its wonted fierceness that fewer grew sick of it and of them many grew well; till the approach of the Winter, when this Feaver almost wholly vanished, and health was rendred to this City and the Country round about fully and wholly.

Thus you have seen from the beginning, progress, and end of this Feaver, at first only a Camp Feaver, but at length became Pestilential, and Epidemical. That at first the Disease began in the Souldiers Camp, may seem to be imputed, not only to their nastiness and stinking smells, but in some sort to a common vice of the Air, for as these Feavers come not every year, their original may be ascribed, partly to the peculiar Constitution of the year. Because, by that means, a more light intemperance of the Air being contracted, tho it did not affect the more healthful Inhabitants, yet in the Army, where evident causes, *viz.* errors in the six non-naturals, very much happen to the general procatartic cause, there is a necessity for these kind of sicknesses easily to be excited. For the constitution of this year, was in the Spring very moist, and slabbery, almost with continual shours, to which a more hot Summer succeeding, and the infection of the Feaverish Contagion here first increasing, still grew worse, and disposed all Bodies the more for the receiving it; wherefore, that this Disease was almost proper to this Region, and at this time Epi-

demical, the seed of it ought to be ascribed to its first rising from the Army, being quartered round about. But forasmuch as it afterwards being made Pestilential, and very Epidemical, it infected most of the people living here, and killed not a few, the reason was, the evil affection of the Air, which because of the intemperance of the year being unwholsom, besides by the continual breathing forth of stinking vapours from the Souldiers Camps, and the quarters of the sick, it became at last so vitious, that the infection of the feaver being dispersed in it, was greatly exalted, and arose almost to the virulency of the Plague. *Diemerbrochius* relates from the like Camp Feaver, arising in the summer at *Spires,* afterwards another Malignant and Pestilential and then the Plague it self to have accrewed. Also, it was a sign that this Feaver of ours, became at last equal to the Plague it self besides the great force of the Contagion and the frequency of Burials, most wicked distempers of the Blood and nervous Liquor, being brought presently upon all by it: because strength being suddenly overthrown the weak intermitting pulse, the creeping forth of measly Blisters, the eruption of Buboes, argued the Coagulation and corruptive disposition of the Blood; besides the Delirium, Madness, Phrensie, Stupefaction, Sleepiness, Vertigo, Tremblings, Convulsive motions and divers other distempers of the Head, shewed the great hurt of the Brain and nervous stock.

James Lind

SECT. II

OF THE JAIL DISTEMPER*

Origin of the Jail Infection unknown; its Source; is diffused by air as a vehicle; its properties in common with the plague and Small-pox; Small distance to which its influence extends; its Self-extinction; method of destroying it in infected places and Substances.

THE *origin* of the jail infection is a point at present entirely unknown. No person has

given us the least satisfactory account how, or where, it is generated. It does not seem to originate in air, and there are many prisons abounding with filth and impurities, perfectly free from it.

In ships also an infection is generally imported from the land, and many, that have been long in a very dirty condition at sea, bring their men quite healthy into the harbours. Indeed I have always observed, that the most healthy ships were such as arrived from a long foreign voyage, the scurvy being the chief, and almost the only complain

* Lind, James, *Essay on the means of preserving the health of seamen,* London, Wilson, 1774, p. 315.

among them; whereas, ships of war, especially when fitted out in the *Thames,* even in times of peace, very often received this infection from *London.*

The clearest idea we can conceive of the manner in which this infection is *communicated* is to suppose there is in all infected places, adhering to certain substances, an envenomed *nidus,* or source of effluvia, corpuscules, or of whatsoever infection may be supposed to consist; and that the *air* according as it is more or less confined, becomes more or less strongly impregnated with them. In this respect, the jail distemper, the plague and small-pox are similar; though the air be the *vehicle* of the infection, by which they are severally communicated, yet none of these infections can be said properly to *reside* in air, but are occasionally sent into it, from substances in which they reside; such becoming always more highly infectious in a close confined place: by confinement in infected cloaths, the infection is *multiplied,* and acts with far greater virulence than when immediately transmitted from the *naked* body. Let us view, in proof of this, the different conditions of ships loaded with men and women, where the passengers are *covered* with tainted rages, and where they are almost entirely *naked.* An example of the former we have in the great mortality from the jail distemper usual in ships carrying *Felons* to *America,* a circumstance universally known and from whence our colonies have frequently suffered by infection: also in the *Dutch,* who are said to send annually 2000 soldiers to *Batavia,* and to lose three fourths of them by the ship fever before they arrive.

To these let us oppose the condition of the poor Negroes, who, in amazing numbers, are yearly shipped from *Guinea* to all the European settlements in America. The *Guinea* ships frequently carry double, or triple the number of either our transport, or the *Dutch East-India* ships, and the poor wretches are crowded together, below the deck, as close as they possibly can lie, with only small separation between the men and women; every night they are shut up under close hatches, in a sultry climate, barred down with iron to prevent an insurrection. They had no bed to lie upon, and scarce any cloaths to cover them; the children, both boys and girls, until a certain age, go quite naked and even the

grown negroes have, for the most part, only a wrapper about their middle. They thus wear nothing capable of *imbibing* or *retaining* infection; and although some have been suffocated by the close confinement, or foul air, though they are subject to the flux, and suffer from a change of climate, yet an infection is scarce among them, cr if any accidental fever, occurring from the change of climate, should become infectious, it is generally much more mild than in the opposite situation, where polluted rags afford it a prompt* receptacle, and prove a constant source of fresh infection. In several other respects, also, besides that of being conveyed by rags and tainted substances, the infection of the jail distemper *agrees* with that of the plague; in common with it, this infection extends to no great distance from its source and is often extinguished without any evident cause.

First. This infection *extends* itself at no great distance; the houses in the neighbourhood of an infected prison, are in no danger of infection from it, provided all communication be cut off.

In the open free air, this infection does not appear to diffuse itself above fifty or sixty

---

* A whole Indian Nation in *Nova Scotia* was not long since almost entirely destroyed by some infected blankets and cloaths. In the year 1746, while the *French* squadrons, under the command of the Duc d'Anville, passed the summer at *Chebucto,* now *Hallifax,* an infectious fever prevailed among them, and cut off a great number of their men. On the return of the squadron to *Europe,* several blankets and old cloaths, which had been used in their tents and hospitals, were unfortunately left behind. These fatal receptacles of disease were soon after eagerly picked up by a party of *Mimack* Indians, who accidentally came to visit the place, and who cloathed themselves with some of them; others they carried home and distributed among their tribe. The unhappy consequence of which was the almost total extinction of the *Mimack* nation; scarce any of them survived. The *English,* upon traveling the country next summer from *Anapolis Royal,* were surprised with finding the dead bodies and skeletons of whole families of that nation lying unburied in their huts, until the neutrals, who also inhabited that country, and the neighbouring Indians informed them, that the Mimacks had been cut off by the *French* blankets. In several of their huts these blankets were found, where not one of the family remained.

This account was given me by a gentleman of veracity, who from being upon the spot, had an opportunity of knowing the circumstances.

feet from its *Nidus;* though even at that distance, a person might run some risque from being exposed to a current of air highly impregnated with the contagion which issued immediately from a door or window, where it had been long pent up.

Secondly. This infection, after every method used to destroy it has proved ineffectual, will often of itself gradually *abate,* and at length entirely *vanish;* this circumstance I often observed in our prisons during the last war, where, after ommitting great ravages among the French prisoners, the infection often stopped of a sudden; and they were sometimes so entirely free from it, that in the month of September, 1762, when I was employed by the Government to muster the prisoners of war in the castles of *Portchester* and *Winchester,* which in the preceding year had suffered much by the jail distemper, I did not find one person labouring under that distemper among 7000 prisoners, many of whom had been confined for several years. But, as this infection often proves highly destructive before the period of self-extinction, it is a satisfaction to know, that in whatever substance, chamber, or prison it is lodged, it may at any time be effectually *destroyed* by the force of *fire.*

1. That a *great* heat, like that of an oven, such as would prove destructive to all animal life, effectually destroys this infection in all substances which can be for some time exposed to it.

2. That an *inferior* degree of heat, in which a man can breathe, will ofen *fail* of destroying it.

Hence the infection may *with certainty* be destroyed in any ship, prison, or situation where the *people* can be *removed,* so that fires may be lighted, and the smoak confined with safety. But in prisons, ships, or places, where the people cannot be removed, and consequently a *sufficient* degree of heat cannot be raised, the application of fire and smoke to remove infection, may prove *ineffectual.* I am confirmed in this assertion by repeated instances of infection in ships both at sea and when lying at Spithead, where every method failed of putting a stop to it as long as the men remained on board. A certain method therefore of destroying infection, in places from whence persons cannot be removed, is a *Desideratum* not yet obtained in physic. I have proposed without success. However, these have been instances of large fires made in ships proving highly serviceable on such occasions, both at sea and in harbours, even while the men continued on board.

William Wood Gerhard

Paris was the medical Mecca of the world in the early years of the nineteenth century and attracted many students from the New World. Among the American students who made this pilgrimage and later achieved great distinction in medicine was William Wood Gerhard. Gerhard was born in Philadelphia in 1805, went to Dickinson College, and then graduated in medicine at the University of Pennsylvania in 1831. Soon after graduation he proceeded to Paris and studied with Louis at *la Pitié.* Louis' influence on American medicine has been described by Osler (*Bull. Johns Hopkins Hosp.* [1897], VII, 161), who remarks that "Wm. W. Gerhard was the most distinguished of the American pupils in Paris between 1830 and 1840." Louis produced a very profound impression upon the young American physician who wrote, "he is a remarkable man, very different from the physicians of England or America, and remarkable even at Paris by the strict mathematical accuracy with which he arrives at his results." While in Paris, Gerhard collected material from which he published important papers on Asiatic cholera, smallpox, tuberculosis, meningitis, and pneumonia in children.

Gerhard returned to Philadelphia in 1832 and became resident physician to the Pennsylvania Hospital. Soon afterwards he demonstrated that the common continued fever in Philadelphia was identical with the typhoid he had seen in Paris, and in 1836 he studied an epidemic of typhus fever which he found to be an entirely different disease. In 1837, he published epochal papers in the *American Journal of Medical Sciences,* pointing out the differences between typhoid fever and typhus fever, "the first in any language which give a full and satisfactory account of the clinical and anatomical distinctions we now recognize." (Waterson)

Gerhard had great success as a lecturer at the Philadelphia Hospital. Stewardson, a fellow-student at Paris wrote, "As a clinical teacher he was remarkably successful and exerted a powerful and commanding influence. . . . Without any pretension to eloquence, he nevertheless riveted the attention of his hearers and stimulated their enthusiasm. Himself deeply interested in his subject, he communicated this interest to his audience by the sheer force of truth. . . . Students saw that truth was his object, not display." Gerhard retired from practice in 1868 and died in Philadelphia in 1872. His work on typhoid and typhus has assured him of a permanent niche in the annals of medical history.

ART. I. ON THE TYPHUS FEVER, WHICH OCCURRED AT PHILADELPHIA IN THE SPRING AND SUMMER OF 1836; ILLUSTRATED BY CLINICAL OBSERVATIONS AT THE PHILADELPHIA HOSPITAL; SHOWING THE DISTINCTION BETWEEN THIS FORM OF DISEASE AND DOTHINENTERITIS OR THE TYPHOID FEVER WITH ALTERATION OF THE FOLLICLES OF THE SMALL INTESTINE. By W. W. Gerhard, M.D., one of the Physicians of the Hospital.*

During a residence of two or three years at Paris, I had studied with great care the pathology and treatment of the disease usually termed, in the French hospitals, typhoid fever or typhoid affection. There is another designation for it, founded on its anatomical characters, and therefore more in accordance with modern medical nomenclature; it is dothinenteritis. This variety of fever which is identical with the disease termed typhus mitior or nervous fever, is frequent at Paris, and is almost the only fever which can be said to be endemic there. Intermittent and remittent fevers are rarely seen, except amongst those individuals who had already contracted some form of these diseases in the malarious districts of France. Some slight fevers, attended with a whitish or yellow tongue and gastric symptoms, occasionally occur; they scarcely assume the form of a fixed disease, and usually disappear under a very simple treatment.

These fevers were the only ones known at Paris for some years past; but in 1813-14 there occurred a severe epidemic fever, char-

acterized by extreme prostration and strongly marked cerebral symptoms. This epidemic was first noticed amongst the troops who returned from Napoleon's unsuccessful campaigns in Germany and the east of France; it afterwards spread amongst the inhabitants of Paris and other large cities, and was every where extremely fatal. No accurate description of this fever is on record, although it was witnessed by several of the most distinguished French physicians. Some of these, more especially Louis and Chomel, are inclined to consider it as identical with the prevailing dothinenteritis, but their opinion is probably erroneous, and the disease, as far as we know, should be classed amongst the forms of continued fever, distinguished by the terms typhus, typhus gravior, petechial or spotted fever, &c.

There, are, however, complete histories of the typhoid fever or typhoid affection, or dothinenteritis, (all names belonging to one disease). It is one of the most frequent and the most severe acute affections observed at Paris, and has been studied with extreme accuracy, more especially by Louis and Chomel, who have both published admirable

*Am. J. M. Sc., 1837, XIX, pp. 289-292; 298-299; 302-303.

descriptions of it. The work of Dr. Louis is especially interesting, and is a model in its kind; he has analyzed the symptoms and pathological phenomena of the fever so accurately and fully, as to surpass any other description of individual diseases. The typhoid fever was placed by this work of Dr. Louis, in the same relation to other fevers that pneumonia holds in reference to the affections of the chest. They are both so well studied, and their symptoms are so well known, that they can serve as types with which other less thoroughly understood affections may be compared.

It affords us, then, great advantages in the investigation of the history of fevers, to begin with the typhoid, as the best known of these affections. Assuming this disease as the basis of our investigations, one great point is gained, and much greater certainty can be given to our ulterior researches, if we compare the symptoms of any fever which is little known and imperfectly described, with those of the typhoid fever, or dothinenteritis, as it is now frequently called from its anatomical lesion.

This inquiry was in accordance with a desire which I had long cherished of investigating the most common fevers in the middle states of America, where, from our geographical position, we witness the fevers observed at the northern, and occasionally those of the southern states. The commercial relations of Philadelphia are so frequent with the whole southern coast of the United States, and the passage to the north so rapid in the summer and autumnal months, that we receive into our hospitals a considerable number of patients taken ill on the coast of North Carolina, Virginia, and even Alabama and Louisiana. There are, therefore, few places where such a study could be pursued to more advantage than at Philadelphia. During the last three years of a constant connexion with our largest hospitals, either as resident or attending physician, I have not lost sight of this object of study, and I have already published in the *American Journal* for the year 1835, some cases of the dothinenteritis as well as of the remittent and intermittent fevers.

Dothinenteritis is by no means a rare disease at Philadelphia, although less common than at Paris. In the essay alluded to, I established the identity of the anatomical

characters and of the symptoms of the fever, occurring at Philadelphia, with that observed at Paris. I also showed that the patients were chiefly those who had resided but a short time in Philadelphia, and that they were taken ill on ship-board, or under some other circumstances causing an abrupt change of food and habits of life. They were also young persons, but few having passed the age of twenty-five years. Both these conditions of age and change of habit are observed to be essential to the development of typhoid fever at Paris.

Having once established the complete identity of a fever which is so common at Paris and so well described, with a similar affection, not unfrequently met with at Philadelphia, I examined the pathological phenomena of our remittent and intermittent fevers of the severe malignant character so frequently observed along the southern coast, and sometimes occurring in those malarious parts of the country which are situated within a short distance of Philadelphia. In all these fevers, the glands of Peyer as well as the other intestinal follicles, were found perfectly healthy; the large intestine was occasionally but not constantly diseased, while the stomach, and to a still greater degree the liver and spleen were invariably found in a morbid condition. If the fever proved fatal in the course of the first fortnight, the liver and spleen were softened as well as enlarged; but if the disease assumed a more chronic form, the viscera were hardened as well as hypertrophied. The latter state was the first stage of these chronic lesions which are formed in the livers of patients long affected with remittents or intermittents, and which continue throughout the course of the ascites, which is so common a consequence of these diseases. I made numerous examinations of the bodies of patients who died of the same variety of malignant remittent and intermittent during the summer of 1835, and still more frequently in the epidemic of 1836, a year in which these diseases have been unusually fatal throughout the southern states. The results of these late examinations have confirmed those already obtained, and showed that the follicles of the small intestines are free from lesions, and that the anatomical character of the disease is to be looked for in the spleen, liver, and stomach.

The bilious and yellow fevers are probably referrible to the same class as the malignant remittents, but in yellow fever the disorganization seems to be most extensive in the stomach, whence arises the black vomit, which forms a characteristic symptom of the disease. Bilious fever, or, in other words, the remittent fever attended with unusual alteration of the liver and a disordered secretion of bile is common with us. Yellow fever is rare, and occurs in an epidemic form at such long intervals, that I have seen but few cases of it.

The typhus fever, which is so common throughout the British dominions, especially in Ireland, is not attended with ulceration or other lesions of the glands of Peyer. From the account of the lesions presented by most of the writers upon the subject, it would seem that there is no constant anatomical lesion, but that the lungs present traces of disease more frequently than any other organ. My own observation of this variety of fever was limited to the examination of the fever patients under the care of the late Dr. Gregory of the Edinburgh infirmary. This observation was not sufficiently long or accurate to enable me to do more than refer to those physicians who have enjoyed extended facilities for the study of this affection. The lesion of the glands of Peyer is now well known to the British physicians, but an error frequently committed by them is that they regard this affection (dothinenteritis) as a mere complication of their ordinary typhus, or a modified form of it. At least I do not at this moment recollect any one who has clearly stated that the two diseases are always distinct, before the publication of a note in the *Dublin Journal,* by Dr. Lombard of Geneva (Sept. 1836).

* * *

The evidence of contagion at the Philadelphia hospital was more direct and conclusive. Three of the principal nurses, and about a dozen assistant nurses, besides a number of patients ill with various diseases were taken with the fever. The three principal nurses belonged, two to the wards for blacks, where there were the greatest number of fever patients, and the third to a ward for whites, where there were several cases. There was only one nurse of a ward in which many of the patients were collected,

who escaped, but several of his assistants and patients were taken ill. Two of the resident physicians in attendance upon the same ward, where the patients were most numerous, were also severely ill with the fever. On the other hand, no nurse from the part of the hospital where there were but few or no typhus cases, suffered, and the number of patients taken ill in the surgical of lunatic wards was very small, not exceeding six in number. The wards in which fever patients were placed did not contain more than a third or a fourth of the population of the hospital, yet the number of cases originating in them after the first introduction of the disease was at least four times as great as in all the other parts of the building. The Almshouse and house of employment, which are separated from the hospital by a space of at least forty feet at the nearest points, furnished five or six cases, probably not more than the same number of poor in any other part of the neighbourhood would have done

* * *

Pathological Anatomy.—Dr. Pennock and myself examined a very large number of the bodies of those patients who died of the fever. Indeed, during nearly the whole epidemic scarcely a single examination was omitted, excepting in cases where it was impracticable from the removal of the body by the friends, immediately after death, or where putrefaction supervended, as it sometimes did almost immediately after dissolution. In this large number of autopsies, amounting to about fifty, there was but in one case, and that doubtful in its diagnosis, the slightest deviation from the natural appearance of the glands of Peyer. In the case alluded to, in which there had been some diarrhoea, the agglomerated glands of the small intestine were reddened and a little thickened; but there was no ulceration and no thickening or deposit of yellow puriform matter in the submucous tissue. The disease of the glands resembled that sometimes met with in small-pox, scarlet fever or measles, rather than the specific lesion of dothinenteritis. In all other cases, the glands of Peyer were remarkably healthy in this disease, as was the surrounding mucous membrane, which was much more free from vascular inection than it is in cases of various diseases not originally affecting the small intestine.

The mesenteric glands were always found of the normal size, varying, as in health, from the size of a small grain of maize to three or four times these dimensions. With the exception of a slightly livid tint, common to them and rest of the tissues, they offered nothing peculiar either in consistence or colour.

The spleen was of the normal aspect, in one half the cases, in the other half it was softened, but not enlarged, and in one case out of five or six, enlarged and softened.

Thus, the triple lesion of the glands of Peyer, mesenteric glands and spleen, constituting the anatomical characteristic of the dothinenteritis or typhoid fever, although sought for with the greatest care, evidently did not exist in the epidemic typhus. Indeed, it was a subject of remark, that in the typhus fever the intestines were more free from lesion than in any other disease accompanied by a febrile movement. This exemption extended to the large intestine until the summer heats began, when a few scattering cases offered some symptoms of diarrhoea, during the prevalence of an epidemic dysentery; and, where they terminated fataly, softening and other signs of inflammation of the mucous coat of the colon were observed.

The fact that the morbid changes pathognomonic of dothinenteritis, are not met with in the typhus fever, would of itself seem conclusive that the two diseases are no more identical than pneumonia and pleurisy. Although, in some respects, the two affections are analogous, and even similar, the radical difference of anatomical lesions is at least as well marked as the distinction between the symptoms. It is, indeed, singular that there should of late be a strong tendency to confound two fevers, which were regarded as entirely distinct by some of the older physicians. The prominent symptoms and difference of treatment being particularly well pointed out by Huxham.

Charles Nicolle

Charles Nicolle was born in Rouen, France, in 1866 and for nearly ten years, from 1895 until 1903, taught in the medical school of Rouen. In 1903 he was appointed director of the Pasteur Institute of Tunis and succeeded in a very short time in raising this institution to the rank of one of the leading centers of bacteriological research in the world. Many students of tropical medicine, especially those from Russia, Sweden, Italy, Greece, Poland, and America, came to work in the Institute. In order to publish their work and maintain a certain *esprit de corps,* Nicolle founded in 1904 the *Archives de l'Institut Pasteur de Tunis,* which has published much of his own best work as well as that of his associates.

Nicolle's contributions to bacteriology and immunity have been numerous and of great importance. He was the first to show that the serum from convalescent measles patients would protect susceptible individuals against an attack. He extended these observations and demonstrated the same property of the serum of patients convalescent from typhus and undulant fever. He found that grippe is due to a filtrable virus and proved that leishmaniasis is transmitted by the dog flea. His most notable researches, however, have been on typhus fever, observations which have been carried on for nearly a quarter of a century. He found that typhus fever could be transmitted to a chimpanzee by the injection of a small quantity of blood from a patient in the acute stages of the disease, and, in 1909, that typhus fever could be transmitted from monkey to monkey by the bite of the body louse.

Nicolle celebrated in 1928 the twenty-fifth anniversary of his appointment as director of the Pasteur Institute of Tunis. The same year he received the Nobel Prize in medicine. He died in 1936.

EXPERIMENTAL TRANSMISSION OF TYPHUS EXANTHEMATICUS BY THE BODY LOUSE

Note by M. M. CHARLES NICOLLE, C. COMTE and E. CONSEIL, transmitted by M. ROUX.*

Study of the recent epidemics of typhus which have raged in Regency, particularly at Tunis, Metlaoui and Redeyef (phosphate company of Gafsa) and on the Kerkennah Islands, have led us to consider an insect as the probable agent in the transmission of the disease.

Typhus in upper Africa, is a result of crowding and poverty; it rages among the people who are the poorest and the least careful of hygienic rules; it is not contagious in a clean house, or in the wards of a well-kept hospital. Under these conditions, only the parasitical insects of the house, clothing and body can be suspected, lice, fleas and bedbugs. The usual time of appearance of typhus (spring) makes the rôle of mosquitoes, ticks and stomox very improbable.

Many observations have led us to limit our hypothesis to the louse. At the hospital of Tunis, the patients on admission are washed and re-dressed with clean clothing; no case of inside contagion has been observed, notably during the epidemics of 1902 and 1906, in spite of the absence of any isolation and the presence of numerous bedbugs in the wards. The only cases of contagion observed have been among the personnel in charge of receiving and disinfecting the personal effects of those admitted. On the Kerkennah Islands, an epidemic foyer of typhus, bedbugs are rare. In Djerid, where the disease appears as elsewhere, there are no *fleas*. These insects multiply on the contrary in the tunnels of the phosphate mines; they attack there both Europeans and natives, and moreover, the latter alone are affected with typhus. Finally two observations are known to us, where, after the duration of ordinary incubation, typhus followed obviously the bite of a *louse*.

These observations were known to us when one of us succeeded in inoculating a chimpanzee with typhus and after passing it through the chimpanzee to a bonnet-macaque

(*macacus sinicus*). Also since the beginning of our investigations, we have attempted the transmission of the disease from monkey to monkey by means of the *body louse*.

Our experiments have been carried out thus: We placed upon bonnet-macaque I, infected with the blood of the chimpanzee at the 16th day of inoculation and during the hours which followed the appearance of the eruption, 29 lice obtained the day before from a man and kept fasting for 8 hours.

In the morning and on the following days, we placed them upon two bonnet-macaques A and B. Monkey A was bitten for 6 consecutive days by 15, then 12, 13, 8, 6 and 3 lice; and monkeys B 12 days by 14, then 15, 13, 9, 5, 5, 6, 5, 5, 4, 2 and 1 louse. Every day after biting, the lice were mixed and kept at a temperature of 16° to 20°.

The two monkeys, A and B, had been previously employed for some experiments upon kala-azar: both of them had recovered at the time of their inoculation and another important fact was that their temperature had been taken twice daily for 5 months (monkey A) and 1 year (monkey B) and had never shown any elevation of temperature.

Monkey A—Nothing noticeable until the 22nd day of the inoculation. On this date, there was an elevation of temperature to 39.2° and 32.9° then a fall the 23rd and 24th day. Then temperature climbed again on the 25th day and reached or passed 40° the 26th, 27th and 28th day. Slow defervescence from the 30th to 34th day. The 39th day, the temperature rose, relapse for five days with a classical fever curve (maximum 40.5° the 41st day). Death the morning of the 44th day.

The general condition was good until the 30th day; on this date depression, the animal ate less, was easier to seize. No eruption. Extreme agitation during the second febrile period. Violet coloration of the lips the last two days. At autopsy, no lesion except an irregular ulceration of the caecum covered

* *Compt. rend. Acad. d. sc.*, Paris, 1909, CXLIX, 486.

with a diphtheroid exudate.

Monkey B.—Nothing until the 40th day of inoculation. The 41st day, an elevation of temperature corresponding to the second attack of fever in Monkey A. The 44th day, temperature of 40° defervescence from the 46th day and the same day, an eruption. The only symptoms observed were some weakness and less appetite; almost immediate return to health.

These experiments show that it is possible to transmit the typhus of the infected bonnet-macaque to a new monkey, by means of the body louse. The application of this finding to the etiology and the prophylaxis of the disease in man, is important. Measures to combat typhus should have as their aim, a destruction of the parasites; they live principally on the body, linen, clothes and bedclothes of the patients.

TYPHOID FEVER

Thomas Willis

CHAP. IX

*Of a Putrid Feaver**

In this Feaver, four times or seasons are to be observed, in which, as it were so many posts, or spaces, its course is performed: These are then, The Beginning, the Augmentation, the Height, and Declination. These are wont to be finished in some sooner, in others more slowly, or in a longer time. The beginning ought to be computed, from the time the Blood begins to be made hot, and its Sulphur to conceive a burning, untill the ardors, and burnings are diffused, thorow the whole mass of Blood. The Increase or Augmentation, is from the time, that the Blood being made hot, and inkindled thorow the whole, burns forth for some time, and its mass is aggravated with the Recrements, or burnt Particles, which increase the fermentation. The state, or standing of the Disease is when (after the Blood has sufficiently burned forth, and its burning now remits) the long vexed Blood, like a noble wrestler, when his adversary is a little yielding, recollecting all his strength, endeavours a bringing under, and a separation of that adust matter, with which it is filled to a plentitude, and also, a Crisis or separation being once or oftener attempted, an expulsion of it forth of doors. The Declination succeeds after the Crisis or secretion, in which the Blood grows less hot, with a languishing fire, and either, (the vital Spirit being as yet strong) overcomes what is left of that adust and extraneous matter and by degrees puts it forth, until it is restored to its former vigour; or, whilst the same Spirit is

too much depressed, the liquor of the Blood, is still stuffed with adust recrements, and therefore becomes troubled and depauperated, that it neither assimilates the nourishing Juice, nor is made fit for an accension in the heart, for the sustaining the lamp of Life.

1. When therefore any one is taken with a putrid Feaver, the first assault is for the most part accompanied with a shivering or horror: for when the Blood begins to grow hot, there is a flux made, and a swelling up of the crude Juice, freshly gathered together in the Vessels, even as in the fit of an intermitting Feaver, heat, and sometimes sweat follow, upon the shivering, by which, the matter of that crude Juice is inkindled, and dispersed: afterwards, a certain remission of the heat follows, but yet from the fire still glowing in the Blood, a lassitude and perturbation with thirst and waking, continually infest: A pain arises in the Head, or Loins, partly from the ebullition of the Blood and partly from the motion of the nervous Juice being hindred; also a nauseousness, or a vomiting offends the Stomach, because the Bile flowing out of the Choleduct Vessels, is poured into it, and a Convulsion from Vapours, and from the sharp Juice brought thorow the arteries, is excited in the Stomach. In the mean time, altho the heat be more increased and inequal, it is not yet strong, because the Blood as yet abounding with crude Juices, is only inkindled by parts: and therefore burns out a little, and then ceases. and at last, returns; like a flame that is made by wet, and moist straw.

* Willis, Thomas, *Practice of physick*. London, Basset, 1684, p. 93.

In this condition for some days, the Disease remains, the Urine is more red than usual, by reason of the Salt and Sulphur being more dissolved and infected with the *serum;* It still retains its Hypostatis or substance, because the Coction and assimilations are not altogether depraved; it appears greater than ordinary, in its sediment, which is yet easily separated, and falls to the bottom of its own accord. At this time, they may let Blood and administer Physick by Vomit, or Purge, so it be done without any great perturbation of the Blood: it often happens, from these kind of evacuations, timely performed, that a greater increase of the Disease is prevented, and the Feaver as it were killed in the shell. The limits of this stadium or space, are variously determined, according to the temper of the sick, and other accidents of the Disease, sometimes, the first rudiments of this Feaver, are laid in a day or two; sometimes the beginning of the Disease is extended to more; if in a corpulent Body full of Spirit, Juice, and hot Blood, or it happen in a youthful Age, and very hot season, if the disposition to a Feaver be potent, and the evident cause coming thereupon be strong, the Feaverish heat, being once begun, quickly invades all the Blood, and on the second or third day, having rooted itself, the Disease arises to its increase; but if the Feaverish indisposition be begun in a less hot Body, a Phlegmatic temper, or a melancholy; and in old age, or a cold season, the entrance is longer and scarce exceeds the limits of this first stadium of space, before the sixth or seventh day.

2. The increase of this Disease is computed from what time, the burning of the Feaver hath possest the whole mass of Blood: that is, the Sulphur, or the oily part of the Blood having been long heated, and growing fervent in parts, at length, like Hay laid up wet, breaks forth, after a long heating, all at once into a flame; the Blood at this time cruelly boils up, and very much inkindled in the Heart, by its deflagration, diffuses as it were a fiery heat thorow the whole Body; and especially in the precordia; hence the sick complain of intolerable thirst, besides a pain of the head, pertinacious wakings, and oftentimes a delirium, Phrensie, and Convulsive motions infest: all food whatsoever is loathsom, either it is cast up again by Vomit, or if retained, being baked by too much heat, it goes into a Feaverish matter; besides, there happens a bitterness of the mouth, an ingrateful favor, a scurfiness of the Tongue, a vehement and quick Pulse, an Urine highly red, and for the most part troubled, full of Contents, without Hypostasis of laudab'e sediment; when the Blood is at this time almost wholly inkindled by its deflagration, it begets great plenty of adust matter (as it were ashes remaining after a Fire) with which the *serum* being very much stuffed, renders the Urine thick, and big with Contents: Also the Blood being filled with a load of this, to a rising up, is irritated into Critical motions, by which this Feaverish matter, (if it may be done) being brought under, and separated, is shut out of doors; and indeed, this state of the Feaver induces that in which a Judgment is discerned, between Nature and the Disease, the strife being as it were brought to an æquilibrium; and therefore the evacuation, which follows from thence, is called the Crisis.

The state, therefore, or height of a putrid Feaver, is that time of the Disease, in which Nature endeavors a Crisis, or an expulsion of the adust matter, remaining after the deflagration of the Blood. To this is required, in the first place, that the Blood hath now for the most part burned forth; because in the midst of its burning, Nature is not at leisure for a Crisis, nor is it ever prosperously endeavored, nor in truth procured by Art with good Success. Secondly, that the spirit of the Blood, doth first, by some means subdue this adust matter, or *Caput mortuum*, separate it from the profitable, and render a period to the expulsion, for otherways, tho a copious evacuation happens, Nature will never bee free from her burden. Thirdly, that this matter be gathered together in such a quantity, that by its turgency, it may irritate Nature to a Critical expulsion. If these rightly concur, a perfect Crisis of the Disease, for the most part succeeds, in which, even as in the Fits of intermitting Feavers, a Flux being arisen, whatsoever extraneous and heterogeneous thing, is contained in the bosom of the Blood, is exagitated, then being separated, and involved with *serum,* it is thrust forth of doors; when anything of these is wanting, the Crisis, for the most part, is in vain, and not to be trusted, and rarely cures the Disease. For if in the midst of the burning, before the Blood hath sufficiently burned forth, an evacuation happens, by Sweat, a Lask, Bleeding, or any other way, the adust matter is not all separated, or else, if for the present, it be drawn away for the greatest part, the Blood more largely flaming out, presently substitutes new, and will renew the Feaver again, that seemed to be vanquished: If that this matter, not being yet overcome, nor brought to a fulness of rising up, be irritated to an expulsion by Nature, an imperfect, and partial Crisis only follows; and when the first indeavor of excretion shall be in vain, rarely a perfect and curatory succeeds after that one time.

The Crisis in a continual Feaver, is almost the same thing, as the Fit of the intermitting Feavers. For as in this, when the mass of Blood is filled to a fulness of swelling up, with the particles of depraved alible Juice, and fitted for maturation, there are made a Flux, secretion, and expulsion out of doors of that matter: so in a continual Feaver, from the deflagration of the Blood, and alible Juice, very many little Bodies of adust matter are gathered together, with which, when the Blood is aggravated, and is at leasure, a little from the burning, it overcomes them, by little and little separates them, and then a Flux being raised up, endeavors to cast them out of doors: wherefore, as the Fits of intermitting Feavers come not but at a set time, and after so many hours, so also the Critical motions, happen from the fourth day to the fourth, or perhaps from the seventh day to the seventh, for this kind of space, the Blood being inkindled burns forth, and with its burning makes an heap of adust matter, as it were ashes, which being troublesom to Nature by their irritation, induces Critical motions.

* * *

14. No less frequent a symptom in Feavers, is a Diarrhea, or Flux of the Belly, which somtime happens about the begining of the Disease, and arises (for the most part) either from the Bile, flowing forth of the Coleduct Vessels, into the *Duodenum;* or from the recrements of the Blood, and Nervous Juice poured forth from the Arteries and the passage of the Pancreas, into the intestines. All the aforesaid humors, (but especially the Choleric) when they are supplied in abundance, often Ferment with the mass remaining of the Chyme, that the same swelling up with a spumous rarefaction, irritates the intestines and provokes to the motion of excretion: somtimes also, about the standing of the Disease, and in the declination of it, a Lask is excited; and so, either Nature being Conquerors, the more thick purgings of the Blood, are this way critically sifted forth; or being overcome, the Flux of the Belly, is the effect and sign, of the Viscera wholly losing their strength and firm tenour. It somtimes happens in a Feaver, that the Belly is always bound, that it is not at all loosened, but by Physick, and tho the sick take nothing but liquid things, for many days, the stools are still of a solid consistence, and hard, this seems for the most part to be done, when the Blood growing sharply and exceeding hot, like fire, consumes the humidities, wherever they flow, and draws to it self, out of the Bowels, the watery matter, by a Copious emission of vapours, and presently makes it to be evaporated outwardly: wherefore, the thicker part, being left in the intestines, is made firm, from the scorching heat as it were a *Caput Mortuum,* remaining after distillation.

A Dyssentery is a distemper, so frequent in continual Feavers, that some years it becomes Epidemical, and not more mild than the Plague, kills many: The cause of it is wont to be, not any humor produced within the Viscera, that corrodes the intestines with its Acrimony, (as some affirm) but a certain infection impressed on the Blood, and so intimately confused with it, that, under the form of a vapour, of a sincere humor, it cannot be pulled away from the Blood: wherefore, the thrusting forwards, towards the intestines, unlocks the little mouths of the Arteries, and makes there little Ulcers, and exudations or flowings forth of the Blood, like as when from the Feaverish Blood, Pustles and inflamations break forth outwardly, with a flowring toward the skin: But it is most likely, these dysenteric distempers, which accompany Malignant, or Epidemical Feavers, arise from a certain coagulation of the Blood, as shall be more fully declared hereafter.

Pierre Bretonneau

CONCERNING THE DISEASE TO WHICH M. BRETONNEAU, PHYSICIAN OF THE HOSPITAL OF TOURS, HAS GIVEN THE NAME OF DOTHINENTERITIS:

By M. TROUSSEAU, D.M.P. former interne of the same hospital.*

Before now works on pathological anatomy and clinical medicine have described perfectly the various changes in the inner gastro-intestinal membrane. The works of Brossais, Petit, Serres, Rayer, Andral, Hutton, Leuret, and Billiard, have accurately pointed out to us the different forms in which inflammation can appear in the digestive tract, but there is something lacking, it seems to me, since none of these authors have attached in a precise fashion a series of symptoms to certain changes; thus under the name of gastritis, enteritis, colitis, vollitis, erythematous, erysipelatous, aphthous and pustulent inflammation, etc., we have confused each in turn and no one has determined but very imperfectly, the common symptoms, or the differential signs of each of these inflammations, moreover, it is possible that the internal tegument, as well as the external, is subject to different and specific inflammation.

The long and useful work of Dr. Bretonneau has finally cleared up this question. Since 1813 he has collected a large number of cases in his civil practice, as in the hospital at Tours, at whose head his merits have placed him.

He has been led to distinguish a disease, the seat of which appears to be exclusively in the glands of Peyer and Brunner, which one finds in the jejunum, ileum and large intestine. He has given this affection the name of dothinenteritis (from δοθιήν-button, postule, furuncle; and ἔντεϱον-intestine). He has indicated the relationships, traced the symptoms and described with precision, the appearance of the disease, which changes on successive days. He has stressed so well, all of the essentials of the diagnosis, that few of his pupils, or of the great number of those who have had knowledge of his researches and ideas, cannot distinguish perfectly well in most cases, from all other forms, this form of enteritis which is so common.

In waiting for this distinguished practitioner to give the final touches to his work, I wish to give a sketch of his labors in order to call attention of physicians to a disease extremely frequent, but badly studied, until the present, and also to assure Dr. Bretonneau the possession of his discovery, which they have already wished to take from him. In the first part of this communication I will describe day by day, the pathological changes which dothinenteritis shows in the glands of Peyer and Brunner. I will describe them from the specimens under my eyes. We possess and we preserve with care, the intestinal tract of a large number of individuals, who have succumbed the same day, or at different times, from this disease, in certain cases, where one cannot accuse the treatment of having produced similar changes.

In this second part I will sketch rapidly the forms and symptoms of the disease, then after having devoted several lines to its resemblances, I will recall the time at which M. Brettonneau himself, made known to the Academy and to a large number of physicians at the capital, the interesting results of his researches; and I will compare finally, the ideas of this physician with those of MM Serres, Broussais, Lerminier, Andral, Rayer, Leuret, Hutin, Beschet.

If dothinenteritis were a disease well-known, if it only showed itself but once and then would not appear except at certain periods, or in distant ages, or on very few individuals, the work of Bretonneau would, without doubt, not be of very great interest; but if one visualizes that this disease is just as common and no less murderous than smallpox, measles and scarlet fever, that few people go to the end of their life without having experienced its attacks, that it enjoys, as well as the cutaneous inflammation, which I am going to describe, the singular character of affecting an individual only once during life, and perhaps of a contagious nature; that it is nothing else than *febris putrid genuina.* The *synchus putris* and *imputris,* the *mucous adynamic* fever of Pinel, prototype of the *gastro enterite* is of Monsieur Broussais, the malady which MM Petit and Serres described under the name of *enteromesenteric fever,* the *typhus mitior,* which showed itself four years ago in Ireland. If

* *Arch. gén de Méd.,* 1826, x, 67.

one recalls that there is not a single hospital in Paris, (except the home for the aged), which, at the moment I speak, has not in its wards a large number of dothinenteritics. If one recalls that dothinenteritis rages constantly in Paris, and in all of the larger cities where the contagious diseases, especially those which do not affect the same individual, but once, find always fresh bodies for their attacks, one will conceive of the importance it is for the practitioner to know the symptoms, course, duration, treatment of this disease and distinguish it with care, from others which attack the digestive tract.

I am going to start with a description, day by day, of the appearance of the glands of Peyer and of Brunner: I will suppose that the inflammation has been entirely limited to them.

5th day of the invasion of the fever: M. Bretonneau has never carried out an autopsy on a dothinenteritic before the fifth day. The glands of Peyer, especially those which border on the ileo-cecal valves, are markedly swollen. Their borders stand up in relief from the mucous membrane of the digestive tract, their surface is a little uneven, they have increased in breadth and length.

The glands of Brunner commence to project within the intestine. It is sometimes possible to distinguish the orifice of the mucous crypts.

The mesentric glands take on a somewhat pinkish tint, their size equals that of a sparrow's egg.

6th day: Most marked tumefaction of the glands of Peyer: the thickness of the plaques which they form is considerable: on placing the open intestine between the eye and the light and looking over the peritoneal surface, one can distinguish the row of follicles, by their much greater capacity. Its tissue is fragile and is broken with ease, sometimes, but very rarely one sees it shrouded with inflammed aureola.

The glands of Brunner, for most part of the size of a grain of hemp, form a very apparent projection, in such a manner that the intestinal membrane or intestine seems to be the seat of extensive pustular eruption.

The size of the mesentric gland is still increased; the tissue of a brighter pinkish color; they are less sticky.

7th day: Now, during the two preceeding days, the inflammation has attacked the mucous crypts, which were not inflamed the day before. But today all which are inflamed are seen, and the eruption, successive like that of smallpox, finally ceases the seventh day. The swelling increases until the 9th day and on that day the glands and lymph glands show the following appearance:

9th day: The glands of Peyer now large, more rounded, showing a projecting and uneven edge, are red fungoid, softened, unequal, but they do not show any traces of erosion.

The same is true of the isolated glands of Brunner.

Those organs are circumscribed by rather extensive inflammatory aureola, of which one can, only rarely, find any traces in the cadaver.

The mesenteric glands have acquired considerable size; they are for the most part the size of a pigeon's egg. I have seen among the anatomic specimens of the 9th day, which Bretonneau has preserved the glands from the end of the ileum, which were the size of a hen's egg. The color is very much darker; the tissue is soft and pulpy.

10th day: One of two things, either the inflammation proceeds to resolution, or it continues to go through various changes. In the first case, which is the more common, the following is the appearance which the glands of Peyer and Brunner and of the mesentary glands show successively.

11th day: The tumefaction of these glands is less and goes on decreasing until the 14th day, which is also true of the lymph glands.

14th day: The isolated and confluent follicles are still a little swollen. The surface is reticulated, shows a little brighter color than the rest of the membrane.

At the close of the third week it is difficult to find any traces of the disease, excepting a slight redness of the places which have been inflamed and the more marked opacity of the intestine.

SECOND CASE—THE INFLAMMATION GOES THROUGH ALL ITS STAGES

10th day: The surface of the glands of Peyer is elevated, rough, the tissue of the follicle is red, thickened, as though cornified.

* * *

15th day: a sort of core begins to detach itself; the covering which encloses it is reversed and shows a large ulcer, in the center of which is a mass of dead tissue adherent to its base. An inflamed aureole surrounds the ulcerated glands.

16th day: the core is entirely detached, yielding to the least effort, leaving in its place a deep excavation, with unequal walls, elevated, reversed; the base of the ulcer rests upon the muscular coat, upon the peritoneum, which they perforate so frequently.

* * *

I would not feel that we had completed the picture of pathological alterations peculiar to the inflammation, some of whose characteristics I have just described, if I did not briefly indicate the point of election of the dothinenteritic eruption. Dr. Bretonneau and after him all of his pupils, who at Tours or Paris or in the army, have carried on researches upon dothinenteritis, have always noted that the last position of the ileum was constantly involved, that the dothinenteritis inflammation would not occupy more than three, six, or ten inches of the small intestine. These were the third, sixth or tenth last inches of the ileum, that the eruption was invariably more confluent when one examined the internal membrane close to the ileo-caecal valve: that the stomach, the duodenum, the first part of the jejunum, have never shown any papillary inflammation in dothinenteritis, that in the large intestine the eruptive dothinenteritis inflammation was more confluent as it approached nearer the cecum; that never, in this disease, had spontaneous performation taken place, elsewhere than in the center of a gland of Brunner or of an ulcerated gland of Peyer.

In indicating, during this short exposé, the anatomic lesions characteristic of inenteritis, I would not wish to say that the gland of Peyer or of Brunner were exclusively affected, but I say and that is what the most careful observation has shown M. Bretonneau, that if in dothinenteritis, the stomach, the small intestine, and the large intestine, have been found sometimes inflamed, independent of the glands of Peyer and Brunner, this inflammation cannot be considered other than an accident consecutive to dothinenteritis itself, an accident which does not hinder this latter disease from taking its course and from presenting the symptoms which characterize it.

Without doubt it would have been better to have let M. Bretonneau himself, publish his ideas on dothinenteritis; this physician has traced with more clearness the picture of the changes which follow this important disease. But it is important, both for the glory of my Master, and for science, to present a glimpse of the important work, to which he has placed his hand. This conscientious practitioner, who believes it would be false to the principles of his profession, if he would establish a law, which was not for him, the expression of the entire truth, carries on each day new researches, adds to them, compares them, and enriches them with new facts and waits before submitting his work to the judgment of the public, until he, himself, judges it worthy of being presented.

Pierre Charles Alexandre Louis

Pierre Charles Alexandre Louis was born in 1787 and graduated at Paris in 1813. After graduation he returned to his home in Aï, uncertain as to his future, when a friend invited him to take a trip to Russia. After traveling in Russia for three years, he settled in Odessa where he practised medicine for four years. He became dissatisfied with the therapeutic methods currently employed in practice and returned to Paris for further study. Presently he obtained a position as assistant to Chomel, renounced all private practice and for six years, until the age of forty, spent his entire time in La Charité Hospital, where he also lived.

The first important publication of Louis was his *Recherches anatomico-pathologiques sur la phthisie* which appeared in 1825. In this work Louis introduced the numerical or statistical method of studying disease. It remains to this day one of the great works on pulmonary tuberculosis. The second great work of Louis was his *Recherches anatomiques, pathologiques et théra-peutiques sur la maladie connue sous les nomes de gastro-entérite, etc.,* which was published in 1828. In this work he described clearly the characteristic pathological lesions of typhoid fever, but he did not clearly differentiate typhoid from typhus fever.

Louis rose rapidly to fame and was especially popular among American

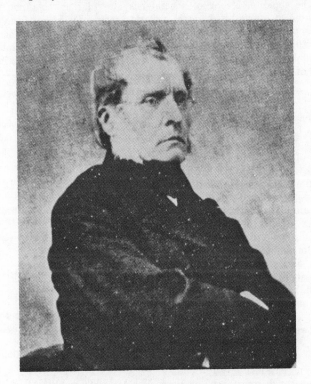

PIERRE CHARLES ALEXANDRE LOUIS (1787-1872)
Kindness of Dr. George Blumer

physicians then studying in Paris, among whom were Oliver Wendell Holmes, Henry I. Bowditch, George C. Shattuck, James Jackson, Jr., Alfred Stillé and W. W. Gerhard. Louis died in 1872.

In 1906, William Osler headed a small group of admirers who gathered in the Montparnasse Cemetery in Paris to lay a wreath on the tomb of Louis. On this occasion Osler delivered a brief address on the importance of Louis to French and to American medicine. "While not sitting with Bichat and Laennec on the very highest seats of our professional Valhalla, Louis occupies a seat of honor and distinction with his friends, Andral and Chomel, and with Bretonneau and Corvisart, with Bright, Addison and Hodgkin, with Skoda and Schoenlein—among the men who gave to the clinical medicine of the nineteenth century the proper methods of work. Louis has special claims to remembrance as the introducer of the numerical method, by which he made his works on typhoid fever and on phthisis storehouses of facts which are consulted today by students of these diseases."

The following selection describes the typical lesions of the small intestine in a patient dying of typhoid fever.

FIRST OBSERVATION*

Diminution of the appetite, feeling of general heaviness during the three first days; considerable diminution of strength, complete anorexia; copious diarrhoea from the beginning; pains in the abdomen seldom; meteorism, delirium, and prolonged somnolency; death on twentieth day. Elliptical patches of the ilium red, and very much ulcerated; mesenteric glands red, voluminous, softened; studded with yellow points; inflammation of the gall-bladder; oedema of the glottis, &c.

A man æt. 23, of medium size, and rather thin, was admitted to the hospital of La Charité, September, 17th, 1824. Had been residing at Paris for six months, and during previous four months, had been occupied in the preparation of warm baths, in various parts of the city, and had always had good nourishment, had not been accustomed to excess of drink, had never ceased from his daily occupation. He said he had been ill, six days. In the beginning; pain in the head; inclination to sleep; indistinct vision; sensation as if dazzled; pain in limbs; general feeling of heaviness; very great sensibility to cold; with extreme heat of skin; urgent thirst; complete anorexia; diarrhoea. These symptoms continued, and the diarrhoea increased so that during the last three days, he had from fifteen to twenty dejections in twenty-four hours. At this time, new symptoms made their appearance; to wit, nausea, vomiting, and pains in the epigastrium; very few colic-pains; and a slight cough commenced on the evening that the patient entered the hospital. All these symptoms had been preceded during three days by a slight diminution of appetite, and a feeling of general languor, or dullness. Our patient had kept his bed from the outset, and had taken only beef-tea for nourishment, and for drink, barley water sweetened with honey, with some wine mingled with it. He had taken also every day, one or two glasses of undiluted wine, and had not perceived any exacerbation of his symptoms, of those particularly which related to the stomach.

*Louis, P.Ch.A., *Anatomical Pathological and Therapeutic Researches upon the Disease known under the Name of Gastro-Enterite, Putrid, Adynamic, Ataxic or Typhoid Fever, etc.* Translated by Henry I. Bowditch, Boston, Butts, 1936, I, p. 3.

Opening of the corpse twenty-three hours after death

EXTERIOR.—Numerous red lines like what would be produced by severe blows with rods, upon the lateral and posterior parts of the body; skin corresponding to the blisters reddish, and a little thickened; subjacent cellular tissue containing fat a little more dense than in the neighboring parts; muscles firm, not sticky, and of a natural color.

* * *

Small intestine was a little more voluminous than natural, and in its interior contained every where a blackish, viscid, stringy matter; under which the mucous membrane was, in the first half, greyish, or slightly shaded with red; of proper thickness, and of a consistence little less than that which is natural to it. Beyond it was of a vivid red, and very much softened, especially in the last five feet, where it could not be raised in strips, and where the subjacent cellular tissue was a little infiltrated. In this same part were seen thirty elliptical patches, some ulcerated others not, but all more or less thickened.* The first three covered about an inch and a half of surface, were whitish, and composed, as in health, of a great number of small grains, very apparent, particularly on the surface of mucous mebrane, that adhered to the subjacent cellular, and being larger than usual, they caused the mucous mem-

* The elliptical patches that are found in the track of the small intestine, especially in the ileum, in the natural state, have been already described minutely in my "Researches upon Phthisis." The reader may consult that description and consequently I have thought it would be useless to repeat it in this work.—Louis

brane at this point to be a millimeter† in thickness. The cellular tissue corresponding to them was of its usual whiteness, and a little thickened. After these patches came two more a little more prominent, of the same structure, of a somewhat vivid red, slightly ulcerated, and under which the submucous tissue was very red, and very thick. Finally, the mucous membrane was entirely destroyed throughout the whole extent of the other patches, and the bottom of the ulcerations, more or less uneven, was formed by the cellular tissue, which was of a deep red color, and about a millimeter thick. This latter tissue itself was more or less largely destroyed, and the muscular membrane laid bare, by the last ten ulcerations. The last, situated near the ilio-coecal valve occupied the circumference of the intestine, and was ten or twelve lines broad. The muscular membrane was laid bare over nearly its whole surface, and at its edge were a great number of membranous slips, which, after repeated washings, had still a gangrenous odor. Much shorter strips were detached from the ulcerations, and floated in the water in which the intestine was placed.

† The reader is probably aware, that there are about twenty-five millimeters in our English inch.—H.I.B.

Large intestine, contained a matter similar to that which was in the small, less viscid and less colored in the rectum than elsewhere. Its mucous membrane was greyish or blackish, except in this last part, where it was of a pale red; it was of double the usual thickness, and of good consistence in the ascending colon; it was thinner and more or less softened thence towards rectum. *Mesenteric glands* greyish, firm, increased in size near duodenum; but they were of a more or less vivid red, moderately softened, and of the size of a filbert, spotted in their interior with a considerable number of yellow points, in the latter half of the intestine. The glands of the mesocolon were blackish, and of the size of a pea. The *spleen* was more than three times its usual size, of an amaranthine red color, very soft, so as to be easily reduced to a pulpy state by pressure. *Liver* soft; rather pale, and its two colors were nearly confounded with each other. The *gall-bladder* was of the size of a goose-egg, and contained a reddish, thin liquid, at the bottom of which was a thin puriform fluid, without sediment. Its mucous membrane was reddish, and whitish; of natural thickness and consistence. Biliary ducts and other organs in the abdomen were in a healthy state.

CERTAIN OTHER INFECTIOUS DISEASES

The following descriptions in this chapter of certain infectious diseases are either recognized classic accounts or the first known account of the disease in question. Sydenham's account of scarlet fever, of measles, and of influenza, while not the earliest, brought, nevertheless, these diseases to the attention of physicians in such a manner as to give them the status of well defined clinical syndromes. The same is true of Heberden's description of chicken-pox and Caius' account of sweating fever. Pfeiffer's account of glandular fever, Winterbottom's reference to sleeping sickness, Baillou's description of whooping cough, Rutty's account of relapsing fever, and the selection of Schönlein are all apparently the first unmistakable descriptions of these diseases. Rheumatic fever, first named by Baillou, was afterwards described by Sydenham, Morton, and Haygarth, all of whom chiselled out more clearly, as it were the clinical features of this disease. Wells and Bouillaud stressed the importance of cardiac involvement in Rheumatic fever. Rush was the first in America to call attention to the importance of focal infection, a discovery whose later recognition and application is distinctly an American achievement. Hodgkin's disease, while a disease of unknown etiology, has been included in this group because of certain affinities with infections. Later discoveries may place it in an altogether different category.

EPIDEMIC CEREBROSPINAL MENINGITIS

Epidemic cerebrospinal meningitis was first clearly described by Gaspard Vieusseux of Geneva in 1806. Vieusseux observed that many of his patients showed purple spots on the skin and at autopsy, marked engorgement of the brain. He noted that the patients complained of violent headache, stiffness of the spine and convulsions. Elisha North of Goshen, Connecticut, observed a similar epidemic in 1807 which he described in a monograph published in 1811, the first published book on this disease.

Gaspard Vieusseux

THE DISEASE WHICH RAGED IN GENEVA DURING THE SPRING OF 1805*

Although the disease which raged during the past spring in Geneva and its suburbs has not been notable for either the number of patients affected or dead, and although it lasted only about three months, it is, none the less, remarkable because of the symptoms which distinguish it from every type of ever which has appeared in the practice of the doctors who have practiced their art in our village for more than thirty years. Whatever has been said upon this subject, whether in the report of the Bureau of Health published by the Prefect of Leman, or in the public papers, is not complete enough, and will have nothing but a passing existence. As there was no mention made of it in our old *Journal of Medicine*, I have thought it a duty to describe the disease in it—the most widely read and the proper vehicle for publication.

It began in a most peculiar and terrifying manner at a very small distance from the town, in a district inhabited by poor people, dirty, and in whom the manner of life favored the development of every contagious disease. It is common enough to see this sort of people attacked by putrid and malignant fevers in spring, when the wind from the southeast prevails and blows far and wide the marshy exhalations of the ditches in this part of the edge of the lake.

At the end of January, in a family composed of a woman and three children, two of the children were attacked and died in less than forty-eight hours. Fifteen days later the disease appeared in another family in the neighborhood, composed of a father, mother, and five infants, four of whom were attacked almost at the same time, and all

died from the tenth to the twelfth of February, after having been sick fourteen to fifteen hours with striking symptoms of malignancy.

One did not realize how much these rapid and numerous deaths could produce terror, although we did not doubt that there was a malignant contagious fever against which one should take the greatest precautions. As a consequence, all the furniture and clothing of the two families were burned. The individuals were transported elsewhere, and their dwellings washed, white-washed, and disinfected with the greatest care.

At the end of fifteen days a young man living in a house nearby was also attacked by the same disease and died between evening and morning, having a purple body, even to the tips of his fingers, for a few hours before his death.

* * *

It commences suddenly with prostration of strength, often extreme; the face is distorted, the pulse feeble, small and frequent, sometimes almost absent, hard and elevated in a small number of cases. There appears a violent pain in the head, especially over the forehead; then there comes pains of the heart, or vomiting of greenish material, of stiffness of the spine, and in infants, convulsions. In the cases which were fatal, loss of consciousness followed. The course of the disease is very rapid, termination by death or by cure. In the first case the disease lasts from twelve hours to five days, but not beyond; and in the cases of cure, it is often also short. Sometimes, moreover, it is prolonged, an follows the course of an ordinary bilious fever; often, also, it takes the type of an intermittent fever, and there have been

Journal de Médicine Chirurgie Pharmacie, etc., 1806, XI, 163.

some of these cases which became fatal which one could have regarded as pernicious fever, in which the first attack carried off the patient.

In most of the patients who died in twenty-four hours or a little after, the body is covered with purple spots at the moment of death or very little time afterwards. Sometimes, indeed, during life there is that which gives it a terrifying aspect, and a greater appearance of malignancy, according to the eyes of the common people, but experience proves that these changes in the color of the body, and these violet or livid spots are frequently found in those who died very promptly, whether there was any malignant fever or not. Besides, one sees the patients with a true malignant fever, but in whom the death is less prompt, as we will see in an example later in which there was no alteration in the body after death.

* * *

Examination of the body showed most frequently a sanguinous engorgement in the brain without any particular alteration of the other viscera. In some of them this engorgement was not considerable and in very small numbers the brain was in its normal state. After this description one sees that this disease has certain singular characteristics, especially in the grave cases. These characteristics are the sudden invasion, the violence of the headache, the vomiting, and especially the rapidity of the termination, either by death or by cure. It forms then, a distinct species, and the name of cerebral malignant, non-contagious fever is that which appears the best. The brain is the only organ in which the post-mortem inspection has shown any alteration; the affection of the other parts appears to come only from the brain, and all the symptoms of it are nervous. At the moment when one sees nothing but yellow fever in all the epidemic diseases, it is not astonishing that one believes one can find a relationship between this disease and that of Geneva. There is the frontal headache, vomiting, and the violence of the disease; but the differences are too marked for one to pause long at this idea of a resemblance with yellow fever. The duration of that disease is generally longer; the vomited material is black; the skin becomes yellow, and the openings of the body shows that the liver is particularly affected with a gangrenous state. The same is true of the stomach and intestines, and the disease is contagious. In the cerebral fever of Geneva the termination is very abrupt, the vomited material is green, or often there is none; the skin does not become yellow, and examination of the body shows nothing but engorgement of the brain; the liver and intestines are healthy, and the disease is not contagious. The violence, the singularity and the uniformity of the symptoms do not deny to this fever the name of an epidemic, since it has raged for three months in all parts of the town and in the country.

Elisha North

Elisha North was born in Goshen, Connecticut, in 1771. He studied medicine first with a local doctor, then with his father and later with Dr. Lemuel Hopkins of Hartford. He began the practice of medicine in his home town and, after accumulating some money, he entered the University of Pennsylvania Medical School in 1793. He did not graduate but returned presently to Goshen, where he again took up the practice of medicine.

North was early interested in Jenner's discovery of vaccination and in 1800, two years after the appearance of Jenner's classic, vaccinated three persons in Goshen, traveling fifty miles to New Haven to obtain fresh vaccine. In 1807 a new disease, spotted fever or epidemic cerebrospinal meningitis, descended on Goshen "like a flood of mighty waters, bringing along with it the horrors of a most dreadful plague." His experience with this epidemic is described in *A Treatise on a Malignant Epidemic commonly called Spotted Fever,* an early American medical classic.

In 1812 North removed to New London, where he became a most active and respected practitioner in physic and surgery, working not only as a general practitioner but as an oculist and surgeon as well. He died in New London in 1843.

SECTION I*
ON THE SYMPTOMS OF THE FIRST SPECIES OF THE FEVER

These are the following: A great, surprising, and sudden loss of strength, is a constant and prominent symptom; a cold surface also mences in the limbs, it soon mounts up to the head. Distress about the precordia, violent and extreme, also universal agony

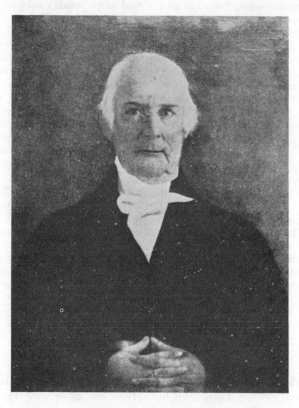

ELISHA NORTH (1771-1843)
Kindness of Dr. Walter Steiner

presents itself, sometimes accompanied with chills, sometimes not. The extremities, in the cold stage, appear of a purplish or livid colour. Violent pain of the head, and many times of the limbs, is among the first symptoms; sometimes one, at other times the other is first attacked. When the pain commences of the whole system, and numbness of the extremities, are often added to the above list of symptoms. The breathing is often laborious, and attended with frequent sighing. Syncope sometimes occurs. The pulse in this, and in all the varieties and stages of this complaint, is soft, weak, and never hard, although sometimes as slow, and even slower than in health; it is often intermitting, fluttering, or totally absent, even in cases in which the patient has afterwards recovered.

*North, Elisha, *A Treatise on a Malignant Epidemic, Commonly Called Spotted Fever*, New York, T. & F. Swords, 1811, pp. 10, 11, 12, 13, 15, 16.

The tongue is generally covered with a white coat; but in some bilious cases it is of a brownish hue; sometimes it has been observed to have a bloodless appearance, which has been considered as almost a certain token of approaching death. The urine deviates but little from health, except a hysteric flow which has sometimes been observed to happen. There is loss of appetite, and sickness at stomach, and vomiting. The worst form this disease ever assumes, particularly in children, is that of coma, or cholera morbus. It frequently assumes the form of a violent mania at the time, or within a few hours of the attack, particularly in sanguine young men. Sometimes delirium is among the first symptoms; sometimes coma; and many times petechia. This symptom does not occur so often as the name which the disease has obtained would lead one to expect: these vary in size, and in colour, from a bright red to a dark purple.

Unless the patient recovers, he commonly dies within the first twelve, twenty-four, or forty-eight hours. Death is ushered in by the gradual giving up of the powers of life, by syncope, by the febrile apoplexy, or by convulsions. In those who recover, the disorder puts on, either before or soon after the expiration of the first forty-eight hours, the form of the second variety of this disease; or, to express myself in the words of others, "runs into the form of a mild typhus of uncertain duration."

As petechiae, when they do occur, may almost always be considered as marking the worst form of this disease, I will now describe them in the words of Dr. Strong. "Blind haemorrhages, or those where the blood flowing from the vessels of the skin, is detained beneath the cuticle, forming petechial spots, were more common:" i.e. more common than other haemorrhage during the first season in which the disease prevailed, that it was considered as one of its most striking characteristicks, and gave rise to the name *petechial*, or *spotted fever*, which has been very generally, though very improperly, applied to the disease. These spots commonly appeared on the face, neck, and extremities, frequently over the whole body. They were generally observed in the early stages of the disease. In size they were various, commonly the head of a pin and a six cent bit would mark the two extremes. These spots were evidently formed by extravasated blood; they did not rise above the surface, and would not recede upon pressure. In colour, they varied from a common to a very dark purple, and the darker the shade, the more fatal the prognosis. These spots, which in 1806-7 marked almost every case, in 1808-9 were rarely observed." In addition to this, I would observe, that in some protracted cases, where the patient has recovered, these spots have sphacelated, and suppurated, and, upon coming out, have left ulcers, which required some time to heal.

* * *

SECTION III
ON THE MORE UNUSUAL SYMPTOMS OF THE FEVER

These are a dilatation, and, in some, a contraction of the pupils of the eyes; redness and suffusion of the eyes; blindness in some, in other double or treble vision; a drawing back of the head, with a kind of clonic spasm of the muscles of the neck; apthae in the throat; an inflammation like erysipelas upon the limbs; swelling like rheumatism of the joints; paralysis of an arm or a leg, or both; carbuncles and buboes; stranguary, and to such a degree as to require the use of the catheter; a violent pain in a finger or toe; hysteric symptoms; pain like cholic of the bowels; a slight cough; oedematous and shining appearance of the skin; transitory and evanescent flushes of heat; erratic pains flying from part to part; a deadly feeling of the stomach; a corpse-like rigidity of the limbs; haemorrhages, which were less frequent, however, than the other symptoms would lead one to suspect; costiveness; and many other symptoms too tedious to relate.

The disease has been observed to assume different shapes, according to the different constitutions of the patient affected with it: Thus women were more liable to hysteric symptoms; in children it sometimes appeared in the form of cholera morbus; and in young men of the sanguine temperament it not unfrequently produced a violent mania.

SCARLET FEVER
Daniel Sennert*

Daniel Sennert, the celebrated German physician of the seventeenth century, was born in Breslau in 1572, the son of a poor cobbler. He lost his father when thirteen years of age but the industry and frugality of his mother made it possible for the boy to continue his studies. In 1593 he entered the Univer-

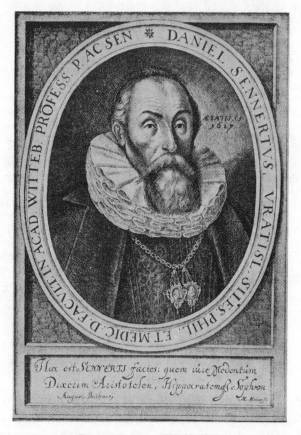

DANIEL SENNERT (1572-1637)
A portrait of Sennert in 1627 drawn by August Buchner
and engraved by Matthew Merian

sity of Wittenberg where he studied philosophy and in 1598 received his Master's degree. He had planned to become a school master but gave up this idea and began the study of medicine. He studied for three years at Leipsic, Jena and Frankfort-on-the-Oder and in 1601 received his doctor's degree at Wittenberg. The following year Sennert was appointed to the chair of medicine at Wittenberg, a position he held for thirty-five years. He showed his courage in numerous occasions when the plague infested Wittenberg, for unlike many other physicians, he remained at his post and treated the sick. On six such occasions Sennert defied the pestilence and treated its victims, but during the seventh invasion of the plague he contracted the disease and died at the age of sixty-five.

Sennert was a famous physician in his time. He was a very industrious writer whose works were widely read, and a very skillful physician whose clientele came from all parts of Europe. He was not an original thinker nor a genius, but a careful and judicious compiler. Although he believed in demons and in witchcraft and was convinced that sorcerers could cause and also cure disease, yet he saw many things clearly and has written some striking accounts of disease. He is usually given the credit for the first clear description of scarlet fever although it seems probable that his brother-in-law, Michael Döring, first observed it in Breslau and called Sennert's attention to the distinctive features of this disease.

Besides these differences there is still another, and moreover more unusual, which I have observed at different times, by what name however I should differentiate it from the others, I have been until now uncertain. For although like erysipelas it attacks almost the entire body, however I did not see adults, as usually happens in erysipelas, but infants alone it attacked. Therefore I should like to refer to measles. And perhaps it is the malady which Forestus, *book 6, observation 59*, calls purpura & rubores as well as ἐρυθήματα (erythemata). Joh. Philippus Ingrassias, *loco citato*, writes that they are called by the Neapolitans Rossania & Rossalia. Spots red & as if on fire which I scarcely dignify by speaking of a swelling, which are throughout the entire body as if some lesser erysipelas had broken out in the beginning, or on the fourth or fifth day of the disease. In its real state the entire body appears red & as if on fire, and also as if it suffered from a universal erysipelas. In declination the redness itself diminishes, & wide red spots again appear as in the beginning, which however disappear the seventh or ninth day with the skin falling off like scales. This disease indeed is grave and dangerous & often lethal.

Now the fever is most intense, the thirst unquenchable, & commonly inflammation of the lungs (whence coughing is excited) of the fauces & of other viscera, delirium & other ills appear. In declination moreover the material is transferred to the joints of the extremities, and excite pain, & redness, as in arthritis. The skin peels like scales, soon the feet swell to the ankles & right on to the calves, they have discomfort in the hypochondrium, respiration becomes more difficult, and besides the abdomen swells, and the patients are restored to their original state of health only with great effort & after a long time, moreover frequently they die. My honored Brother-in-law the most Illustrious Master Michael Döring observed this, he wrote in letters delivered to me that, a certain boy of Breslau after this disease had swelling of the feet, the legs, the scrotum, the abdomen and face, with a marked and lasting swelling of the knees, irregular fever, cough, which was slight; he expectorated foam at least & mucus, with the greatest difficulty in respiration. This boy on the seventh day, before he died, after the greatest difficulty in respiration, a sensation of oppression in the chest, and stertor, he coughed up pus & black blood from a ruptured abscess in the lungs, & then on the 7th day from this paroxysm, when the same symptomes returned, he died.

On opening the body the entire cavity of the chest was filled with yellow fluid, and the lungs were seen everywhere livid & gangrenous; & the left contained within a large abscess. On opening the abdomen all the intestines floated in a similar fluid; the omentum was seen to be nearly consumed. The liver because of the person, was of great size and pale. It is no wonder that both such ills and symptoms, indeed painful joints, & swellings, swelling of the abdomen & similar things followed this disease. For while smallpox is apt to break out not only in the external parts but moreover on the surface of all the viscera: the same moreover can happen in Rossalia; & just as the whole body

---

* Sennert, Daniel, *De febribus libri IV,* Venice, Junta & Herty, 1641, p. 178.

without is inflammed, so indeed the internal viscera without doubt are inflamed, and it is doubtless true of the lungs. The same thing happens moreover, without doubt in the other organs; when the material pushed to the external parts first produces arthritic pains, then hydropic swellings, and the viscera themselves are injured.

Thomas Sydenham

The writings of Thomas Sydenham, often called the "Father of English Medicine" and the "English Hippocrates," are better known than the events

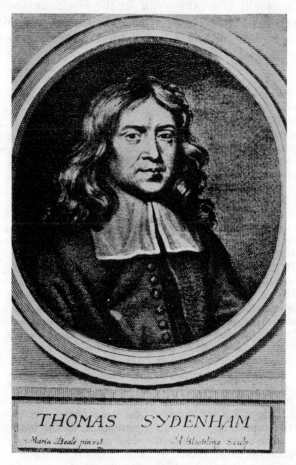

THOMAS SYDENHAM (1624-1689)
From the portrait by Maria Beale—etched by Blooteling.
Frontispiece to *Observationes Medicae*, 1676

of his life. Lettsom remarks that his biography "scarcely enlarges beyond the information that he was a soldier; that he told Sir R. Blackmore, who inquired of him the best books to study in order to acquire medical knowledge, to peruse Don Quixote; that he pursued some short studies; and that he died a martyr to the gout."

Sydenham was born at Winford Eagle in 1624 and at the age of eighteen, entered Magdalen Hall at Oxford. Soon afterwards, the Civil War broke out in England, and Sydenham left Oxford to serve in the army of Parliament with the rank of captain. In 1647, he returned to Oxford as a student of medicine and, six months later, was created bachelor of medicine by the order of the Earl of Pembroke, chancellor of the university. This was a highly irregular procedure since he had not taken a degree in arts and had studied medicine only a few months. The conferring of this medical degree really marked the beginning of Sydenham's medical studies instead of their completion. Later he went to Montpelier, where he studied under Barbeyrac, a physician of great repute in France as a teacher and consultant. He began practice in London about 1661 and in 1663 became a licentiate of the Royal College of Physicians. In 1667, he obtained the degree of M.D. at Cambridge, where his son was a student. He never applied for a fellowship in the Royal College of Physicians but Munk says his name was always mentioned with respect by the college. He died in 1689 and was buried in St. James Piccadilly.

Sydenham stands out as the greatest representative of the practical medicine of practical England. He was primarily a great physician, was little concerned with the vague scientific theories of the time, but relied upon his powers of observation and his vast fund of experience. He had little interest in the theories of the iatro-physicists who sought to explain disease on a mechanical basis, or in the speculations of the iatro-chemists who saw in every disease only a disturbance in the acid-alkali balance. Instead, he stressed careful observation and accurate note taking at the bedside. "I have been very careful," he says, "to write nothing but what was the product of faithful observation and neither suffered myself to be deceived by idle speculation, nor have deceived others by obtruding anything upon them but downright matter of fact." As a medical practitioner he did the best he could for his patients and although he was not free from the abuses of the polypharmacy prevalent in his day, there were many cases in his practice where, he says "I have consulted my patients safety and my own reputation most effectually by doing nothing at all." In the field of therapeutics Syndenham was noteworthy for his championship of quinine, or Jesuits bark, in the treatment of malarial fevers—a drug whose introduction was stoutly resisted by many physicians of his time. He denied that the stars either produced diseases or influenced their course but was convinced of the rôle played by climate and weather. His treatise on epidemic diseases and on gout were his masterpieces and his accounts of scarlet fever and measles stamp him as an accurate and careful observer. All of his writings bear the impress of the Hippocratic spirit and method and this is the secret of his influence upon English medicine and upon the medicine of the world. During his lifetime, Sydenham was less esteemed at home than abroad. His own colleagues bestowed no honors upon him, but abroad, his name was mentioned in learned circles with admiration and respect. Although he was not a member of the Royal Society and his connection with the College of Physicians was a loose and nominal one, it is noteworthy that two of his closest friends were the chemist Robert Boyle and the physician-philosopher John Locke, both of whom influenced his thought and were influenced by him. Sydenham's fame spread rapidly after his death, as his writings became widely read, and the verdict of the eighteenth and of the succeeding centuries was well expressed by Albrecht von Haller when he asserted that the writings of Sydenham mark an epoch in the history of medicine.

The selections in this work on scarlet fever, measles, and gout are from the edition of his writings published by the Sydenham Society in 1850. His account of influenza is from an American edition of his works edited by Benjamin Rush and published in Philadelphia in 1809 by B. and T. Kite.

CHAPTER VII
ON THE SCARLET FEVER*

This attacks infants most, and that towards the end of summer. Shivers and chills at the commencement; but no great depression. The whole skin is marked with small, red spots, more frequent, more diffused, and more red than in measles. These last two or three days. They then disappear; leaving the skin covered with branny *squamulæ*, as if powdered with meal.

℞ Hartshorne,
   Gasciogne's powder, āā ℨss;

The Works of Thomas Sydenham, translated by R. G. Latham, M.D., London Sydenham Society, 1850, ii, p. 242.

Cochineal, gf. i j;
White sugar, ℨj.
Mix, and make into a very fine powder. Divide into twelve papers. Take one every six hours. Wash down with two or three spoonsfuls of—

℞ Black-cherry water,
   Aqua lactis alexeteria aa ℥iij;
   Syrup of lemon-juice, ℨj.
Mix, and make into a julip.

Apply also a blister to the neck. Order, too, a paregoric of syrup of poppies to be taken every night. Purge when the symptoms have ceased.

SMALLPOX AND MEASLES
Rhazes

Abu Becr Mohammed Ibn Zacariya Ar-Razi, better known as Rhazes, was born in the town of Raj in Khorasan, Persia, in 860 A.D. He received a good education in philosophy, philology, and mathematics and was an accomplished musician. He did not begin the study of medicine until he was thirty years of age, and decided to study medicine one day after he had by chance visited the hospital at Bagdad and been impressed by the misery he saw there. Rhazes studied at Bagdad and later went to Palestine, Egypt, and Spain where he studied with the greatest physicians of his age. After his return home, he soon became celebrated as a physician, teacher, and writer. He was a most voluminous writer and wrote at least 200 books, not on medicine alone, but also on mathematics, physics, chemistry, and astronomy.

According to accounts, he presented to the Prince Al-Mansur a book on chemistry which pleased the prince so much that he presented Rhazes with a purse of 1000 dinars and asked him to demonstrate one of the chemical experiments. The experiment was, however, a failure, and this enraged the prince so that he struck the unfortunate author on the head with his whips, injuring his eyes so that he developed cataracts and became blind. A surgeon offered to operate upon Rhazes but the latter asked him how many tunics the eye possessed. The surgeon admitted that he did not know, whereupon Rhazes declared, "Whoever does not know that shall lay no instruments upon my eyes." Later he declined operation, remarking that he had already seen too much of the world. He died in 932 A.D. in abject poverty, having given away all his wealth to his poor patients.

Rhazes was a follower of Galen in theory but a true disciple of Hippocrates in the simplicity of his treatment and in his insistence upon bedside observation. He was often called the Arabian Hippocrates and his writings stamp him not as a theorist or dogmatic systematizer but as a great clinician. His book on therapeutics was the standard work for more than six centuries and his account of smallpox and measles "is the first authentic account in literature" and "is so vivid and complete that it is almost modern." (Garrison)

CHAPTER II*

A SPECIFICATION OF THOSE HABITS OF BODY WHICH ARE MOST DISPOSED TO THE SMALL-POX; AND OF THE SEASONS IN WHICH THESE HABITS OF BODY MOSTLY ABOUND

The bodies most disposed to the Small-Pox are in general such as are moist, pale, and fleshy; the well-coloured also, and ruddy, as likewise the swarthy when they are loaded with flesh; those who are frequently attacked by acute and continued fevers, bleeding of the nose, inflammation of the eyes, and white and red pustules, and vesicles; those that are very fond of sweet things, especially, dates, honey, figs, and grapes, and of all those kinds of sweets in which there is a thick and dense substance, as thick gruel, and honey-cakes, or a great quantity of wine and milk.

(2) Bodies that are lean, bilious, hot, and dry, are more disposed to the Measles than to the Small-Pox; and if they are seized with the Small-Pox, the pustules are necessarily either few in number, distinct, and favorable, or, on the contrary, very bad, numerous, sterile, and dry, with putrefaction, and no maturation.

(3) Lastly, those bodies that are lean and dry, and of a cold temperament, are neither disposed to the Small-Pox nor to the Measles; and if they are seized with the

Small-Pox, the pustles are few, favorable, moderate, mild, without danger, and with a moderate light fever from first to last, because such constitutions extinguish the disease.

(4) I am now to mention the seasons of the year in which the Small-Pox is most prevalent; which are, the latter end of the autumn, and the beginning of the spring; and when in the summer there are great and frequent rains with continued south winds, and when the winter is warm, and the winds southerly.

(5) When the summer is excessively hot and dry, and the autumn is also hot and dry, and the rains come on very late, then the Measles quickly seize those who are disposed to them; that is, those who are of a hot, lean, and bilious habit of body.

(6) But all these things admit of great differences by reason of the diversity of countries and dwellings, and occult dispositions in the air, which necessarily cause these diseases, and predispose bodies to them; so that they happen in other seasons besides these. And therefore it is necessary to use great diligence in the preservation from them, as soon as you see them begin to prevail among the people; as I shall mention in the sequel.

* A Treatise on the Small-Pox and Measles, by Abú Becr Mohammed Ibn Zacariyá Ar-Rázi (commonly called Rhazes). (London, Sydenham Society, 1848), p. 32.

* * *

CHAPTER III

ON THE SYMPTOMS WHICH INDICATE THE APPROACHING ERUPTION OF THE SMALL-POX AND MEASLES

The eruption of the Small-Pox is preceded by a continued fever, pain in the back, itching in the nose, and terrors in sleep. These are the more peculiar symptoms of its approach, especially a pain in the back, with fever; then also a pricking which the patient feels all over his body; a fullness of the face, which at times goes and comes; an inflamed colour, and vehement redness in both the cheeks; a redness of both the eyes; a heaviness of the whole body; great uneasiness, the symptoms of which are stretching and yawning; a pain in the throat and chest, with a slight difficulty in breathing, and cough; a dryness of the mouth, thick spittle, and hoarseness of the voice; pain and heaviness of the head; inquietude, distress of mind, nausea, and anxiety; (with this difference, that the inquietude, nausea, and anxiety are more frequent in the Measles than in the Small-Pox; while, on the other hand, the pain in the back is more peculiar to the Small-Pox than to the Measles;) heat of the whole body, an inflamed colour, and shining redness, and especially an intense redness of the gums.

(2) When, therefore, you see these symptoms, or some of the worst of them, (such as the pain of the back, and the terrors in sleep, with the continued fever,) then you may be assured that the eruption of one of these diseases in the patient is nigh at hand; except that there is not in the Measles so much pain of the back as in the Small-Pox; nor in the Small-Pox so much anxiety and nausea as in the Measles, unless the Small-Pox be of a bad sort; and this shows that the Measles come from a very bilious blood.

(3) With a respect to the safer kind of the Small-Pox, in this it is the quantity of the blood that is hurtful rather than its bad quality; and hence arises the pain of the back, from the distension of the large vein and artery which are situated by the vertebrae of the spine.

MEASLES

Thomas Sydenham

CHAPTER XIV

ON THE MEASLES*

The measles generally attack children. On the first day they have chills and shivers, and are hot and cold in turns. On the second they have the fever in full—disquietude, thirst, want of appetite, a white (but not a dry) tongue, slight cough, heaviness of the head and eyes, and somnolence. The nose and eyes run continually; and this is the surest sign of measles. To this may be added sneezing, a swelling of the eyelids a little before the eruption, vomiting and diarrhoea with green stools. These appear more especially during teething-time. The symptoms increase until the fourth day. *Then*—or sometimes on the fifth—there appear on the face and forehead small red spots, very like the bites of fleas. These increase in number, and cluster to-gether, so as to mark the face with large red blotches. They are formed by a small papulae, so slightly elevated above the skin, that their prominence can hardly be detected by the eye, but can just be felt by passing the fingers lightly along the skin.

2. The spots take hold of the face first; from which they spread to the chest and belly, and afterwards to the legs and ankles. On these parts may be seen broad, red *maculæ, on*, but not *above*, the level of the skin. In measles the eruption does not so thoroughly allay the other symptoms as in small-pox. There is, however, no vomiting after its appearance; nevertheless there is slight cough instead, which, with fever and the difficulty of breathing, increases. There is also a running from the eyes, somnolence, and want of appetite. On the sixth day, or thereabouts, the forehead and face begin to

* *The Works of Thomas Sydenham*, translated by R. G. Latham, M.D., London, Sydenham Society, 1850, ii, p. 250.

grow rough, as the pustules die off, and as the skin breaks. Over the rest of the body the blotches are both very broad and very red. About the eighth day they disappear from the face, and scarcely show on the rest of the body. On the ninth, there are none anywhere. On the face, however, and on the extremities—sometimes over the trunk—they peel off in thin, mealy squamulae; at which time the fever, the difficulty of breathing, and the cough are aggravated. In adults and patients who have been under a hot regimen, they grow livid, and afterwards black.

℞ Petoral decoction, Oiss;
   Syrup of violets,
   Syrup of maidenhair āā ℥iss

Mix, and make into an apozem. Of this take three or four ounces three or four times a day.

℞ Oil of sweet almonds, ℥ij;
   Syrup of violets,
   Syrup of maidenhair, aa ℥j;
   Finest white sugar, q.s.

Mix, and make into a linctus; to be taken often, especially when the cough is troublesome.

℞ Black-cherry water, ℥ij;
   Syrup of poppies, ℥j.

Mix, and make into a draught; to be taken every night, from the first onset of the disease, until the patient recovers: the dose being increased or diminished according to his age.

3. The patient must keep his bed for two days after the first eruption.

4. If, after the departure of the measles, fever, difficulty of breathing, and other symptoms like those of peripneumony supervene, blood is to be taken from the arm freely, once, twice, or thrice, as the case may require, with due intervals between. The pectoral decoction and the linctus must also be continued; or, instead of the latter, the oil of sweet almonds alone. About the twelfth day from the invasion the patient may be moderately purged.

5. The diarrhoea which follows measles is cured by bleeding.

Henry Koplik

Henry Koplik was born in New York City in 1858 and graduated in medicine from Columbia University in 1881. He was for twenty-five years attending physician at Mt. Sinai Hospital, and in 1896 described the initial eruption of measles on the mucous membrane, a phenomenon which has since been known by his name and has been of great diagnostic importance in the early recognition of this disease. He established the first depot for pasteurized milk in America and made numerous contributions to the literature of pediatrics. He died on April 30, 1927 in New York.

THE DIAGNOSIS OF THE INVASION OF MEASLES FROM A STUDY OF THE EXANTHEMA AS IT APPEARS ON THE BUCCAL MUCOUS MEMBRANE*

It is indeed very late in the day to describe something connected with the diagnosis of the exanthemata. It will be seen from what follows that one of the most, if not the most, reliable sign of the invasion of measles has fully failed to receive due attention. My experience leads me to believe that the sign to be described is fairly ignored. This has led me to describe it here. Its importance in making a positive diagnosis of measles cannot be over-estimated. The text-books on diseases of infancy and childhood describe the appearances of the exanthema of measles both on the skin and also in fragmentary ways on the mucous membranes. Scant attention is given to the most important elements of the eruption as it appears on the mucous membrane of the inside of the cheeks and on that of the lips. A thorough understanding of the eruption on the buccal mucous membrane will aid in separating an invading measles from a mass of eruptions resembling measles which appear on the skin in infancy and childhood. Any positive sign of the invasion of any infectious or contagious disease is a step to proper isolation and prophylactic hygiene.

The eruption of the exanthemata of

* Koplik, Henry, *Arch. Pediat.* 1896, xiii, 918.

measles on the buccal mucous membrane, its spread and decline, forms a sort of cycle which can be verified by any one who will study it. The height of the eruption is reached just as the skin eruption has appeared and is spreading. When the skin eruption of measles is at its efflorescence, the eruption on the buccal mucous membrane has begun its decline. I have looked in all the classical text-books, but fail to find any extended mention of these facts, or any minute description of the buccal eruption. Starr, in his article in the *American Text-Book,* on Diseases of Children, does not enter at all into the eruption to which I refer. J. Lewis Smith, in the edition of 1878, does not mention it. Beginsky, in his text-book, speaks of a "red spotted appearance of the pharynx," quoting Mettenheimer and Rehn. Barthez and Rilliet simply mention a redness of the throat as preceding the eruption on the skin, quoting Heim and Despine. Bednar makes no mention of the eruption. Osler (edition of 1892), speaking of the invasion of measles says: "Examination of the throat may show a reddish hyperaemia, or in some instances, a distinct punctiform rash. Occasionally this spreads over the whole mucous membrane of the mouth with the exception of the tongue."

Again in the paragraph on diagnosis and differential diagnosis, the rash on the mucous membrane is not made use of in the differential tests.

Henoch describes the eruption on the mucous membrane of the mouth thus: "Before the end of the second day, you may observe, especially in robust children, on the hard and soft palate, a diffuse redness, spotted in places. More often the pale mucous membrane shows the so-called palate exanthema to a greater or less extent, punctate or star shaped red spots. These, when distinctly visible, may be considered a positive evidence of beginning measles."

There is nothing especially distinctive about the eruption in the pharynx, or on the hard or soft palate in measles. The throat, in the beginning, is reddened, the fauces, the soft palate, may be spotted, but this is also the case in many affections, such as grippe, Rötheln, catarrhal angina, and scarlet fever. In the latter the redness is diffuse, not spotted. The first twenty-four to forty-eight hours of the invasion of measles is marked by a suffusion, slight or marked, of the eyes, and the conjunctiva at the nasal canthus is not only reddened, but distinctly redundant. There is, at this stage, a slight febrile movement; there may be a cough or some little sneezing; the mother has noticed nothing except that the infant or child has a slight fever. At this period the eruption on the skin has not made its appearance. In the majority of cases there is no suggestion of any exanthema. In a few cases there is an indistinct spotting around the lips and alae nasi, but no eruption.

The Mouth.—If we look in the mouth at this period, we see a redness of the fauces; perhaps, not in all cases, a few spots on the soft palate. On the buccal mucous membrane and the inside of the lips, we invariably see a distinct eruption. It consists of small, irregular spots, of a bright red color. In the centre of each spot, there is noted, in strong daylight, a minute bluish white speck. These red spots, with accompanying specks of a bluish white color, are absolutely pathognomonic of beginning measles, and when seen can be relied upon as the forerunner of the skin eruption. These bluish white specks have, I believe, been described by French writers, though the author has described them to students before he has seen mention of them elsewhere. No one, however, has to my knowledge called attention to the pathognomonic nature of these small bluish white specks, and their background of red irregular shaped spots. They cannot be mistaken for sprue, because they are not as large nor as white as sprue spots. These specks of bluish white, surrounded by a red area, are seen on the buccal mucous membrane and on the inside of the lips, not on the soft or hard palate. Sometimes only a few red spots, with the central bluish point, may exist, six or more, and in marked cases they may cover the whole inside of the buccal mucous membrane. If these bluish white specks, on a red spotted background, are at the height of their development, they never become white opaque as sprue, and in this respect, when once seen, are diagnostic, nor do they ever coalesce to become plaque like in form. They retain the punctate character. I have noted and demonstrated these spots on the buccal mucous membrane when the other symptoms were so slight that physicians have doubted the diagnosis. I have been invariably confirmed in my diagnosis by the subsequent appearance of the skin eruption.

Cycle.—The eruption just described is of

greatest value at the very outset of the disease, *the invasion*. As the skin eruption begins to appear and spreads, the eruption on the mucous membrane becomes diffuse, and the characters of a discrete eruption disappear and lose themselves in an intense general redness. When the skin eruption is at the efflorescence, the eruption on the buccal mucous membrane has lost the characters of a discrete spotting and has become a diffuse red background with innumerable bluish white specks scattered on its surface.

The buccal eruption begins to fade even while the skin exanthema is at its height, or at least while it is running a late course. The mucous membrane retrogrades to the normal appearances long before the eruption on the skin has disappeared. This being the case, it will be seen that the buccal eruption is of greatest diagnostic value at the outset of the disease, *before* the appearance of the skin eruption and at the outset and height of the skin eruption.

MUMPS
Hippocrates
BOOK I—OF THE EPIDEMICS*
SECTION I—CONSTITUTION FIRST

1. In Thasus, about the autumnal equinox, and under the Pleiades, the rains were abundant, constant, and soft, with southerly winds; the winter southerly, the northerly winds faint, droughts; on the whole, the winter having the character of spring. The spring was southerly, cool, rains small in quantity. Summer, for the most part, cloudy, no rain, the Etesian winds, rare and small, blew in an irregular manner. The whole constitution of the season being thus inclined to the southerly, and with droughts early in the spring, from the preceding opposite and northerly state, ardent fevers occurred in a few instances, and these very mild, being rarely attended with hemorrhage, and never proving fatal. Swellings appeared about the ears, in many on either side, and in the greatest number of both sides, being unaccompanied by fever so as not to confine the pa-

tient to bed; in all cases they disappeared without giving trouble, neither did any of them come to suppuration, as is common in swellings from other causes. They were of a lax, large, diffused character, without inflammation or pain, and they went away without any critical sign. They seized children, adults, and mostly those who were engaged in the exercises of the palestra and gymnasium, but seldom attacked women. Many had dry coughs without expectoration, and accompanied with hoarseness of voice. In some instances earlier, and in others later, inflammations with pain seized sometimes one of the testicles, and sometimes both; some of these cases were accompanied with fever and some not; the greater part of these were attended with much suffering. In other respects they were free of disease, so as not to require medical assistance.

INFLUENZA
Thomas Sydenham

41.[1] In the following year, viz. 1679, these intermittents reappeared at the beginning of July and increasing every day proved very violent and destructive in August. But having already treated of these at large, I shall only observe, that they gave way to a new epidemic which proceeded from the manifest qualities of the air in November.

42. For at the beginning of this month a cough arose, which was more epidemic than any I had hitherto observed; for it seized nearly whole families at once. Some required little medicine, but in others the cough occasioned such violent motion of the lungs, that sometimes a vomiting and vertigo ensued. On the first days of the disorder, the cough was almost dry and the expectoration not considerable, but afterwards the matter in some measure increased. In short, from the smallness of the expectoration, the violence of the cough and the duration of the

* *The Genuine Works of Hippocrates*, translated by Francis Adams, New York, Wm. Wood, n.d., Vol. I, p. 293.

[1] *Works of Sydenham, Thomas*, with notes . . . by Benjamin Rush, Philadelphia, Benj. and Thos. Kite, 1809, p. 215.

coughing fits; it seemed greatly to resemble the convulsive hooping cough of children, only it was not so severe. But it was attended with a fever and its usual concomitants, in which particular it exceeded the convulsion cough, for I never knew that accompanied with those symptoms.

43. Though coughs are common at the beginning of winter, yet every body wondered to find them so frequent this year; which I conceived proceeded chiefly from this cause: the month of October having been wetter than usual (for it seldom ceased raining), the blood, corresponding with the season, drank in abundance of crude, watery particles, by reason that perspiration was stopt upon the first coming of the cold, whence nature endeavoured to expel them, by means of a cough, through the branches of the pulmonary artery, or, as some will have it, through the glands of the windpipe.[2]

44. When there is occasion for medicine, I am sure the cure is best attempted by evacuation, namely by bleeding and purging; for the redundant serous particles cannot be so

[2] The disease under consideration appears to have been the influenza. Our author ascribes it to what he calls a manifest quality of the atmosphere, but its existing independently of its sensible qualities, and its not occurring uniformly in such weather as our author has mentioned, renders it probable that it depends upon an insensible matter in the air, and hence the rapidity with which it spreads through whole countries, and sometimes over half the globe. In no instance do the contagious diseases spread with the twentieth part of the rapidity of the influenza. The small pox was fifty years in affecting every part of Europe after its importation from the east, and we find from our author's account of that disease, that it was several years before it affected all the inhabitants of the compact city of London.

commodiously expelled by any other method, as by these two evacuations, which greatly empty the veins.

45. For as to pectorals, setting aside their pleasing the patient, I own I do not conceive how they can contribute to remove the cause of the cough; since their whole operation seems to consist, either in thickening the matter when it is too thin to be expectorated, or in attenuating it when, by reason of its viscidity, it comes up with difficulty. This I certainly know, that it is lost time to give such medicines, and that sometimes the blood is so impoverished by the retention of the serious particles which are prejudicial to nature, and further that the lungs, irritated by the violence of the cough, are so shaken by the great and almost continual motion, that a consumption is often occasioned thereby, from which the patient should be freed by hastening the cure. Nor are sudorifics much safer; for sometimes they cause a fever, and sometimes also the particles of the blood, which are easily inflamed, are so thrown upon the pleura, that a pleurisy is occasioned, which happened to great numbers in the course of this epidemic cough, and was very dangerous.

46. Accordingly I took away a moderate quantity of blood from the arm, and applied a sufficient large and strong blister to the neck, in order to make a revulsion of part of the peccant matter. Afterwards I exhibited a lenient cathartic every day, made an infusion of sena and rhubarb, with manna, and solutive syrup of roses, till the symptoms abated considerably, or a perfect recovery ensued; or if draughts were disagreeable, I directed two scruples of the greater pil. cochia, to be taken every morning at five o'clock, sleeping upon them.

SWEATING FEVER

John Caius

John Caius was born at Norwick in 1510, and entered Gonville Hall, Cambridge, as a scholar in 1529. In the bursar's account, while he was a student there we find his name spelled in at least ten different ways—Keese, Kees, Keyes, Keis, Cais, Kaius, Keyse, Cayus, Keysse, and Caius. These spellings indicate that he pronounced his own name "Keyes," and as such was always known among his contemporaries. At the time of Caius' entrance at Cambridge the English Reformation was not yet victorious, and the student body consisted of two groups, the monks, who were soon to disappear, and the resident fellows and masters of arts, who sympathized with the reformers. The students were a very studious lot who took their pleasures, not in games, but in disputations, and who spent their slender allowances not on clothes, but upon books.

Caius took his B.A. degree in 1532 and apparently looked forward to entering the priesthood. However, his lack of sympathy with the Reformation caused him to study medicine instead. Although he was later physician to Edward VI and Queen Elizabeth, he seems to have remained at heart a Roman Catholic and was frequently denounced as a "papist."

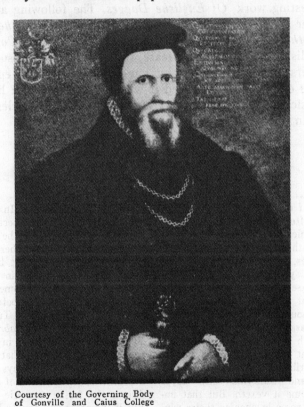

Courtesy of the Governing Body
of Gonville and Caius College

JOHN CAIUS (1510-1573)
From the portrait presented by Dr. Caius to the Gonville
and Caius College. Artist unknown

In 1539, Caius left England and went to Padua to study medicine. There he became acquainted with Vesalius, who was preparing his *De Fabrica Humani Corporis* and lived in the same house with him for eight months. He received his M.D. at Padua in 1541 and remained at the University for two years as professor, an unique distinction for a foreigner. He returned to England in 1544 and began practice at London three years later. He was admitted to membership in the College of Physicians in 1547 and in 1555 became its president.

In London he erected a monument in St. Paul's Cathedral to the memory of Linacre, and in 1557, while physician to Queen Mary, he endowed his old college at Cambridge and changed its name from "Gonville Hall" to "Gonville and Caius College." The following year he became master of his old college and held this position until a year before his death, which occurred in 1573. He was buried in the college chapel under a monument he himself had designed, with the well known epitaph: *Fui Caius* (I was Caius).

Caius, while master of the college, obtained permission to take the bodies of two malefactors annually for dissection and was thus a pioneer in advancing the study of anatomy in England. He published several medical works and an interesting work, *Of Englishe Dogges.* The following account of the sweating fever is taken from his *A boke or counseile against the disease commonly called the sweate or sweatyng sicknesse made by Jhon Caius doctour in phisicke,* published in 1552. This disease, sweating fever, the "sudor Anglicus" of later writers, has been thought by some to have been an epidemic of influenza, while others have identified it with miliary fever. In his account of the sweating sickness, Caius makes no reference to miliary vesicles, a characteristic finding in miliary fever.

THE BOKE OF JHON CAIUS
AGAINST THE SWEATYNG SICKNES

In the yere of our Lorde God M.CCCC.-lxxxv. shortly after the vij. daye of august, at whiche tyme kynge Henry the seuenth arriued at Milford in Walles, out of France, and in the firste yere of his reigne, ther chaunced a disease among the people, lastyng the reste of that monethe & all september, which for the soubdeine sharpenes and vn-wont cruelnes passed the pestilence. For this commonly geueth iij. or iiij. often vij. sum-tyme ix. as that firste at Athenes whiche *Thucidides* describeth in his seconde boke, sumtyme xj. and sumtyme xiiij. dayes respecte. to whome it vexeth. But that immediately killed some in opening theire win-dowes, some in plaieng with children in their strete dores, some in one hour, many in two it destroyed, & at the longest, to thē that merilye dined, it gaue a soroful Supper. As it founde them so it toke them, some in sleape some in wake, some in mirthe some in care, some fasting and some ful, some busy and some idle, and in one house sometyme three sometime fiue, sometyme seuen some-tyme eyght, sometyme more some tyme all, of the whyche, if the haulfe in euerye Towne escaped, it was thoughte great favour. How, or wyth what manner it toke them, with what grieffe, and accidentes it helde theym, here-after thē I wil declare, whō I shal come to

The begin-nyng of the disease

shewe the signes thereof. In the mene space. know that this disease (because it most did stand in sweating from the beginning vntil the endyng) was called here, the Sweating sickenesse: and because it firste beganne in Englande, it was named in other countries, the englishe sweat. Yet some coniecture that it, or the like, hath bene before seene among the Grekes in the siege of Troie. In thēperor Octauius warres at *Cantabria*, called nowe Biscai, in Hispaine: and in the Turkes, at the Rhodes. How true that is, let the authours loke: how true thys is, the best of our Chronicles shewith, & of the late begonne disease the freshe memorie yet confirmeth. But if the name wer now to be geuen, and at my libertie to make the same: I would of the manner and space of the disease (by cause the same is no sweat only, as herafter I will declare, & in the spirites) make the name *Ephemera*, which is to sai, a feuer of one natural dai. A feuer, for the feuor or burning, drieth & sweating feure like. Of one naturall day, for that it lasteth but the time of xxiiij. houres. And for a distinction from the commune *Ephemera*, that Galene writeth of, comming both of other causes, and wyth vnlike paines, I wold putte to it either Eng-lishe, for that it followeth somoche English menne, to whō it is almoste proper, & also began here: or els pestilent, for that it cōmeth by infection & putrefaction, otherwise then doth the other *Ephemera*. Whiche thing I suppose may the better be done, because I se straunge and no english names both in Latine and Greke by commune vsage taken for Englishe. As in Latin, Feure, Quotidiā, Tertian, Quartane, Aier, Infection, Pestilence, Uomite, Person, Reines, Ueines, Peines, Chamere, Numbre, &c. a litle altered by the commune pronunciation. In Greke, Pleuresie, Ischiada, Hydrops, Aposthema, Phlegma, and Chole: called by the vulgare pronunciatiō, Schiatica, Dropsie, Impostume, Phleume, & Choler: Gyne also, and Boutyre, Sciorel, Mouse, Rophe, Phrase, Paraphrase, & cephe, whereof cometh Chaucers couercephe, in the romant of the Rose, writtē and pronoūced comōly, kerchief in yᵉ south, & courchief in the north. Thereof euery head or principall thing, is commonlye called cephe, pronoūced & writtē, chief. Uery many other there be in our commune tongue, whiche here to rehearse were to long. These for an example shortelye I haue here noted. But for the name of this disease it maketh now no matter, the name of Sweat beyng cōmōly vsed. Let vs therfore returne to the thing, which as occasiō & cause serued, came againe in M.D.vi. the xxii. yeare of the said Kyng Henry the seuenth. Aftre that, in the yeare M.D.xvii. the ix. yeare of Kyng Henry the viii, and endured from July, vnto yᵉ middest of Decēbre. The iiii tyme, in the year M.D.xxviii. the xx. yeare of the saied Kyng, beginning in thende of May, & continuing June and July. The fifth tyme of this fearful *Ephemera* of Englande, and pestilent sweat, is this in the yeare M.D.L.I. of oure Lorde God, and the fifth yeare of oure Souereigne Lorde king Edwarde the sixth, beginning at Shrewsbury in the middest of April, proceeding with greate mortalitie to Ludlowe, Prestene, and other places in Wales, then to Westchestre, Couentre, Oxenfoorde, and other tounes in the Southe, and such as were in and aboute the way to London, whether it came notablie the seuenth of July, and there continuing sore, with the losse of vii C. lxi. from the ix. day vntil the xvi. daye, besides those that died in the vii. and viii. dayes, of whō no registre was kept, for that it abated until the xxx. day of the same, with the losse of C.xlii. more. Then ceassing there, it wente from thence throughe al the east partes of England into the Northe vntill the ende of Auguste, at whiche tyme it di-

minished, and in the ende of Septembre fully ceased.

This disease is not a Sweat onely, (as it is thought & called) but a feuer, as I saied, in the spirites by putrefaction venemous, with a fight, trauaile, and laboure of nature againste the infection receyued in the spirites, wherevpon by chaunce foloweth a Sweate, or issueth an humour compelled by nature, as also chanceth in other sicknesses whiche consiste in humours, when they be in their state, and at the worste in certein dayes iudicial, aswel by vomites, bledinges, & fluxes, as by sweates. That this is true, the self sweates do shewe. For as in vtter businesses, bodies yᵗ sore do labour, by trauail of the same are forced to sweat, so in inner diseases, the bodies traueiled & labored by thē, are moued to the like. In which labors, if nature be stōg & able to thrust out the poisō by sweat (not otherwise letted) yᵉ persō escapeth: if not, it dieth. That it is a feuer, thus I haue partly declared, and more wil streight by the notes of the disease, vnder one shewing also by thesame notes, signes, and short tariance of the same, that it consisteth in the spirites. First by the piene in the backe, or shoulder, peine in the extreme partes, as arme, or legge, with a flusshing, or wind, as it semeth to certeine of the pacientes, flieng in the same. Secondly by the grief in the liuer and the nigh stomacke. Thirdely, by the peine in the head, & madnes of the same. Fourthly by the passion of the hart. For the flusshing or wynde comming in the vtter and extreame partes, is nothing els but the spirites of those same gathered together, at the first entring of the euell aire, agaynste the infection thereof, & flyeng thesame from place to place, for their owne sauegarde. But at the last infected, they make a grief where thei be forced, which cōmonly is on tharme or legge (the fartheste partes of theire refuge) the backe or shulder: thrieng ther first a brūt as good souldiers, before they wil let their enemye come further into theire dominion. The other grefes be therefore in thother partes aforesaid & sorer, because the spirites be there most plentuous as in their founteines, whether alwaies thinfection desireth to go. For frō the liuer, the nigh stomack, braine, and harte, come all the iij. sortes, and kyndes of spirites, the gouernoures of oure bodies, as firste spronge there. But from the hart, the liuish spirites. In putrifieng wherof by the euel aier in bodies fit for it, the harte is oppressed. Whereupon also foloweth a maruelous heauinesse, (the fifthe token of this disease), and a desire to sleape, neuer, contented, the senses in al partes beynge as they were bounde or closed vp, the partes therefore left heuy, vnliuishe, and dulle. Laste foloweth the shorte abidinge, a certeine Token of the disease to be in the spirites, as wel may be proued by the *Ephemera* that Galene writethe of, whiche because it consistethe in the Spirites, lasteth but one natural day. For as fire in hardes or straw, is sone in flambe & sone oute, euen so heate in the spirites, either by simple distemperature, or by infection and putrefaction therin conceyued, is sone in flambe and sone out, and soner for the vehemencye or greatnes of the same, whiche without lingering, consumeth sone the light matter, contrary to al other diseases restyng in humoures, wherein a fire ones kindeled, is not so sone put out, no more than is the same in moiste woodde, or fat Sea coles, as well by the particular Example of the pestilence, (of al others most lyke vnto this) may be declared, whyche by that it stãdeth in euel humors, tarieth as I said, sometyme, from iiij. vii. ix. & xj. vntill xiiij dayes, differentlie from this, by reason thereof, albeit by infection most lyke to this same. Thus vnder one laboure shortelie I haue declared—both what this disease is, wherin it consisteth, howe and with what accidentes it grieueth and is differente from the Pestilence, and the propre signes, and tokens of the same, without the whiche, if any do sweate, I take theym not to Sweate by this Sickenesse, but rather by feare, heate of the yeare, many clothes, greate exercise, affection, excesses in diete, or at the worst, by a smal cause of infection, and lesse disposition of the bodi to this sicknes. So that, insomuche as the body was nat al voide of matter, sweate it did when infection came: but in that the mattere was not greate, the same coulde neyther be perilous nor paineful as in others, in whom it was greater cause.

CHICKEN POX

William Heberden

CHAPTER 96

VARIOLAE PUSILLAE. THE CHICKEN POX*

The chicken pox and swine pox differ, I believe, only in name: they occasion so little danger or trouble to the patients, that physicians are seldom sent for to them, and have therefore very few opportunities of seeing this distemper. Hence it happens that the name of it is met with in very few books, and hardly any pretend to say a word of its history.

But though it be so insignificant an illness, that an acquaintance with it is not so much use for its own sake, yet it is of importance on account of the small pox, with which it may otherwise be confounded, and so deceive the persons, who have had it, into a false security, which may prevent them either from keeping out of the way of the small pox, or from being inoculated. For this reason I have judged it might be useful to contribute, what I have learned from experience, towards its description.

These pocks break out in many without any illness or previous sign: in others they are preceded by a little degree of chillness, lassitude, cough, broken sleep, wandering pains, loss of appetite, and feverishness for three days.

In some patients I have observed them to make their first appearance on the back, but this perhaps is not constant. Most of them are of the common size of the small pox, but some are less. I never saw them confluent, nor very numerous. The greatest number, which I ever observed, was about twelve in the face, and two hundred over the rest of the body.

On the first day of the eruption they are reddish. On the second day there is at the top of most of them a very small bladder, about the size of a millet-seed. This is sometimes full of a watery and colourless, sometimes of a yellowish liquor, contained between the

* Heberden, William, *Commentaries on the History and Cure of Diseases,* Boston, Wellys and Lilly, 1818, p. 361.

cuticle and skin. On the second, or, at the farthest, on the third day from the beginning of the eruption, as many of these pocks, as are not broken, seem arrived at their maturity; and those which are fullest of that yellow liquor, very much resemble what the genuine small pox are on the fifth or sixth day, especially where there happens to be a larger space than ordinary occupied by the extravasated serum. It happens to most of them, either on the first day that this little bladder arises, or on the day after, that its tender cuticle is burst by the accidental rubbing of the clothes, or by the patient's hands to allay the itching which attends this eruption. A thin scab is then formed at the top of the pock, and the swelling of the other part abates, without its ever being turned into pus, as it is in the small pox. Some few escape being burst; and the little drop of liquor contained in the vesicle at the top of them grows yellow and thick, and dries into a scab. On the fifth day of the eruption they are almost all dried and covered with a slight crust. The inflammation of these pocks is very small, and the contents of them do not seem to be owing to suppuration, as in the small pox, but rather to what is extravasated immediately under the cuticle by the serous vessels of the skin, as in a common blister. No wonder therefore that this liquor appears so soon as on the second day, and that upon the cuticle being broken it is presently succeeded by a slight scab: hence too, as the true skin is so little affected, no mark or scar is likely to be left, unless in one or two pocks, where, either by being accidentally much fretted, or by some extraordinary sharpness of the contents, a little ulcer is formed in the skin.

The patients scarce suffer any thing throughout the whole progress of this illness, except some languidness of strength and spirits and appetite, all which may probably be owing to the confining of themselves to their chamber. I saw two children ill of the chicken pox, whose mother chose to be with them, though she had never had this illness. Upon the eighth or ninth day after the pocks were at their height in the children, the mother fell ill of this distemper then beginning to show itself. In this instance the infection lay in the body much about the same time that it is known to do in the small pox.

Remedies are not likely to be much wanted in a disease attended with hardly any inconvenience, and which in so short a time is certainly cured of itself.

The principal marks, by which the chicken pox may be distinguished from the small pox are.

1. The appearance on the second or third day from the eruption of that vesicle full of serum upon the top of the pock.

2. The crust, which covers the pocks on the fifth day; at which time those of the small pox are not at the height of their suppuration.

Foreign medical writers hardly ever mention the name of this distemper; and the writers of our own country scarce mention any thing more of it, than in name. Morton speaks of it as if he supposed it to be a very mild genuine small pox. But these two distempers are surely totally different from one another, not only on account of their different appearances above mentioned, but because those, who have had small pox, are capable of being infected with chicken pox; but those, who have once had the chicken pox, are not capable of having it again, though to such, as have never had this distemper, it seems as infectious as the small pox. I wetted a thread in the most concocted pus-like liquor of the chicken-pox which I could find; and after making a slight incision, it was confined upon the arm of one who had formerly had it; the little wound healed up immediately, and shewed no signs of an infection. From the great similitude between the two distempers, it is probable, that, instead of the small pox, some persons have been inoculated from the chicken pox, and that the distemper which has succeeded, has been mistaken for the small pox by hasty and unexperienced observers.

There is sometimes seen an eruption, concerning which I have been in doubt, whether it be one of the many unnoticed cutaneous diseases, or only, as I am rather inclined to believe, a more malignant sort of chicken pox.

This disorder is preceded for three or four days by all the symptoms which forerun the chicken pox, but in a much higher degree. On the fourth or fifth day the eruption appears, with very little abatement of the fever; the pains likewise of the limbs and back still continue, to which are joined pains of the gums. The pocks are redder than the chicken pox, and spread wider, and hardly rise so high, at least not in proportion to their size. Instead of one little head or vesicle of a serous matter, these have from four to ten or twelve. They go off just like the chicken pox, and are distinguishable from the small pox by the same marks; besides which the continuance of the pains and fever after the eruption, and the degree of both these, though there be not above twenty pocks, are, as far as I have seen, what never happen to the small pox.

Many foreigners seem so little to have attended to the peculiar characteristics of the small pox, particularly the length of time, which it requires to its full maturation, that we may the less wonder at the prevailing opinion among them, that the same person is liable to have it several times. Petrus Borellus* records the case of a woman, who had this distemper seven times, and catching it again died of it the eighth time. It would be no extravagant assertion to say, that here in England not above one in ten thousand patients is pretended to have had it twice; and wherever it is pretended, it will always be as likely that the persons about the patient were mistaken, and supposed that to be the small pox, which was an eruption of a different nature, as that there was such an extraordinary exception to what we are sure is so general a law.

* *Hist. and Obs. Rar. Med. Phys.,* centur. iii obs. 10.

GLANDULAR FEVER

Dr. Emil Pfeiffer (Wiesbaden)

A LECTURE READ AT THE NATURFORSCHER VERSAMMLUNG IN COLOGNE*

The object of the communication to which I wish to direct your attention for a short time, is a disease which appears very frequently in children. I would not venture to speak of it here, except that the medical literature, and especially the textbooks of pediatrics, say nothing whatsoever concerning it. It is not my intention to present you a complete and exhaustive picture of this disease, since up to this time the pathological anatomical findings are lacking and bacteriological reports as well. My purpose is only to sketch for you the clinical picture, as a foundation to which further observations and contributions can be added. Without doubt this clinical picture, like so many of our clinical pictures, includes different disease-processes and bacteriological and pathological investigations are necessary before we can separate forms which differ in etiology and in anatomical findings.

I present to you the most commonly observed picture of the disease.

You are called to see a child 5, 6, or 8 years old, which became sick during the night or on the evening before, with high fever, pains in all extremities, and great uneasiness. Perhaps it has also vomiting and loss of appetite.

Inquiries into the history show no indica-

tions of any especial injury which could have produced it, nor have they enjoyed heavy food or an excess of food nor have they been chilled or exposed to the weather, had excessive exercise or anything of the sort. Also no contact with any patient suffering from a contagious disease can be proved.

The fever is marked—between 39 and 40 C; the tongue is a little coated, the fauces highly reddened but without any membrane. Constipation. All organs are normal, but over the neck there is a great tenderness, not only in swallowing, but also in moving and, during the investigation, we find numerous swollen and painful lymph glands around the entire neck, but especially around the sterno-mastoid and the nape of the neck. The following day the fever has often disappeared and there is nothing abnormal present except the more or less numerous enlarged and painful lymph glands on the neck. The child is again frisky, but still holds its neck a little stiff or complains of slight pains on swallowing. After a few days, the glands have all gone down and everything has returned to normal.

This is the course of a large number of cases and if one does not know the disease, and, the day before, has shown an anxious face and has thought of all the possible terrible infectious diseases, he is, on the following day, astonished and somewhat chagrined.

Besides the light cases, which perhaps form

* Pfeiffer, Emil, *Jahrb. f. Kinderh.,* 1889, xxix, 257.

the so-called "febricula" of the old authors, there is moreover a whole series of cases which last longer and the disease in such cases can prolong itself 8 or 10 days. In these cases, the fever does not disappear on the second day, but continues for several days at the original level, the glands swelling up, first on one side of the neck and then, the following day, those on the other side begin to be painful and to enlarge: other glands in the neck are also involved, the mucosa of the throat becomes red and there is slight pain on swallowing, also a light cough may appear and symptoms of a cold appear. On the third or fourth day, every time, the liver and spleen are definitely enlarged, both palpable and, in the majority of cases, there is paain in the lower abdomen, which, every time, is precisely in the midline and exactly in the middle between the umbilicus and symphysis. This pain is more commonly spontaneous than induced by pressure.

Aside from the appearance in the glands and the fever, there are no further signs: neither the throat, nor digestive organs, nor the lungs, nor the skin show any especial disturbances. The light angina shows no tendency to the formation of a membrane and is never severe enough to explain the high fever; the appetite is not so diminished as to cause one to think of a stomach complaint, the stools are constipated, no diarrhoea. The lungs are quite normal and no skin eruptions are seen.

The glands which swell up in these cases, besides the liver and spleen, are only the glands of the neck, especially of the nape, the axillary and inguinal glands I have never found swollen. The light, irritating cough and the pain on swallowing, as well as the pain between the umbilicus and symphysis, suggest that also the retro-esophageal, retro-tracheal, and mesenteric lymph glands are swollen; however there is no certainty concerning this, as they never become palpable.

The chronic cases give rise to more errors, false diagnoses, and difficulties than the light cases. If one will only pay attention to the enlargement of the glands, so the onset of a severe illness like scarlet or thyroid will not be feared. The enlargement of the glands of the neck—this characteristic symptom makes such a fear groundless. Many similar cases, however, may be regarded as an abortive typhoid.

The course of the disease is always favorable. Even in the severe cases recovery comes in a few days, although the child often remains for some time pale and anemic. The glands never go on to suppuration.

Clinical experience characterizes this disease in question as an infectious disease, because it appears in epidemics and indeed in house epidemics. If also at certain times in a large group of houses, several cases appear simultaneously, so one cannot call it an epidemic and speak of the disease as an infectious disease, since this can appear in any disease. But the appearance of definite house epidemics, family epidemics, speaks for the infectious character of the disease. I will describe for you, as an example, the course of a family epidemic which I observed in the course of this year in the family of a worker.

As I visited the family daily for the electrical treatment of the nervous disease of the wife, so one day in the month of January. the 13-year old son was presented to me, who had not been entirely well for several days and had been absent from school. He showed clearly swollen and slightly painful lymph glands on the neck behind the sternomastoid. There was no fever present. However he complained of a disagreeable scratching of his neck and a sensation of cold. The symptoms disappeared in a few days, the glands became painless and gradually disappeared and the boy returned to school.

On the 26th of January the eldest son, 16 years old, became ill with chills and fever, loss of appetite, weakness in his extremities and nervous, and an estimation of the temperature in the evening showed 39.6 C. in the axilla. Examination the following day showed, aside from the fever, no local findings except the swelling and pain of several neck glands behind the sternomastoid on the right side. The loss of appetite and pain in the extremities continued until January 29, when the temperature became normal. The 30th of January the temperature was again elevated, numerous painful and large lymph glands appeared in the left side of the neck behind the sternomastoid muscle, the spleen and liver definitely enlarged and there was a distinct spontaneous pain between the umbilicus and symphysis. The first of February the temperature again became normal and remained for several days subnormal. At the same time there appeared a striking weakness and a general loss of energy for about 10 to 14 days, just as after a severe infectious disease. The boy in question had recovered two years previously from typhoid fever.

On January 30th, 5 days after the eldest brother, the youngest daughter, 10 years old, became sick, also feverish, with definite gastric disturbances, weakness, chills, and fever. Here also the lymph glands of the neck were swollen and painful and the spleen and liver on the fourth day became enlarged. The patient complained of no pain between the umbilicus and symphysis.

During this time, the 11-year old son of the family also became ill, although he was not confined to bed. He only missed school 3 or 4 days, he complained of similar symptoms like his older brothers and sister, especially scratchings in the neck and a cough. The cervical lymph glands were swollen and painful.

The curves show the fever in the 16-year old boy and the 10-year old girl.

In this house epidemic, the four children of the family became ill and so uniformly, varying only in the degree, that we must assume here a common cause. The different beginnings of the disease speaks for a longer lasting activity of the cause of the disease and most of all for the presence of some infectious material.

This is the usual course of house epidemics. In certain cases one must be careful not to diagnose this described disease only from the existence of enlarged cervical glands. In many children, especially young children, the cervical glands are constantly enlarged, but entirely painless. Only when in a fever the lymph glands enlarge, so to say, under the eyes of the observer, and especially when they become quickly painful, has one the right to think of the described disease as glandular fever. One is sure only when the lymph glands which were previously swollen like a rosary back of the sternomastoid, re-

turn completely to normal and in a few days or weeks.

The lymph glands in front of the sternomastoid also frequently take part in the process; however, nothing characteristic in their enlargement, since they also enlarge in many other diseases and become painful, for example in sore throat, in stomatitis, etc.

Whether we are dealing here with an especial disease, a disease *sui generis*, or whether the glandular fever is only an abortive condition of some other disease, it is for the present undetermined, and further observation is necessary.

Abortive typhoid comes to consideration only in those cases which last a considerable time, but even in them there is no reason to think of the typhoid process. The observation of the 16-year old patient mentioned above, who two years previously had had a characteristic attack of typhoid fever, speaks very decidedly against such a suggestion. The prodromal appearances were absent, the gradual climbing and falling of temperature were absent, there was no headache, no bronchitis, and especially no diarrhoea.

The abortive diphtheria, that is, one without a membrane, could only be assumed if the lymph glands near the tonsils were involved. The lymph glands in the back of the neck never swell in diphtheritic processes and one would not think here of a typical case of diphtheria.

One would think first of an abortive scarlet fever, abortive measles or chickenpox, since in these diseases the lymph glands are usually markedly swollen. Still, in all the cases of simple glandular fever observed up to this time, the possibility of an infection with these diseases cannot be entertained.

The therapy of glandular fever consists of rubbing the swollen glands with oil or packing the neck in cotton, and rest in bed in severe cases.

WHOOPING COUGH

Guillaume Baillou

CONSTITUTIO AESTIVA
ANNI DOMINI 1578*

Now the beginning of summer has been

* Ballonius, Gulielmus, *Epidemiorum et Ephemeridum libri duo. Opera omnia*, Venice, Jeremia, 1736, I, p. 155.

discussed before. At the close of summer almost the same diseases prevailed as before. The summer was burning & hot. Fevers attacked boys of four months, of ten months and a little older, countless numbers of whom died. Principally that common cough, which is usually called *Quinta* or *Quintana,* which has been mentioned before. Serious are the symptoms of this. The lung is so irritated so that every attempt to expell that which is causing trouble, it neither admits the air nor again easily expells it. The patient is seen to swell up & as if strangled holds his breath tightly in the middle of his throat. Why it is commonly called *Quinta,* is not without uncertainty. They think the word is formed from onomatopaea, from the sound & rattling which those coughing make. Others do not derive it from this, but think the cough is called *Quintana* in Latin because it is repeated at certain hours. This indeed experience proves to be true. For they are without this troublesome coughing for the space of four or five hours at a time, then this paroxysm of coughing returns, now so severe that blood is expelled with force through the nose & through the mouth. Most frequently an upset of the stomach follows, nor have I read any author, who has made mention of this cough.

And they doubt whether from the head, or from the body of the lung itself or from some other place, the serum or acrid fluid, or lymph or bestial distillation is wont to trickle down. It seems to be from the lung itself. For we have seen so many coughing in such manner, in whom after a vain attempt semiputrid matter in an incredible quantity was ejected. So it seems very likely that this matter which is present & collected there is the cause of this very cough. To others it seems to be from the head itself, as if liquified by some effusion, as Hippocrates says; What if from elsewhere? For there are two remarkable passages in Galen & Hippocrates, from which a proof of these points can be elicited: Galen in his *Epidemics* assigning the causes of a dry cough, states the first cause to be irritation of the gullet & throat. Second a disturbance of the apparatus serving respiration. Third, thickness of the humor. Fourth, thinness of the humor. Then concerning thin humor he wrote thus: Now a thin humor running down into the throat & the trachea into the lung, that is, it is prevented from being spread out and divided or before it is poured out and dispersed (for the interpreters carelessly omit the elegant word φθάνει) before it is excluded by the blast of air excited by the cough which happened to

the Thasions since with the head full of dryness, thus the distillation was transmitted to all parts of the thorax. . . .

Conforming to these ideas Hippocrates wrote: Erysipelas may be in the lungs when it is dried too much from heat, from fevers, work and intemperance. For then it draws too much blood to itself, mostly from the great veins. For these are themselves near & rest upon it: then it draws the blood out most thinly and feebly. When it draws it, an acute fever comes from it, a dry cough, fullness in the chest, acute pain in the anterior & posterior parts, greatest around the spine with the large veins becoming too heated. They vomit sometimes a somewhat bloody at other times a rather bluish material. They vomit phlegm & bile & become breathless. In this place moreover he explains the nature of this most distressing cough, which is called *Quinta.* And the cause of the cough is not from the head, as is thought by many, but sometimes from the lung itself, sometimes from adjacent parts. That it may be from the lung itself, the enormous amount of putrid and semi-putrid phlegm which is coughed out proves: for if the bestial distillation were the sole cause of this annoying cough, which is commonly called *Quinta,* such an incredible amount of material would not have been expelled.

However, I do not deny that sometimes something flows from the head which irritates or from the head which irritates the matter collected in the abdomen from behaving in the same manner as that material which is in the stomach? But that which is in the abdomen, if at any time it is stirred, causes griping, & pricking in the belly, dysentery, diarrhoea, slight ulcerations. So also it causes irritation in the lung, it irritates as it is moved, & makes man subject to coughing, excites true coughing & a useless desire to cough. Therefore those err who refer the cause of the cough to the head.

* * *

The little daughters of Doctor Richer & Doctor Rose & Joannes Connart were seized with a steady fever with coughing (which they call *Quinta*). There was associated both cough & fever until emaciation. The symptoms were extraordinary. A melting nearly reached them like that which was mentioned before, indeed the hot and acrid distillations caused a thinning of the body. Beyond hope they recovered.

* * *

The son of Doctor Conart suffered from this common cough, which is called Quinta. Continued fever. An incredible amount of putrid phlegm was brought up from the lungs by coughing. It is no wonder, if the boys unable to expectorate die from the force of such coughing. For they were oppressed by both the amount & the heaviness of the peccant matter.

RHEUMATIC FEVER

Guillaume Baillou

DESCRIPTION OF THE FIRST AFFECTION WHICH IS GIVEN THE NAME OF RHEUMATISM*

BEFORE we place this affection in a class of diseases or symptoms (since it causes its effects by the primary disease and the symptoms produced by it is commonly & very badly confused) just as what it is, we shall explain by what and in what manner it arises: we shall point out the train of pains & symptoms also present, not neglecting some examples of those whom we see attacked by this affection, & by what manner these may be met and considered: for thus the treatment itself leads in some degree to its knowledge & understanding.

It is proper to note especially in this place that two groups of patients that are affected. This is fundamental in the discussion

In the first place moreover it is proper to observe the persons in whom this affection takes hold, & in what way they are attacked, & how the blood is affected. Two kinds of persons, experience teaches, are attacked especially by this affection, one of them healthy, seen in the fullness of health but soon attacked by the disease; when now this disease attacks, a spontaneous lassitude precedes it & the blood is diseased, & indeed this is found to be the case, as was noted by Hippocrates, they are obviously sick as soon as they are attacked. The other kind of persons usually attacked by this affection, are those who at the time are really sick, indeed especially with a chronic disease, which has now desisted or seems dissolved by a false & hasty crisis, but however it survives and is not destroyed: the case of President Greyotte demonstrates this, whom this type of disease attacked most severely.

Now concerning other kinds of patients.

*Baillou, Guillaume, *Liber de rheumatismo. Opera Medica omnia*, Geneva, De Tournes, 1762, p. 314.

Among the patients now who are tried so by this grave disease, a great many are either cacochymic or not so much caco-chymic as plethoric & full blooded, in whom either on account of a checking of its dispersion or from some other cause, produces disease of the blood, indeed especially those persons are subject to this disease who are apt to be attacked by the putrid synochus fever. For since there is movement & corruption of the blood in synochus, the blood itself does the same in this fever, but in a different manner, for neither is the fever evident, but in a certain measure confined, so that instead of the synochial fever in which the blood is inflamed evenly & feverish, this affection advances almost without fever. For we see among the patients, very many certainly attacked by fever, in one way or another, although their blood is pure; on the contrary, others in whom the humors are putrid, in some manner of which I am ignorant, are seen to be free from fever: for they are seen to fever anyhow with a fever which is perceived. And this type of men are seized with this disease concerning which this discussion is undertaken.

Chyle

* * *

On the other hand the method by which this affection attacks which is falsely called catarrh: (for the name catarrh signifies distillation from the head) it seems better to speak of the other as rheumatism, is as follows. But in order that it be better understood it is proper to recall the previously mentioned hypothesis of the difference of the people who are attacked by this disease for it appears in the same manner in the healthy and in the ill, but different and of another kind in the body affected. The whole body becomes painful, the face in some becomes red, the pain rages especially about the joints, so that indeed neither the foot nor the hand, nor the finger can be moved in the least without pain & outcry: moreover in the same way the greater pain lies in the joints because that part is endowed with greater and more exquisite sensation. For the causes of the pains present equally either in the part, or in the whole body, that part pains most which has the more delicate sense, as Galen wrote on pains in the head. When the hand is pressed on the parts, the sensation & feeling, (even if you touch it lightly) is of a definite severe heat. If you examine the pulse, the fever is seen to be little or nothing: & indeed there is neverless fever but not very great: which if it becomes greater should have been indeed a continued putrid fever besides the heat is perceived to be severe, &

Fever (which is to be noted) the disease is brought on by purgation, a custom in those diseases which consist in inflammation. The fever which is present in the state of the body, whence Galen formerly considered the seat of origin, as we taught in the treatise on causes, which fever does not have obvious exacerbations. Indeed the pains are worse at night, the patients cannot sleep, partly because they are unable to be moved from their position & from that posture they first usually lie and recline, they remain in it & are scarcely moved or touched without excruciating or terrible pain, there is a contraction & a certain sensation of stinging, moreover there is a fullness & cacochymia: from which things those who

suffer from this affection, although bled copiously & frequently, this is obviously corrupted & dissolved into a putrid serum. Finally all kinds of muscles and nerves are replaced by serum and putrid blood which makes in these same parts an abscess or some kind of inflammation whence the pain arises. For such pains are formed on account of the sharpness of the matter, & because nature chooses to deposit this substance not yet mild, not as yet prepared for the passages in the skin. And although the arthritis is in a certain part, this rheumatism itself is in the entire body; with pain, tension and a somewhat sharp feeling, others say with the sensation of heat (as already mentioned). Both are very severe: but the arthritic pain recurs at certain times and at certain periods: this rheumatism is not the same as in those who sin in their way of life, so that the nerves become infirm & with increasing cacochymia at length can have an arthritic habitus or diathesis. And indeed those who suffer rheumatism three or four times (unless they guard themselves or take care) can scarcely escape the arthritic torment, so that this rheumatism is like a prodrome & preparation for arthritis. This affection can not be better explained and described, than by stating the analogy and affinity which there is between this & arthritis: and very many indeed of the physicians who are not yet familiar with this affection, have given it the name of universal arthritis. And the treatment which we shall propose a little later, will teach us from what humor the principle comes.

Thomas Sydenham
CHAPTER V*
RHEUMATISM

1. This disease may come on at any time. It is commonest, however, during the autumn, chiefly attacking the young and vigorous. It generally originates in some such cause as the following. The patient has been heated by either some over-violent exercise, or by some other means, and has taken

cold upon it. The sad list of symptoms begins with chills and shivers; these are followed immediately by heat, disquietude, thirst, and the other concomitants of fever. One or two days after this (sometimes sooner) the patient is attacked by severe pains in the joints, sometimes in one and sometimes in another, sometimes in his wrist, sometimes in his shoulder, sometimes in the knee—in this last joint oftenest. This pain changes its place from time to time, takes the joints in turns,

* Sydenham, Thomas, *Medical Observations. The Works of Thomas Sydenham* translated by R. G. Latham, M.D., London, Sydenham Society, 1848, I, p. 254.

and affects the one that it attacks last with redness and swelling. Sometimes during the first days the fever and the above-named symptoms go hand in hand; the fever, however, gradually goes off whilst the pain only remains; sometimes, however, it grows worse.

The febrile matter has, in that case, been transferred to the joints. This is clearly proved from the fact of the fever being frequently lit up afresh after the driving of the morbific matter by the unseasonable use of external remedies.

Richard Morton

CHAPTER XI

OF A CONSUMPTION PROCEEDING FROM THE GOUT, AND FROM A RHEUMATISM*

There is a colliquation in a Gout and Rheumatism
In a Gout and Rheumatism, especially that which is true and Humorose (which is caused by a sharp Ferment supplied from the Nerves) there is such an evident Colliquation in the whole Mass of Blood, that no Body can reasonably think it strange, that a Consumption should arise from these Distempers (but especially when they are Stubborn, and Chronical, and return often). And hereupon it is an easy Matter to observe, that a Rheumatick Pain, coming from the taking of Cold, seldom, if ever, is wont to seize upon the Joynts without a Pulmonary Cough. And as I have seen that great Man, the Lord *Bridgman,*

In Rheumatic pains there is a cough
Mr. *Philips,* and Mr. *Tibs,* and many others, after frequent and long Fits of the Gout and Rheumatism, die at last of a Consumption or *Asthama;* so I have likewise observed, that some times an Acute and Fatal Consumption has followed upon the first Fit of a Rheumatism.

This Consumption, when it seizes them from the first invasion of a Rheumatism, happenes sometimes to be Acute, for this Reason: because it proceeds from a Colliquation of the Humours in an

This Consumption is sometimes acute
Acute Fit of a Humorose Rheumatism. And therefore because it partakes of the Nature of an ordinary Consumption, it ought to be treated wholly in the general Method, that is, with the Use of Lubricating, Incrassating, Opiate, and other Pectoral Medicines. And indeed it has been my Practice, and that with very good Success, to prescribe in every

* Morton, Richard, *Phthisiologia or a Treatise of Consumptions,* London, Smith and Walford, 1694, p. 276.

Rheumatick Fit the plentiful Use of Pectoral, Lubricating, and Incrassating, *Apoaemes* and *Linctuses,* tho' there be no urgent Cough, nor difficulty of Breathing, not only to temper and soften the Blood, but likewise to prevent a Consumption, which uses often to be the Effect of a Rheumatism.

* * *

HISTORY 2

Mrs. *Covert,* a Virgin, about the Eighteenth Year of her Age, fell into a continual Fever, which at length was follow'd by another that was intermittent, which continued for the space of Eleven or Twelve Months. But this went away of its own accord, only a Humorose Rheumatism succeeded to it. But the Fever and Rheumatism in process of time being (I know not by what means) in some measure overcome, yet the poor Virgin remained continually Hetical, Coughing, Shortbreath'd, very much Emaciated, and pale as if she had no Blood in her, presenting in a manner an *Hippocratical* Face. Moreover the Tendons of her Muscles were almost universally stiff, by reason of a preternatural thickness and hardness in them, the Trophies of her former Rheumatism, so that all her joynts, not only the lesser ones of her feet and hands, but also the larger being plainly unable to do their Office, or least doing it with a great deal of difficulty and Pain, she continued almost always fixed to her Chair or Bed like an Image. She was likewise many times seized with wandering and shifting, spasmodick and dreadful pains up and down and all about her Breast, and troubled with Hysterical Faintings, and Fits of Fever often returning at uncertain times. To all these Symptoms there were joined a continual languishing Weakness, a want of appetite, and a Suppression of her Courses. The universal Habit of her Body too seemed to me to be very Scorbutical. A case verily (if any is so) very deplorable, which yet (with the Blessing of God) I did help by our Art in the following manner.

* * *

Mrs. Lane, a Barber's Wife, whose Husband lived in *Cow-Lane,* being about Five and Thirty Years old, when she had lived in a Consumptive State, Emaciated and Coughing, for several Years past, fell in the Month of April, 1684 into a true Rheumatism, with violent Pains, and Inflamed Swellings, which yet were moving frequently from one Joint to another, with Fever likewise, that was evidently of a remitting kind, accompanying of it, which had the Type of a *Tertian* (which I have very often observed to be the Nature especially peculiar to a Rheumatick Fever). In which case whenever a new Fever-Fit seized the patient, the Rheumatick Pain and Swelling, which before were almost quited, are wont to be renewed in the parts that were before affected, or else by a *Metastasis* of the Matter (as the Ancients love to speak) to be translated to some other Joynts. But the Fits were very long, lasting for the space of Twelve to Sixteen Hours, and attended with a want of Sleep, Light headaches, great Tumbling and Tossing, Heat and a very Feverish Pulse, All which Symptoms used to be followed, and go off with great Sweats. But at the beginning of every Fit I observed that her Rheumatick Pains always grew more sharp in the Joints affected, or else seized some other Joints that were free before. So that a new Rheumatism seemed to come with every Fever Fit. Being called in the time of her Fit, I endeavored to satisfy the present indications with *Bleeding, Blisters, an*

Anodyne Draught, Tincture of Roses, a Pectorial Linctus and a Pearl Julip. And indeed all the Symptoms going off at the end of the Fit, when I came to see my Patient the next day, I reckoned the Distemper was overcome, and removed with those things I had ordered, till at length by the return of the Fever, and Rheumatism the next Night, I plainly understood how vainly I had hirtherto flattered myself. And therefore according to the urgency of the Symptoms that indicated it, I bled her again, ordering the repetition of the *Hypnotick* Draught, and likewise the Application of an Anodyne Cataplasin to the Joints, that were affected with extreme Pain from the Rheumatism for two or three times, to be plainly a *Tertian;* and that notwithstanding the Method I had before prescribed, all things continually grew worse, the very system of the Nerves being now at length seized with Spasms, but especially in the time of the Fit her Mouth being likewise ulcerated with a Thrush, being by a happy conjecture, I betook myself in his deplorable case to the use of the *Pervian Bark,* prescribing a Dram to be given every third or fourth Hour, when her Fit was off. With the use of which, in the space of Twenty Four Hours, she was freed both from her Rheumatism and Fever, without any other remedy and she was well after her manner, that is Consumptively, but yet she was less oppressed in her Lungs, than she had been before she fell sick. But as soon as she got rid of her Pain and Fever, she wholly neglected her Chronical Consumption (which likewise seemed to be helped with the Bleedings, the use of the Bark, and the other Medicines before prescribed) refusing all sorts of Medicines; thereupon after a Year or two she died of that Chronical Consumption of the Lungs.

John Haygarth

John Haygarth, one of the most prominent medical figures of his time, was a native of Yorkshire, England, and was brought up in the same neighborhood as John Fothergill, Anthony Askew, and John Dawson. Haygarth was born near Sedbergh in 1740 and after finishing the famous Grammar School of Sedbergh proceeded to St. John's College, Cambridge, where he received his M.B. in 1766. After further study at London and Edinburgh, Haygarth was appointed physician to the Chester Infirmary and settled in that city.

In Chester he began immediately to make careful notes on all the patients, these notes forming later the basis of many of his important observations. John Fothergill, then at the height of his reputation, came every year for two months to his estate in Cheshire, where young Haygarth visited him and discussed medical problems with him. Haygarth early became interested in contagious diseases and in 1777 read a paper before the Royal Society proposing that the spread of contagious diseases be checked by isolation. In 1784 he

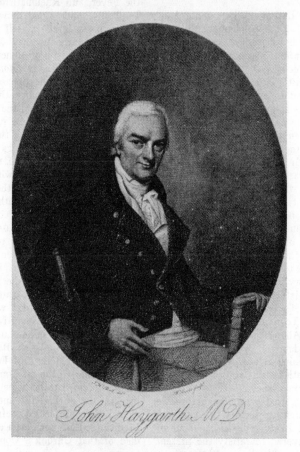

JOHN HAYGARTH (1740-1827)
Frontispiece to *A clinical history of diseases* (London, 1805)
From an etching by W. Cooke

published an *Inquiry how to Prevent the Small-Pox,* which attracted much attention and was translated into French and German. Six years, however, before the publication of his *Inquiry* he had established a "society for promoting inoculation and preventing the casual Small-Pox in Chester" which had done such remarkable work in checking smallpox that it had attracted national attention. This Smallpox Society recommended inoculation every two years and certain rules of prevention in the intervals.

After Jenner's discovery of vaccine inoculation, Haygarth turned his attention to other matters and became interested in typhus fever plague and yellow fever. In 1798 he removed to Bath, where he set to work analysing his clinical records, the result of which he published in 1805, with the title, *(1) A Clinical History of the Acute Rheumatism, (2) A Clinical History of the Nodosity of the Joints.*

Haygarth died near Bath in 1827 at the age of 87. His name is still venerated in Chester, the city of his adoption, where he spent the most active years of his professional life.

OF THE ACUTE RHEUMATISM OR REUMATIC FEVER. SECTION I

This History is intended to be arranged in two Sections. The former is written in so popular and plain a manner, as to be intelligible to the patients themselves. The latter Section will consist of *Proofs* and *Illustrations* which are more particularly submitted to the judgment of the medical read. To this division the Tables, the Cases, and other details of facts and authorities, will be consigned for the sake of reference; which to some readers will afford but dry and dull entertainment. However, physicians who possess a truly professional spirit of improvement will find the arrangement of facts the most satisfactory, interesting, and instructive part of these pages. By a comparison of the data with the conclusions, they will have an opportunity thoroughly to examine, whether a true foundation is laid of practical knowledge.

Among the higher and middle ranks of society I have noted and classed the cases of 10,549 patients, from 1767 to 1801 inclusive, others undoubtedly have been omitted from the hurry of professional duties and different causes but in what proportion cannot be ascertained. However, as these omissions were accidental, and as they did not exclude any particular disorder, except what was very slight or desperate, an impartial view of medical facts is exhibited whence true conclusions may be drawn by fair induction.

The term Rheumatism, both in common and medical language, includes a great variety of disorders, which ought to be distinguished from each other by different names. After separating from it the Nodosity of the Joints, Tic douloureux, Sciatica, Lumbago, and other

diseases, which Nosologists have placed under this denomination, there still remain 470 cases of Rheumatism. This disease is generally classed with fevers, and yet only 170 (about one-third of them) had any fever. These last are the cases which come under the title of acute Rheumatism, and exclusively form the subject of the following pages.

II

The Rheumatick Fever, in common with most others, begins with chilly fits; succeeded by increased heat; frequent pulse; thirst; loss of appetite; and prostration of strength. The symptom peculiar to this disease is an inflammation of the joints, which often increases to great violence, with swelling, soreness to the touch and sometimes redness of the skin. It attacks most, if not all, the joints of the body in different patients, often two, three or more joints at a time, leaving some and going to others in succession, frequently returning again to each of them several times during the disease. The muscles are sometimes affected, but less generally and severely than the joints. The patient being unable to find an easy place for the diseased limbs often remaining restless and watchful for many days and nights together. Sweats appear spontaneously, or are easily excited by remedies, frequently to a profuse degree. The urine is, at first, high-coloured, and lets fall a red sediment. The blood is generally covered with an inflammatory crust.

(margin note: Description of Acute Rheumatism)

Exposure to cold or moisture is the chief cause of the acute Rheumatism.

This is very formidable and extremely painful disease, generally continues for many weeks; more or less, according to the magnitude of the malady, and the efficacy of the

* John Haygarth, M.D., *A Clinical History of Diseases, Part First being* 1. *A Clinical History of the Acute Rheumatism.* 2. *A Clinical History of the Nodosity of the Joints,* London, Cadell and Davies, 1805, p. 13.

remedies which are employed to remove it. The consequences of this disorder are often painfully felt for many years.

V

More Males are attacked with the acute Rheumatism than Females, in the proportion of 98 of the former to 73 of the latter, or nearly as 4 to 3, probably because Male and Female patients men are more exposed to cold and rain than women. On communicating this observation to a very intelligent physician, who resided for several years at Rotterdam, he made the following remark: " 'what confirms this idea' is that in Holland the Rheumatism among Females is comparatively seldom; though the air is extremely moist. They are much more domesticated than in this country, and their 'dress much warmer.' "

VIII

Exposure to cold and moisture is a principal cause of the acute Rheumatism, and many other especially inflammatory diseases. For this reason we cannot be too minute and diligent in our endeavours to investigate the circumstances in which this enemy of mankind produces such injurious effects. In 6 cases Rheumatism is ascribed to having caught cold. The following circumstances are specified in what manner cold had been caught in 23 instances. It is observable that in most of them, in 20 out of 23 examples, dampness or moisture is particularly mentioned. Useful instruction may hence be derived in what circumstances there is danger in order to avoid the mischief.

William Charles Wells

William Charles Wells was born in Charleston, South Carolina, in 1757, the son of Robert Wells, who had immigrated from Scotland. His father was an ardent loyalist and made his son wear a cotton coat and a blue bonnet so he might not be mistaken for an American.

William Wells served an apprenticeship with Dr. Gardner, of Charleston, from 1771 to 1775 and began his medical studies in Edinburgh, where he lived from 1775 to 1778. He attended the lectures of Dr. William Hunter in London, studied for a year at St. Bartholomew's Hospital, and then served in a Scottish regiment which was in Dutch service. In 1780 he returned to Edinburgh, where he graduated the same year. Two years later he went to Saint Augustine, Florida, where he set up a printing press and commenced the publication of a weekly newspaper. In 1784, he returned to England and began practising in London. He was physician to St. Thomas' Hospital from 1800 until his death in 1817.

Wells was a very original thinker and made important observations in physics, biology, and medicine. In his classic *Essay on Dew,* published in 1814, he explained correctly the manner in which dew is formed and for this contribution was awarded the Rumford Medal by the Royal Society. In 1813 he proposed the theory of natural selection, which contained the germ of the thought later developed by Charles Darwin in his *Origin of the Species.*

Two of Wells's medical papers were of great importance in the development of medicine. In 1810, he published what is perhaps the earliest account of the cardiac complications of rheumatic fever and in 1811 he described albuminous urine in cases of dropsy. These papers were published in the *Transactions of the Society for the Improvement of Medical and Chirurgical Knowledge.*

ON RHEUMATISM OF THE HEART*

Dr. David Pitcairn, about the year 1788, began to remark, that persons subject to rheumatism were attacked more frequently than others, with symptoms of an organic disease of the heart. Subsequent experience having confirmed the truth of this observation, he concluded, that these two diseases often depend upon a common cause, and in such instances, therefore, called the latter disease rheumatism of the heart. He communicated what he had observed to several of his friends, and to his pupils at St. Bartholomew's Hospital, to which he was then Physician; but no notice, I believe, was taken of his remark in any book, before it appeared in the second edition of Dr. Baillie's Morbid Anatomy, which was published in 1797. No similar observation, as far as I know, is to be found in any book written before that time. Morgagni, indeed, and Dr. Ferriar of Manchester, has given cases of rheumatism existing with an organic disease of the heart, but it is evident that they considered the concurrence of the two diseases as merely accidental; and it is very probable, that similar cases occur in other authors who wrote before Dr. Baillie, though I have not met with them.

* * *

CASE I

Mr. T. M. came from Scotland in April, 1798, to reside in Berkshire, being then in his eighteenth year. He was of a fair complexion, short stature, and a habit rather full than muscular. From the age of nine years he had been every year attacked with acute rheumatism. Four of the attacks had been very severe, each of them confining him to bed for several weeks; the others seldom kept him at home longer than a week, though the redness, swelling, and pain of the joints did not leave him for two or three weeks more. While he was labouring under this disease, the pains often shifted in the most sudden manner; and, in the greater fit of it, he was often distressed with a sense of oppression in his chest, frightful dreams, and despondency of mind. In November 1797, he had likewise had a slight spitting of blood.

* Wells, William Charles, *Tr. Soc. Improve. Med. and Chir. Knowledge*, London, cxi, 372.

Four weeks after he came to Berkshire, he fell into a small pond of water, while attempting to leap over it, and wetted his lower limbs as far up as the middle of his thighs. He pursued, however, his exercise, and suffered his clothes to dry upon him. The following day, while walking on the streets of Oxford, he was suddenly seized with a trembling and coldness, principally affecting his lower limbs, with faintness, giddiness, sickness at the stomach, and a sense of oppression in his chest. He afterwards became warm, and then began to feel a palpitation of his heart, and a beating in is head. In the progress of his illness, he was frequently attacked with breathlessness, a sense of choking, and a feeling as if he were about to expire. In the night time he used to be warm, and to sweat. After he had been affected in this way about three weeks, he came to London and consulted me. At his first visit, I did not become acquainted with all the circumstances which I have mentioned; and as I found his pulse frequent, and tongue white, and was told by him that he was worse every day at ten o'clock in the forenoon, I thought it probable that his disease was a tertain fever, which had not yet fully intermitted. As I learned, however, when I saw him next, that the beating in his chest was never absent, though at some times much greater than at others, and that he had been much subject to rheumatism, I began to suspect, that his disease might be nothing except what I had learned from Dr. Baillie's publication. I carried him therefore, to Dr. Pitcairn, who confirmed my conjecture, and was fearful that he would not recover.

Mr. M. went again into the country; but I had frequent letters respecting him, and once visited him there. I think it, however, unnecessary to say more upon his case, than, that, after he had laboured under the palpitation four months, he was attacked with pains, swellings, and redness of his joints, which continued about six weeks, but were not so severe as to confine him to bed; that during this time the palpitation began to lessen, but that it did not entirely leave him before the end of the second year from its commencement. Mr. M. during his illness was several times seen by Dr. Bourne of Oxford. He was seen also by Dr. James Russell, of Edinburgh, who had often attended him in sickness in Scotland, and, having been called by business to Birmingham, had afterwards extended his journey to Berkshire to visit him.

Since his recovery I have met with him frequently, and have several times applied my hand to the region of his heart, without feeling there any unusual beating. But he says, that exercise is now more apt to excite palpitation than formerly, and that he sometimes experiences it without any apparent cause. He thinks too, that it occurs oftener while he is affected with rheumatism of the joints, which continues to attack him every year, than at any other time. Before the palpitation comes on, he is seized with a gnawing pain in the region of the heart, and a sense of suffocation. In two or three minutes these symptoms either disappear or become less; the palpitation then begins, and lasts about the same time. Such attacks, however, do not happen oftener than twice or thrice in the year.

I may add, that in the course of my correspondence with the relations of Mr. M. I learned, that one of his uncles, whom he resembles in external appearance, after being severely afflicted with rheumatism, became, when about sixteen or seventeen years old, subject to violent papitation of the heart, and some time after died suddenly; and that, his body being opened, the heart was found enlarged.

CASE II

Martha Clifton, aged nearly fifteen years, was admitted into St. Thomas's Hospital, on the 18th of February, 1802, after labouring under acute rheumatism about sixteen days. Her pulse was small, but the heart struck the ribs with such force, that its beats could be reckoned by applying the hand to the right side of the chest. About two or three years before, she had likewise been affected with acute rheumatism, during the presence which she had been troubled also with a violent beating of her heart. In the interval between the two attacks of rheumatism, she had experienced no palpitation in her chest. The account of what I did not observe myself I received from the patient, and her mother; but those, who are conversant with the business of an Hospital, know that little dependance is to be placed upon the accuracy of patients or their friends, when they speak of symptoms which have formerly occurred. She remained at the Hospital eleven weeks, and was then taken away by her relations, for the purpose of being sent into the country. The pains in her limbs were nearly gone, and the palpitation of her heart was much diminished.

Many of the tendons of the superficial muscles in this patient were studded with numerous small hard tumours, an appearance I have observed only in one other person, a thin and feeble man forty-one years old, who also laboured under rheumatism.

Jean Bouillaud

Jean Bouillaud was born in 1796 in the small hamlet of Bragette near Angoulême. His father was a tile maker, who by economy and hard work, saved up enough money to send his son to the lycée at Angoulême. After graduation at the lycée he decided to study medicine on the advice of his uncle, and started for Paris with a slender stock of money and a letter of recommendation to Percy. Young Bouillaud was not received cordially by the great Percy, and in his letters home he complained of the hardness of Paris, of his isolation, and of the high rents, his lodgings costing him twelve francs ($2.40) a month. He began his medical work at the Cochin Hospital, but shortly afterwards, Napoleon returned from Elba and young Bouillaud with patriotic enthusiasm rushed to the colors and enlisted in a hussar regiment. With the cessation of hostilities he returned to Paris, where he took his M.D. in 1823, and in 1825 at the age of twenty-nine became a member of the Academy of Medicine.

Bouillaud's rise was truly phenomenal. In 1826 he became professor agrégé and in 1831 became professor of medicine, to the great delight of the students who carried him about in triumph on their shoulders. He was a very popular teacher and carried on investigations of great value. His *Traité cliniques des maladies du cœur*, dedicated to his old uncle, was a classic work, and his recog-

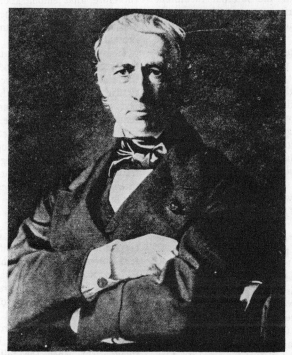

Courtesy of Dr. J. D. Rolleston

JEAN BOUILLAUD (1796-1881)
Portrait by C. H. Lehman, 1875

nition of the relationship between rheumatic fever and endocarditis may be ranked with the greatest discoveries in clinical medicine. Bouillaud died suddenly in 1881 at the age of eighty-five.

NEW RESEARCHES ON ACUTE ARTICULAR RHEUMATISM IN GENERAL*
PRELIMINARY CONSIDERATIONS

On a first view of the subject, it would seem that nothing could be more forbidding, or, one might say, more worn out, than a history of rheumatism in particular. It is not so, however, and I venture to hope that the researches which constitute the object of

this work will offer some interest and novelty. They will prove, if I am not much deceived, that upon this subject, as well as upon many others, there was something for us yet to glean after our predecessors; and that it was destined to be submitted to that great law of progress and reform, which animates, fecundates, and governs in medicine as in all other things.

* Bouillaud, J., *New Researches on Auricular Rheumatism,* translated by James Kitchen, M.D., Philadelphia, Baillière, 1837.

The newest and most curious point of view of these researches is, without doubt, that coincidence of inflammation of the sero-fibruos internal and external tissues of the heart (rheumatismal endocarditis and pericarditis) with acute articular rheumatism.

Inflammation of the internal membrane of blood-vessels aften accompanies acute articular rheumatism, and I intend, hereafter, to treat of this point, which is, in some measure, extension of that which is now about to occupy us.

It is now about three years since observations collected with care presented to me this important connexion. I will, however, state upon what occasion I was led to fix my attention on the leading fact which occupies us. In auscultating the sounds of the heart in some individuals still labouring under, or convalescing from, acute articular rheumatism, I was not a little surprised to hear a strong file, saw, or bellows sound (*bruit de rape, de scie ou de soufflet*); such as I had often met with in chronic or organic induration of the valves, with contraction of the orifices of the heart. Now nobody would suspect an affection of this kind amongst the majority of persons who suffered with rheumatism and were submitted to our examination. Many of them were for the first time affected with articular rheumatism, and had hitherto enjoyed the most perfect health. I then called to mind other cases of acute disease of the heart, during the course of which I had heard the bellows and file sounds, and I resolved to explore, attentively, the heart and its functions in all those affected with rheumatism whom I should meet with. Thanks to this exploration, I soon discovered that an acute affection of the heart, in cases of acute articular rheumatism associated with violent fever, was not a simple accident, a rare or as it were fortuitous complication, but in truth the most usual accompaniment of this disease.

* * *

CHAPTER I. PART FIRST, II

The number of separate observations, contained in the two chapters of the above mentioned treatise consecrated to pericarditis and endocarditis, amount to ninety-two, viz. thirty-seven of pericarditis and fifty-five of endocarditis. Now, of these ninety-two observations, we have thirty-one in which pericarditis and endocarditis coincided with articular rheumatism, viz. seventeen of pericarditis and fourteen of endocarditis. Thus, then about one half of the cases of pericarditis and one fourth of those of carditis existed in rheumatic individuals. It follows, therefore, that among about a third of the individuals affected with pericarditis and endocarditis, articular rheumatism was also present.*

It is demonstrated by these calculations that inflammation of the pericardium and of the endocardium has coincided with an articular rheumatism in a third of the cases. But we are far from asserting, that in the remaining two thirds there did not exist articular rheumatism. In fact, many of these cases are deficient in etiological details; and it appears probable enough, that amongst these last a certain number belonged also to the list of rheumatic pericarditis and endocarditis.

* * *

V. What then, we shall be asked, are the certain indications of the inflammation of the sero-fibrous tissue of the heart (pericarditis and endocarditis)? As I have exposed them at length in the *Clinical Treatise of Diseases of the Heart,* I shall be content here to repeat those which are most evident.

The existence of pericarditis is certain in the individual affected with acute articular rheumatism, when the following symptoms are present: a dull sound over the precordial region, much more extended than in the normal condition (double, triple in every direction); arched form of same region; remote beatings of the heart, but little or not at all sensible to the touch, sounds of the heart, distant, obscure, accompanied by different abnormal sounds, some rising from the rubbing of the opposite coats of the pericardium against each other; others from the complication of pericarditis with valvular endocarditis; a pain more or less acute at that region of the heart; palpitations, irregularities, inequalities, and intermissions of the pulse are sometimes conjoined with the above symptoms.

The coincidence of endocarditis with acute articular rheumatism is, to our minds, certain, when the following signs are present.

Bellows, file, or saw sound in the pre-

* See observations of the Traité Clinique des Maladies du Cœur, etc.

cordial region, with a dulness of this part on percussion, to an extent much more considerable than that in the normal state, and which also, sometimes present, but in a less degree than in pericarditis with effusion, an elevation or abnormal arching; the movements of the heart elevate with force the precordial region; and they are aften irregular, unequal, intermittent, and accompanied at times with a vibratory trembling. The pulse is hard, strong, vibrating, unequal and intermittent, like the beating of the heart.

It appears from the above that there are signs common to pericarditis and endocarditis, and that the differential physical signs are not always well marked. Cases, also, presented themselves in which it is difficult enough to determine whether there is pericarditis of endocarditis, and whether one of these affections, once well recognized, exists alone or combined with the other. These are the cases in which pericarditis may be present without an evident effusion, and with a production only of false membranes. Then, indeed, the beatings of the heart are sensible to the touch, as in simple endocarditis, and the saw and bellows sound, the vibratory trembling of the precordial region, may be present in this case as in endocarditis. After all, this distinction may be thought really more curious than useful. It is enough for the practitioner to know that one of the two exists, since the treatment is essentially the same, whether there be only pericarditis or endocarditis, or whether there be endo-pericarditis.

RELAPSING FEVER

John Rutty

John Rutty was born in Wiltshire, England, in 1698 and received his M.D. at Leyden in 1723. The following year he settled in Dublin where he practised until his death in 1775. He was a very devout Quaker, lived sparely, sometimes dined on nettles and frequently practised rigid abstinence from food and drink. Boswell's *Life of Samuel Johnson* contains the following interesting entry for September 19, 1777.

"He was much diverted with an article which I showed him in the *Critical Review,* giving an account of a curious publication entitled *A Spiritual Diary and Soliloquies by John Rutty, M.D.* John Rutty was one of the people called Quakers, a physician of some eminence in Dublin. This Diary, which was kept from 1753 to 1775, the year in which he died, exhibited, in the simplicity of his heart, a minute and honest register of the state of his mind, which though frequently laughable enough, was not more so than the history of many men would be if recorded with equal fairness. . . . Johnson laughed heartily at this good Quietist's self condemning minutes."

In this diary Rutty accuses himself of irritability, of too much love for materia medica, meteorology and good food. In addition to the famous diary, Rutty wrote several books on medical subjects, one of which, a "Chronological History . . . of the Diseases in Dublin," in 1770, contains the first clear description of relapsing fever.

THE WEATHER*

August. The first nine days variable, and the winds N.N.W.E., and S.E. From the ninth to the twentieth fair, and the winds E. and S.E. thence to the end rainy, and mostly S.W. and it concluded N.W. and cold, wet and windy.

The latter part of July and the months of August, September, and October, were in-

* Rutty, John, *A chronological history of the weather and seasons and of the prevailing diseases in Dublin,* London, Robinson and Roberts, 1770, p. 75.

fested with a fever, which was very frequent during this period, not unlike that of the autumn of the preceding year; with which compare also the years 1741, 1745, 1748. It was attended with an intense pain in the head. It terminated sometimes in four, for the most part in five or six days, sometimes in nine, and commonly in a critical sweat: it was far from being mortal. I was assured of seventy of the poorer sort at the same time in this fever; abandoned to the use of whey and God's good providence, who all recovered. The crisis, however, was very imperfect, for they were subject to relapse, even sometimes to the third time; nor did their urine come to a complete separation.

Divers of them, as their fever declined, had a paroxysm in the evening, and in some there succeeded pains in the limbs.

SLEEPING SICKNESS

Thomas M. Winterbottom

Thomas Winterbottom was born in South Shields, England, in 1766. He studied first at Edinburgh and later at Glasgow, where he graduated in 1792. After graduation he was appointed physician to the colony of Sierra Leone and practised in Africa for four years. He then returned to his native town, where he succeeded to the practice of his father and began the arduous life of a country doctor. He retired after twenty years of hard work, which brought him not only an ample fortune, but the esteem and love of his town and of the neighbouring country as well. An accomplished scholar and linguist, he spent his days with his books, interrupting his studies once a year for an extended tour on the Continent. His last illness was long and painful, and the extraordinary and unexpected protraction of his life led him to remark that he never remembered being "so out in his prognosis before." He died in 1859, in his ninety-fourth year, twenty-seven years after his retirement from medical practice.

In 1803 he published his best-known work, *An Account of the Native Africans in the Neighborhood of Sierra Leone.* This book contains probably the earliest account in English of sleeping sickness or trypanosomiasis.

The Africans* are very subject to a species of lethargy, which they are much afraid of, as it proves fatal in every instance. The Timmanees call it marree, or, 'nluoi, and the Bulloms, nagónlôc, or kadeera: it is called by the Soosoos, kee kollee kondee, or sleepy sickness, and by the Mandingos, seenoyúncaree, a word of similar import. This disease is frequent in the Foola country, and it is said to be much more common in the interior parts of the country than upon the sea coast. Children are very rarely, or never, affected with the complaint, nor is it more common among slaves than among free people, though it is asserted that the slaves from Benin are very subject to it. At the commencement of the disease, the patient has commonly a ravenous appetite, eating twice the quantity of food he was accustomed to take when in health and becoming very fat. When the disease has continued some time, the appetite declines, and the patient gradually wastes away.

Squinting occurs sometimes, though very seldom, in this disease, and in some rare instances the patient is carried off in convulsions. Small glandular tumors are sometimes observed in the neck a little before the commencement of this complaint, though probably depending rather upon accidental cir-

* Winterbottom, Thomas, *An Account of the Native Africans in the Neighborhood of Sierra Leone,* London, Hatchard and Mawman, 1803, p. 29.

cumstances than upon the disease itself. Slave traders, however, appear to consider these tumors as a symptom indicating a disposition to lethargy, and they either never buy such slaves, or get quit of them as soon as they observe any such appearances. The disposition to sleep is so strong, as scarcely to leave a sufficient respite for the taking of food; even the repeated application of a whip, a remedy which has been frequently used, is hardly sufficient to keep the poor wretch awake. The repeated application of blisters and of setons has been employed by the European surgeons without avail, as the disease, under every mode of treatment, usually proves fatal within three or four months. The natives are totally at a loss to what cause this complaint ought to be attributed;

sweating is the only means they make use of, or from which they hope for any success: this is never tried but in incipient cases, for when the disease has been of any continuance they think it in vain to make the attempt. The root of a grass, called by the Soosoos kallee, and the dried leaves of a plant, called in Soosoos fingka, are boiled for some time in water, in an iron pot; when this is removed from the fire the patient is seated over it, and is covered over with cotton cloths, a process which never fails to excite a copious perspiration. This mode of cure is repeated twice or three times a day, and is persisted in for a considerable length of time, until the disease is carried off, or appears to be gaining ground. No internal medicines are given in the complaint.

SCHÖNLEIN'S DISEASE
Johann Lukas Schönlein

Johann Lukas Schönlein was born at Bamberg in 1793 and took his doctor's degree at Würzburg in 1816. He became Privatdozent in Medicine at Würzburg, full professor in 1824, and remained there until 1833, when he went to Zürich as Professor of Medicine. He remained in Zürich for six years and then accepted the chair of medicine at Berlin, where he was active until 1859. His death occurred in 1864. While in Würzburg, Schönlein rapidly achieved the reputation of being the first clinician in Germany and gave courses in physical diagnosis in his clinic. He pointed out to his students the fine râles in pneumonia, the metallic sounds in pneumothorax, and the murmur over the femoral arteries in aortic insufficiency.

In Zürich, Schönlein's reputation grew steadily, and in 1835 he was called to Brussels to attend the Queen of the Belgians. The King was very much pleased with Schönlein and made him many flattering offers to remain in Brussels as the royal physician. Finally the King asked him what he still wished. "The Lake of Zürich," Schönlein answered.

In Berlin, Schönlein was the real founder of modern clinical teaching in Germany. His lectures were given in the German language and at his clinic at the Charité he introduced such modern methods as percussion and auscultation, chemical and microscopic examinations of the blood and urine.

Schönlein suffered for many years from a goitre which gradually increased in size. Virchow relates that while in Berlin, it often interfered with his speaking, and that when he leaned over the bed to examine a patient, he became quite cyanotic. After his resignation in Berlin, Schönlein retired to his old home Bamberg where he spent the last five years of his life quietly with his books. He amassed an extensive library containing many old and valuable editions and also assembled a large collection of rare coins. He was a very liberal contributor to various charities, libraries and schools and to the

Catholic Church. Considered the first citizen of Bamberg, there was universal sorrow at his death and almost the entire population of the city followed his body to the cemetery.

Schönlein first described peliosis rheumatica (Schönlein's Disease), he discovered the parasitic nature of favus and introduced the terms "typhus abdominals," "typhus exanthematicus," "tuberculosis" and "hemophilia." The

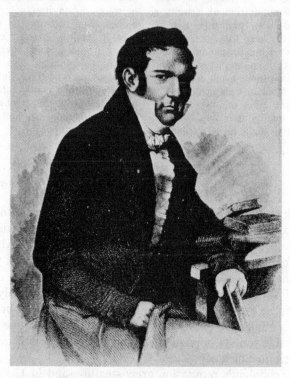

JOHANN LUKAS SCHÖNLEIN (1793-1864)
An engraving by Carl Mayer. Reproduced from the fifth
edition of Schönlein's *Allgemeine und specielle Pathologie
und Therapie*

following account of peliosis rheumatica is translated from Schönlein's *Allgemeine und specielle Pathologie und Therapie, nach dessen Vorlesungen niedergeschrieben und heraus gegeben von einigen seiner Zuhörer* (General and Special Pathology and Therapy written down from his lectures and published by some of his pupils), St. Gallen, 1841.

SECOND FORM*
PELIOSIS RHEUMATICA (PEL. CIRCUMSC.)

The spots never run together, as they often do in Werlhof's disease.

Appearances.—The patients have either suffered earlier from rheumatism or rheumatic symptoms appear at the same time, gently periodic sticking pains in the joints (in the ankles and in the knees, seldom in

* Schönlein, J. L., *Allgemeine und speicelle Pathologie und Therapie. Zweiter Teil*, IV Ed., St. Gallen, Comptoir, 1839, p. 42.

the hand and shoulder joints), which are oedematous, swollen and very painful when moved; the characteristic spots of the disease appear in the majority of cases first on the extremities and particularly on the lower ones (seldom the upper ones), and here only up to the knee. The spots are small, the size of a lentil, a millet seed, bright red, not elevated above the skin, disappearing on pressure of the finger; they became gradually a dirty brown, yellowish, the skin over the spots appears somewhat branny, the eruption comes by fits and starts, often throughout several weeks. Every slight change in temperature, for instance going around in a room that is a little cooled off, can produce a new eruption. The disease appears usually with fever; the fever has a remitting type. Towards evening the appearances are most marked; in the morning there is a letting-up of the signs. Not often separation in the urine.

Diagnosis.—This disease has been confused with morbus maculosis Werlhoffi; the absence of the so-called purpuric signs in the mouth, where there are absolutely no changes, the absence of all hemorrhages, the character of the exanthema (it is limited to one extremity, or appears here first, and never becomes very large, is bright red, never blue, livid); the affection of the joints, which is absent in Werlhof's disease, and the absence of nervous symptoms, the great depression of spirits, the weakness, clinch.

Etiology.—The disease is found especially in individuals with soft, vulnerable skin, who have suffered previously from a cold, or in those who, as the result of a cold, show both the symptoms of peliosis and those of rheumatoid arthritis.

Terminations. 1) In Healing.—The fever disappears through the skin and urine crises, but the exanthema usually remains after the crisis, so that its disappearance must be considered the crisis of the exanthema. Very slight relapses appear, often following the slightest chilling.

2) In Another Disease.—If the exanthema are driven from the skin, then it may attack the inner organs, the heart and large vessels. Under such conditions, a chronic inflammation appears in these organs (affinity with impetigo-like forms).

3) In Death.—Only as the result of this change.

Prognosis.—Is very favorable.

Therapeutics.—Bathing is bad; for this reason the diagnosis from the Werlhof's disease is so necessary. The principal thing here is the regulation of the diet. The patients must be kept in an even, warm temperature and dare not, so long as the affection persists, leave their beds. As food, gruel, cooked vegetables, and as drinks, lukewarm simple lemonade (which also works on the skin and intestines) cream of tartar water. If no crises comes through the skin, ammonium acetate, with equal parts of elder tea and Dover powders. For the intestinal secretion: if there is constipation, gentle cathartics; dandelion extract with rhubarb and tartar, so that daily 2-3 mushy stools follow. Also when the exanthema has disappeared, the patient must keep thus in an even temperature and take light aromatic tonic medicines, calamus with ammonia, ammonium succinate and slightly bitter tea with card, bened. or vermouth.

FOCAL INFECTION

Benjamin Rush

Edouard Rist remarks in his interesting essay *Qu'est ce que la médicine?*, that "in every country, our confreres have their phantoms and their ghosts. For the Englishman it is uric acid, for the German the exudative diathesis, for the American focal infection." Although we admit that focal infection has at times been almost done to death by its friends, yet it remains a very solid contribution to medicine. As a distinctively American contribution, it is of interest to note that one of the great pioneer American physicians, Benjamin Rush, was one of the first physicians to recognize the relationship between apical infections and arthritis.

Benjamin Rush was born near Philadelphia in 1745 on a homestead founded by his grandfather, a Quaker gunsmith, who had come to America with William Penn. He graduated at Princeton in 1760 and the following year was apprenticed to Dr. John Redmond, of Philadelphia, who, Rush wrote in his memoirs, had "the most extensive business of any Physician in the city." From February 1761 to 1766, he "was absent from his master's business but eleven days and never spent more than three evenings out of his house." After six years of apprenticeship, Rush went to Edinburgh, where he received

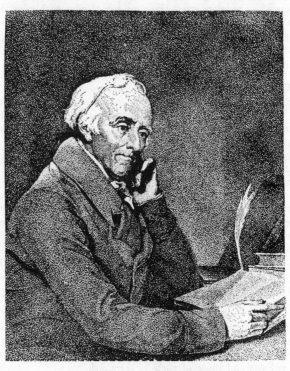

BENJAMIN RUSH (1745-1813)
Portrait by Sully. From the engraving by Edwin. From
American Medical Biography by James Thacher (Boston,
1828)

the degree of M.D. in 1768. Later he went to London and Paris, returning to Philadelphia the same year. He gradually built up a practice, of which he says in his memoirs, "in the year 1775 it was worth about 900 pounds a year, Pennsylvania currency."

Rush's reputation grew steadily. Becoming interested in national affairs, he published in 1771 a pamphlet against slavery which excited the ire of many slave-holders in the colonies. He became a close friend of Benjamin Franklin and, as a member of Congress from Pennsylvania, was one of the signers of the Declaration of Independence. He served as Surgeon General of the Middle Department in the War of the Revolution, but broke with Washington at Valley Forge.

Rush's constant excursions into politics, his crusades against slavery, war, alcoholism, and the death-penalty, injured his practice, as he tells us that from the year 1797 his medical practice "sensibly declined. I have had no new families except foreigners and many of my old patients deserted me." In 1799, owing to the depleted state of his affairs, he felt compelled to apply to the President of the United States for the office of Treasurer of the Mint. Rush received this appointment from President Adams, although there were forty other applicants for the position. Rush died in 1813 from typhus fever.

Benjamin Rush is regarded as the outstanding American physician of his time. His descriptions of dengue, yellow fever, and his treatise on insanity are classics. Rush Medical College was named in his honor, although Rush himself received this honor posthumously, since he died nearly twenty years before Cook County was incorporated, with Chicago, a tiny village, as its county seat.

AN ACCOUNT, &c.

Some time in the month of October, 1801, I attended Miss A. C. with rheumatism in her hip joint, which yielded for a while, to the several remedies for that disease. In the month of November it returned with great violence, accompanied with a severe toothache. Suspecting the rheumatic affection was excited by the pain in her tooth, which was decayed, I directed it to be extracted. The rheumatism immediately left her hip, and she recovered in a few days. She has continued ever since to be free from it.

Soon after this I was consulted by Mrs. J. R. who had been affected for several weeks with dyspepsia and toothache. Her tooth, though no mark of decay appeared in it, was drawn by my advice. The next day she was relieved from her distressing stomach complaint, and has continued ever since to enjoy good health. From the soundness of the external part of the tooth, and the adjoining gum, there was no reason to suspect a discharge of matter from it had produced the disease in her stomach.

Some time in the year of 1801 I was consulted by the father of a young gentleman in Baltimore, who had been affected with epilepsy. I inquired into the state of his teeth, and was informed that several of them in his upper jaw were decayed. I directed them to be extracted, and advised him after to lose a few ounces of blood, at any time when he

felt the premonitory symptoms of a recurrence of his fits. He followed my advice, in consequence of which I had lately the pleasure of hearing from his brother that he was perfectly cured.

I have been made happy by discovering that I have only added to the observations of other physicians, in pointing out a connection between the extraction of decayed and diseased teeth and the cure of general diseases. Several cases of efficacy of that remedy in relieving headache and vertigo are mentioned by Dr. Darwin. Dr. Gater relates that Mr. Petit, a celebrated French surgeon had often cured intermitting fevers, which had resisted the bark for months, and even years, by this prescription; and he quotes from his works two cases, one of consumption, the other of vertigo, both of long continuance, which were suddenly cured by the extraction of two decayed teeth in the former, and of two supernumerary teeth in the latter case.

In the second number of a late work, entitled *Bibliothèque Germanique Medico Chirurgicale*, published in Paris by Dr. Bluver and Dr. Delaroche, there is an account, by Dr. Siebold, of a young woman who had been affected for several months with great inflammation, pain, and ulcers, in her right upper and lower jaws, at the usual time of the appearance of the catamenia, which at that period were always deficient in quantity. Upon inspecting the seat of those morbid affections, the doctor discovered several of

---

* Rush, Benjamin, *Medical Inquiries and Observations*, III Ed., Philadelphia, Benj. and Thos. Kite, 1809, Vol. I, p. 351.

the molars in both jaws to be decayed. He directed them to be drawn, in consequence of which the woman was relieved of the monthly disease in her mouth, and afterwards had a regular discharge of her catamenia.

These facts, though but little attended to, should not surprise us, when we recollect how often the most distressing general diseases are brought on by very inconsiderable inlets of morbid excitement into the system. A small tumor, concealed in the fleshy part of the leg, has been known to bring on epilepsy. A trifling wound with a splinter or a nail, even after it has healed, has often produced a fatal tetanus. Worms in the bowels have produced internal dropsy of the brain, and a stone in the kidney has excited the most violent commotions in every part of the system. Many hundred facts of a similar nature are to be met with in the records of medicine.

When we consider how often the teeth, when decayed, are exposed to irritation from hot and cold drinks and ailments from pressure by mastication, and from the cold air, and how intimate the connection of the mouth is with the whole system, I am disposed to believe they are often the unsuspected causes of general, and particularly of nervous diseases. When we add to the list of those diseases the morbid effects of the acrid and putrid matters, which are sometimes discharged from the carious teeth, or from the ulcers in the gums created by them, also the influence which both have in preventing perfect mastication, and the connection of that animal function with good health, I can not help thinking that our success in the treatment of all chronic diseases would be very much promoted, by directing our inquiries into the state of the teeth in sick people, and by advising their extraction in every case in which they are decayed. It is not necessary that they should be attended with pain, in order to produce disease, for splinters, tumors and other irritants before mentioned, often bring on disease and death, when they give no pain, and are unsuspected causes of them. This translation of sensation and motion into parts remote from the place where impressions are made, appears in many instances, and seems to depend upon an original law of the animal economy.

HODGKIN'S DISEASE
Thomas Hodgkin

Thomas Hodgkin was born at Tottenham in 1798 and took his medical degree at Edinburgh in 1823. He became a member of the College of Physicians in London in 1825 and soon afterwards proceeded to the Continent, spending much time in France and Italy. Upon his return to England, he joined the group at Guy's Hospital, becoming curator of the pathological museum and demonstrator in pathology. He did an enormous amount of work at Guy's Hospital in collecting specimens and labelling them, this work forming the basis of his *Lectures on the Morbid Anatomy of the Serous and Mucous Membranes*.

Hodgkin was lecturer on pathology at Guy's Hospital for ten years, but resigned his chair after an unsuccessful candidature for the position of assistant physician. He continued to practice medicine in London, but being very generous by nature and careless in collecting fees, gradually dropped out of practice and devoted the latter years of his life to philanthropic work. He formed a deep and lasting friendship with Sir Moses Montefiore, the Jewish philanthropist, and while traveling with him in the Orient died at Joffa of dysentery in 1866, at the age of sixty-eight. He was buried at Joffa, his tomb bearing over it an obelisk of granite with an inscription setting forth his splendid character and attainments and also the note, "This tomb is erected by Sir Moses Montefiore, Bart., in commemoration of a friendship of more than forty years and of many journeys taken together in Europe, Asia, and Africa."

Thomas Hodgkin was a consistent member of the Society of Friends. He always wore their characteristic dress and employed their distinctive forms of speech, both in his conversation and his writings. He wrote an account of insufficiency of the aortic valves three years before Corrigan's classic paper, and described first a simultaneous enlargement of the spleen and lymph glands, a morbid entity later called by Wilks in 1865 "Hodgkin's Disease," by which

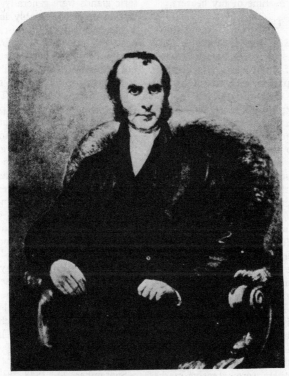

Courtesy of Guy's Hospital Reports
THOMAS HODGKIN (1798-1866)
From the portrait in the possession of Mrs. Lucy Hodgkin.
Artist unknown

name it has since been known. In his *Lectures on the Morbid Anatomy of the Serous and Mucous Membranes,* published in 1836, he shows a clear understanding of acute appendicitis and its complications.

ON SOME MORBID APPEARANCES OF THE ABSORBENT GLANDS AND SPLEEN*

By Dr. Hodgkin. Presented by Dr. R. Lee

Read January 10th and 24th, 1832

The morbid alterations of structure which I am about to describe are probably familiar to many practical morbid anatomists, since they can scarcely have failed to have fallen under their observation in the course of ca-

* *Med. Chir. Tr.*, London, 1832, XVII, 68.

daveric inspection. They have not, as far as I am aware, been made the subject of special attention, on which account I am induced to bring forward a few cases in which they have occurred myself, trusting that I shall at least escape severe or general censure, even though a sentence or two should be produced from some existing work, couched in such concise but expressive language, as to render needless the longer details with which I shall trespass on the time of my hearers.

CASE I

November 2, 1826. Joseph Sinnot, a child of about nine years of age, in Lazarus's ward, under the care of J. Morgan. His brother, his constant companion with whom he had habitually slept, died of phthisis a few months previously; he was much reduced by an illness of about nine months, during which he had been subject to pain in the back, extending around to the abdomen. On his admission, his belly was much distended with ascites. He had also effusion into the prepuce and scrotum. On the latter was a large ulcer induced by a puncture made to evacuate the fluid.

Head.—There was a considerable quantity of serous effusion under the archnoid and within the ventricles. There were a few opake spots in the arachnoid, but this membrane was in other respects healthy. The pia mater appeared remarkably thin and free from vessels. The substance of the brain was generally soft and flabby, but no local morbid change was observed.

Chest.—The pleura on the right side had contracted many strong and old adhesions, in addition to which there were extensive marks of recent pleuritis. On the left, the pleura was nearly or quite free from adhesions, but there was some fluid effused into the cavity. There was some little trace of a tubercular cicatrix at the summit of the right lung, but the substance of both lungs was generally light and crepitant, with a very few exceedingly small tubercles scattered through them.

The mucous membrane exhibited an excess of vascularity; the bronchial glands were greatly enlarged and much indurated.

The heart appeared healthy.

Abdomen.—There was an extensive recent inflammation of the peritoneum, in the cavity of which there was a copious sero-purulent effusion, and the viscera were universally overlayed with a very soft light yellow coagulum, too feeble to effect their union. though evidently having a tendency to do so. The mucous membrane of the stomach and intestines was generally pale and of its ordinary appearance, but in some few spots it was softened and readily separated itself from the subjacent coat. The contents of the intestines were copious and of an unhealthy character, overcharged with bile. The mesenteric glands were generally enlarged, but one or two very considerably so, equalling in size a pigeon's egg, of semi-cartilaginous hardness and streaked with black matter. The substance of the liver was generally natural. but contained a few tubercles somewhat larger than peas, white, semi-cartilaginous. and of uneven surface. The pancreas was firmer than usual, more particularly at its head, which was somewhat enlarged. The spleen was large and contained numerous tubercles. The absorbent glands about both the two last-mentioned organs were much enlarged. Both kidneys were mottled with a light colour, but were free from induration. A continuous chain of much enlarged indurated absorbent glands of a light colour accompanied the aorta throughout its course closely adherent to the bodies of the vertebrae, and extended along the sides of the iliac vessels as far as they could be traced in the pelvis. None of these vessels had been sufficiently compressed to occasion the coagulation of the contained fluids. The coats of the thoracic duct, which was large, were perfectly transparent and healthy.

CASE II

September 24, 1828. Ellenborough King. aged ten years, was admitted into Luke's ward on the sixth of August, 1828, under the care of Dr. Bright. He was the youngest of six children, of whom the first five were reported to be all healthy. This child had also been healthy till about thirteen months ago, when his strength, flesh, and healthy appearance began to fail. He was at that time living in the west of England. A tumor was observed in the left hypochondrium in the situation of the spleen, the glandulae concatenatae on the right side were observed to be considerably enlarged, but under the treatment employed, these tumors, as well as that in the situation of the spleen, were at times very considerably reduced in size.

It does not appear that he was ever subject to hemorrhage, nor till very lately to dropsical effusion; his appetite was generally good. After his admission into the hospital the tumor on the left side was observed to extend considerably below the left hypochondrium, but was reported not to be so large as it had formerly been. The glands on the left side of the neck were swollen, as well as those on the right, the abdomen was somewhat distended and there was considerable œdema of the scrotum.

The head was not opened.

The glands in the neck had assumed the form of large smooth ovoid masses connected together merely by loose cellular membrane and minute vessels: when cut into they exhibited a firm cartilaginous structure of a light colour and very feeble vascularity, but with no appearance of softening or sappuration. Glands similarly affected accompanied the vessels into the chest, where the bronchial and mediastinal glands were in the same state and greatly enlarged. There were some old pleuritic adhesions. The substance of the lungs was generally healthy. There was a good deal of clear serum in the pericardium, but this membrane, as well as the heart, was quite healthy.

In the peritoneal cavity there was a considerable quantity of clear straw-coloured serum mixed with extensive, recent thin diaphanous films. The mucous membrane of the stomach and intestines was tolerably healthy.

The mesenteric glands were but slightly enlarged, and but little if at all indurated; but those accompanying the aorta, the splenic artery, and the iliacs were in the same state as the glands of the neck.

The liver contained no tubercles, and its structure was quite healthy. The pancreas was rather firm, and the glands situated along its upper edge, were, as before stated, greatly enlarged. The spleen was enlarged to at least four times its natural size, its surface was mammillated, and its structure thickly sprinkled with tubercles, presenting the same structure as the enlarged glands already described.

II. DISEASES OF METABOLISM

DIABETES MELLITUS

Diabetes has a long and interesting history. The Papyrus Ebers, one of the most venerable of medical documents refers to polyuria by which the ancient Egyptian physicians may have meant diabetes. Aretaeus the Cappadocian has left a very accurate account of diabetes, giving a most vivid description of this disease. Paracelsus' description of diabetes, although couched in some-

Facsimile of a page from the *Papyrus Ebers*

what fantastic language, is quite clear and, if we substitute sugar for salt, has a surprisingly modern ring.

Thomas Willis discovered that the urine in diabetes was sweet "as if imbued with sugar or honey." This simple observation differentiated diabetes mellitus from diabetes insipidus and introduced the modern era in the study of diabetes. Matthew Dobson extended the observations of Willis and proved that the sweetish taste of diabetic urine was produced by sugar. In the following century Mering and Minkowski made an epoch-making discovery when they discovered that removal of the pancreas produced a fatal diabetes in dogs, and

Eugene Opie, by his pathological studies focussed attention upon the Islands of Langerhans as the seat of the disturbance.

The final landmark in the history of diabetes was the discovery of insulin by Banting and Best.

One of the most interesting clinical signs, seen in severe diabetes, is the characteristic air hunger, described by Adolf Kussmaul, an observation which chronologically preceded those of Mering and Minkowski, Opie, and Banting and Best. A very interesting although unusual complication is a skin eruption, xanthoma diabeticorum, first described by Thomas Addison.

Papyrus Ebers

The Papyrus Ebers, which dates from approximately 1500 B.C., is one of the oldest of all medical documents. It was obtained by Georg Ebers in Luxor in 1872 and a complete translation by Joachim appeared in 1890. This document, which was written a thousand years before the birth of Hippocrates. contains what is thought to be the first reference to diabetes mellitus. The following translation is from the version of Joachim. An English version by Cyril P. Bryan was published in 1930, and a new translation into English by Ebbell appeared in 1937.

A medicine to drive away the passing of too much urine:

Prescription:		Prescription:	
Cakes		Branches of Qadet plant	1/4
Wheat grains	1/8	Grapes	1/8
Fresh grits	1/8	Honey	1/4
Green lead earth	1/32	Berries from üan tree	1/32
Water	1/3	Sweet beer	1/6
Let stand moist; strain it; take it for 4 days.		Cook: fitler and take for 2 days.	

Prescription:		Prescription:	
Sebesten	1/8	Cakes	1/8
Wheat grains	1/8	Honey	1/32
Green lead earth	1/32	Water	1/3
Cakes	1/32	Filter and take 1 day.	
Water	1/2		

Aretaeus the Cappadocian

Aretaeus the Cappadocian has left behind no information regarding his life activities. It is probable that he lived in the second century of the Christian era and was a contemporary of Galen. From his name, he was presumably a native of, or at least practised for a time in Cappadocia, a mountainous region in Asia Minor near the river Euphrates. He wrote in Greek and the first modern edition of his works was a Latin translation by Junius Paulus Crassus, Professor at Padua, which was printed at Venice in 1552. In this book the following selections are from the English translation of Francis Adams, published in 1856.

The Chapter "de diabetes" is generally considered the first accurate account of diabetes that has come down to us from ancient times. His remarks concerning the name of the disease is interesting, for after noting that water goes through these patients, he concludes that the name is derived from the Greek διαβήτης, "a siphon," from διαβαίνειν, "to go through."

Aretaeus recognized the murmur of heart disease, "A noise of the heart" and describes "rhogmoi" (râles) of the chest in asthma. His writings were neglected for many centuries but he is now universally regarded as one of the great medical writers of antiquity. He excels in the description of morbid conditions such as diabetes, tetanus, epilepsy, and pneumonia. Many of his aphorisms deserve to rank with those of Hippocrates. These two are characteristic: "It is impossible to make all the sick well, for the physician in that case would be superior to the gods; but the physician can secure respite from pain and intervals in disease and can render disease latent." "One must be fertile in expedients and not be satisfied to apply his mind entirely to the writings of others."

CHAPTER II*
ON DIABETES

Diabetes is a wonderful affection, not very frequent among men, being a melting down of the flesh and limbs into urine. Its cause is of a cold and humid nature, as in dropsy. The course is the common one, namely, the kidneys and the bladder; for the patients never stop making water, but the flow is incessant, as if from the opening of aqueducts. The nature of the disease, then, is chronic, and it takes a long period to form; but the patient is short-lived, if the constitution of the disease be completely established; for the melting is rapid, the death speedy. Moreover, life is disgusting and painful; thirst unquenchable; excessive drinking, which, however, is disproportionate to the large quantity of urine, for more urine is passed; and one cannot stop them either from drinking or making water. Or if for a time they abstain from drinking, their mouth becomes parched and their body dry; the viscera seem as if scorched up; they are affected with nausea, restlessness, and a burning thirst; and at no distant term they expire. Thirst, as if scorched up with fire. But by what method could they be restrained from making water? Or how can shame become more potent than pain? And even if they were to restrain themselves for a short time, they become swelled in the loins, scrotum, and hips, and when they give vent.

they discharge the collected urine, and the swellings subside, for the overflow passes to the bladder.

If the disease be fully established, it is strongly marked; but if it be merely coming on, the patients have the mouth parched, saliva white, frothy, as if from thirst (for the thirst is not yet confirmed), weight in the hypochondriac region. A sensation of heat or cold from the stomach to the bladder is, as it were, the advent of the approaching disease; they now make a little more water than usual, and there is thirst, but not yet great.

But if it increase still more, the heat is small indeed, but pungent, and seated in the intestines; the abdomen, shrivelled, veins protuberant, general emaciation, when the quality of urine and the thirst have already increased; and when, at the same time, the sensation appears at the extremity of the member, the patients immediately make water. Hence, the disease appears to me to have got the name *diabetes*, as if from the Greek word διαβήτης (*which signifies a siphon*), because the fluid does not remain in the body, but uses the man's body as a ladder (διαβάθρη), whereby to leave it.[1] They

---

* The Extant Works of Aretaeus, the Cappadocian. Edited and Translated by Francis Adams, LL.D., London, Sydenham Society, 1856, p. 338

[1] Altogether, this interpretation is so unsatisfactory, that I was almost tempted to alter the text quite differently from Wigan and Ermerins, and to read ὁκοῖόν τις διαβησείων when the passage might be rendered thus: "it got the name of diabetes, as if signifying one having a frequent desire of descending, because the fluid does not

stand out for a certain time, though not very long, for they pass urine with pain, and the emaciation is dreadful; nor does any great portion of the drink get into the system, and many parts of the flesh pass out along with the urine.

The cause of it may be, that some one of the acute diseases may have terminated in this; and during the crisis the diseases may have left some malignity lurking in the part. It is not improbable, also, that something pernicious, derived from the other diseases which attack the bladder and kidneys, may sometimes prove the cause of this affection. But if anyone is bitten by the dipsas,[2] the affection induced by the wound is of this nature;

for the reptile, the dipsas, if it bite one, kindles up an unquenchab'e thirst. For they drink copiously, not as a remedy for the thirst, but so as to produce repletion of the bowels by the insatiable desire of drink. But if one be pained by the distention of the bowels and feel uncomfortable, and abstain from drink for a little, he again drinks copiously from thirst, and thus the evils alternate; for the thirst and the drink conspire together. Others do not pass urine, nor is there any relief from what is drank. Wherefore, what from insatiable thirst, an overflow of liquids, and distension of the belly, the patients have suddenly burst.

Paracelsus

LIBRI SECUNDI DE TARTARO
TRACTATUS III. CAP. II. DE DIABETICA*

Diabetes is due to a dry salt dissolved & divided by the ingress of a sharp salt in the midst of the principal parts. This salt is lasting, permanent and fixed. Signs: Thirst of a chronic kind, pain in the back (which for the most part begins in the neck) swelling of both feet, much urine, yellow & very red, rapid pulse and pains in the thigh, that is in the hip. Cure by anodynes: salt divided alone is curative.

ANNOTATIONES

Diabetic passion, etc. The urine has nitric properties: for it ought so to be considered, otherwise, nothing is said, what I say is to be respected: for it is known what the urine is & from whence. Therefore the urine is passed, & the salt divided, that is, what is there is like Saltpeter (dissolved by the alum from the urine is saltpeter. And indeed from the

urine besides the armorer could get Saltpeter. Thus too, it is in the body: moreover when the salt in the urine comes to the kidneys, it irritates them, indeed the tartar in the fluid, & that dissolved from the alum, its principle penetrates into the kidneys, slips in) & makes the kidneys thirsty. Now the thirst always comes from the salt, thus this salt makes the kidneys salty. Moreover those other members which ought to be humid, by the power of attraction draw the humidity & that attraction 's through the salt. And where there is humidity, they are contended: but in the kidneys this dissolved alum permits little humidity; therefore it is not possible to drink enough, & as man always drinks, he floods the kidneys, which they do not excrete through the urine; for the expulsive force is not able to expell so much, therefore it does not all go into the urine, but goes into other members: thus the humor comes & swells the feet. Some call it dropsy but it is not: but the power of expelling is not able to expell it by the urine, but it drips downwards through the pores of the flesh, and, heavy, it all goes downward & swells the feet, and the expulsive power is not able to expell it, so they are saturated, the expulsive force not being able to expell all, therefore it went to this place. The remedy is, to fast two days, so that the expulsive power may be able to expell the rest: therefore I say when the power of expulsion

---

remain in the system, but uses the man's person as a ladder for its exit." At all events, the reading of Wigan and Ermerins, seems inadmissible; for how can the two comparisons, to a siphon, and to a ladder, be admitted together? It is possible, however, that διαβάθρη is faulty, and that we ought to read διαβήτη.

[2] The dipsas was a species of viper. See Paulus Aegineta, ii, p. 185.

* Dritter Theil Der Bücher und Schrifften des Edlen Hochgelehrten und Bewehrten Philosophi und Medici Philippi Theophrasti Bombast von Hohenheim Paracelsi gennant, Frankfort, Wechels, 1603, p. 170.

is not able to expell, it goes to the feet and makes a swelling. Therefore old men & strollers avert the swelling & when it comes it goes to the kidneys & death comes. Diabetes then appears when the salty essence settles in the kidneys, and salts them.

The signs of diabetes then are these: thirst of a chronic state, that is they have the thirst daily, & afterwards the feet swell and it is from the diabetes. Then pains in the spine, and this pain begins in the neck, spots come in the head and back, & go to the hips, are the principle symptoms of diabetes: also equal swellings in the feet, much urine yellow and very red, that is the urine per se reddish & when put on cloth and dried, the cloth is yellow. Indeed it is yellow that it stains like gall. Also, the pulse is fast, & there are pains in the hips, that is, the hips act as if they were lame, & when they sit down and walk about they have pain, until they exercise themselves a little, is a sign of diabetes, if moreover there is thirst.

The treatment of the diabetes should be with anodynes: for the dissolved salt & alum should be overcome, since arsenic, which is of itself a great poison, when placed on an ulcer with oil added it heals for it restrains the power of the oil: & thus this salt should be restrained & not cause the liver to cool. Drink julep for the thirst but the salt ought to be gotten rid of in diabetes, besides the application of anodynes: for the vapor in anodynes penetrates & is powerful, not otherwise. Moreover if thou takest crude mercury, and make a mouth over it, in two hours thou seest not the fumes, at once the teeth ache and thou feelest salt from the vapor, & thus the diabetic substance cannot go back into the kidneys but the vapor is sufficient, when thou appliest they feel it, just as the Naegelein Blumen, they emit strength with odor, when they are dried they emit no odor & now moreover are without value. Thus the vapor from anodynes flow to the kidneys & extinguish thirst & the crude salt or crude alum produces pain, etc.

Thomas Willis

Thomas Willis was born in 1621 at Great Bedwyn in Wiltshire and received his primary education at a private day school. In 1636 he entered Christ Church, Oxford, and took his master's degree in 1642. In the Civil War he joined the army of King Charles I and became a soldier in the garrison of Oxford, which remained loyal to the Royalist cause. The garrison, however, surrendered in 1646 and the same year Willis took his bachelor of medicine degree and began practice at Oxford. During the Cromwellian occupation of Oxford, Willis remained faithful to the King and to the Church of England, and set aside a room in his house where the services of the Church were held twice daily. He found time during this period to write and publish his dissertations on Fermentations, Fever, and Urines.

After the Restoration, Willis was rewarded by being appointed Sedleian Professor of Natural Philosophy at Oxford. His predecessor, Dr. Crosse, was, we are told, "ejected." The same year, he was granted the degree of Doctor and soon afterwards became a member of the Royal Society. In 1667 Willis removed to London and began to practise there, and was so successful that "never any physician before went beyond him or got more money yearly than he." Soon afterwards he became a Fellow of the Royal College of Physicians and was appointed physician to the King.

"He was a plain Man, a Man of no Carriage, little Discourse, Complaisance or Society, yet for his deep Insight, happy Researches in natural and experimental Philosophy, Anatomy, and Chymistry, for his wonderful Success and Repute in his practice, the natural smoothness, pure elegancy, delightful, unaffected neatness of *Lat.* Stile, none scarce hath equall'd, much less out-done him, how great soever." (Anthony à Wood *Athenae Oxonienses*).

Willis died in 1675 and was buried in Westminster Abbey, the cost of his funeral amounting, we are told, to £470 4s. 4d. without the gravestone.

Willis was endowed with remarkable powers of careful clinical observation

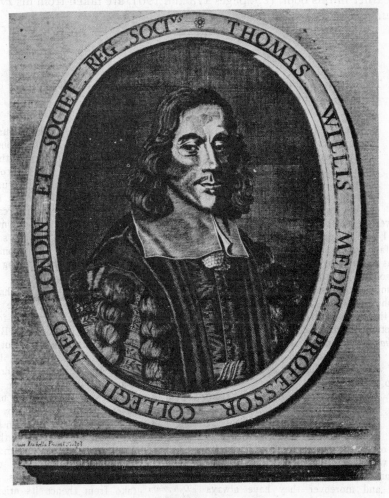

THOMAS WILLIS (1621-1675)
A copper engraving at the age of forty-five by Isabella Piccini. From the frontispiece of *Opera omnia* (Geneva, 1694)

and was the first to note the sweetish taste of diabetic urine. He also described myasthenia gravis and in his *De febribus* wrote early accounts of epidemics of typhus fever and of typhoid fever. In his *Anatomy of the Brain* he described most accurately the anatomy of the nervous system and arterial circle at the base of the brain, the "circle of Willis." His *Pharmaceutica rationale* enjoyed a great reputation in his day, but of this work Sir William Osler said: "It is

as dead as Willis. It gives me a shudder to think of the constitution our ancestors had, and of how they withstood the assaults of the apothecary."

The following account of diabetes is from Willis' *Pharmaceutice rationalis
or an Excercitation of the Operations of Medicines in Humane Bodies,* published in London in 1679. The account of typhus fever and of typhoid fever,
found earlier in this book (*c.f.* pages 178 and 190), are taken from his *Practice
of Physick,* London, 1684.

CHAP. III*

OF THE TOO MUCH EVACUATION BY URINE, AND ITS REMEDY; AND ESPECIALLY OF THE
DIABETES OR PISSING EVIL, WHOSE THEORY AND METHOD OF CURING,
IS INQUIRED INTO

*The
Diabetes
formerly
rarely
and not
yet well
known*

The *Diabetes* was a Disease
so rare among the Ancients, that
many famous Physicians made no
mention of it; and *Galen* knew
only two sick of it: But in our
Age given to good fellowship and
gusling down chiefly of unallayed
Wine; we meet with examples and instances
enough, I may say daily, of this Disease. But
yet as familiar as it is, and though it be
known as to its Type, its causes and the formal reason notwithstanding, is almost altogether unknown. That I may be so bold to
Philosophize, or rather to conjecture concerning these; we will first of all give you
a description of this Disease, as to all or the
chief *Phaenomena* of it: Then we will endeavour diligently to find out from the
fault, of what part or humour every of them
single do arise.

*Its
descrip-
tion*

Diabetes is called so from
διαβαίνω *Transeo,* or passing
through too swift a passage of the
matter that is drunk, also a *pro-
fluvium* or thorow-flux of Urine. Those labouring with this Disease, piss a great deal
more than they drink, or take of any liquid
aliment; and moreover they have always
joyned with it continual thirst, and a gentle,
and as it were hectick Fever. But that as
many Authors affirm the drink to be little or
nothing changed, is very far from truth; because the Urine in all (that I have known
who hath hapned to have it, and I believe to
be so in all) very much differing both from
the drink taken in, and also from any hu-

* Willis, Thomas, *Pharmaceutice Rationalis or
an Excercitation of the Operations of Medicines
in Humane Bodies,* London, Dring, Harper and
Leigh, 1679, p. 79.

mour that is wont to be begot in our Body,
was wonderfully sweet as it were imbued with
Honey or Sugar. The occasion of the foresaid error (as I suppose) was the colour of
the Urine, which always appears crude, and
watry as of those labouring with a *Pica* or
with the Dropsie. That we may carefully
search out the reasons of these Symptoms,
we must first inquire from whence so quick
and copious an excretion of Urine comes, and
then we will proceed to the shewing of the
remaining Reason of this Disease.

*Its cause
is not the
attraction
of the
Reins*

It no way pleases us that some
do assign for the cause of the
Diabetes, the attracting force of
the Reins: because the Blood is
not drawn to the Reins but driven
thither by the motion of the Heart. Further
neither doth the *Serum* seem to be drawn or
emulged from the Blood washing thorow
them, but to be separated (as we have already more clearly shewed) partly by straining, and partly by fusion or a certain kind of
precipitation: wherefore we believe the *Diabetes* to be rather and more im-

*But
rather
a
Deliquium
of the
Blood*

mediately an affection of the
Blood than of the Reins, and to
take from thence its origin, for
as much as the mass of Blood is
as it were melted, and is too
copiously fused into serosity: which easily
appears truly from the quantity of the Urine
increased into so great immensity which cannot proceed but from a melting and consumption of the Blood. Wherefore also the
remaining Blood, its *Serum* going away so
plentifully, become more crass or thick, and
more apt to be coagulated, as may be argued
from the swift working Pulse: for the Heart
is therefore more rapidously moved, that

whilst it exagitates the Blood more than usual, it might preserve it from Coagulation. Further that the fluidity of this, apt to be dangerous by reason of the too great loss of the serous Liquor, might be continued, potulent matter is most plentifully taken in an huge thirst provoking to it, and besides the Humours that are within the solid parts are supped up from the Blood, yea their fillings are melted for the reparation of this; hence it is that those labouring with this Disease are exceeding thirsty, and quickly grow lean.

The Conjunct cause is chiefly in the Blood — Therefore, that I may endeavor to shew the conjunct cause and formal Reason of the *Diabetes*, I am led to believe the *Crasis* or mixtion of the Blood to be so laxed and as it were dissolved that the watry Particles cannot be contained by the more thick, but that they quickly sliding from their embraces, and being imbued with saline Particles, do run forth thorow the most open Passages of the Reins. But in the mean time other humors both from without and from within for the moystning the Blood, and hindring it from coagulation, are conveyed into it; and the *praecordia* are urged even with a mighty force into a more rapid motion. . . .

* * *

The evident causes of the Diabetes — So much concerning the formal Reason and causes, to wit, the conjunct and more remote, of the Disease of the *Diabetes*, as to the evident, causes, to wit, the occasions by which the acid juices, which excite the fusion to coagulation of the Blood, are begot in our Body, these are of a various kind and original. An ill manner of living, and chiefly an assiduous and immoderate drinking of Cider, Beer, or sharp Wines; sometimes sadness, long grief, also convulsive affections, and other inordinations and depressions of the animal spirits are want to beget and cherish this morbid Disposition. I knew one using Rhenish Wine for his ordinary drink twenty days together, that contracted an incurable *Diabetes*, of which he dyed within a month, notwithstanding all the remedies and councels of a great many famous Physicians. I remember two Women obnoxious to convulsive and hypochondriack Affections, to whom accrued from thence a great flood of Urine and languor, and wasting away of the Flesh. The theory of this Disease being now ex-

The explication of notable symptoms in the Diabetes — plicated, there remains yet for us to shew the reasons of the known symptoms, I suppose some of them to be manifest enough out of the premises, to wit, wherefore there is so swift and copious an excretion of urine in the *Diabetes*: But that the sick are fevourish, and very thirsty, the reason is partly, because the humours and the juices by which both the Blood and the solid parts are moystned and refreshed, are by a too continual expense drawn forth by the *Diuresis*, or urinary evacuation, wherefore the throat is dry, and the *Praecordia* are greatly heated; and partly because the Heart by the urgent instinct of Nature, and the Lungs are provoked into a more rapid motion, that the Blood being deprived of the moystning *Serum*, might be hindered from coagulation or concretion or growing together, and might be continued in its Circulation.

From whence the often and copious pissing

But it seems more hard to unfold, wherefore the Urine of the sick is so wonderfully sweet, or hath an honied taste; when rather on the contrary if according to our *Hypothesis* the fusion of the Blood and (which therefore follows) the profusion of the Urine happens by reason of the combination of Salts, the Liquor certainly impregnated with these would be rather salt than sweet. But it is easy to unfold this in declaring first of all that the urine is deprived of its salt taste, for as much as many Salts that are of divers Nature are combined in it. For this appears by a manifold experiment in Chymistry, that if Salts that are of a divers Nature, as fixed and volatile, be mixed with an acid thing, the acrimony of either is diminished or lost; wherefore we need not wonder that the urine of those labouring with the *Diabetes* is not salt. But why that it is wonderfully sweet like Sugar or hony, this difficulty is worthy of explanation.

From whence the Fevour with thirst and languishing

Wherefore the urine of the sick is sweet like honey

The honied taste is not from the nutritious juice, but from combinations — Some would think this effect to arise from this, that together with the Blood running forth thorow the Reins, both the recent nutritious Liquor, and the melting of the solid parts are sent away, wherefore it should seem not improbable that this sweetness should be procured from these fat juices being mixed with Stale. But indeed from that mixture only a soft taste like milk or broth or flesh, pleasingly soft, but not sweet like hony should arise, yea but to this which is not only grateful but in a manner pricking, Saline spiculas or little stingings together with sulphureous sweetings (as I have else where shewed) ought to concur. Wherefore as we have shewed Sugar and Hony to be made sweet deservedly by the concretions of saline Sulphurs, so it may be suspected of the Urine in the *Diabetes,* that with the salts combined in the Serum sulphureous Particles picked forth of the Colliquation of the solid parts, do grow together.

Prognos-ticks of the Disease As to the fore-knowledge, this Disease at first is often easily cured, but being confirmed most rarely or with difficulty. For as much as the disposition of the Blood being but a little laxed, is reduced without great trouble, but that being very much loosed so that very many parts separate the one from the other, it scarce or never can be restored.

As to what belongs to the Cure, it seems a most hard thing in this Disease to draw propositions for curing, for that its cause lies so deeply hid, and hath its origin so deep and remote. For what is commonly thought, that the Reins, and the other solid parts, containing or transmitting the *Serum* and the Blood are in the fault, because that they send away too hastily their contents, and for that cause astringing Medicines are chiefly and altogether to be insisted on: I say both reason and experience doth contradict both this *Hypothesis* and practice, for that few or none are cured by this Method: and it is highly improbable (if I may not say impossible) for that *Diuresis* to proceed from such a cause.

Matthew Dobson

Matthew Dobson was born in Yorkshire, England, the son of a nonconformist minister. He was originally destined for the ministry but, finding medicine more to his liking, he entered the University of Edinburgh, where he graduated in 1756. He began practice in Liverpool and was appointed physician to the Liverpool Infirmary, a position he filled from 1770 to 1780. His health failing, he moved to Bath, where he died in 1784.

Few details of Dobson's life have been preserved and Williams states that the only known portrait of him was destroyed. We know that he was a friend of John Fothergill, that he was a member of the Medical Society in London, and that he was elected a Fellow of the Royal Society. The Medical Society was a very select body, "the number of members was probably never more than a handful," meeting on alternate Monday evenings at the Mitre Tavern in Fleet Street. The society published a selection of the papers read before it, and six volumes of its *Medical Observations and Inquiries* were published between 1757 and 1784, the society disbanding in 1784.

Dobson was filled with the true spirit of science and was a pioneer in medical research at Liverpool. He was the first to demonstrate the presence of sugar in the urine of diabetes and his paper describing this most important discovery was presented before the Medical Society by his friend Fothergill. Dobson was very much interested in chemistry and his *Medical Commentary on Fixed Air* (carbonic acid gas), contains many interesting observations on air, renal stones, and putrefaction.

XXVII. EXPERIMENTS AND OBSERVATIONS ON THE URINE IN A DIABETES;

By Matthew Dobson, M.D., of Liverpool

Communicated by Dr. Fothergill*

Some authors, especially the English, have remarked that the urine in the diabetes is sweet. Others, on the contrary, deny the existence of this quality, and frequently exclude it from being a characteristic of the disease. So far as my own experience has extended,

MEDICAL

OBSERVATIONS

AND

INQUIRIES.

BY

A SOCIETY OF PHYSICIANS IN LONDON.

VOLUME V.

LONDON:

Printed for T. Cadell, in the Strand.

MDCCLXXVI.

Title page of *Medical observations and inquiries by a Society of Physicians in London.* Volume V (London, 1776)

and I have met with nine persons who were afflicted with the diabetes, the urine has always been sweet in a greater or less degree, and particularly so in the case of the following patient.

Peter Dickonson, thirty-three years of age, was admitted into the public hospital in Liverpool, October 22, 1772. His disease was confirmed diabetes; and he passed twenty-eight pints of urine every twenty-four hours. He had formerly enjoyed a good state of health; nor did it appear what had been the

* *Med. Obs. & Inq.,* London, 1776, v. 298.

remote causes of this indisposition, except that he came from a part of Lancashire where agues were rather frequent; that about eleven years before, when a soldier, and quartered in Essex, he had a quartan ague for 12 months, and that after he was dismissed from the army; he had sometimes been exposed to hard labour when very hungry. The disease had now continued for more than eight months.

He first observed that he was very thirsty, that he drank large quantities of water, and made large quantities of urine. There was a great uneasiness about the stomach, with a perpetual gnawing sense of hunger; the palms of his hands and the soles of his feet were frequently hot, and the heat was generally increased in the evening and the beginning of the night. He lost strength and flesh; his skin was always dry, and his hands, from being plump and soft and moist, became wasted, dry, and hard.

When he came to the hospital he was emaciated, weak, and dejected; his thirst was unquenchable; and his skin dry, hard, and harsh to the touch, like rough parchment, the cuticle being raised in a kind of small branny scales. The pulse was generally from 80 to 90. But at irregular intervals of 10 or 15 days, there were feverish paroxysms; his nights were restless, with much heat and a parched tongue; and the pulse, at these times, rather hard, and from 115 to 120.

* * *

The urine had a sweetish smell, and was very sweet to the taste. It had sometimes a degree of opaqueness much resembling a dilute mixture of honey and water; it was more frequently, however, perfectly transparent, and almost colourless. These changes I have often observed, without there being any alterations in the other sensible qualities of the urine, or the state of the disease.

* * *

EXPERIMENT I

Some of this patient's urine, which was quite transparent and of a very pale straw colour, sweet and not the least urinous to the taste, was set by in an open vessel to observe its spontaneous changes. This was in the month of November, when Fahrenheit's thermometer stood about 52 during the warmest part of the day.

In 24 hours, a separation began to take place; some wooly clouds appeared, which gradually subsiding, covered the bottom of the vessel with a loose white precipitate. At the same time, air bubbles were detached, which carried small portions of the wooly clouds to the surface, where they remained suspended. This intestine motion continued for several days, and produced a thin head on the surface of the urine, much resembling that which is formed on the surface of fermenting liquors. On shaking the vessel, the intestine motion was increased, and a vinous smell was easily distinguished. Soon after this fluid became sourish; and the resolution going on, the next change was to the keen smell of vinegar.

The further and last change was to the putrid and offensive.

EXPERIMENT II

Eight ounces of blood taken from the arm of this patient, exhibited, after standing a proper time, the following appearances. The *crassamentum* had a slight buff, a due degree of firmness, and was in the usual proportion to the *serum*. The *serum* was opaque, and much resembled common cheese whey; it was sweetish, but I thought not so sweet as the urine.

EXPERIMENT III

The urine of this patient, exposed to a boiling heat, suffered no degree of coagulation.

EXPERIMENT IV

Neither was it coagulated, on being mixed with the mineral acids.

EXPERIMENT V

Two quarts of this urine were, by a gentle heat, evaporated to dryness, under the inspection of Mr. Poole, apothecary to the hospital, and Mr. Walthall, one of the house apprentices. There remained, after the evaporation, a white cake which weighed ℥ iv. ℥ ij and ℈ ij. This cake was granulated, and broke easily between the fingers; it smelled sweet like brown sugar, neither could

it from the taste be distinguished from sugar, except that the sweetness left a slight sense of coolness on the palate. It had no saltness, nor was there any effervescence, on the addition of the acid elixir of vitriol; but on the addition of a more concentrated vitriolic acid, an effervescence ensued, and some fumes arose which had the pungent smell of the marine acid.

EXPERIMENT VI

The same experiment was repeated after the patient was so far recovered as to pass only 14 pints of urine in the 24 hours, to have a moist and soft skin, and to have gained flesh and strength. There was now a strong urinous smell during the evaporation, and the residuum could not be procured in a solid form, but was blackish and much resembled very thick treacle.

These experiments suggest the following

OBSERVATIONS AND QUERIES

1. That the fluid which was separated by the kidneys of this patient, had very little of the nature or sensible qualities of urine, but contained a substance which readily passed through the vinous, acetous, and putrefactive fermentations.

2. That it partook more of the nature of chyle or milk, than of any other animal fluid. Both are sweet to the taste, and both soon run into the state of fermentation.

3. It appears from Experiment V that a considerable quantity of saccharine matter off by the kidneys, in this case of diabetes, and probably does so in every instance of this disease, where the urine has a sweet taste. From Experiment II it further appears, that this saccharine matter was not formed in the secretory organ, but previously existed in the serum of the blood.

* * *

5. This idea of the disease, also, well explains its emaciating effects, from so large a proportion of the alimentary matter being drawn off by the kidneys, before it is perfectly assimilated, and applied to the purposes of nutrition. The *diabetes* proves, in some cases, a very rapid consumption; I have known it terminate fatally in less than five weeks. In others, it becomes a chronic complaint.

Thomas Addison
ON A CERTAIN AFFECTION OF THE SKIN
Vitiligoidea-a. Plana, B. Tuberosa
With Remarks and Plates*

On the 18th August, 1848, a patient was admitted into the hospital, under the care of Dr. Hughes, for diabetes. The following is an outline of his history at the time:—John Sheriff, aet. 27, of middle stature; by occupation a tailor, residing near Kingsbridge, in Devonshire. About six months before he began to pass on unusual quantity of water, feeling at the same time weak and feverish, with a dry, harsh skin. On admission he presented the ordinary symptoms of diabetes; he voided four pints and a half of urine daily, sp. grav. 1050. The treatment pursued was various, but without any obvious improvement. On the 25th January of the following year (1849), the quantity of urine was seven pints and a half, sp. grav. 1042. At this time an eruption somewhat suddenly appeared on the arms, at first apparently of a lichenous character. In the course of ten days it had extended over the arms, legs, and trunk, both anteriorly and posteriorly, also over the face and into the hair; it consisted of *scattered tubercles of various sizes*, some being as large as a small pea, together with shining, colourless papules. They were most numerous on the outside and back of the fore-arm, and especially about the elbows and knees, where they were confluent. Along the inner side of the arms and thighs they

were more sparingly present, and entirely absent from the flexures of the larger joints. Besides the compound character produced by the confluence of two or three tubercles, many of the single ones had also a compound character, or appeared to have such, as shown by the prominent whitish nodules upon them. Some looked as if they were beginning to suppurate, and many were not unlike the ordinary Molluscum, but when incised with a lancet they were found to consist of firm tissue, which, on pressure, gave out no fluid save blood. They were of a yellowish colour, mottled with a deepish rose-tint, and with small capillary veins here and there ramifying over them. They were accompanied with a moderate degree of irritation, hence the apices of many were rubbed and inflamed. The nature of the eruption gave rise at the time to much discussion. On its first appearance, some suspected it to have a secondary venereal affection; but there was nothing in the case, nor indeed in the character of the eruption, when carefully examined, to support this view. The only cutaneous affection with which we could associate it, was that of a young woman, whose case we have given above, where the tubercles had occurred in the face only. The eruption continued almost stationary from the end of January to the beginning of March, when many of the tubercles began to subside, having no obvious change in the texture of the skin. At the end of March the patient left the hospital, and the further course of the case was not ascertained.

* From a *Collection of the Published Writings of the late Thomas Addison, M.D., Physician to Guys Hospital.* Edited, with introductory prefaces to several of the papers, by Dr. Wilks and Dr. Daldy. London, The New Sydenham Society, 1868, p. 157.

Adolf Kussmaul

Adolf Kussmaul was born in 1822 near Karlsruhe and, after the completion of his medical studies in Heidelberg, served for two years as an army surgeon. He then practised as a county doctor for several years but, deciding to enter an academic career, matriculated at Würzburg, where he received his doctor's degree. He went to Würzburg primarily to attend the lectures of a young German pathologist, Rudolf Virchow, whose fame was rapidly spreading throughout the medical world. Kussmaul was later professor of medicine successively at Heidelberg, Erlangen, Freiburg, and Strassburg. After his retirement at Strassburg, he retired to his beloved Heidelberg to spend the evening of his life. He died in 1902 at the age of eighty.

Kussmaul's name is remembered by medical historians as the author of *Jugenderinnerungen eines alten Arztes* (The Recollections of the Youth of an Old Physician), one of the most interesting and fascinating medical autobiog-

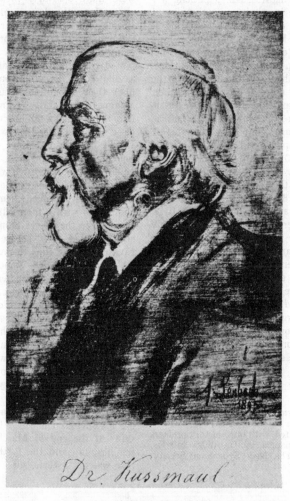

ADOLF KUSSMAUL (1822-1902)
A portrait by Franz von Lenbach, 1895

raphies that has ever been written. Kussmaul lived in one of the most interesting epochs of modern history. He saw the invention of the steam railway, the development of electricity as a motive power and as a source of light, the discovery of the phonograph, and, in his own medical field, the introduction of asepsis into surgery, the birth of the new science of bacteriology, the beginning of metabolic studies in medicine, and the discovery of the x-rays.

Kussmaul's scientific studies were of first rank. He was the first to describe periarteritis nodosa and progressive bulbar paralysis; the first to diagnose mesenteric embolism; to attempt eosophagoscopy, and gastroscopy; to practise gastric lavage for dilatation of the stomach; and to employ thoracentesis. Perhaps, his name is best known for his description of a peculiar type of respiration association with diabetic coma—"Kussmaul's air-hunger." The following extract is a translation of his description of air hunger.

CONCERNING A PECULIAR MODE OF DEATH IN DIABETICS, CONCERNING ACETONEMIA, THE GLYCERIN TREATMENT OF DIABETES AND THE INJECTION OF DIASTASE INTO THE BLOOD IN THIS DISEASE

By Prof. Dr. Kussmaul, in Freiburg i. Br.*

Since I have seen three diabetics in the course of a year die, with remarkably similar symptoms in which there was a *peculiar comatose condition preceded and accompanied by dyspnoea,* I believe that it is not merely a play of chance, but am of the opinion that it has to do with a form of death in diabetes which is rarely observed and bears the closest relationship to the disturbances in the metabolism in diabetes. I will now describe the three observations in the same order that they came to me.

First Observation

A blooming, well built, well nourished, in spite of great activity—yes, fat,—thirty-five year old woman, the mother of several children, was treated for a long time for falling of the uterus and ulcers of the cervix. She lived in happy circumstances. She noticed first in the summer of 1869 that her urine left white spots on her linen. Since the summer of 1872, her thirst, already strong, showed a great increase, she complained of a feeling of weakness and became breathless on climbing stairs or running about rapidly. The diabetes was first diagnosed at the end of December 1872, by a chemical examination of the urine. During the winter she became strikingly thin and in the spring of 1873, the weakness and loss of weight continued, although the patient was still corpulent.

On the 16th of May 1873, the patient took a stroll of two hours, after which she returned home very tired. On the 17th and 18th of May she did not complain more than usual. On the night from the 18th to the 19th of May, she slept well until 2 o'clock in the morning. Then she awakened with *great*

Deutsch. Arch. f. klin. Med., 1874, XIV, 1-46.

shortness of breath, complaint of *severe pains in the hypogastrium* and feeling very sick. Her condition rapidly became so disturbing that her family physician asked me to come to a consultation.

As I came to the patient about eleven o'clock in the morning, I found her lying in bed, but in the *greatest uneasiness,* throwing herself here and there and begging for help, in the fear of death. She seemed *very pale, face and body cool, extremities cold, pulse very small,* easily compressed, *very fast* (135 to 140), *breathing loud, rapid* (36), *and the respiratory movements strikingly large.* Powerful costal abdominal inspirations alternating with powerful expirations. The extension of the thorax was in all directions. She complained of a very great feeling of oppression and very severe pains in both sides of the hypogastrium. She made the remark that she expected her periods. Her abdomen was soft, could be very deeply pressed in without feeling anything unusual; deeper pressure in the hypogastrium was painful. The heart sounds were weak, respiratory sounds loud, pure, and there were no whistling crackles, wheezes or râles to be made out. Her mind was perfectly clear. Disturbed by great thirst, she drank a great deal of spring water. She urinated much, the straw yellow urine containing much sugar but no albumin. Warm foot and hand baths, salts, ashes, synapisms, warm cloths laid on the abdomen, subcutaneous morphine injections of 0.008 of morphine acetate at 10:45, produced not the slightest improvement.

* * *

On the 20th of May I found the patient very ill, throwing herself around on the bed, complaining of great oppression, pale and slightly cyanotic, respiration 36 to 40. All the respiratory muscles in the greatest activity, pulse smaller and very active (140). head and body warmer than on the day before. Also, on the morning of the 20th. auscultation showed no crackles and no râles. About mid-day, the patient took leave from her children. She sank soon afterwards into a *stuporous condition, in which the great loud breathing continued,* and died at 9 o'clock at night.

* * *

These conditions, with which all the patients reached the terminal stage, were essentially as follows:

1. A *dyspnoea of an unusual kind.* There is nothing here, as in ordinary dyspnoeas, to indicate that the air has to overcome the slightest obstacle on its way into or out of the lungs; on the contrary, it comes in and out with the greatest ease; the thorax widens itself splendidly in all directions, without any evidence of pulling in of the lower end of the sternum or the intercostal spaces, and a complete inspiration followed each complete respiration; down to the deepest part of the lungs, one hears a pure, loud and sharp vesicular breathing (so-called puerile breathing); and that all points to the highest degree of air hunger (Lufthunger), as does the oppressive pain of which the patient complains, as well as the tremendous activity of the respiratory muscles, which are so readily seen, the loud noise which the mighty respiratory and even stronger expiratory air stream produces in the larynx. Never, however, is there a real stridor—that whistling which comes only with stenosis of the larynx and

of the trachea. On the contrary. the expiratory breath sounds are often groaning; also, when the patients are either unconscious or in deep coma and when the air goes in unhindered, the venous blood flows easily into the thorax; only when later edema appears in the lungs or if previously large areas of the lungs are destroyed by phthisis, then. instead of a pale color. the bluish tint appears in the face; the swelling up of the veins in the neck was not noticed in these cases and could only, if at all, appear shortly before death; even in the cadavers of cases I and III, there were absolutely no symptoms of congestion in the kidneys and lungs.—*This great breathing* (grosse Athmung) was in my cases, strange to say, *as a rule increased at the same time;* the first patient breathing in the first 24 hours, 36 to 40 times per minute, whether the respiration with the onset of coma became slower, was not noticed; the second patient, who went into coma earlier and whose respiration was not counted before, breathed 20 times per minute, later only 15 or 16 times; while with the third patient, the frequency of respiration before coma was 23 to 24, at the beginning of coma 36, later 24 to 20. The breathing furthermore, proceeded *with great regularity*, was not interrupted and showed no sudden changes in rate. In deep coma, a long pause separated expiration from inspiration, in cases II and III.—In spite of the great distress, the dyspnoea did not become orthopnoea, because the patients were too weak to hold themselves up. The contrast of the general weakness with the strength of the respiratory movements is one of the most remarkable characteristics in this picture.

* * *

Kussmaul later on in this article draws the following conclusions:

1. This dyspnoea is not the product of a reflex excitation of the respiratory centers from the vagus or the laryngeal nerve, but is a result of a direct central stimulation.

2. It is not the result of a lack of oxygen in the respiratory center, either the result of a stagnation of a slow flow of blood in the capillaries or the result of an inability of the red blood cells to hold oxygen.

3. It is not the result of an inordinate

increase of carbon dioxide in the blood.

4. It must have its cause in an intoxication of another sort which stands in close relationship to the chemical disturbances of the body in diabetes; concerning the nature of this toxic agent we cannot say anything for a certainty; acetonemia in the form as it is described by Kaulich, does not explain it. However, it is necessary to prove first the correctness of Kaulich's view.

Oskar Minkowski

Oskar Minkowski was born in 1858 at Alexoten in the province of Kovno, Russia. He finished the gymnasium at Königsberg and studied medicine at Strassburg and Freiburg. Returning to Königsberg, he took his doctor's degree under Naunyn and became an assistant in Naunyn's clinic. When Naunyn was called to Strassburg in 1888 as Kussmaul's successor, Minkowski accompanied his chief to the Alsatian university. In 1905 Minkowski was appointed

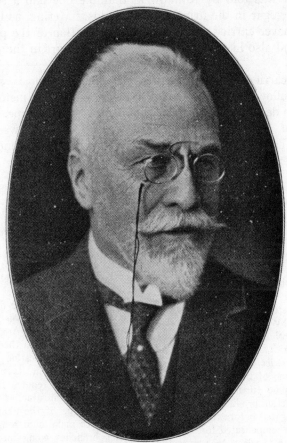

Courtesy of "Münchener Medizinische Wochenschrift"
OSKAR MINKOWSKI (1858-1931)

professor of medicine at Greifswald and in 1909 became professor at Breslau. He retired from the latter position in 1926 as emeritus professor and lived in retirement at Wiesbaden, until his death in 1931.

Naunyn in his *Memoirs* refers to Minkowski in terms of the highest praise. "Minkowski is a man of unusual intelligence. The freedom, clarity, and mobility of his mind, based upon the rapidity and accuracy of his observations and his grasp of things, qualified him for critical judgment as well as scientific investigations. In experimental work, his manual dexterity is of great service.

The ease with which he finds himself at home in so many different fields, is astonishing. . . . He was—this still to-day makes me indignant—nearly fifty years old, when he received his first call" (to a professorship).

In 1889 Minkowski and von Mering, Naunyn tells us, had an argument as to whether a dog would survive the extirpation of the pancreas. A few days later Minkowski carried out an extirpation of the pancreas with von Mering as assistant. Von Mering left the city immediately and upon his return twenty-four hours later was told by Minkowski that the dog had a severe diabetes with 5 per cent sugar in the urine. Naunyn adds, "Mering, as long as he was in Strassburg, never carried out himself an extirpation of the pancreas or attempted one, and also in general took a very small part in the pursuit of this problem."

Minkowski carried out very important studies on acidosis, on the changes in metabolism following extirpation of the liver, and on the metabolism of uric acid. In 1900 he described hemolytic jaundice for the first time. The discovery that removal of the pancreas produced a fatal diabetes was perhaps the greatest single contribution to the study of diabetes and one of the most brilliant discoveries in medicine.

From the Laboratory of the Medical Clinic in Strassburg, i. E.

DIABETES MELLITUS AFTER EXTIRPATION OF THE PANCREAS*

By J. v. Mering and O. Minkowski

* * *

II

The different circumstances which contribute most to the success of the operation, have already been stressed by different quarters, particularly by *Martinotti.* They are particularly: *Control of hemorrhage, avoidance of necrosis of the duodenum and the carrying out of a strict antisepsis.*

As far as checking of hemorrhage is concerned, this causes no further difficulties if all vessels whose section produces any hemorrhage are doubly ligated before they are cut. The loss of time is compensated for, because one can then, up to the last, look over the field of operation and carefully remove the entire organ.

The second condition is usually easily taken care of. Difficulties have been largely because of the anatomical relationships. As is known, the pancreas in dogs consists of two parts, one running horizontally and the other vertically. The first one lies close to the large vessels of the spleen, from which it receives a few branches; with care the vessels can be very easily removed from it.

*Arch. f. exper. Path. u. Pharmakol. 1889-90, XXVI, 375.

The latter part, for approximately 5 to 10 cm., is in a very close relationship to the duodenum. In this part, which is grown around the intestine, the ducts merge, and here run the common vessels for the duodenum and pancreas (Art. und Ven. pancreaticoduodenalis). Farther away the pancreas leaves the intestine and lies, freely movable, shut up in its mesentery.—It is now necessary to remove the larger vessels which feed the intestine, as much as possible from the tissue of the pancreas. Here it is necessary to make numerous ligations of the smaller branches going into the pancreatic tissue. This part of the operation, in certain cases, is more or less difficult, according to the individual variations in the relationship and course of the vessels; very rarely, however, are these difficulties insurmountable.

It is very much more difficult, however, to follow the third condition, the carrying out of strict antisepsis. It might appear, at first, striking, that one often sees the most complicated wounds of animals heal up without any antisepsis whatever, and it is perhaps exactly on this point that most of the attempts at total extirpation of the pancreas fail. The striking feature in this case is that the dogs, after complete removal of the pancreas, are diabetic and, just like a diabetic man, show a diminished tendency to the healing of wounds and a lessened resistance against the pus producers which invade. The following is well adapted to demonstrate the importance of this condition: We have, in all of our operations, carried out the antiseptic rules just as strictly as these are carried out today by surgeons in laparotomies on men. In all animals which are not diabetic, even when the injuries in the abdomen are severe, the wounds heal by primary intention. In diabetic animals, with the observation of the same rules, we were able only once among twenty, to get complete healing. Almost without exception, we had to fight infection of the operation wound, abscesses, etc.[1] and often the animals died from peritonitis.

Furthermore, in regard to the operation, it should be noted that it is advisable, if possible, to remove the organ, in a single piece, because one, in this way avoids most easily leaving certain lobes of the gland in the abdomen. Also, it is advisable to operate upon fasting dogs, since this makes the carrying out of the operation markedly easier.

All of the operations were carried out in deep anaesthesia.

III

As far as the results of extirpation of the pancreas are concerned, we have already mentioned the most important: *After complete removal of the organ, the dogs became diabetic.* It has not to do simply with a transient glycosuria, but a genuine *lasting diabetes mellitus,* which in every respect corresponds to the most severe form of this disease in man.

The appearance of such diabetes, after complete extirpation of the pancreas, comes *without exception,* unless the animals have died from the immediate effects of the operation. Only in three of twenty-one dogs upon which we have, up to the present time, carried out this operation, did we miss the excretion of sugar. These animals all died within the first twenty-four hours, without having emptied any urine. In the bladder, we found at autopsy, only a small amount of urine, which contained no sugar; however,

this urine could have been secreted before the operation. In the other eighteen cases, there was regularly a very large amount of sugar in the urine.

The *excretion of sugar* began 4 to 6 hours after the operation, usually later, often not until the following day. The first portion of urine contained, as a rule, only very small traces of sugar, which could scarcely be estimated. After 24 to 48 hours, the excretion of sugar reached its height, climbed up from 5 to 11 per cent, without the animals having received any nourishment whatever. Indeed, after a seven day fast, the sugar did not disappear from the urine, although the amount of sugar excreted in the urine did become gradually less with long continued feasting. With a very liberal diet, large amounts of sugar were constantly excreted in the urine. For example, one dog weighing 8 kilograms, on a diet of meat and bread, excreted daily, for a long time, 70 to 80 grams of sugar.

The excreted sugar proved to be fermentable dextrorotatory glucose. The comparative estimation of the sugar content with a polariscope and titration with Fehling's solution, proved that no other type of sugar was present in the urine in any important amounts.

Besides the constant excretion of sugar, we also noted in the operative animals all the other symptoms which appear in the severe form of diabetes mellitus in man:

Immediately after the extirpation of the pancreas, the dogs—unless they were affected with some complicated disease—showed an abnormal *hunger* and an abnormally increased *thirst.* With an extraordinary greediness, they threw themselves at any time upon the food which was offered them, even when they had, only a short time before, been amply fed, and all the time they looked around for every drop of water they could get hold of. Often enough, they swallowed their own feces, which, to be sure, as will be mentioned later, usually contained large amounts of undigested food stuffs.

Corresponding to the increased amount of water taken in, there was also a marked *polyuria.* One dog of 7 kilograms weight, excreted daily 1000 to 1200 cc. of urine; another weighing 10 kilograms, 1600 to 1700 cc. in 24 hours. If the water intake was limited, so, naturally, the amount of urine became smaller.

In spite of the rich, yes, excessive, feeding, one notices an extraordinarily quick *emacia-*

---

[1] In one case, Dr. E. Levy grew Staphylococcus pyogenes albus in pure culture in the blood of such dogs.

tion and a rapid *loss of strength*. In the third week after the operation, the muscle-weakness was already so far developed that the animals could not go any further.

Sooner or later, there appeared in certain cases, besides the sugar in the urine, also large quantities of *acetone, diacetic acid,* and *oxybutyric acid,* those substances which are so frequently found in the urine in severe cases of diabetes mellitus. Acetone, as a rule, could be demonstrated a few days after the operation in a distillate of the urine by means of the *Lieben* test or the *Legal* reaction. Later on, the amount increased rapidly and then the urine gave an increasingly positive *Gerhard* iron chloride reaction. The values for the sugar obtained by the use of the colorimeter, were always lower than those obtained from titration, which points to the presence of laevo rotatory substance. In fact, from the acid ethereal extract of a 24 hour urine specimen of a dog in which the pancreas had been extirpated 14 days previously, we obtained 3 to 4 grams of acid which could be identified as oxybutric acid because of its specific laevo rotation, as well as the fact that on distillation with sulphuric acid, it yielded carbonic acid.

The sugar content of the blood was very markedly increased. In one case, we found, on the sixth day after operation, 0.3%, with a urine sugar of 7.1%; in another case, on the 27th day after the removal of the pancreas, it was 1.46%, with a sugar excretion of 7.5% in the urine.

The *glycogen content* of the organ was reduced early down to minimal traces. In the first of the animals just mentioned, which, after feeding with meat and milk, was killed on the 6th day after the operation, we found in the liver a quantity that could not be estimated, in the muscles, still 0.248% glycogen. In the second dog, on the 27th day, with the same feeling, we found, both in the liver and in the muscles, only traces of glycogen that could not be estimated.

The diabetes continues until the death of the animal. The greater part of the operated animals died, to be sure, in the course of the first week after the operation: Some from necrosis of the duodenum, which could not always be avoided; others from peritonitis, which, as a rule, results from the poor healing, purulent abdominal wound. On two occasions, the abdominal wound broke open and the intestines protruded so that it was

necessary to kill the animal. Three dogs died from the results of intussusception of the intestine with necrosis of the intussusceptum; one of these on the 12th day after operation, which he had stood perfectly well. Only in five dogs, was there a more or less perfect healing of the operative wound. None of them lived longer than four weeks. They died, partly from inanition, partly with the appearance of lung disease; one as the result of an accidental complication—perforation of a round ulcer of the stomach.

At the autopsy we could regularly confirm the complete absence of the pancreas. Further, we could convince ourselves that there were no other injuries present—Aside from the complicating disease in certain cases, one of the constant and striking findings in the organs was a high grade fatty degeneration of the liver. The fat content of this organ was approximately 30 to 40 per cent of the fresh substance.

IV

It would seem most important, first to decide the question whether the diabetes followed the removal of the pancreas and is to be regarded as a direct result of the abolition of the function of the pancreas, or whether other lesions produced through the operation are to be regarded as the final cause of the excretion of sugar. Particularly in regard to the observation of Klebs and Munk, we must keep the possibility in mind, whether here the nervous apparatus, especially a disturbance of the slower complexes, might not play a rôle.

However, the production of such nervous lesions is impossible, because of the nature of the operation, which is limited essentially to the shelling out of the pancreas from its peritoneal covering and the separation of the same from the intestine. Also, as is already mentioned, there are never anywhere any secondary injuries found at autopsy which would be of any importance.[1] However, it seems to us desirable to get still more varied proof of the importance of the function of the pancreas in the production of diabetes.

We severed, therefore, in the next experiment, the entire mesentery from the pancreas, so that the pancreas was left in connec-

[1] In one case, Professor von Recklinghausen had the kindness to carryout the autopsy and found that the solar plexus was undamaged.

tion only with the duodenum. This dog did not become diabetic.

In two other cases, we ligated the excretory ducts of the pancreas with double ligatures and separated it from the duodenum, leaving only connection with the mesentery. These animals, also, did not become diabetic.[2] One of these was killed six weeks later; there was already a markedly advanced atrophy of the glands. The second one is still living and in good condition.

Still more convincing are the results of partial extirpation:

If the pancreas is only partly extirpated, diabetes does not follow. We have a partial extirpation carried out in such a manner that in every case another piece of the pancreas was left behind. The secondary wounding which, here particularly could be of importance, would surely appear in one or more of the extirpations. In spite of this, we never

[2] In one case, the first portion of urine excreted, showed a positive sugar reaction; the urine voided later was sugar free. The transient glycosuria was perhaps the result of the disturbance of the circulation in the pancreas.

noticed any excretion of sugar in the urine, neither either traces nor transient. Only after the rest of the pancreas was removed, did the animals become diabetic.

* * *

We also wish to note that the appearance of diabetes is by no means the only disturbance which follows the extirpation of the pancreas.

The absorption of fat and the utilization of protein in the intestine is influenced in the highest degree by the removal of this organ. Dogs in whom the pancreas is completely removed, after feeding with a diet rich in fat, pass large amounts of undigested fat in their feces, often, indeed, pure; at times fluid and, after cooling, a hardened fat, which entirely covers the fecal masses. Furthermore the large amount of feces by meat diet, the large content of same in unchanged meat fibers, proves that the protein digestion in the intestine is markedly impaired. These relationships, however, will be studied later through more exact quantitative analyses.

Eugene Lindsay Opie

Eugene Lindsay Opie was born at Staunton, Virginia, in 1873, and was educated at the Johns Hopkins University, taking his A.B. in 1893, and his M.D. in 1897. While an instructor in the department of pathology at Johns Hopkins, he described hyaline degeneration of the islands of Langerhans in cases of diabetes mellitus. This very important discovery attracted attention to the islets as the probable source of an internal secretion, lacking in diabetes mellitus. The same observation was made independently shortly afterwards by Ssobolew. Opie's discovery led Sir Edward Sharpley-Schafer to postulate in 1916 the theory that diabetes is due to the lack of a hypothetical internal secretion—insulin.

Opie was a member of the Rockefeller Institute for Medical Research from 1904 until 1910, when he became professor of pathology at the Washington University. He held the latter chair until 1923, when he accepted the chair of pathology at the University of Pennsylvania, resigning this position in 1932 to become professor of pathology in Cornell University.

ON THE RELATION OF THE CHRONIC INTERSTITIAL PANCREATITIS TO THE ISLANDS OF LANGERHANS AND TO DIABETES MELLITUS*

By Eugene L. Opie, M.D., Instructor of Pathology, Johns Hopkins University

(From the Pathological Laboratory of the Johns Hopkins University and Hospital)

* * *

HYALINE DEGENERATION OF THE PANCREAS

In the study of lesions of the pancreas the greatest interest centres in their relation to the disease diabetes mellitus. Before discussing the possible relationship of changes affecting the islands of Langerhans to this disease, I shall describe a very remarkable lesion cf the organ occurring in a girl, who, for two years before death, had suffered from diabetes. For the tissues from the case I am indebted to Dr. Flexner, who has kindly placed them at my disposal.

The pancreas is the seat of a lesion which obliterates the vascular supply of a considerable proportion of the parenchyma. Of special interest is the fact that the process, though not confined to the islands of Langerhans, has so completely altered them that in no part of the gland are they recognizable. That intact islands are not discoverable is surprising when we find a considerable proportion of the parenchyma very slightly changed.

CASE XVII.—*Summary of clinical history.*—Female, aged 17 years. As a child the patient has never been healthy and when 17 months old her parents state that she suffered from an abscess of the abdominal wall near the liver. The onset of symptoms of the fatal illness occurred two years before death with extreme thirst and polyuria; sugar was found in the urine and has been constantly present in large amount until death. Record of the quantity has not been preserved. Upon diabetic diet the sugar diminished in geries of tortuous hyaline columns between which are compressed lines of cells apparently of parenchymatous origin.

Much clearer pictures are obtained in sections from the tail of the gland where self-digestion is least advanced. Here in preparations stained with haematoxylin and eosin these structures form sharply defined areas (Plate XXVIII, Fig. 4), taking a bright eosin stain in marked contrast to the general ground of glandular tissue, which contains

* *J. Exper. M.*, 1900-1901, v, 419.

many nuclei staining deeply. Their structure is as follows: Course, tortuous hyaline columns separate strands of tissue, containing nuclei and representing in part at least capillary endothelium, from compressed rows of epithelial cells, evidently atrophied parenchymatous cells. The hyaline material lies immediately outside the capillary wall, between capillary and parenchyma. Occasionally the lumen of the capillary is visible and may contain shadows of red corpuscles.

The hyaline material has at times an indistinctly striated appearance, the striation being parallel to the course of the capillaries. A zone near the capillary endothelium, but not in immediate contact with it, often contains a deposit of calcium salts and stains deeply with haematoxylin. The epithelial cells between the tortuous hyaline columns form compressed rows varying in width. The cell-bodies are diminished in size and at times are hardly recognizable. The cells are usually arranged in columns giving no indication of acinar arrangement, but rarely within such an area or more frequently at its periphery is amount but did not disappear. Marked loss of body-weight was not noted. Death occurred with coma which appeared suddenly and lasted hardly more than twenty-four hours.

Autopsy.—The only lesion noted was that affecting the pancreas. The entire organ was preserved for microscopic study.

Microscopic examination of the pancreas.—The organ is in large part self-digested and stained specimens have a blurred appearance, cell protoplasm and nuclei staining with almost equal intensity. In the tail, however, several areas where the tissue is well preserved give a clear histological picture of the lesions which are present. The interstitial tissue is increased only in localized areas. Throughout the organ, readily distinguishable even in the most digested portions of the gland, are very conspicuous, sharply defined, round, or oval, hyaline areas embedded in the parenchyma. They vary considerably in size. Where the parenchyma stains deeply with haematoxylin these bodies stand out conspicuously as almost completely unstained areas formed by a confound a double row of cells about a well-marked lumen.

The hyaline material does not stain by Weigert's method for the staining of fibrin. Reactions for amyloid were not obtained with specimens hardened in alcohol. When sections are stained with phosphomolybdic acid haematoxylin, the hyaline takes a peculiar bright-blue stain in marked contrast to the deep blue-black of the fibrous tissue.

no increase of interstitial tissue and the blood-vessels are normal. In a section of the kidney a small collection of lymphoid cells is present at one point. Otherwise no change is noted.

The very remarkable lesion just described has apparently obstructed the vascular supply of a very large proportion of the gland-parenchyma. New-formed hyaline material is deposited between the capillaries and the parenchyma-cells (Plate XXVIII, Fig. 4). This material has a homogeneous hyaline ap-

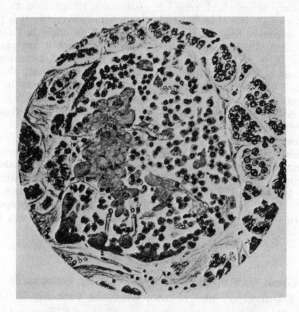

A plate from Opie's article on the Islands of Langerhans

In general the parenchyma in which the hyaline masses lie is not markedly changed. The cells are somewhat smaller than usual and in material hardened in Flemming's solution are found to contain numerous fat droplets. The interstitial tissue is not as a rule increased. In the tail the parenchyma, representing several groups of lobules, has been almost completely replaced by the hyaline structures described, between which is fibrous tissue containing only a few atrophied acini composed of low cubical cells about a distinct lumen. Islands of Langerhans of normal structure are not found. The blood-vessels outside the hyaline areas show no change.

Microscopic examination of other organs. —The liver is normal in appearance; there is

pearance and stains deeply with acid dyes. The tissue which was studied was hardened in 95 per cent alcohol and the absence of reactions for amyloid was not conclusive. That the lesion is not this form of degeneration is shown by the absence of similar change in other organs which, much more frequently than the pancreas, are the seat of amyloid degeneration. I have found in the literature no reference to a similar lesion of the gland.

In the tail of the pancreas areas of hyaline transformation are larger and more numerous than elsewhere, involving at least two-thirds of the sectional area. Though the remainder of the parenchyma is in a fair state of preservation, islands of Langerhans are not found. This fact is especially remarkable when we remember that the interacinar islets are normally most abundant in this part of the organ. It is evident, therefore, that the lesion implicates these structures, but that it is not confined to them is shown by the extent and abundance of the affected areas. Often they correspond in size and shape to the islands, but they may be several times as large. The occurrence of epithelial cells arranged about a lumen, particularly at the periphery of the altered tissue, shows that acini as well as interacinar islets are affected. In the head and body of the gland, areas of hyaline transformation are less abundant and smaller, usually corresponding in size to islands of Langerhans. Unfortunately, self-digestion of these parts of the organ prevents the recognition of very early stages of the lesion and their relation to the various histological elements.

Of present importance is the fact that the islands of Langerhans are destroyed or at least isolated from their vascular supply, while a considerable part of the secreting parenchyma is not markedly changed. The occurrence of diabetes mellitus under these conditions is of interest and will be now discussed.

I have examined microscopically the pancreas from eleven cases of diabetes, and in four instances such marked change was found that one could not doubt the relationship of the general disease to the lesion of the organ. The limited number of cases makes far reaching conclusions impossible. Nevertheless, several facts of considerable interest appear.

Where (Case XVII) the pancreas was found to be the seat of advanced hyaline degeneration, the islands of Langerhans were universally involved in the process so that structures recognizable as interacinar islets were not discoverable. It is probable that the lesion had its origin in these bodies, though with its advance it has passed their limits. On the other hand, a considerable proportion of the secreting tissue, though the seat of fatty degeneration, was in a fair state of preservation and there was no hyaline deposit about its blood-vessels. Where the histological picture was not obscured by self-digestion, which is itself evidence of functional activity, the gland-cells were relatively normal in appearance. In this case fatal diabetes followed a lesion which had in great part obliterated the islands of Langerhans, though a considerable proportion of the intervening parenchyma was relatively intact.

Sir Frederick G. Banting

Frederick Grant Banting was born at Alliston, Ontario, in 1892. He was educated at the University of Toronto, where he took his M.D. in 1916. He served with the Canadian army overseas in the World War and in 1920 settled down to practise in London, Ontario. Banting was an orthopedic surgeon, but obtained a position at the University of Western Ontario as a demonstrator in physiology. He became interested in the problem of extracting the active principle of the islands of Langerhans—Sharpey-Schafer's hypothetical insulin. Banting became so engrossed with this idea that he gave up his practise at London and went to Toronto to work on the problem in Professor J. J. R. Macleod's laboratory. At Toronto, he met a second-year medical student, Charles H. Best, with whom he started work in May, 1921. Before the end of the year, insulin was discovered and, the following year, was introduced into practice.

The Nobel Prize for medicine in 1923 was divided between Banting and Macleod for the discovery. In 1930 the magnificent Banting Institute of the University of Toronto was dedicated, and the dedication was the occasion of a world-wide homage to the man who discovered insulin at the age of thirty. In 1934 the title of knighthood was conferred on Banting. The following selection contains the conclusions at the end of Banting and Best's paper in which they demonstrated the presence of insulin in the pancreas. Banting was killed in a flying accident February 21, 1944.

THE INTERNAL SECRETION OF THE PANCREAS*

By F. G. Banting, M.B., and C. H. Best, B.A.

In the course of our experiments, we have administered over seventy-five doses of extract from degenerated pancreatic tissue to ten different diabetic animals. Since the extract has always produced a reduction of the percentage sugar of the blood and of the sugar excreted in the urine, we feel justified in stating that this extract contains the internal secretion of the pancreas. Some of our more recent experiments, which are not

Sir Frederick G. Banting (1892-1944)
Photograph by Ashley and Crippen

yet completed, give, in addition to still more conclusive evidence regarding the sugar retaining power of diabetic animals treated with extract, some interesting facts regarding the chemical nature of the active principle of the internal secretion. These results, together with a study of the respiratory exchange in diabetic animals before and after administra-

* J. Lab. & Clin. M., 1922, VII, 265.

tion of extract, will be reported in a subsequent communication.

We have always observed a distinct improvement in the clinical condition of diabetic dogs after administration of extract of degenerated pancreas, but it is very obvious that the results of our experimental work as reported in this paper do not at present justify the therapeutic administration of degenerated gland extracts to cases of diabetes mellitus in the clinic.

CONCLUSIONS

The results of the experimental work reported in this article may be summarized as follows:

Intravenous injections of extract from dog's pancreas, removed from seven to ten weeks after ligation of the ducts, invariably exercises a reducing influence upon the percentage sugar of the blood and the amount of sugar excreted in the urine.

Rectal injections are not effective.

The extent and duration of the reduction varies directly with the amount of extract injected.

Pancreatic juice destroys the active principle of the extract.

That the reducing action is not a dilution phenomenon is indicated by the following facts (1) hemoglobin estimations before and after administration of extract are identical; (2) injections of large quantities of saline do not effect the blood sugar.

Extract made 0.1 per cent acid is effectual in lowering the blood sugar.

The presence of extract enables a diabetic animal to retain a much greater percentage of injected sugar than it would otherwise.

Extract prepared in neutral saline and kept in cold storage retains its potency for at least seven days.

Boiled extract has no effect on the reduction of blood sugar.

We wish to express our gratitude to Professor Macleod for helpful suggestions and laboratory facilities and to Professor V. E. Henderson for his interest and support.

THYROID DISEASE

The frequent occurrence of goitres among the inhabitants of certain countries has long been known. Pliny the Elder (23-79 A.D.) referred to them as often occurring in certain districts of Switzerland, and other writers have made similar references from time to time. The first clinical description of cretinism was apparently that of Paracelsus, published in 1603 and followed shortly by the description of Felix Platter. Somewhat later, in 1657, the account of Wolfgang Hoefer appeared. It is sometimes incorrectly stated that Hoefer was the first to describe cretinism. These three descriptions of cretinism follow. The observations of Curling demonstrated the relationship of the absence of the thyroid to cretinism, a relationship later emphasized by George Murray's article, which is of especial interest since it details the life history of the first case of myxedema treated with thyroid extract.

Exophthalmic goitre apparently was not recognized until more than a century later. This disease is commonly called Graves' disease or Basedow's disease, but there is no question that it was first recognized and described by Parry. Parry's observation was made in 1786, Graves' in 1835, and Basedow's in 1840. Flajani's claims have been advanced by some who assert that he described the disease in 1800, but impartial observers who read his description will have much difficulty in being sure that Flajani was actually describing exophthalmic goitre. Osler was unquestionably right when he said that if any one's name were attached to the disease it should be that of Parry.

MYXEDEMA

Paracelsus

Aureolus Philippus Theophrastus Bombastus von Hohenheim, better known as Paracelsus, was born in 1493 near Zürich, Switzerland, the son of Dr. Wilhelm von Hohenheim, a learned and cultured physician. His true name was Theophrastus Bombast von Hohenheim, the names Philippus and Aureolus being later additions. The name Paracelsus was probably one of his own making, indicating, according to some, his equality with Celsus, while others consider it to be simply a latinized form of Hohenheim. Paracelsus was one of the most remarkable characters in the history of medicine. At the age of sixteen he entered the University of Basle, but dissatisfied there, he went to the Abbot of Sponheim, with whom he studied chemistry. Tiring of the good abbot's search for the philosopher's stone, he went to the mines of Tyrol. Here he studied the physical and chemical properties of ores and metals, mineral waters, the diseases of miners and the accidents that befall them. He then travelled widely over Europe, consorting with all sorts and conditions of men, and was accused of being addicted to low company. His usual method of self-education, he defended by retorting, "Whence have I all my secrets, out of what writers and authors? Ask rather how the beasts have learned their arts. If nature can instruct animals, can it not much more men?"

Paracelsus was appointed town physician of Basle in 1526 and gave some lectures at the University. These lectures were given not in Latin, but in German, and instead of being commentaries on Galen and Avicenna, were recitals of his own experiences. The storm soon broke, Paracelsus was forced to flee and, for a decade, was a wanderer. He died in Salzburg in 1541. Some assert his death was due to a fracture of the skull received in a tavern brawl, while others believe his death was due to natural causes and point out that he

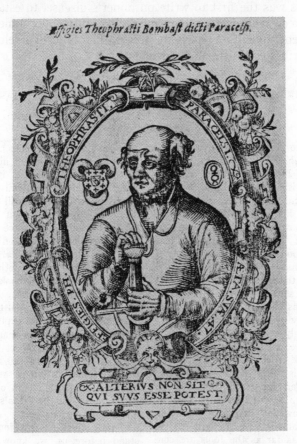

PARACELSUS AT THE AGE OF FORTY-SEVEN
Reproduction of a woodcut from Paracelsus' *Operum Medico-Chimicorum Sive Paradoxorum* (Frankfort, 1603). This is a variant of the engraving by Augustin Hirschvogel

made his will three days before his death, stating that he was "weak in body and sitting in a camp-bed, but clear in mind." Paracelsus was pictured by the poet Browning as a sensitive, superrefined soul filled with mysticism and, by his enemies, as a lying, cheating, bragging, hard-drinking bully. He seems to have been neither, but rather an original, unusual thinker, somewhat quarrelsome by disposition, but possessed of great courage. His medical views, far in advance of his age, show him to have been an acute observer and a profound thinker.

Many of Paracelsus' writings are difficult to read and even more difficult to understand. His language is largely allegorical, mystical, and symbolic, well understood perhaps by the alchemists of his day, but exceedingly difficult for the modern reader. His vocabulary is so complex and obscure that one of his disciples wrote a *Dictionarium Paracelsicum* to assist the reader in understanding his works.

Paracelsus was the first to write on miner's disease, to establish the relationship between cretinism and endemic goitre, to employ mineral baths, and to note the geographic differences in disease. The following selection from his writings describes cretinism and endemic goitre.

DE GENERATIONE STULTORUM, LIBER THEOPHRASTI TRACTATUS I

PROLOGUE*

It is greatly to be wondered at, while God redeemed so high and dearly with his death and shedding of blood man, allows the same be born as foolish men: who cannot recognize or understand his death. his teaching, his signs, his work, his good deeds to man, and is robbed of all reason and the wisdom that belongs thereto. Therefore also since man is the image of God, so he should be burdened with a fool, idiots, simple unknowing men and appear: so therefore man is the noblest creature of all, should also stand before all creatures alike as base, so however all creatures are happy that they have no fools among them, only man.

Now there are many causes for this and they will not be discussed in the prologue. This, however, is the great thing, that God does not consider the person, but died for many, that is to say they are all well redeemed. That however said above that fools, simpletons are among men, is hard to find the cause for: as far as the fools are concerned, it is easy to think what of whatever temperament man may be master, these things to search out. Then also, when a thing is born that is hard for what birth gives who can take it or put it away. It is all the more difficult when fools are born and there is no disease, they are incurable, we have no stone or herbs with which to make them bright.

Besides, so Christ healed many sick, possessed, and lepers and all sorts of misery. But to restore fools, there nothing has been found. From its nature it is not possible. There must be a great Arcanum that could

heal such things as fools have, but nothing is there. A great mystery hid in nature itself should be investigated: it is curious that no other becomes foolish only man and he is the noblest creature, still they have such faults and blemishes. But these things are all to be untangled, since it happened, so should one philosophize on things that happen.

Of pharmacy there is nothing to say, therefore it is lacking in the book of this tract and in other tracts alone they appear, to relate the cause and customs, not to pass for understanding but rather to explain to those who presume to know what man is and of what he is, and that he reflect that his wisdom before God is nothing, but that we are all in our wisdom like fools: and so much we imagine and think out in our bestial intelligence, is all like these fools, and that Christ alone must be our helper, otherwise we are all fools. Therefore the fools, our brothers, stand before us, we know we are friends, and one in blood: Also in our reason of the same blood as our wisdom before God. Also brothers, one who is a fool and the other clever: now there is blood there, also a reason, one is as noble as the other, also one with bestial intelligence is as clever to God as the other. And he who has redeemed the clever, has also redeemed the fool, as the fool also the clever.

LIBER PRIMUS

TRACTATUS I

Paragraph 7.
But to speak of these creatures that they

* Paracelsus, *Opera Omnia*, Strassburg, Zetzner, 1603, II, p. 174.

174

DE GENERATIONE
STVLTORVM, LIBER
THEOPHRASTI.

TRACTATVS I.

Prologus.

Ich ist groß zuverwundern/ dieweil vnd Gott den Menschen so hoch vnd thewr erlöst hat/ mit sein Tod vnd Blutvergiessen/ denselbigen jetzt zu einem Vnweisen Menschen geboren werden: der sein Nammen sein Tod sein Leib sein Zeichen/ seine Werck/ sein Gutthat gegen Menschen beschehen/ nit kann erkennen noch verstehn/ ist aller Vernunfft/ Weißheit so darzugehört beraubt: Darzu auch dieweil der Mensch an Bildung Gottes ist/ soll also mit einem Narren/ Thoren/ einfältigen/ vnwissenden Menschen behafft seyn vnd erscheinen: So doch der Mensch die Edleste Creatur ist vber all/ soll also vor allen Creaturen gleich als schandlich stehn/ so doch auch alle Creaturen gefreyet sind/ vnd sein Narren vnter jhnen haben/ allein der Mensch. Nun aber der vrsach seind viel/ hie in der Leerred nit not zuerzehlen: Daß ist aber ein groß/ daß Gott die Person nicht ansicht/ für viel gestorben/ Narren die alle wol erlöst. Das aber vber daß/ Narren/ Thoren sind vnder den Menschen/ ist schwer die vrsach zufinden/ Das aber die Natur antrifft ist leicht zufinden/ welcher Natur der Mensch wol mag Meister seyn/ die ding zuergründen. Darzu auch/ daß ein ding geboren wird/ daß ist schwer/ dann was die Geburt gibt/ wer kans nemmen/ oder hinweg thun? Dester schwerer ist es/ daß Narren geboren werden/ vnd sein Kranckheit ist/ sind vnheilbar/ haben kein Gestein noch Kreutter/ darmit sie möchten witzig werden. Darzu auch/ so hatt Christus viel Krancken/ Beschire/ vnd Aussetzen/ auch allerley Ellend gewendt. Aber von Narren widerzubringen/ da ist nichts erfunden worden. Der Natur ist es nit müglich. Es muß auch ein groß Arcanum seyn/ daß die ding so die Narren an jhn haben/ wenden möcht/ aber nichts ist da. Darumb so muß es ein groß Mysterium han/ das verborgen ist in der Natur dasselbige zu ergründen: Sonderlichen in dem/ daß so gar sein Creatur narret wirdt/ allein der Mensch/ vnd ist die Edlest Creatur/ die doch gar solt on Gebresten seyn vnd Mangel. Aber die ding sind alle außzuschlahen/ dieweil vnd es beschicht/ so muß man von beschehenen dingen Philosophieren. Bey der Arßney aber ist nichts zu reden/ darumb so wird das Buch desselbigen Tractats mangeln/ vnd in den andern Tractaten allein jhr herkommen/ Vrsprung vnd Sitten zu erzehlen: Nicht sie zuerkennen geben/ aber darbey zuverstendigen ein jeglichen/ der die ding für sich nimbt/ daß er wisse was der Mensch sey vnd worauß er sey: Vnd daß er bedenck/ daß sein Weißheit nichts sey vor Gott/ sondern daß wir all in vnser Weißheit gleich den Narren seinde: Vnd so viel wir in vnserer viehischen Vernunfft ersinnen vnnd erdencken/ das alles gleich diesen Narren ist/ vnd daß allein Christus muß vnser Helffer seyn/ sonst sind wir alle Narren. Darumb stehnd die Narren/ vnsere Brüder/ vor vns/ zugleicher weiß wie wir Freund seind vnd eins im Blut: Also seind wir auch in vnserer Vernunfft desselbigen Bluts mit vnser Weißheit vor Gott. Also so zwen Brüder werend/ einer wer ein Narr/ der ander fast Witzig: nuhn ist ein Blut da/ also auch ein Vernunfft/ einer ist als Edel als der ander: Also auch einer in viehischer Vernunfft als Witzig für Gott/ als der ander: Vnd der den Witzigen erlöst hat/ hat auch den Narren erlöst/ alß den Narren/ also den Witzigen.

LIBER PRIMVS.

TRACTATVS I.

Dieweil jhm nuhn Gott fürgenommen hatt den Menschen zubeschaffen/ vnnd denselbigen nach seiner Bildniß/ vnd auch den selbigen zusetzen in Ebron/ darumb so hatt der Mensch müssen rein beschaffen seyn/ von wegen der statt darein (er) gesetzt ist worden. Wiewol das ist/ daß er auß dem Limbo ist gemacht worden/ vnd derselbig Limbus ist all Creaturen Art vnd Eigenschafft gesehn/ vn in jhm gehabt/ darumb auch der Mensch Microcolmus geheissen soll werden. Auß solche vrsachen hatt aber Gott den Menschen so rein behalten/ daß derselbigen Eigenschafft/ so auß dem Limbo geborn ist/ seine gebüret noch herfür kriechen hat/ sondern gantz lauter/ vnd hat jhm also ein lautern Menschen in das Paradeiß gesetzt/ vnd gebracht: wiewol mit allen dingen bestecket/ aber Vnwissentlich. Dann so einer nit weiß das/ das in jhm ist/ so kan ers nit thun/ vnd thuts nit: Jetzt ist dieser Rein/ vnd Pur/ wiewol doch das in jhm ist. Als ein Junkfrawen dieweil sie nit weiß/ daß sie ein Fraw seyn mag/ vnd was es ist/ dieweil ist sie Rein/ wiewol sie dasselbia ist. Also auch was Adam ein Mensch mit sampt der Eua/ in denen aller Creaturen art warend/ aber sie wustens nit darumb so warend sie Rein. Also kam Adam. Rein in das Paradeiß. Dann das Paradeiß Ebron was ein Statt da kein Vnlauterer/ sein Bypiß geschehen mag noch kan: aber dieweil der Mensch auß der Welt war/ vnd auß der Welt in das Paradeiß gefürt/ vnd jhm da die Heimligkeit eyngeben/ da nam jhm der Leutarban ein Ur.

A page from Paracelsus' *Opera omnia* (Strassburg, 1603), describing cretinism and endemic goitre perchance also have defects in body, that is they carry growths with them, such as goitres and the like: this perhaps is not a characteristic of fools, but also of others, however it fits most of them. This is the same cause that not only their reason is deformed but also their body is deformed and hung with unnatural things. But they come from heating and mineral waters, they give birth to goitres of a peculiar kind, and then such configurations also are numerous and commonly mostly where such regions are. Therefore on account of such deformities every one should know that we are no more of the image of God but outrage the same. And however that is, that Christ has carried the likeness, but was not weighted down with the load, with which we the children of Eve are oppressed. The difference produces in us great astonishment, for we men carry an image in which the nature also the blood and flesh of all kinds of beasts reconcile: and is in it so we let some of the bestial in us. So then we call the nature of the fools bestial and in beasts rule the Vulcani.

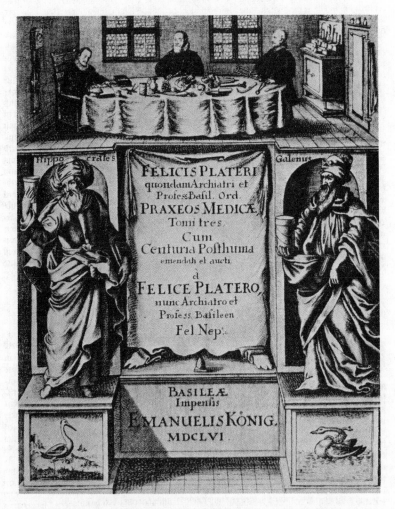

Title-page from Felix Platter's *Praxeos medicae* (Basle, 1656)

Felix Platter

Felix Platter, or Platerus, was born in 1536, at Basle, the son of a distinguished father. He studied medicine at Montpellier and in 1556 received the degree of bachelor of medicine. He returned to Basle the following year, where he received the degree of doctor of medicine, and although only twenty-one, was elected member of the "consilium medicum." In 1571 he was appointed to the chair of medicine in the University of Basle, a position he held forty-three years, until his death in 1614. At the same time, he became archiater or city physician, a position which made him the director of all the hospitals in

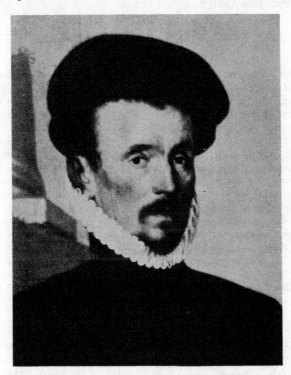

FELIX PLATTER (1536-1614)
From a painting by Hans Bock. In the Naturhistorisches
Museum, Basle. Kindness of Dr. Arnold Klebs.

Basle as well as director of public health. During the epidemic of plague in 1563-64 he displayed great courage and ability. Although the plague carried off his servant and a young man living in his home and attacked his father, mother, and their entire household, he remained at his post and fought the pestilence. On four later occasions, in 1576, 1582, 1593, and 1609, he faced the same epidemic, but neither he nor his wife were attacked.

Platter is best remembered by medical historians as the man who first described in 1614 thymic death in an infant and who was among the earliest to give an accurate clinical picture of cretinism, noting its relationship to goitre. Platter's description of thymic death appeared in his *Observationum in hominis affectibus* and his description of cretinism is found in his *Praxeos medicae,* the first volume of which appeared in 1602. Many editions of his *Praxeos medicae* were printed and for more than a century it was one of the best and most widely used medical textbooks.

Platter's memoirs have been preserved in the University of Basle and give a most interesting account of medical education and medical practice in the sixteenth and seventeenth centuries. Dr. Charles Greene Cumston published in the *Johns Hopkins Hospital Bulletin* (1912), XXIII, 105, a very interesting series of extracts from this diary, and this brief biography of Platter was prepared largely from this source.

DE MENTIS ALIENATIONE*
CAPUT III

Stulti-
tia

Simple mindedness, Failing, Silliness, Infantilism, and not alone in *boys,* who are moreover deprived of judgment, & *old people,* who are said to become childish (although in these it is rather debility than depravity) but at *all ages,* all men are labeled with this name, when all their human actions are seen to be simple: as *Erasmus when failing, Brand on the ship of fools,* in all kinds of men they appear clearly: moreover with propriety it is applied to those who are truly born simple and insipid, for soon in these infants we see the indications of simple mindedness, gesticulating, they rather act like the rest of infants, nor do they obey easily, or are they docile, so that they neither learn to speak sensibly much less to attend to other duties, in which any industry is required. Wherefore the *disease is frequent* in certain *regions,* in the beginning they write of Egypt, & in *Valesia Canton Bremis,* as indeed I have seen it myself, & in the *Carinthia valley* called Bintzgerthal, many *infants* are wont to be afflicted: who besides their *innate simple mindedness,* the *head is now and then misformed, the tongue immense and tumid, dumb, a struma often at the throat,* they show a *deformed appearance:* & seated in *solemn stateliness, staring, and a stick resting between their hands, their bodies twisted variously, their eyes wide apart,* they show *immoderate laughter & wonder at unknown things.*

Wolfgang Hoefer

Wolfgang Hoefer was born in 1614 at Freising in Bavaria. His father was professor of medicine at the University of Ingolstadt, where the son graduated in 1653. Very little is known regarding the life of Wolfgang Hoefer except that he practised in Straubing, Linz, and Raab, and later was called to Vienna as a k.k. Hofrath (court physician), where he died about 1681.

Hoefer wrote but one book, *Hercules medicus,* which was first published at Vienna in 1657, and contains a noteworthy account of cretinism. The following selection is translated from the edition of 1675 published in Nuremberg.

STULTITIA*

Though feeble-mindedness be indeed so common to so very many inhabitants of the

* Platter, Felix, *Praxeos Medicae,* Basle, King, 1656, Vol. I, p. 81.
* Hoefer, Wolfgang, *Hercules Medicus Sive Locorum communium liber,* Nuremberg, Michael and Johann Fred, Endte, 1675, p. 56.

Alps & endemic, some ascribe it to the air, others to the water, others to food and upbringing. Beware that thou believest the first, otherwise you will be deserving of the same reply given to a certain person who facetiously attacking the foolishness of these men, blamed bitingly the defect on the air, which is often said of the place, & enjoyed the same air as the guest: 'Go speedily, good man, lest infected by the same air thou thyself become foolish with us.'

Not the second, since for most of the inhabitants of the Alps the drinking waters are most healthy and still the foolish are as numerous as possible. Therefore the third: to food & education. And this opinion is

proper provision with food melancholy & gloomy their spirits are of necessity made stupid & foolish. Strumae also are produced from exactly this cause.

While indeed the children are thus neglected & sit down by themselves at leisure Hocken übereinander benm Ofen like dogs devouring bits of food with full throats, they stretch the skin & glands around the throat,

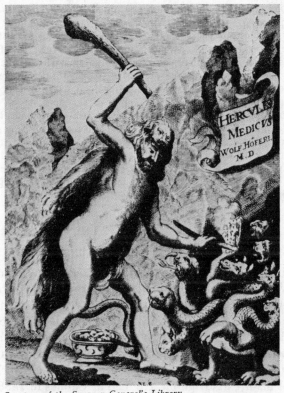

Courtesy of the Surgeon General's Library

Frontispiece from Wolfgang Hoefer's *Hercules Medicus,*
first edition, 1657

proved by other things in my examination of their Diet and mode of life. For this is a Class who are delighted with foods giving much excrement, giving little nourishment, and offended by the opposite: therefore most voracious & never satisfied, save with an abdomen strained to the bursting point. The children stuffed at least four times daily, all winter at home, which for them is very long, they lie at the oven. They teach them neither letters, nor morals, nor labors, nor moreover repeated prayers so that above all with im-

they enlarge, & their heads are filled with harsh vapors from the same food, which is turned into liquid & flowing down either it is imbibed by the glands or they form new glands & monstrous strumae.

To be sure moreover there is no denying, that such Hernias of the throat, called Bronchocele or struma, can be contracted by these inhabitants of the Alps themselves, through the drinking of water infected with mercury, which by its own singular quality produces rheumatism, torments of the throat

& teeth, and produces tumors, as Reusner rightly thought *tract. de scorbuto*. Indeed the inhabitants themselves when asked advise strangers that they abstain from those springs for they had been taught by experience, by the casting of staffs, which a little afterwards drawn out were deformed with many knots, & were uneven. Forsooth indeed such springs are most rare, it is my judgment to give assent to the first allegation & demonstrated view. This one thing added: through such a kind of life the power of generation itself is not taken away from them: consequently moreover by the hereditary evil parents transmit foolishness to their own offspring.

As said above, these corrupted people of the Alps are offended by better & more finer food. One sole example may be cited here, which although most distasteful to others, they however hold as a delicacy, & call by their own idiom Muncken. They cook oats just as it is, ground in the mill in a frying-pan with water, sprinkled with a little salt, until it assumes the form of peeled barley. Then they pour into the middle by a hole made sufficiently large melted lard zerlaffen Schmalz from which with a shell they separate from time to time a portion of the porridge which clings tenaciously & devour it. And moreover they use such foods as is customary the most excrementous, the greater part of which is passed by the belly & the lesser part for example yields nutriment.

Now if, contrary to custom, they approach a more noble table if they are fed with food great in nutriment & poor in excrementitous materials, they ingest just as much of the more delicate food as of the accustomed. Now the stomach and the second and third parts devoted to digestion form from the better food which is supplied in abundance more of the substance of alimentation than of excrement, & if suddenly not without any offence to reason & deliberation, they are fed with food more proper for the body, they are obviously injured and fall into disease. Of this fate I can relate several histories but enough said of these things.

Thomas Blizard Curling

Thomas Blizard Curling, who first noted myxedema, was born in 1811 and at the age of twenty-one was appointed assistant surgeon to the London Hospital. He received this appointment through the influence of his uncle, Sir William Blizard, whose private medical school later became the London Hospital Medical School. He was assistant surgeon for fifteen years and then full surgeon for a period of twenty years. He retired from his position at the London Hospital in 1869 and a few years later retired from all work and spent the last ten years of his life at Brighton. He died at Cannes in 1888.

Curling, in 1842, pointed out the association between severe skin burns and ulcers in the duodenum. He wrote a prize essay on tetanus, and books on diseases of the testes and of the rectum. His paper on *Two Cases of Absence of the Thyroid Body,* which appeared in 1850, described quite accurately the clinical picture of cretinism twenty-three years before the appearance of Gull's paper.

The British Medical Journal, in an obituary notice, said, "Mr. Curling was by nature somewhat cold and did not lay himself out either to make friends or to obtain praise. His character was, however, one of singular honesty and straightforwardness, and he had a kind heart. He secured and kept the deep respect of all who knew him."

TWO CASES OF ABSENCE OF THE THYROID BODY, AND SYMMETRICAL SWELLINGS OF FAT TISSUE AT THE SIDES OF THE NECK, CONNECTED WITH DEFECTIVE CEREBRAL DEVELOPMENT

By Thomas Blizard Curling, F.R.S., Surgeon to, and Lecturer on Surgery at, The London Hospital

Received May 13th.—Read June 25, 1850*

The imperfect state of our knowledge of the office of the thyroid body, and the assistance often derived from facts, even of a negative character, in physiological investigations, independently of other circumstances of interest, lead me to consider the two following cases deserving of record.

CASE I.—In July 1849, Dr. Little invited me to see a case of what he considered *cretinism,* at the Idiot Asylum at Highgate; and to examine some swellings at the sides of the neck, the nature of which were doubtful, but which had been suspected to be enlargements either of the lobes of the thyroid body, or of the lymphatic glands. The inmate was a female child, of stunted growth, ten years of age, and a native of Lancashire. She measured two feet six inches in height. Her body was thick, and her limbs disproportionately large and long. The dorsal surface of the body and limbs hairy. The head was heavy looking, the forehead flat, and the fontanelles closed. The countenance had a marked and very unpleasant idiotic expression. The mouth was large, and the tongue thick and protuberant. At the outer sides of the neck, external to the streno-cleido mastoid muscles, there were two tolerably symmetrical swellings, which had a soft, doughy, inelastic feel. Similar swellings, but smaller and less defined, were observed in front of the axilla. No enlargement existed in front of the neck, nor could the thyroid gland be perceived. The child had very little power of locomotion; but could manage to walk from chair to chair with a little assistance. She had no power of speech. She was able to recognise her parents, and evinced some manifestations of the exercise of the will. She seemed to direct the resident medical officer to be seated, and helped herself to mount on his knee.

I am indebted to Dr. Little for the following additional particulars: she had a severe attack of erysipelas whilst in the institution, after temporary recovery from which her mind seemed more developed. A considerable abscess formed in the thigh, which discharged copiously during many weeks. The wound healed; but erysipelas subsequently reappeared, accompanied with glossitis and stomatitis, from which she died exhausted six months after the commencement of her illness, and about fifteen months after admission into the asylum.

The body was examined twenty-four hours after death by Mr. Callaway, who has favoured me with the following particulars. The body was much emaciated. The swellings in the neck were much less in size than what they had been prior to her illness. They were composed of fat, and occupied the posterior triangle of either side of the neck, dipping downwards behind the clavicles, and filling the axillae. They could be traced extending slightly over the infraspinal muscles, and the lowest angle of scapula. They were not enveloped in capsule, but consisted of fat of a loose lobular structure, which seemed under the microscope to be made up of connecting tissue and fat globules. There was not the slightest trace of a thyroid body.

CASE II.—In November 1849, a female infant, aet. six months, was sent to me by a surgeon for examination, on account of some anomalous swellings in the neck. The parents were healthy. The mother was 28 years of age, and this was her second child. The infant was plump, but had a marked idiotic expression,—a large face with a small head, and very receding forehead. The tongue was large and protruding from the mouth. On the sides of the neck, beyond the sterno-cleido mastoid muscles, were two soft symmetrical swellings, having a doughy feel, and incompressible. They were of an oval shape, lying obliquely across the sides of the neck, and extending from the edges of the trapezii to the middle of the clavicles. I was at once struck with the strong resemblance which this case presented, both in respect to the tumours and the general aspect, to the idiot at Highgate. The mother described the child to me as being helpless with its lower limbs: that is to say, as not being so strong as her former child. She afterwards became

* *Med-Chir. Trans.*, London, 1850, XXXIII, 303.

ill, refused to take nourishment, and died convulsed December 7th. On dissection of the body next day, nothing abnormal was observed in the brain, except a remarkably small development of the anterior lobes of the cerebrum. A very careful examination was made of the neck, but no thyroid nor trace of this gland could be discovered. The swellings in the neck were found to consist of superficial collections of fat tissue, without any investing envelope, and loosely connected to the surrounding parts.

I am not acquainted with any case on record in which a deficiency of the thyroid gland has been observed in the human body. But apart from the interest which must attach to the cases just related, from their great rarity, the development of adipose tissue forming symmetrical swellings in the neck, cannot fail to add to their importance; for it is highly probable, that this abnormal secretion of fat was dependent on the absence of those changes which result from the action of the thyroid, or on some imperfection in the assimilating processes, consequent on the want of this gland: and the facts here detailed may not be without significance in directing the researches of future inquirers into the use of this body. In countries where cretinism and bronchocele prevail, it was long supposed, that there was some connection between the defective condition of the brain, and the hypertrophy of the thyroid. Pathologists have recently been inclined to view the coincidence of these two affections as accidental, or as having no direct relation. In the foregoing cases we have examples of a directly opposite condition, viz., a defective brain, or cretinism, combined with an entire absence of the thyroid, which may be regarded as tending to confirm the more modern opinion respecting the connection between cretinism and bronchocele.

Sir William Gull

William Withey Gull was born at Colchester, England, on December 31, 1816, the youngest of eight children. His father, John Gull, was a barge owner and died of cholera in 1827, leaving his family in straitened financial circumstances. Gull's mother was a remarkable woman and instilled into her son habits of perseverance and industry. In his later years he often said that his real education had been given him by his mother. After attending several small private schools, he resolved to study medicine and, in 1837, at the age of twenty-one, obtained an apprenticeship at Guy's Hospital which brought him two rooms, a salary of £50 a year, and every opportunity for study. He became so attached to this institution that for fifteen years he lived within its walls or in adjacent lodgings. In 1841 he became M.B. of London University and in 1846 M.D. He taught successively materia medica, natural philosophy, physiology, and comparative anatomy at Guy's Hospital, and in 1856 became lecturer on medicine, a position he held until 1867. He was elected a Fellow of the Royal Society in 1858 and received the degree of D.C.L. from Oxford, LL.D. from Cambridge and Edinburgh. In 1872 he was created a baronet in recognition of his services to the Prince of Wales when the latter was ill of typhoid fever. He subsequently became physician to the Prince of Wales and to Queen Victoria. Sir William Gull died in 1890.

Sir William Gull was of medium height, of great strength and vigor, and in face, form, and manner resembled very much Napoleon the First. He was a brilliant, forceful speaker, and his addresses bristled with aphorisms and epigrams. His impartial attitude in medicine was expressed when he said: "We have no system to satisfy, no dogmatic opinions to enforce. We have no ignorance to cloak, for we confess it." He was never tired of exposing the prevalent polypharmacy and remarked, "I do not say that no drugs are useful; but there is not enough discrimination in their use."

"If I am anything, I am a clinical physician," said Gull of himself. Nowhere is his keenness of perception and the accuracy of his pathological views better shown than in his paper, *A Cretinoid Condition in Adult Women*—almost the

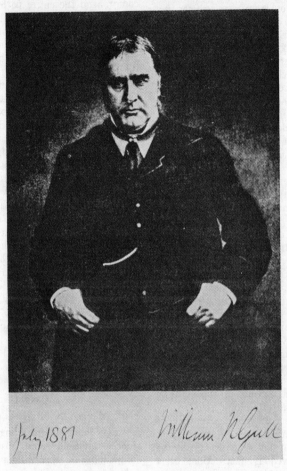

July 1881   William W. Gull

SIR WILLIAM GULL (1816-1890)
From *A Collection of the Published Writings of
William Withey Gull* (London, 1896)

last paper he wrote. While this was not the first paper describing myxedema, it remains one of the striking descriptions of this malady and one of the earliest ones to point out its cause.

———

XXXVII.—ON A CRETINOID STATE SUPERVENING IN ADULT LIFE IN WOMEN*

By SIR WILLIAM W. GULL, Bart., M.D., Read October 24, 1873

The remarks I have to make upon the above morbid state are drawn from the observation of five cases. Of two of these I am able to give many details, but the three

* *Tr. Clin. Soc.*, London, 1873, VII, 180-185.

others were only seen by me on one or two occasions.

CASE I

Miss B., after the cessation of the catamenial period, became insensible more and more languid, with general increase of bulk. This change went on from year to year, her face altering from oval to round, much like the full moon at rising. With a complexion soft and fair, the skin presenting a peculiarly smooth and fine texture was almost porcelainous in aspect, the cheeks tinted of a delicate rose-purple, the cellular tissue under the eyes being loose and folded, and that under the jaws and in the neck becoming heavy, thickened, and folded. The lips large and of a rose-purple, alæ nasi thick, cornea and pupil of the eye normal, but the distance between the eyes appearing disproportionately wide, and the rest of the nose depressed, giving the whole face a flattened broad character. The hair flaxen and soft, the whole expression of the face remarkably placid. The tongue broad and thick, voice gutteral, and the pronunciation as if the tongue were too large for the mouth (cretinoid). The hands peculiarly broad and thick, spade-like, as if the whole texture were infiltrated. The integuments of the chest and abdomen loaded with subcutaneous fat. The upper and lower extremities also large and fat, with slight traces of oedema over the tibiae, but this not distinct, and pitting doubtfully on pressure. Urine normal. Heart's action and sounds normal. Pulse, 72; breathing 18.

Such is a general outline of the state to which I wish to call attention.

On the first aspect of such a case, without any previous experience of its peculiarity, one would expect to find some disease of the heart leading to venous obstruction, or a morbid state of the urine favouring oedema. But a further inquiry would show that neither condition was present; nor, when minutely studied, is the change in the body which I have described to be accounted for from either of these points of view.

Had one not proof that such a patient had been previously fine-featured, well-formed, and active, it would be natural to suppose that it was an original defect such as is common in mild cretinism. In the patient whose condition I have given above, there had been a distinct change in the mental state. The mind, which had previously been active and inquisitive, assumed a gentle, placid indifference, corresponding to the muscular languor, but the intellect was unimpaired. Although there was no doubt large deposit of subcutaneous fat on the extremities, chest and abdomen, the mere condition of corpulency, obesity, or fatness, would not in any way comprehend the entire pathology.

It is common to see patients with a very superabundant accumulation of fat in the subcutaneous adipose tissues, and on that ground more inactive, without the change in the texture of the skin, in the lips and nose, increased thickness of tongue and hands, &c, which I have enumerated. The change in the skin is remarkable. The texture being peculiarly smooth and fine, and the complexion fair, at a first hasty glance there might be supposed to be a general slight oedema of it, but this is not confirmed by a future examination, whilst the beautiful delicate rose-purple tint on the cheek is entirely different to what one sees in the bloated face of renal anasarca. This suspicion of renal disease failing, any one who should see a case for the first time might suppose that the heart was the faulty organ, and that this general change in the features and increase of bulk were owing to venous congestion. But neither would this be confirmed by an exact inquiry into the cardiac condition.

I am not able to give any explanation of the cause which leads to the state I have described. It is unassociated with any visceral disease, and having begun appears to continue uninfluenced by remedies.

CASE II

P. M., æt. 40, a married woman, having had five children, and living in good circumstances, came under my observation in 1866, complaining of general languor.

Heart normal. Pulse, 60. Catamenia too profuse. There had been gradual and general increase of bulk. The features had become broad and flattened, the skin was peculiarly fair and fine and soft, with a very delicate rose-bloom on the cheeks. The cellular tissue about the eyes was thrown into folds, giving the impression, when cursorily looked at, of being oedematous. The eyes were bright, the lips were thickened, and of a light rose-purple. Tongue large, the speech guttural, and, as in the former case, as if the tongue were rather unwieldly. The sounds and impulse of the heart were normal, urine normal. In fine, there was no discoverable change in any of the viscera, and the morbid state complained of seemed to be some primary change in the integuments, the muscles, and the nervous tissues of the cerebro-spinal system. This change continued to advance, so that in 1873 I made the following notes:—

"Tongue large; false teeth cannot be worn, as tongue bitten by them. Lips large, thick, of a light rose (venous) tint. Features broad. Tissue under eyes loose, suggesting oedema. Fine delicate rose-tint on cheeks. Hair soft. Neck thick. Skin and subcutaneous textures lying in resisting folds. Hands broad and spade-like, the textures suggesting oedema, but not pitting. Much subcutaneous fat on chest, abdomen, and extremities. Thighs 39 inches in circumference. Mind generally placid and lazy, but liable to being occasionally suddenly ruffled. Heart's action and breathing normal. Urine normal. Catamenia continue rather profuse."

The following is from a letter written by me on this case March 7, 1873, and fairly expresses my views of it at that time, which was seven years after my first observation of it.

'I believe it to be a rare form of constitutional disorder, without any internal visceral disease, but characterised by great inaptitude to spontaneous exertion both of mind and body. The deposit of fat and the changes in the skin and connective tissues correspond to a languid condition of the venous circulation, but without any tendency to oedema, or any sign of cardiac defect.

'No doubt, under the stimulus of external circumstances, there is a response of mental activity which seems to prove that the mind requires but an exertion of the will to work up to its normal level. Though this be theoretically possible, I doubt if it be practically so in this state. The peculiar condition of the nervous system will, I believe, be best understood by reference to the external condition of the frame; for although I do not think the nervous centres have undergone any discoverable anatomical change, nor is there any evidence that the intellect is materially injured, I believe the nervous power is upon the whole lessened, and hence have arisen the changes in the temper, and the attacks which have been described to me.

"The best suggestions I can make are to let events take their course very much, maintaining the strength by simple regimen and fresh air, and by the occasional or more or less continuous use of such remedies as quicken the peripheral venous circulation. Hot-air bath, or warm bath, frictions, &c, but the general good effect will, I think, be limited."

To those about such a patient the whole morbid condition is likely to be attributed to indolent habits, and the apparent incapacity for exertion to be deemed dependent upon mere inertness of the will. No doubt extreme circumstances have a distinct influence upon these as upon other patients, but I believe the disinclination to mental or muscular activity is largely pathological.

There is certainly a degree of habitual and mental indifference, though this may under occasional circumstances be obviated, since the intellect seems to be unimpaired. It will be noticed that I have designated this state *cretinoid*. My remarks are rather tentative than dogmatical, my hope being that once the attention of the profession is called to these cases, our clinical knowledge of them will in proportion improve. That the state is a substantive and definite one, no one will doubt who has had fair opportunity of observing it. And that it is allied to the cretin state would appear from the form of the features, the changes in the lips and tongue, the character of the hands, the alterations in the condition of locomotion, and the peculiarities, though slight, of the mental state; for, although the mind may be clear and the intellect unimpaired, the temper is changed.

In an interesting Paper* on sporadic cretinism occurring in England, my friend Dr. Fagge has given a case which began as late as the eighth year, in a subject previously healthy and well developed; and he states that in this case the physical configuration was alone manifested, or at any rate that any change in the mental powers was doubtful; and he adds it may therefore be interesting to speculate as to what character would be present should the disease, if that be possible, arise still later in the course of adult life.

In the same paper we find that "in the report of the Sardinian Commission it is stated that, according to information received from medical men practising in infected districts, and according to all those who have written on this degeneration, there is no example in which, after the seventh year, a

* *Med. Chir. Transactions,* 1871.

healthy child has become a cretin." And the Commission further quote with approval the statement of Maffei (who practised for a long time where cretinism was endemic, and who therefore had good opportunities of observing it), "that the period within which cretinism may commence is limited by the fourth year of life. . . . It must indeed be mentioned that Rösch has recorded two cases in which the disease is said to have begun respectively at five years of age, and between seventeen and eighteen years."

It is to be borne in mind that these statements are applicable only to endemic cretinism, and therefore the objections from the experience of those who have observed only the endemic cases will be of less value.

The occasional occurrence of cretinism in children of healthy parents, and living in healthy districts in this country, is now well known. But our experience as to its development at different periods of childhood is of the most limited kind. The whole information on the point is contained, I believe, in Dr. Fagge's Paper, and is illustrated by the second case given.

In the cretinoid condition in adults which I have seen, the thyroid was not enlarged: but from the general fulness of the cutaneous tissues, and from the folds of skin about the neck, I am not able to state what the exact condition of it was. The supra-clavicular masses of fat first described by Mr. Curling, and specially drawn attention to by Dr. Fagge as occurring in cases of sporadic cretinism in children, did not attract my attention in adults. The masses of supra-clavicular fat are not infrequent in the adult, without any associated morbid change whatever.

George Redmayne Murray

George Redmayne Murray was educated at Eton, Cambridge, and University College Hospital, London. After postgraduate study in Berlin and Paris, he became professor of comparative pathology at Durham University. Later he was appointed professor of medicine at Victoria University, Manchester, and consulting physician to the Manchester Royal Infirmary and the Royal Victoria Infirmary at Newcastle. Dr. Murray saw service during the World War, rising to the rank of colonel, and has led a most active professional life. His story of the life history of the first myxedematous patient treated with thyroid extract is a fitting climax to this most interesting chapter of glandular hypofunction.

THE LIFE-HISTORY OF THE FIRST CASE OF MYXOEDEMA TREATED BY THYROID EXTRACT*

By GEORGE R. MURRAY, M.D., D.C.L., F.R.C.P., Professor of Systematic Medicine in the Victoria University and Physician to the Royal Infirmary, Manchester. Lately Colonel A.M.S. and Consulting Physician in Italy.

The development of the principles and practice of endocrinology during the last thirty years has been rapid and progressive. The practice of this branch of medicine has unfortunately not always been based on sound physiological principles, so that glandular extracts have been given indiscriminately in many conditions with disappointing results. In the case of some preparations there is little evidence that the hormones they are supposed to contain are able to exert their

normal physiological action when given by mouth. It therefore may be of interest to complete the life-history of the first case of myxoedema successfully treated by thyroid extract—it has recently terminated at the age of 74—as the results obtained in this case not only afforded definite proofs that the thyroid gland produced an internal secretion, but showed that the thyroidal insufficiency of myxoedema in man could be made good by maintaining an adequate supply of thyroidal hormones from an external source.

* Brit. Med. Jour., 1920, I, p. 359-360.

During the war we learned to appreciate more fully the value of the collective investigation of disease for which the aggregation of large numbers of men under military discipline and the co-operation of groups of medical officers provided the opportunity. A striking example of the results to be obtained by this method had, however, already been furnished by the publication, in 1888, of the report of the special committee which was appointed by the clinical society[1] in 1883 to investigate the relation of myxoedema and allied conditions to the thyroid gland. The history of the subsequent developments of the treatment of these maladies as a direct result of the work of this committee has just been so clearly given by Mr. Stephen Paget[2] that further reference to it is not necessary. It is, of course, well known that the experimental work of Sir Victor Horsley, which was undertaken at the request of this committee, first definitely proved that myxoedema, cretinism, and cachexia strumipriva were due to loss of function of the thyroid gland. Although at that time it had not been proved that this function was to provide an internal secretion, he suggested that grafting a portion of healthy thyroid gland would be a rational method of treating these maladies.[3] The striking improvement which followed the adoption of this method in Bettencourt and Serrano's[4] case led me to suggest and carry out the treatment of myxoedema by thyroid extract in the case whose complete life history I now wish to record as an example of the value of observation of individual cases over long periods of time in the elucidation of certain problems in medicine.

Mrs. S., aged 46, was shown at a meeting of the Northumberland and Durham Medical Society on February 12th, 1891.[5] She had had a family of nine children, of whom six were living. At the age of 40 she had a miscarriage, after which she had menstruated once, at the age of 42. When she was 41 or 42 years of age her relations had noticed that she was becoming slow in speech and action, and she

herself began to find that it required a great effort to carry on her ordinary housework. The features gradually became enlarged and thickened and the hands and feet increased in size and changed in shape, so that at the time of this meeting she presented the typical features of an advanced case of myxoedema of at least four years' duration. After showing the patient, I stated my intention of treating her with thyroid extract, and described the principles upon which this treatment was based and the reason for expecting that it would be successful. The treatment was not commenced until two months later, and the following note taken on August 13th, 1891, describes her condition at that time:

She complained of a languor, a disinclination to see strangers, and great sensitiveness to cold. The temperature is subnormal, and varies between 96.6° and 97.2° in the month. The pulse varies between 60 and 70. The face is blank and expressionless and the features are notably thickened. This change is well seen in the alae nasi and lips. The subcutaneous connective tissue of the eyelids is so swollen that she finds it difficult to look upwards. There is also considerable swelling beneath the eyes and of the cheeks. The hands and feet are both enlarged; the former have that peculiar shape which has been described as spade-like. The skin is very dry, there is no perspiration and the superficial layers of the epidermis are continually being shed as a fine white powder. The hair is very fine in texture, and a considerable quantity of it has been lost. She is slow in answering questions; all her actions are slow and are performed with difficulty. The speech is remarkably slow and drawling and the memory is bad. No thyroid gland can be felt in the neck. The urine contains no albumin or sugar.

The experimental nature of the treatment was explained, and the patient, realizing the otherwise hopeless outlook, promptly consented to this trial. In order to insure that the extract was properly prepared, the thyroid gland was removed from a freshly killed sheep with sterilized instruments and conveyed at once in a sterilized bottle to the laboratory where the glycerin extract was prepared, as elsewhere described.[6] This extract was afterwards included in the British Pharmacopoeia of 1898 as "liquor thyroidei."

At that time care in obtaining the actual

[1] Clinical Society's Transactions, Supplement to Vol. XXI.

[2] Sir Victor Horsley, A Study of His Life and Work, by Stephen Paget, pp. 52-67.

[3] British Medical Journal, February 8, 1890, p. 287.

[4] La Semaine Médicale, August 13, 1890.

[5] Transactions of the Northumberland and Durham Medical Society, February 1891.

[6] British Medical Journal, October 10, 1891.

thyroid gland was necessary, as was shown by the experience of the late Dr. Michell Clarke, who, in the course of a discussion on a paper read by me at the annual meeting of the British Medical Association at Nottingham in 1892,[7] stated that he had carried out the treatment without any benefit in two cases. Several years later, Dr. Clarke kindly told me he had subsequently discovered that his want of success was due to the fact that the butcher had been supplying thymus instead of thyroid gland for the preparation of the extract. Even in recent years some thyroid preparations have proved to be inactive. In the treatment of this first case, a hypodermic injection of 25 minims of extract was given twice a week at first, and later on at longer intervals. The patient steadily improved, and three months later, on July 13th, the condition was thus described:

The swelling has gradually diminished, and has practically disappeared from the backs of the hands, the skin over them being now loose and freely movable. The lips are much smaller. The swelling of the upper eyelids has diminished so much that she can look upwards quite easily. The swelling beneath the eyes and of the cheeks has also much diminished. The face consequently, as a whole, has greatly improved in appearance and has much more expression, as many of the natural wrinkles, especially about the forehead, have returned. The speech has become more rapid and fluent, the drawl being scarcely noticeable at the present time. She answers questions much more readily, the mind has become more active, and the memory has improved. She is more active in all her movements, and finds that it requires much less effort than formerly to do her housework. She now walks about the streets without any hesitation without a companion.

She has menstruated normally during the last six weeks at the regular interval. For the last four weeks the skin has been much less dry and she perspires when walking. The hair remains as before. She is no longer so sensitive to cold. Unfortunately, owing to circumstances, a daily record of the temperature has not been kept, but out of four

observations that have been made lately, about 11 A.M., three times the temperature has been 98.2° F. and once 97.4°.

After this, the injections were given at fortnightly intervals, and later on, when the oral administration had been shown by Dr. E. L. Fox and Dr. Hector Mackenzie[8] to be equally efficient, she took 10 minims by mouth six nights a week, so that 1 drachm was consumed in the course of each week. On this dose she remained in good health, and free from the signs of myxoedema. I have only seen this patient once during the last eleven years, but Dr. Helen Gurney, medical registrar at the Royal Victoria Infirmary, Newcastle, has kindly kept her under observation, and has informed me that she continued to take liquid thyroid extract regularly until early in 1918, when it became difficult to obtain, so that she was given dry thyroid extract in a tablet instead. She enjoyed excellent health until early in 1919, when she developed oedema of the legs, and died in May of that year at the age of 74 from cardiac failure.

This patient was thus enabled, by the regular and continued use of thyroid extract, to live in good health for over twenty-eight years after she had reached an advanced stage of myxoedema. During this period she consumed over nine pints of liquid thyroid extract or its equivalent, prepared from the thyroid glands of more than 870 sheep.

The results obtained in this case show that:

1. The thyroid is purely an internal secretory gland.

2. The symptoms of myxoedema can be entirely removed, and the patient maintained in good health, by the continuous administration of thyroid extract.

The functions of this gland in man can be fully and permanently carried on by the continued supply of thyroidal hormones obtained from one of the lower animals.

The duration of life need not be shortened by atrophy of the thyroid gland provided this substitution treatment is fully maintained, and so under these circumstances the prognosis of myxoedema is very good.

[7] *Ibid.,* August 27, 1892.

[8] *Ibid.,* October 29, 1892.

HYPERTHYROIDISM

Caleb Hillier Parry

Exophthalmic goitre, which is usually called Graves' disease in England and Basedow's disease on the Continent, was first described by Caleb Hillier Parry in 1825. Since Osler particularly called attention to Parry's priority, many textbooks now refer to the disease as Parry's disease. Parry was born in Gloucestershire, England, in 1755, and studied medicine in Edinburgh, where he graduated in 1777. He was a fellow schoolboy of Edward Jenner,

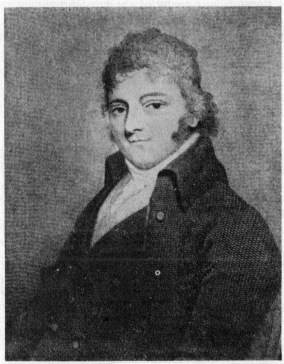

Kindness of Sir Humphry Rolleston

CALEB HILLIER PARRY (1755-1822)
From an engraving by Philip Audinet from a miniature
sketch by John Hay Bell, 1804

with whom he maintained a lifelong friendship. Jenner dedicated his epochal *Inquiry into the Causes and Effects of the Variolae vaccinae* to "C. H. Parry, M.D., at Bath, My Dear Friend." Parry, after settling in Bath, gradually acquired a very large practice and became the most prominent physician at that fashionable health resort.

Parry wrote one of the early accurate accounts of angina pectoris, attributing the malady to disease of the coronary arteries. His most important contribution to medicine was his description of eight cases of exophthalmic goitre in his *Unpublished Medical Writings*, which was published three years after his death. The first case was observed in 1786, preceding Flajani's publication fourteen years, Graves' publication forty-nine years, and Basedow's account fifty-four years.

Parry was a very cultivated man and interested in many things outside of the field of medicine. He was engaged upon some experiments upon the cause and nature of the arterial pulse when he was stricken by apoplexy in 1816. In these experiments, which were carried out upon sheep and rabbits, Parry came to the conclusion that the pulse wave is due to the impulse given by the impact of the left ventricle during systole. He died in 1822, six years after his first apoplectic stroke. As the most prominent consultant at Bath, Parry was brought into relationship with many of the most prominent men in England. His practice, at first small, grew rapidly, and in a few years he amassed a comfortable fortune. Once, while walking home with a companion after a long morning's work, his friend remarked that his waistcoat pockets, cut large according to the fashion of the day, seemed quite full, possibly of guineas. "Yes" Parry replied, "I believe there are ninety-nine; I may make it a round sum before I get home."

DISEASES OF THE HEART*

ENLARGEMENT OF THE THYROID GLAND IN CONNECTION WITH ENLARGEMENT OR PALPITATION OF THE HEART

Case I.—There is one malady which I have in five cases seen coincident with what appeared to be enlargement of the heart, and which, so far as I know, has not been noticed, in that connection, by medical writers. This malady to which I allude is enlargement of the thyroid-gland.

The first case of this coincidence which I witnessed was that of Grace B., a married woman, aged thirty-seven, in the month of August, 1786. Six years before this period she caught cold in lying-in, and for a month suffered under a very acute rheumatic fever; subsequently to which, she became subject to more or less of palpation of heart, very much augmented by bodily exercise, and gradually increasing in force and frequency till my attendance, when it was so vehement, that each systole of the heart shook the whole thorax. Her pulse was 156 in a minute, very full and hard, alike in both wrists, irregular as to strength, and intermitting at least once in six beats. She had no cough, tendency to fainting, or blueness of the skin, but had twice or thrice been seized in the night with a sense of constriction and difficulty of breathing, which was attended with a spitting of a small quantity of blood. She

described herself also as having frequent and violent stitches of pain about the lower part of the sternum.

About three months after lying-in, while she was suckling her child, a lump of about the size of a walnut was perceived on the right side of her neck. This continued to enlarge till the period of my attendance, when it occupied both sides of her neck, so as to have reached an enormous size, projecting forwards before the margin of the lower jaw. The part swelled was the thyroid gland. The carotid arteries on each side were greatly distended; the eyes were protruded from their sockets, and the countenance exhibited an appearance of agitation and distress, especially on any muscular exertion, which I have rarely seen equalled. She suffered no pain in her head, but was frequently affected with giddiness.

For three weeks she had experienced a considerable degree of loss of appetite and thirst, and for a week had oedematous swelling of her legs and thighs, attended with very deficient urine, which was high coloured, and deposited a sediment. Until the commencement of the anasarcous swellings, she had long suffered night sweats, which totally disappeared as the swellings occurred. She was frequently sick in the morning, and often threw up fluid tinged with bile. . . .

* Parry, Caleb Hillier, *Collections from the Unpublished Medical Writings,* London, Underwoods, 1825, Vol. II, pp. 111-120.

Case 2.—Aug. 22, 1803. Elizabeth S., aged twenty-one, was thrown out of a wheel chair in coming fast down hill, 28th of April last, and very much frightened, though not much hurt. From this time she has been subject to palpitation of the heart, and various nervous affections. About a fortnight after this period she began to observe a swelling of the thyroid gland, which has since varied at different times, so as to be once or twice nearly gone. It is now swelled on both sides, but more especially the right, without pain or soreness on pressure. The pulsation of the carotids is very strong and full on both sides; but evidently in the greatest degree on the right. Menses regular; and bowels uniformly open. She voluntarily tells me that she used to be very subject to headache, which has ceased ever since the commencement of these swellings. Pulse 96, small, hard, and regular.— Mitt^r Sanguis è Brachio ad $\frac{3}{3}$x.

Her head was much relieved by the bloodletting, and the swelling of the thyroid gland was evidently diminished.

On the 25th, she was ordered to take thrice a day a teaspoonful of a mixture of Tincture of Digitalis thirty drops, Syrup of Squills an ounce and a half.

Aug. 31. The medicine made her sick on the second day, but she has continued it ever since without the same effect. Her bowels have been regularly purged once or twice a day, but the palpitation of the heart has been frequent, especially on exercise, which much fatigues her. Swelling of the thyroid, and beating of the carotids, much as before. Pulse 96, Mitt^r Sanguis ad $\frac{3}{3}$x. Pergat in usu Syrupi, 4ter in die.

Sept. 7. Bowels open. No sickness, Palpitation somewhat better. Swellings nearly as before, that on the right being still the largest, and the pulsation of the carotid on that side the greatest.—Pergat.

Sept. 14. All complaints nearly gone. Bowels open without sickness. Pulse about 72, and slightly irregular as to the force of the strokes. Pulsation of the carotids still too strong. Swellings lessened. Menses adsunt.—Pergat in usu Syrupi.

Sept. 24. Yesterday morning she was seized with giddiness and sickness without vomiting. Bowels open yesterday and frequently today. On the 14th ultimo, she was menstruating, and continued to do so for three or four days, during which the swelling of the thyroid almost disappeared; but has

since returned, and the beating of the carotid is very strong. She has at this time some catarrh with sore throat.—Pergat in usu Syrupi.

Oct. 1. The symptoms of catarrh are gone; and the swellings are again very much lessened, though the pulsation of the carotids, especially the right, is still too strong. That of the heart, on exercise, is much diminished. Two stools daily, less loose than before.— Pergat in usu Syrupi cum Tincturæ Digitalis 3j. . . .

Case 3.—Mrs. K., aged about fifty, a very thin woman, had for many years laboured under violent and often irregular action of the heart, accompanied with more or less of shortness and difficulty of respiration. During several aggravations of this disease I attended her, and found her heart violently palpitating, so as to reach 136 beats in a minute; extending its throbbing both downwards and on the right of the thorax, far beyond the due limits, and swelling in a preternatural degree all the arteries which were capable of being felt, and more especially the carotids. The pulse was often unequal both as to frequency and strength. The respiration was greatly hurried, and the head was affected with throbbing pains. The urine was often defective. All muscular exertion aggravated the symptoms, which were occasionally relieved by bloodletting, Squills, Digitalis, and aperients. Still, however, much of the malady continued, and I could never perceive that the pulse was reduced below 120 in a minute.

Mrs. K. was also long affected with an extremely large swelling of the thyroid gland, which began at a period, the relation of which to the commencement of the disorder of the heart, she was unable to recollect.

My last attendance on her was in June 1813; on the 24th of which, at eight in the morning, I was called to visit her, and found her in bed. Her pulse was 132 in a minute, and very full, hard, and strong, both in the radials and carotids. The beating of the heart extended all over the thorax, and even into the right hypochondrium. The respiration was 24 in a minute, with grunting expiration, and with no elevation of the diaphragm during inspiration. She had occasional cough, with yellowish brown mucous expectoration. The thyroideal swellings projected before the carotids, and involved the sterno-mastoid muscles from their lower insertion to nearly two-thirds of their length upwards. The carotids were driven somewhat forward, and much enlarged; and the external jugulars were swelled and prominent. For about a fortnight she had been affected with an oedematous swelling of her legs, which had gradually increased. The abdomen was also tense, but not fluctuating, and she suffered considerable pain about the navel, where there was soreness on pressure. The bowels had however been open during the night, with griping. The quantity of urine had not exceeded a teacup full in the last forty-eight hours. Some medicines were given, which it is needless to specify, as the patient died at five o'clock the next morning. A dissection was not permitted.

Case 4.—A woman servant, unmarried, and about thirty years of age, whom, during a space of several months, I had at various times seen labouring under a palpitation of the heart, which always more or less existed, and was accompanied with a very quick and irregular pulse, great hurry in breathing on any exertion, and an extremely strong beating of the carotid arteries, began at length to have enlargement of the thyroid gland, which had not existed more than a fortnight, when I last saw her, and which was much increased from the time when it was first noticed.

Case 5.—During my attendance on this patient, I was consulted by a married Lady, of about forty years of age, from the North of England, who was supposed to be in consumption. She had in fact a very quick pulse, with great shortness and difficulty of breathing, and frequent cough, attended with copious expectoration. She had also an extremely large swelling of the thyroid gland on each side of the neck, with a considerable dilatation of the carotid arteries. The cough having been removed in about a fortnight by blood-letting, Squills, and Citrate of Potash, which were ordered when she first consulted me, I had an opportunity of discovering, at my second visit, that she was afflicted with a most laborious action of the heart, which, from the extent of the pulsation, seemed much enlarged, and suffered a great aggravation of symptoms from any muscular exertion.

This inordinate action of the heart has been of long duration, and considerably preceded the commencement of the thyroideal swelling.

The patient did not remain at Bath long enough for me to know the result of the disease, which, doubtless, would ultimately prove fatal.

My attendance on the three last patients having occurred at the same time, first suggested to me the notion of some connection between the malady of the heart and the bronchocele. I mentioned that opinion to Mr. G. Norman, surgeon, to whom I shewed the lady last mentioned. Shortly afterwards I expressed the same opinion to Mr. Cruttwell, surgeon, to whom it then occurred that he was attending a patient with a similar coincidence, and that in her the bronchocele succeeded to the affection of the heart.

Case 6.—Anne P., aged about thirty, a married woman, thin, and with a very long neck, who has never had a family, five years ago, at Christmas, when affected with chilblaines, for their relief kept her feet in cold water for a quarter of an hour, which made her feet extremely cold. Half an hour afterwards she was seized with a pain about the region of the heart, which was extremely violent; but unaccompanied with cough, fever, or palpitation. Ever since that period she has been subject to attacks of similar pain, which recur frequently. She has also frequent palpitations, which come on more especially after walking or any hurry; though sometimes without any apparent cause whatever. She is often affected also with oppression of breathing, which is sometimes accompanied with globus hystericus, and obliges her to lie rather high in bed. All pressure about the thorax is uneasy to her; but she lies best on her left side. She is free from cough. At this moment she complains of violent pain on the sternum towards the lower part, which is not sore on pressure. Pulse 112, and weak. Respiration 22. Extremities cold. Skin pale. She is sleepy during the day, but sleeps little at night. Tongue rather furred. Appetite irregular. Urine very various as to appearance. Menses, since the commencement of the malady, defective.

During the palpitation, and indeed at other times, she has long had a violent beating in her head, and a throbbing in her neck. This day fortnight she had an unusual degree of this throbbing, accompanied with a great aggravation of a distracting pain in the head, to which she has been subject ever since she began to be ill, and which is always greatly increased by coming out of the air into a warm room. During the more violent accessions of this affection of the head, she cannot bear the least conversation, and feels as if she should die. The evening after the last described aggravation, the thyroid gland began to swell at its lower part before, and the swelling has now diffused itself to a considerable degree on each side, without soreness on pressure. The beating of the carotids is very strong.

Robert James Graves

Robert James Graves was born in 1795 in Dublin and was descended from a colonel in Cromwell's cavalry who had acquired an estate in Limerick County after the conquest of Ireland. His father was a minister and Robert, after taking his degree at Dublin, studied in London, Edinburgh, and on the Continent. He had a great talent for languages and once was imprisoned for ten

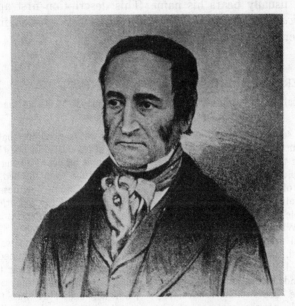

ROBERT JAMES GRAVES (1795-1853)
From the *Medical History of the Meath Hospital* by Lambert H. Ormsby, Dublin, Fannon Company, 41 Grafton St., 1892. Kindness of George Blumer.

days in an Austrian prison as a German spy, the authorities insisting that no Englishman could possibly speak German so perfectly. In Italy he made the acquaintance of the celebrated painter Turner, and it is said that the two traveled together for months without either inquiring the name of the other. Graves returned to Dublin in 1821 and immediately became a leader in his profession. He was a handsome man and possessed of much charm and brilliance in conversation. He was very much dissatisfied with the state of medical teaching as he found it in Dublin and in Edinburgh. The teaching was largely didactic, so that a student could obtain his degree without ever having attempted the diagnosis of a patient or without having watched methods of treatment. Graves was much impressed by what he had seen upon the continent, and it is largely due to his initiative that bedside teaching was introduced in the British Isles. At first, however, his ideas of having advanced students take histories and examine and keep records of patients met with both opposition and ridicule.

Graves was much opposed to the low caloric diets in vogue for the treatment of typhoid and other fevers. One day while passing through the hospital wards, he was struck by the splendid appearance of a patient who was convalescing from typhoid fever. "This is all the effect of our good feeding," he exclaimed; "and lest, when I am gone, you may be at a loss for an epitaph for me, let me give you one in three words: HE FED FEVERS!"

Graves, however, is probably best remembered by his description of the disease which usually bears his name. This description first appeared in the *London Medical and Surgical Journal* in 1835. Graves died in 1853, seventeen years after the appearance of this paper.

NEWLY OBSERVED AFFECTION OF THE THYROID GLAND IN FEMALES*

From the Clinical Lectures delivered by Robert J. Graves, M.D., at the Meath Hospital, during the Session of 1834-5

I have lately seen three cases of violent and long continued palpitations in females, in each of which the sample peculiarity presented itself, viz. enlargement of the thyroid gland; the size of this gland, at all times considerably greater than natural, was subject to remarkable variations in every one of these patients. When the palpitations were violent the gland used notably to swell and become distended, having all the appearance of being increased in size in consequence of an interstitial and sudden effusion of fluid into its substance. The swelling immediately began to subside as the violence of the paroxysm of palpitation decreased, and during the intervals the size of the gland remained stationary. Its increase of size and the variations to which it was liable had attracted forcibly the attention both of the patients and of their friends. There was not the slightest evidence of any thing like inflammation of the gland. One of these ladies, residing in the neighbourhood of Black Rock, was seen by Dr. Harvey and Dr. William Stokes, another of them, the wife of a clergyman in the county of Wicklow, was seen by Dr. Marsh, and the third lives in Grafton Street. The palpitations have in all lasted considerably more than a year, and with such violence as to be at times exceedingly distressing, and yet there seems no certain

*Graves, R. J., *London Med. & Surg. Jour.*, 1835, VII, pt. 2, pp. 516, 517.

grounds for concluding that organic disease of the heart exists. In one the beating of the heart could be heard during the paroxysm at some distance from the bed, a phenomenon I had never before witnessed, and which strongly excited my attention and curiosity. She herself, her friends, and Dr. Harvey all testified the frequency of this occurrence, and said that the sound was at times much louder than when I examined the patient, and yet I could distinctly hear the heart beating when my ear was distant at least four feet from her chest! It was the first or dull sound which was thus audible. This fact is well worthy of notice, and when duly considered appears to favour the explanation lately given by Magendie of the causes of the sounds produced during the heart's action, for none of those previously proposed seem to me capable of accounting for a sound so loud and so distinct. But to return to our subject. The sudden manner in which the thyroid in the above three females used to increase and again diminish in size and the connection of this with the state of the heart's action, are circumstances which may be considered as indicating that the thyroid is slightly analogous in structure to the tissues properly called erectile. It is well known that no part of the body is so subject to increase in size as the thyroid gland, and not infrequently this increase has been observed to be remarkably rapid, constituting the different varieties of bronchocele or goitre. The enlargement of the thyroid, of which I am now speaking, seems to be essentially different from goitre in not attaining a size at all equal to that observed in the latter disease. Indeed this enlargement deserves rather the name of hypertrophy, and is at once distinguishable from bronchocele by its becoming stationary, just at that period of its development when the growth of the latter usually begins to be accelerated. In fact, although the tumour is very observable when the attention is directed to it, yet it never amounts to actual deformity. The well known connection which exists between the uterine functions of the female and the development of the thyroid observed at puberty, renders this affection worthy of attention, particularly when we find it so closely related by sympathy to those palpitations of the heart which are of so frequent occurrence in hysterical and nervous females.

Another fact well worthy of notice, is that females liable to attacks of palpitations almost invariably complain of a sense of fulness, referred to the throat, and exactly corresponding to the situation of the thyroid. This sensation only continues while the paroxysm of palpitation lasts, and frequently is so urgent as forcibly to attract the patient's notice, who now complains of its inducing a sense of suffocation. Here the interesting question occurs whether this feeling of something that impedes the respiration at the bottom of the throat, during the hysterical fit, and which has been included under the general term *globus hystericus*,—the question arises, I say, whether this feeling is always of purely nervous origin. To me it appears probable that it is often induced by the pressure arising from a sudden enlargement of the thyroid, which enlargement subsides as soon as the fit is over. Of this I am certain, that the lump in the throat, of which females complain, is often exactly referred to the situation of the thyroid; and indeed I have been told by other practitioners, upon the accuracy of whose observations I can rely, that this swelling in the throat of females during the hysteric paroxysm has more than once excited their wonder. It is obvious, gentlemen, that if palpitations depending on functional disease of the heart are capable of exciting this swollen state of the thyroid, we may expect to observe the tumefaction of this gland also where the palpitation depends on organic disease of the heart, as in the following case detailed to me by a friend.

A lady, aged twenty, became affected with some symptoms which were supposed to be hysterical. This occurred more than two years ago; her health previously had been good. After she had been in this nervous state about three months it was observed that her pulse had become singularly rapid. This rapidity existed without any apparent cause, and was constant, the pulse being never under 120, and often much higher. She next complained of weakness on exertion, and began to look pale and thin. Thus she continued for a year, but during this time she manifestly lost ground on the whole, the rapidity of the heart's action having never ceased. It was now observed that the eyes assumed a singular appearance, for the eyeballs were apparently enlarged, so that when she slept or tried to shut her eyes, the lids were incapable of closing. When the eyes were open, the white sclerotic could be seen, to a breadth of several lines, all around the cornea. In a few months, the action of the heart continuing with increasing violence, a tumour, of a horseshoe shape, appeared on the front of the throat and exactly in the situation of the thyroid gland. This was at first soft but soon attained a greater hardness though still elastic. From the time it was first observed, it has increased little, if at all, in size, and is now about thrice the natural bulk of the fully developed gland in a female after the age of puberty. It is somewhat larger on the right side than on the left. A circumstance well worthy of notice has been observed in this young lady's case, and which may serve to throw some light on the nature of this thyroid tumefaction. The circumstance I allude to is, that from an early period of the disease a remarkable disproportion was found to exist between the beats of the radial and of the carotid arteries, the pulsations of the former being comparatively feeble, while those of the latter were violent, causing a most evident throbbing of the neck, and accompanied by a loud rustling sound. In about fourteen months the heart presented all the signs of Laënnec's passive aneurism; the tumour in the neck is subject to remarkable variations in size, sometimes diminishing nearly one half. None of her family have had goitres, nor was she ever in any of the usual localities of the disease.

Carl A. von Basedow

Carl A. von Basedow was born on March 28, 1799, in Dessau, and studied medicine at the University of Halle. He early showed a great interest in surgery, and after his graduation spent two years in Paris, years devoted mainly to the study of surgery at the Charité and the Hôtel Dieu. Returning to Ger-

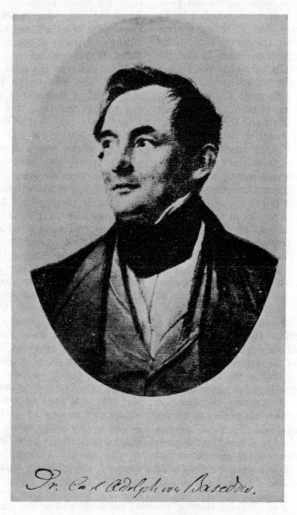

CARL A. VON BASEDOW (1799-1854)
From *Münchener Medizinische Wochenschrift*

many in 1822, he settled in the town of Merseburg, where he practised for 32 years, leading the active and often arduous life of a general practitioner, surgeon, and "Kreisphysicus" (district physician). He seems to have been much interested in pathology and, in 1848, published the autopsy findings in one of his cases of *Glotzaugencachexie* (exophthalmic cachexia), probably the first protocol of an autopsy on a case of recognized exophthalmic goitre. This intense interest in pathology led directly to his death in 1854, which was due to a septic infection, the result of a scratch received while performing an autopsy on the body of a typhus fever victim.

In 1840 his article on *Exophthalmos durch Hypertrophie des Zellgewebes in der Augenhöhle* (Exophthalmos due to hypertrophy of the cellular tissue in the orbit) appeared, which described clearly the so-called "Merseburg Triad" —struma, exophthalmos, and palpitation of the heart. Although later studies have shown that physicians elsewhere, notably Parry and Graves, described the condition before Basedow, yet, on the continent of Europe, it was the great achievement of Basedow to point out this striking disease to his confreres.

"All over Europe, every year, such cases came to the important clinics and before the eyes of the busy, clear-eyed practitioners and then again, unnoticed and not understood, disappeared from their view, until the isolated doctor of a little town in Thuringia had his attention attracted and, with one stroke, recognized the syndrome and sketched clearly the specific disease picture." (Sudhoff)

The following account is from Basedow's article entitled, *Exophthalmos durch Hypertrophie des Zellgewebes in der Augenhöhle,* which appeared in *Wochenschrift für die gesammte Heilkunde,* Berlin, March 28, 1840. This article appears in two issues of the *Wochenschrift* and occupies seventeen pages. Basedow describes in this report three cases. The following description is the history of the first case:

Madame F., brunette, well built, of a decided phlegmatic temperament, suffered as a child with frequent attacks of *Rheumatismus articularis,* in the years of puberty a number of times from *Angina tonsillaris;* lost her mother from *Carcinoma uteri.* The, menses appeared in the 14th year, she was married in 1828, in her nineteenth year, became a mother, nursed her child, and in 1830 after the weaning of her boy and after the menses had appeared again, made a trip to her parents in Leipzig. She became sick there, felt heaviness in her extremities, had continual pressure of the stomach, compression of the chest and suffered suddenly twice in one day from an attack of *Vomitus cruentus* so strong that the loss of blood produced unconsciousness, fainting, and she seemed to be in great danger of her life. After six weeks' treatment, however, she came back to Merseburg and seemed to feel healthy and straightened out in every particular. In November 1831, she bore a second son; she remained healthy; in 1833 she gave birth to a daughter, which she nursed for three quarters of a year, but after weaning, she took to her bed for six weeks because of *Rheumatismus acutus febrilis.* Her health seemed to have been en-

tirely restored. She was again the mother of a fourth child, she nursed it. However, after weaning, the menses were very scanty and then, because of a bad error in diet which she committed during one period, they were entirely suppressed. Madame F. felt herself very exhausted, suffered from an obstinate diarrhoea, had night sweats, lost a great deal of weight; at which time the eyeballs began to protrude from the *Orbita.* The patient complained of shortness of breath; she had a very rapid, small pulse (in the left hand the radial pulse was absent for as long as I have known her); a resounding heart beat, she could not hold her hand still, spoke with striking rapidity; and she liked to seat herself (because she always felt burning hot) with naked breasts and arms, in a cold draft. She showed unnatural excitement and carelessness about her condition. She went around a great deal, without being at all disturbed about her striking appearance in company. She satisfied without any afterthoughts her various strong appetites, slept well, however with open eyes.

Sometime in 1837 however, all of these symptoms increased in intensity, after the patient had taken, without results, medicines to bring back the menses, to relieve the *Erethismus* in the lesser circulation and for the regulation of her digestion.

Her arms, neck, breast, also the breast glands, were markedly emaciated, abdomen unusually full and thick. It showed by a closer examination through percussion most certainly however no *Tympanites,* no hydrops. The legs became, from the lower third of the thighs to the extremities, very fat, however not edematous, the cellular tissue seemed rather brawny, such as is often found in *Chlorosis,* on pressure leaves no dent and after acupunctur produces no falling out of *Serum.*

In the neck there appeared a strumous swelling of the thyroid gland; the area of pulsation of the heart was now broadened, pointing to enlargement, there was a sawing sound audible in the carotids, the pulse was more frequent and smaller, the hastiness of speech and the unnatural excitement of the patient still more increased, night sweats, very offensive; urine scanty and red and, considering the continued diarrhoea, the appetite was always too strong. As far as the eyes were concerned, they were pushed out so far that one could see below and above the *Cornea,* the *Albuginea,* three lines wide; the eyelids were pushed wide from one another; could not be closed with every effort. The patient slept with eyes entirely open.

The condition of the *Bulbi* was not changed, movement toward the side was more difficult, the cleanness of the *Cornea,* the texture of the *Albuginea,* and the position and movement of the *Iris* were entirely normal, pupils clear; one could, however, not push back the tense-feeling *Bulbus.* The patient complained not at all of pain, said only that she felt a stretching in her eyes, suffered often from a flow of tears, also from small inflammations which were limited to the connective tissue, were easy to heal and were apparently due to the inability of the eye to cool. The vision of the eyes was not influenced in the least and showed only short-sightedness, which she had had from childhood.

For a long time, the rumor was widespread in our town that this patient was crazy and was soon going to be taken to an asylum, and in fact she had an unfriendly attitude towards the physician; she never had, however, and that I can assure you, any insane ideas; she never showed any abnormal desires and if her astonishing carelessness over her truly sad condition seemed to be the result of her phlegmatic temperament, so the hastiness of her speech, the uncertain holding of her body and her hands, the tendency to go about naked or very lightly dressed, were undoubtedly symptoms of her heart disease.

We placed leeches on her breasts every eight days, used Adelheidbrunnens (already we had given her *Lapis infernalis* with good effect, three times daily, ¼ grains for the suspected hypertrophy of her heart and the hypertrophy of her glandular system). Then we saw real improvement, the menses began again, the diarrhoea disappeared, the patient was no longer so hasty and spoke noticeably quieter and also the *Exophthalmos* was diminished.

In the autumn of 1837, the menopause appeared and again the former miserable condition; again after four weeks use of the spring waters of Heilbronn there was a marked improvement.

In the winter of 1837, Madame F. was seized with epidemic gastric nervous fever, she withstood it, contrary to my expectations, but after this however, sunk again into her old calamities and for the third time we tried with her the Adelheids spring. She followed this treatment for eight weeks and again she was very much improved after the third and fourth bottles. A very definite improvement in health now came. Now she menstruates regularly, the swelling of the hip and the *Struma* have disappeared for the most part; the sweats have ceased, the body, breast and arms are all well nourished and only the abdomen is still too fat; digestion is normal; the circulation however not so, since the pulse is still frequent and small; the pulsation of her heart is still heard over too wide an area. In spite of this, however, she complains of no catches or shortness of breath while climbing stairs or taking walks. The *Exophthalmos,* however is only slightly diminished and during the last relapse often had to be treated by a soft *Taraxis* which hindered the cooling off of the eyeballs; however the appearance of the *Bulbus* is normal and the vision is not damaged.

* * *

DIE GLOTZAUGEN

From *Wochenschrift für die gesammte Heilkunde*, Berlin, December 2, 1848
By Dr. von Basedow in Merseberg

This article is a brief summary of his experiences with this new disease and the following paragraph is interesting because he recommends the use of iodine. Basedow refers to the condition as "Glotzaugencachexie."

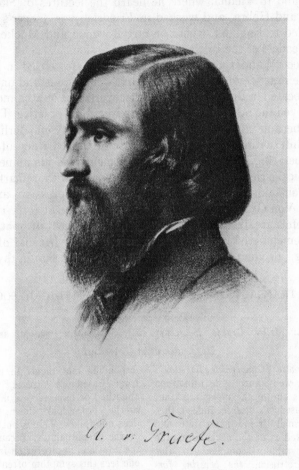

ALBRECHT VON GRAEFE (1828-1870)
Drawing by R. Lehman

This disease has a great deal of similarity with *Chlorosis*, not only because of the uncertainty of cure, although cures often seem to be easily produced in *Chlorosis*. . . . It also resembles it in the character of the remedies employed. In my experience, the best remedies are a combination of iron with *Calomel, Iodine, Aloes, Rhubarb*, and the Adelheid spring water.

Albrecht von Graefe

Albert von Graefe, the "creator of modern ophthalmology," was born in 1828, the son of a well-known and highly respected surgeon, Carl Ferdinand von Graefe, professor of surgery at the University of Berlin. Young von Graefe was a brilliant student, finished the Gymnasium with honors, and began the study of medicine when he was not quite sixteen years of age. He received his doctor's degree in 1847, at the age of nineteen. Among his teachers were Johannes Müller, Schönlein, Virchow, DuBois-Reymond, and Traube—all at the height of their activity and reputation. After his graduation in medicine, von Graefe went to Prague, to work with Arlt; to Paris, where he studied with Desmarres; and to Vienna, where he heard the lectures of Skoda, Oppolzer, Rokitansky, and Hebra, and worked in Friedrich von Jaeger's eye clinic. He then proceeded to England, where he met Bowman and Mackenzie and other outstanding leaders of the British medical profession.

After three "Wanderjahre," Albrecht von Graefe settled in Berlin in 1850 and began the practice of ophthalmology in a very simple and unassuming way. The year he located in Berlin, Helmholtz discovered the ophthalmoscope and von Graefe employed the new instrument constantly in his practice. Two years later, von Graefe became a Privatdozent at the University of Berlin and rapidly achieved an international reputation because of the accuracy of his diagnoses, his skill in operating,, the results of his treatment, and his numerous contributions to medical science. He was a man endowed with remarkable personal charm, with an unusual clarity of perception and expression, and with prodigious energy. Von Graefe died in 1870 at the early age of forty-two.

Von Graefe's greatest achievements were in the field of ophthalmology but his name is remembered by the physician particularly because of his discovery of the "lid lag," or von Graefe's sign, a very important sign in thyrotoxicosis.

THE TRANSACTIONS OF THE BERLIN MEDICAL SOCIETY*
Meeting of March 9, 1864

Chairman: Mr. v. *Graefe;* Secretary: Mr. *Schweigger;* Present as a Guest:

Dr. *Knock* of St. Petersburg

1. Mr. v. *Graefe: Concerning Basedow's Disease.*—As is well known, the protrusion of the eyeball is one of the most important symptoms of Basedow's disease. Indeed, this, with the abnormally rapid heart rate and the strumous swelling of the neck, forms the characteristic symptom complex. In this exophthalmic protrusion, *the pressing forward of the axis* has been emphasized too much and not enough attention has been paid to another symptom, which has value in its earlier phases and mild degrees of illness. This consists in the *disturbed relationship between the movement of the lid and the elevation and sinking of the level of vision.*

When normal individuals elevate or lower their glance, the upper eyelid makes a cor-responding movement. In patients suffering from Basedow's disease, this is entirely abolished or reduced to a minimum. That is, as the cornea looks down, the upper eyelid does not follow. This is not the direct result of the exophthalmos; because in tumors of the orbit and in protrusion from other causes, one sees this symptom often absent, although the movements of the lids are interfered with to a very marked degree. On the other hand, it is present in the slightest degrees of exophthalmos in Basedow's disease, even when the protrusion of the eyeball does not exceed physiological limits. When the protrusion of the eyes is slight and symmetrical in both eyes, it is difficult to say whether it is pathological; it varies also in normal individuals according to the amount of adipose cellular tissue within the orbital fossa. In these slight degrees, this symptom we point out is therefore doubly valuable.

* von Graefe, Albrecht, *Deutsch. Klinik,* 1864, XVI, 158.

Another proof that this symptom is not dependent upon the exophthalmos, consists in the fact that it may disappear in the course of Basedow's disease, either spontaneously or as the result of treatment, while the exophthalmos itself persists. Furthermore, I met with a very remarkable case, where the symptoms suddenly disappeared after an injection of morphine: the lid then sank again without showing evidence of any change in the exophthalmos. Therefore it is obviously to be considered as a peculiar *disturbance in the innervation of muscles of the lid*. It is possible that, as with morphine, certain other substances affecting nervous activity, for example, electricity, might cause the symptom to disappear without any influence upon the exophthalmos.

Concerning the further interpretation of the symptom, I can only present hypotheses. It is probable that, to a certain extent, it has to do with that part of the levator innervated by the sympathetic, which was discovered by *H. Müller,* since that part probably regulates the movement of the lid with the field of vision.

In the practical aspect this symptom should be emphasized, because it helps in the diagnosis of mild degrees of illness which are not so uncommon in the female sex and for whom the therapy is more effective than in the severe cases. The strumous swelling is commonly absent in this mild type. The entire symptom complex is composed of the rapid heart action, without change in the size of the heart or in the heart valves, and this symptom of the eyes. Such a case I present to you here, in order to demonstrate the symptom. The relief which patients experience in their eye symptoms depends entirely upon the fact that when the lid remains behind on looking down, this is very disagreeable and the eye is more exposed when one reads or works.

TETANY

John Clarke

John Clarke, the son of a well known surgeon of the same name, was born at Wellingborough, Northamptonshire in 1761. He was educated at St. Paul's School and at St. George's Hospital London. He settled down to practice in London and became lecturer on obstetrics in the medical school of Dr. William Hunter. He rapidly acquired a large practice and was for many years regarded as the leading obstetrician of London. While at the height of his success, he abruptly gave up the practice of obstetrics, moved to another part of the city and devoted himself to diseases of women and children. His *Commentaries on Some of the Most Important Diseases of Children,* whose completion was prevented by his death, contains what is probably the first account of infantile tetany. John Clarke died in 1815. His younger brother, Sir Charles Mansfield Clarke, was a very distinguished obstetrician.

CHAP. IV

ON A PECULIAR SPECIES OF CONVULSION IN INFANT CHILDREN*

There is one case of convulsive affection, which is more apt to be overlooked than any other, because the symptoms are not at first very violent, so as to attract the attention of parents or nurses. It is often mistaken and treated as some other disease, even by medical men; and the true character of it has been little known, even to practitioners generally conversant with infantile disorders: it is therefore less likely to be detected by those who have bestowed little or no attention upon them.

This convulsive affection occurs by paroxysms, with longer or shorter intervals be-

* Clarke, John, *Commentaries on Some of the Most Important Diseases of Children,* London, Longman, Herst, Rees, Orme and Brown, 1815, pp. 86-90.

tween them, and of longer or shorter duration in different cases, and in the same case at different times.

It consists in a peculiar mode of inspiration, which it is difficult accurately to describe.

The child having had no apparent warning, is suddenly seized with a spasmodic inspiration, consisting of distinct attempts to fill the chest, between each of which a squeaking noise is often made; the eyes stare, and the child is evidently in great distress; the face and extremities, if the paroxysm continues long, become purple, the head is thrown backward, and the spine is often bent, as in opisthotonos; at length a strong expiration takes place, a fit of crying generally succeeds, and the child, evidently much exhausted, often falls asleep.

In one of these attacks a child sometimes, but not frequently, dies.

They usually occur many times in the course of the day, and are often brought on by straining, by exercise, and by fretting, and sometimes they come on from no apparent cause.

They very commonly take place after a full meal, and they often occur immediately upon waking from sleep, though before the time of waking the child had been lying in a most tranquil state. As the breathing is affected by these paroxysms, the complaint is generally referred to the organs of respiration, and it has been sometimes called chronic croup; but it is very different from croup; and is altogether of a convulsive character, arising from the same causes, and is relieved by the same remedies as other convulsive affections.

Accompanying these symptoms, a bending of the toes downwards, clinching of the fists and the insertion of the thumbs into the palm of the hands, and bending the fingers upon them, is sometimes found, not only during the paroxysm, but at other times.

Clenching the fist with the thumb inserted into the palm of the hand, often exists for a long time in children, without being much observed, yet it is always to be considered as an unfavorable symptom, and frequently is a forerunner of convulsive disorders, being itself a spasmodic affection.

It rarely happens that a child recovers from an attack of this sort, unless the progress of the disorder has been interrupted by a timely application of proper remedies, without a general convulsion. Then the friends become alarmed, and a disease, which had existed for two or three months, is for the first time considered to be important enough to require medical assistance, after all the farago of popular medicines, such as fit drops, soot drops, assafoetida, &c. have been ineffectively applied.

Convulsions of this description seldom, if ever, occur after the expiration of the third year of a child's life, and not often in children which have lived by sucking, till they have teeth, and have never taken animal food till the dentes cuspidati have come through the gums; this, however, is liable to some exception.

A long and very attentive consideration of this kind of convulsion, has led the writer to conclude, that in every case of convulsion (be the remote cause whatsoever it may) the brain is at the time organically affected, either directly or indirectly; directly when convulsions arise from phrenitis, hydrocephalus, or on the sudden retiring of cutaneous eruptions, or of inflammation of the mucous membrane of the eyelids and eyes, or when they appear on the accession of some cutaneous disease, attended with febrile symptoms, especially scarlet fever, small-pox, and (sometimes, though less frequently,) of measles: indirectly, as when they are occasioned by an overloaded stomach or by indigestion, by peripneumony, by inflammation, or suppuration in the cavity of the pericardium, by glandular or other humors pressing on the large vessels leading to the lower extremities, or when they take place in the progress of infantile fever, or in marasmus.

GOUT

Thomas Sydenham

5.* Concerning this disease, in its most

* *The Works of Thomas Sydenham*, translated by R. G. Latham, M.D., London, Sydenham Society, 1850, II, p. 124.

regular and typical state, I will first discourse; afterwards I will note its more irregular and uncertain phenomena. These occur when the unseasonable use of preposterous medicines has thrown it down from its original *status*. Also when the weakness and languor of the patient prevent it from rising to its proper and genuine symptoms. As often as gout is regular, it comes on thus. Towards the end of January or the beginning of February, suddenly and without any premonitory feelings, the disease breaks out. Its only forerunner is indigestion and crudity of the stomach, of which the patient labours some weeks before. His body feels swollen, heavy and windy—symptoms which increase until the fit breaks out. This is preceded a few days by torpor and a feeling of flatus along the legs and thighs. Besides this, there is a spasmodic affection, whilst the day before the fit the appetite is unnautrally hearty. The victim goes to bed and sleeps in good health. About two o'clock in the morning he is awakened by a severe pain in the great toe; more rarely in the heel, ankle or instep. This pain is like that of a dislocation, and yet the parts feel as if cold water were poured over them. Then follow chills and shivers, and a little fever. The pain, which was at first moderate, becomes more intense. With its intensity the chills and shivers increase. After a time this comes to its height, accommodating itself to the bones and ligaments of the tarsus and metatarsus. Now it is a violent stretching and tearing of the ligaments—now it is a gnawing pain and now a pressure and tightling. So exquisite and lively meanwhile is the feeling of the part affected, that it cannot bear the weight of the bedclothes nor the jar of a person walking in the room. The night is passed in torture, sleeplessness, turning of the part affected, and perpetual change of posture; the tossing about of the body being as incessant as the pain of the tortured joint, and being worse as the fit comes on. Hence the vain effort, by change of posture, both in the body and the limb affected, to obtain an abatement of the pain. This comes only towards the morning of the next day, such time being necessary for the moderate digestion of the peccant matter. The patient has a sudden and slight respite, which he falsely attributes to the last change of position. A gentle perspiration is succeeded by sleep. He wakes freer from pain, and finds the part recently swollen. Up to this time, the only visible swelling had been that of the veins of the affected joint. Next day (perhaps for the next two or three days), if the genera-

tion of the gouty matter had been abundant, the part affected is painful, getting worse towards evening and better towards morning. A few days after, the other foot swells, and suffers the same pains. The pain in the foot second attacked regulates the pain in the one first attacked. The more it is violent in the one, the more perfect is the abatement of suffering, and the return of strength in the other. Nevertheless, it brings on the same affliction here as it had brought on in the other foot, and that the same in duration and intensity. Sometimes, during the first days of the disease, the peccant matter is so exuberant, that one foot is insufficient for its discharge. It then attacks both, and that with equal violence. Generally, however, it takes the feet in succession. After it has attacked each foot, the fits became irregular, both as to the time of their accession and duration. One thing, however, is constant— the pain increases at night and remits in the morning. Now a series of lesser fits like these constitute a true attack of gout—long or short, according to the age of the patient. To suppose that an attack two or three months in length is all one fit is erroneous. It is rather a series of minor fits. Of these the latter is milder than the former, so that the peccant matter is discharged by degrees, and recovery follows. In strong constitutions, where the previous attacks have been few, a fortnight is the length of an attack. With age and impaired habits gout may last two months. With *very* advanced age, and in constitutions *very* much broken down by previous gout, the disease will hang on till the summer is far advanced. For the first fourteen days the urine is high-coloured, has a red sediment, and is loaded with gravel. Its amount is less than a third of what the patient drinks. During the same period the bowels are confined. Want of appetite, general chills towards evening, heaviness, and a troublesome feeling at the parts affected, attend the fit throughout. As the fit goes off, the foot itches intolerably, most between the toes; the cuticle scales off, and the feet desquamate, as if venomed. The disease being disposed of, the vigour and appetite of the patient return, and this in proportion to the violence of the last fits. In the same proportion the next fit either comes on or keeps off. Where one attack has been sharp, the next will take place that time next year—not earlier.

ADDISON'S DISEASE AND PERNICIOUS ANEMIA
Thomas Addison

Thomas Addison was born of humble parents near Newcastle, about 1793. He graduated at Edinburgh in 1815, where he acquired a reputation as a classical scholar, taking down his lecture notes in Latin. He came to London soon after graduation and first worked with the great dermatologist, Batemen, becoming very skillful in the diagnosis of skin diseases. Later, he became attached to Guy's Hospital, where he was soon recognized as one of the most brilliant members of that very able group of physicians. In 1837, he was selected as the colleague of Richard Bright in the chair of medicine.

Addison was, in person, a great contrast to Bright. Bright was the son of wealthy parents, had had all the advantages of travel and education, and was handsome, cheerful, sociable, and popular in all circles. Addison, on the other hand, was of humble origin, had no independent means, and was compelled to work hard for his livelihood during these early formative years—years which Bright spent at Cambridge, on the Continent, attending lectures at Berlin and Vienna, or travelling in Hungary. Addison lacked Bright's cheer and charm, he was blunt, and had the reputation of being haughty and arrogant. Much of his hauteur, however, was a cloak for his innate shyness. He confessed in after years that he never rose to speak at the students' medical society "without feeling nervous," yet his listeners would depart with the feeling that he had spoken to them in a tone of bluster.

Addison's name has come down to us because of its association with Addison's disease, which was described in a paper which he read before the South London Medical Society in 1849. In his introduction to *The constitutional and local effects of disease of the suprarenal capsules,* he describes a condition far more prevalent and of greater clinical importance than what we now call Addison's disease. This condition is pernicious anemia, also called Addison's anemia or Addison-Biermer anemia.

The following two selections are from Addison's treatise on *Disease of the Suprarenal Capsules,* which appeared in 1855. The third selection which appeared earlier in the book is from a paper entitled, "On a certain affection of the skin; vitilgoidea--α. Plana, β. Tuberosa," which was originally published in 1850 in Guy's Hospital Reports, and contains the first description of xanthoma diabeticorum.

Addison did not marry until he was fifty. Just before the ceremony a storm, unknown to the wedding party, blew part of the church roof upon the altar and the fact was not discovered until they entered the church. "Good God," exclaimed Addison, "is this not ominous"? However, Addison survived his wedding thirteen years, dying in 1860.

One characteristic of Addison should be mentioned: "He has also been known, after seeing a patient within the radius of eight or ten miles, to remember on his near approach to London, thinking over the case on his way, that he had omitted some seemingly important inquiry, and to have posted back some miles for the purpose of satisfying his mind on the doubt which had occurred to it."

ON THE CONSTITUTIONAL AND LOCAL EFFECTS OF DISEASE OF THE
SUPRA-RENAL CAPSULES*

As a preface to my subject, it may not be altogether without interest or unprofitable to give a brief narrative of the circumstances and observations by which I have been led to my present convictions.

For a long period I had from time to time met with a very remarkable form of general anaemia, occurring without any discoverable cause whatever—cases in which there had been no previous loss of blood, no

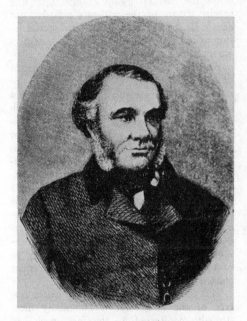

THOMAS ADDISON (1793-1860)

Frontispiece to *A Collection of the Published Writings of Thomas Addison* (London, 1868)

exhausting diarrhoea, no chlorosis, no purpura, no renal, splenic, miasmatic, glandular, strumous, or malignant disease.

Accordingly, in speaking of this form in clinical lecture, I perhaps with little propriety applied to it the term "idiopathic," to distinguish it from cases in which there existed more or less evidence of some of the usual causes or concomitants of the anaemic state.

The disease presented in every instance the same general character, pursued a similar

* *A Collection of the Published Writings of the late Thomas Addison, M.D.,* London, New Sydenham Society, 1868, p. 211.

case last examined, the heart had undergone course, and with scarcely a single exception, was followed, after a variable period, by the same fatal result.

It occurs in both sexes, generally, but not exclusively, beyond the middle period of life, and, so far as I at present know, chiefly in persons of a somewhat large and bulky frame, and with a strongly-marked tendency to the formation of fat.

It makes its approauch in so slow and insidious a manner that the patient can hardly fix a date to his earliest feeling of that languor which is shortly to become so extreme. The countenance gets pale, the whites of the eyes become pearly, the general frame flabby rather than wasted; the pulse, perhaps, large, gut remarkably soft and compressible, and occasionally with a slight jerk. especially under the slightest excitement; there is an increasing indisposition to exertion, with an uncomfortable feeling of faintness or breathlessness on attempting it; the heart is readily made to palpitate; the whole surface of the body presents a blanched, smooth, and waxy appearance; the lips, gums, and tongue seem bloodless; the flabbiness of the solids increases; the appetite fails; extreme languor and faintness supervene, breathlessness and palpitations being produced by the most trifling exertion or emotion; some slight oedema is probably perceived about the ankles; the debility becomes extreme. The patient can no longer rise from his bed, the mind occasionally wanders, he falls into a prostrate and half-torpid state, and at length expires. Nevertheless, to the very last, and after a sickness of, perhaps, several months' duration, the bulkiness of the general frame and the obesity often present a most striking contrast to the failure and exhaustion observable in every other respect.

With perhaps a single exception the disease, in my own experience, resisted all remedial efforts, and sooner or later terminated fatally.

On examining the bodies of such patients after death I have failed to discover any organic lesion that could properly or reasonably be assigned as an adequate cause of such serious consequences; nevertheless, from the disease having uniformly occurred in fat people, I was naturally led to entertain a suspicion that some form of fatty degeneration might have a share, at least, in its production; and I may observe that, in the such a change, and that portion of the semi-lunar ganglion and solar plexus, on being subjected to microscopic examination, was pronounced by Mr. Quekett to have passed into a corresponding condition.

Whether any or all of these morbid changes are essentially concerned—as I believe they are—in giving rise to this very remarkable disease, future observation will probably decide.

The cases having occurred prior to the publication of Dr. Bennett's interesting essay on "Leucocythaemia," it was not determined by microscopic examination whether there did or did not exist an excess of white corpuscles in the blood of such patients.

* * *

The leading and characteristic features of the morbid state to which I would direct attention are, anaemia, general languor and debility, remarkable feebleness of the heart's action, irritability of the stomach, and a peculiar change of colour in the skin, occurring in connection with a diseased condition of the "supra-renal capsules."

As has been observed in other forms of anaemic disease, this singular disorder usually commences in such a manner that the individual has considerable difficulty in assigning the number of weeks, or even months, that have elapsed since he first experienced indications of failing health and strength; the rapidity, however, with which the morbid change takes place varies in different instances.

In some cases that rapidity is very great, a few weeks proving sufficient to break up the powers of the constitution, or even to destroy life, the result, I believe, being determined by the extent, and by the more or less speedy development of the organic lesion.

The patient, in most of the cases I have seen, has been observed gradually to fall off in general health; he becomes languid and weak, indisposed to either bodily or mental exertion; the appetite is impaired or entirely lost; the whites of the eyes become pearly; the pulse small and feeble, or perhaps somewhat large, but excessively soft and compressible; the body wastes, without, however, presenting the dry and shrivelled skin and extreme emaciation usually attendant on

protracted malignant disease; slight pain or uneasiness is from time to time referred to the region of the stomach, and there is occasionally actual vomiting, which in one instance was both urgent and distressing; and it is by no means uncommon for the patient to manifest indications of disturbed cerebral circulation.

Notwithstanding these unequivocal signs of feeble circulation, anaemia and general prostration, neither the most diligent inquiry nor the most careful physical examination tend to throw the slightest gleam of light upon the precise nature of the patient's malady; nor do we succeed in fixing upon any special lesion as the cause of this gradual and extraordinary constitutional change.

We may, indeed, suspect some malignant or strumous disease—we may be led to inquire into the condition of the so-called blood-making organs—but we discover no proof of organic change anywhere—no enlargement of spleen, thyroid, thymus, or lymphatic glands—no evidence of renal disease, of purpura, of previous exhausting diarrhoea, or ague, or any long-continued exposure to miasmatic influences; but with a more or less manifestation of the symptoms already enumerated we discover a most remarkable and, so far as I know, characteristic discoloration taking place in the skin—sufficiently marked, indeed, as generally to have attracted the attention of the patient himself or of the patient's friends.

This discoloration pervades the whole surface of the body, but is commonly most strongly manifested on the face, neck, superior extremities, penis, and scrotom, and in the flexures of the axillae and around the navel.

It may be said to present a dingy or smoky appearance, or various tints or shades of deep amber or chestnut-brown; and in one instance the skin was so universally and so deeply darkened that but for the features the patient might have been mistaken for a mulatto.

In some cases the discoloration occurs in patches, or perhaps rather certain parts are so much darker than others as to impart to the surface a mottled or somewhat chequered appearance; and in one instance there were, in the midst of this dark mottling, certain insular portions of the integument presenting a blanched or morbidly white appearance, either in consequence of these portions having remained altogether unaffected by the disease, and thereby contrasting strongly with the surrounding skin, or, as I believe, from an actual defect of colouring matter in these parts. Indeed, as will appear in the subsequent cases, this irregular distribution of pigment-cells is by no means limited to the integument, but is occasionally also made manifest on some of the internal structures.

We have seen it in the form of small black spots, beneath the peritoneum of the mesentery and omentum—a form which in one instance presented itself on the skin of the abdomen.

This singular discoloration usually increases with the advance of the disease; the anaemia, languor, failure of appetite, and feebleness of the heart, become aggravated; a darkish streak usually appears on the commissure of the lips; the body wastes, but without the emaciation and dry, harsh condition of the surface, so commonly observed in ordinary malignant diseases; the pulse becomes smaller and weaker; and without any special complaint of pain or uneasiness the patient at length gradually sinks and expires.

In one case, which may have been said to have been acute in its development, as well as rapid in its course, and in which both capsules were found universally diseased after death, the mottled or chequered discoloration was very manifest, the anaemic condition strongly marked, and the sickness and vomiting urgent; but the pulse, instead of being small and feeble, as usual, was large, soft, and extremely compressible, and jerking on the slightest exertion or emotion, and the patient speedily died.

My experience, though necessarily limited, leads to the belief that the disease is by no means of very rare occurrence, and that were we better acquainted with its symptoms and progress, we should probably succeed in detecting many cases which in the present state of our knowledge, may be entirely overlooked or misunderstood; and, I think I may with some confidence affirm, that although partial disease of the capsules may give rise to symptoms, and to a condition of the general system extremely equivocal and inconclusive, yet that a more extensive lesion will be found to produce a state which may not only create a suspicion, but be announced with some confidence to arise from the lesion in question. When the lesion is acute and rapid,

I believe the anaemic prostration and peculiar condition of the skin will present a corresponding character, and that whether acute or chronic, provided the lesions involve the entire structure of both organs, death will inevitably be the consequence.

If this statement be correct—and I quite believe it to be so—the chief difficulty that remains to be surmounted by further experience in this, I fear, irremediable disease, is a correct and certain diagnosis—how we may at the earliest possible period detect the existence of this form of anaemia, and how it is to be distinguished from other forms of anaemic disorder.

As I have already observed, the great distinctive mark of this form of anaemia is the singular dingy or dark discoloration of the skin; nevertheless, at a very early period of the disorder, and when the capsules are less extensively diseased, the discoloration may, doubtless, be so slight and equivocal as to render the course of the anaemic condition uncertain.

Our doubts, in such cases, will have reference to the sallow anaemic conditions resulting from miasmatic poisoning or malignant visceral disease; but a searching inquiry into the history of the case, and a careful examination of the several parts or organs usually involved in anaemic disease, will furnish a considerable amount of at least negative evidence; and when we fail to discover any of the other well-known sources of that condition, when the attendant symptoms resemble those enumerated as accompanying disease of the capsules, and when to all this is super-added a dark, dingy, or smoky-looking discoloration of the integument, we shall be justified at least in entertaining a strong suspicion in some instances, a suspicion almost amounting to a certainty in others.

It must, however, be observed, that every tinge of yellow, or mere sallowness, throws a still greater doubt over the true nature of the case, and that the more decidedly the discoloration partakes of the character described, the stronger ought to be our impression as to the capsular origin of the disorder. The morbid appearances discovered after death will be described with the cases in which they occurred; but I may remark that a recent direction (March, 1855) has shown that even malignant disease may exist in both capsules, without giving rise to any marked discoloration of the skin; but in the case alluded to, the deposit in each capsule was exceedingly minute, and could not have seriously interfered with the functions of the organs; extensive and fatal malignant disease had, however, affected other parts.

PAGET'S DISEASE
Sir James Paget

James Paget was born at Yarmouth in 1814, the fifth son of a prosperous brewer and ship owner. At the age of sixteen he was apprenticed to Charles Costerton, an active and prominent surgeon of that city, and at the age of twenty-one, entered St. Bartholomew's Hospital. Two years later he passed the examinations of the College of Surgeons and established himself in London. For many years he taught anatomy and physiology in the College of Surgeons and did not enter private practice until 1851, fifteen years after his graduation.

Paget's rise in his profession was rapid and he tells us that his income soon exceeded £10,000 a year. He enjoyed a very large consulting practice and worked on an average of sixteen hours a day. His consulting practice forced him to travel from 5,000 to 8,000 miles a year. He was created a baronet by Queen Victoria in 1871, and the same year retired from active service at St. Bartholomew's Hospital, which he had served faithfully for twenty-eight years. In 1878 he gave up operating, but for ten years longer he had a very heavy consulting practice. He died in 1899, in his eighty-first year, and his funeral service was held in Westminster Abbey in the presence of an immense throng of mourners.

Paget was admired and worshipped by his patients and trusted by every member of his profession. He had a great capacity for friendships and apart from his hosts of friends in the medical profession, numbered among his close friends Gladstone, Cardinal Newman, Ruskin, Tennyson, Robert Browning, George Eliot, Tyndall, Huxley, Darwin, and Pasteur. He was, during his active career, a very hard worker and found relaxation in books and music. He had a profound knowledge of old Italian music and he had a deep veneration for Bach. A man of deep religious convictions, he never told a story or joke, making jest of sacred words.

Paget's love for brevity was well known to his friends. He never used two words when one was sufficient. Once he was challenged to a sort of contest in brevity, and accepted the challenge. His adversary was a Yorkshireman, who came into his consulting room, and merely thrust out his lips, saying "What's that?" "That's cancer," he answered. "And what's to be done with it?" "Cut it out." "What's your fee?" "Two guineas." "You must make a deal o' money at that rate." And there the consultation ended.

"To be brief" he said, "was to be wise; to be epigrammatic was to be clever." He had a dislike for cleverness and for proverbs. One of his favorite sayings was "as false as most proverbs."

Paget had the rare gift of being able to turn swiftly from work to play and enjoyed his holidays like a schoolboy. He was profoundly indifferent to politics, national or medical, and all his actions were guided by the most scrupulous sense of honor. Richard Owen said of him in 1851 that he had his choice either to be the first physiologist of Europe, or to have the first surgical practice in London, with a baronetcy. One of his sons became the Bishop of Oxford and another was Stephen Paget, the well-known surgeon and writer, author of *Confessio Medici.*

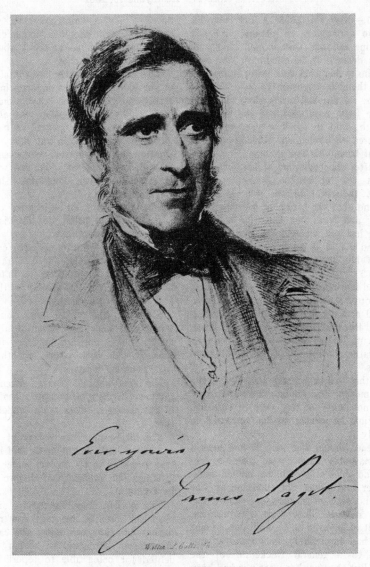

SIR JAMES PAGET (1814-1899)
From a portrait by George Richmond, 1867

On November 14, 1876, he communicated to the Royal Medico-Chirurgical Society his paper *"On a form of chronic inflammation of the bones 'osteitis deformans,' "* since known as Paget's disease. The same name, Paget's disease, is also applied to cancer of the nipple, first described in 1873 by Sir James Paget in the *St. Bartholomew Hospital Reports.*

ADDITIONAL CASES OF OSTEITIS DEFORMANS*

By Sir James Paget, Bart., D.C.L., LL.D., F.R.S., Sergeant Surgeon to
H.M., the Queen, &c.

Received April 17—Read June 13, 1882

CASE 1.—May 29, 1878. A lady aet. 65, having no appearance of general ill-health and looking her age, complained chiefly of what she deemed to be rheumatic and neuralgia pains in her back and lower limbs. She ascribed them to exposure to cold thirteen years ago; for she had rarely since that time been free from pain, and had lost strength and health; and in the last year or more, had suffered with what she considered to be attacks of bronchitis and asthma.

Soon after the beginning of her pain, that is, about ten or twelve years ago, her daughters thought that she was losing in height, and that the shape of her head was changing; and from that time she had been becoming less tall, till now she had lost four inches and a half in height, and stooped so low with her head forward and her chin raised.

She had marks of slight gouty affections in some knotted knuckles, and frequent flatulence and occasional excess of lithic acid in the urine. But she had never had fever, ague, or any acute illness, and had borne five children in rather hard labours, without ill consequences.

Her father had been gouty and died in old age; her mother died young after parturition. She did not know of any case of scrofula, consumption, or cancer having occurred in her family.

Her head, though she said it had always been remarkably large, was certainly enlarged, and chiefly by convex bossed additions over and about the junction of the frontal and sagittal sutures and above the temporal sutures. They were symmetrical, and might be guessed to be additions of one third or half an inch in thickness, perhaps additions to a general thickening of the cranium. But they neither were nor had been associated with headache or any other local trouble, and sight, hearing, and the other senses were unimpaired.

The dorsal spine was curved, inclining a little to the right, without any compensating curve to the left below it. The curve pro-

duced a low stooping posture, with very prominent right shoulder, and might be estimated as shortening the trunk about two or two and a half inches.

The ribs were nearly horizontal, flattened at the sides, and, even in deep inspirations, nearly motionless. The respirations were almost wholly diaphragmatic, with elevation of the sternum. They appeared to be sufficient during quietude, but in any hurry or mental emotion, or any unusual exertion, great distress of breathing was felt, and walking upstairs seemed even dangerous; she was always carried up.

The lumbar spine appeared of natural form, so did the pelvis, and likewise all parts of the upper extremities.

The femora were exceedingly curved outwards and forwards; the left rather more than the right. Their shafts felt in their whole length, especially, I think, in their lower half, large, rounded, thickened.

Similarly the tibiae were curved forwards and were very large in their whole length. Their anterior surfaces felt nearly twice as wide as in nature, smooth, and with large rounded margins.

The feet and all of the articulations of the lower limbs appeared quite healthy. None of the enlarged bones were tender on pressure.

The likeness of the forms of the trunk and lower limbs in this case, and in the first case recorded in my former paper, was very striking. The similarity of disease could not be doubted.

The patient lived two years and a half after this note of her case was made, and during this time was under the care of Dr. Haynes, of Stansted, to whom I am indebted for being able to report that little change ensued in the bones of the lower extremities; that the skull became more deformed, especially with a broad, high boss along the upper middle line; and the spine more curved and prominent in its dorsal part. Death ensued in consequence of Bright's disease and valvular disease of the heart, with extreme anasarka. It did not appear

* Med. Chir. Trans., London, 1882, LXV, 225.

due in any degree to the disease of the bones, unless it were that the difficulty of breathing was aggravated by the deformity of the chest.

There was no indication of cancerous disease of any part.

Examination after death was not allowed.

ACHONDROPLASIA

Samuel Thomas von Soemmerring

Samuel Thomas von Soemmerring was born in 1755 at Thorn, in Poland. His father was a physician who instilled early in him an interest in medicine and frequently took his young son to autopsies. Soemmerring entered the University of Göttingen in 1774 as a student of medicine, finding time also to

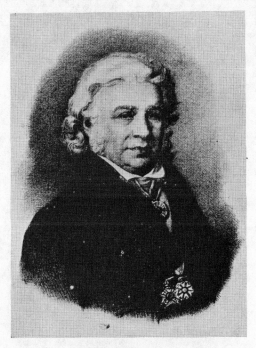

SAMUEL THOMAS VON SOEMMERRING (1755-1830)
A portrait by Thelot

study languages intensively, and to learn the art of engraving. Both of these accomplishments were in later years of great service to him.

Soemmerring as a student began independent research in anatomy and received his degree in 1778, presenting as a thesis a remarkable paper on the cranial nerves, giving a classification which eventually superseded that of Willis. His father had destined him for the practice of medicine but, seeing his scientific bent, furnished him with the means for travel and further study. Soemmerring proceeded to London, where he studied under William and John Hunter; then to Edinburgh, where he worked in anatomy with Munro. On his return to Germany, Soemmerring was appointed a teacher of anatomy in the college at

Kassel. Here he pursued anatomical investigations with great industry and became a friend of the poet Goethe.

In 1784, Soemmerring became professor of anatomy at the University of

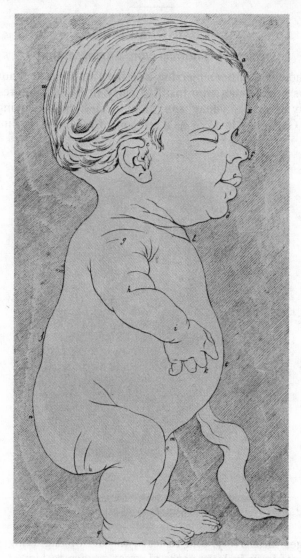

ILLUSTRATION OF ACHONDROPLASIA
From Soemmerring's *Abbildungen und Beschreibungen einiger Misgeburten die sich ehemals auf dem anatomischen Theater zu Cassel befanden* (Mayence, Universitätsbuchhandlung, 1791)

Mayence, holding that position until 1795. During this period, Soemmerring published his anatomical researches on the nervous system, his studies of monsters and his great work on anatomy, which is noteworthy for its accurate, clear pictures, drawn under his direction by Christian Köck. "Soemmerring was

himself a good artist and endowed with an artistic sense for the beautiful."
(Choulant)

From 1795 to 1797 Soemmerring practised medicine in Frankfort and was especially active in spreading the method of vaccination against smallpox recently introduced by Jenner. Soemmerring returned to Mayence in 1797 and resumed his anatomical research, but, five years later, went to Munich. Here he continued his anatomical studies and also became interested in astronomy, paleontology, and physics. In astronomy he made important studies on sun spots and on meteors, in paleontology he studied fossils particularly, and in physics he is remembered by his invention of an electric telegraph, one of the forerunners of the present day instrument. In 1828 he celebrated the fiftieth anniversary of his doctorate and received testimonials of esteem and veneration from the scientific world, a celebration in which his old friend Goethe joined. He died in 1830 at Frankfort.

Among Soemmerring's important discoveries was his description of achondroplasia, which appeared in his *Abbildungen . . . einiger Missgeburten*, published at Mayence in 1791.

ELEVENTH TABLE

Paragraph 76

I add further the picture of a child from the *Kaltschmied* collection, which has a very unusual, peculiar appearance.

It is of the female gender, weighs three pounds, six lothe. It is very fat and round; but the upper and lower extremities are very much too short. The umbilical cord is still fresh.

In order to compare it better with a normal child, I will set down the measurements.

In. Lines

The length from the top of the forehead to the bridge of the nose, or a-b, is	1	10
From the bridge of the nose to the upper lip, or b-c	..	11
From the upper lip to the chin, or c-d	..	9
From the tip of the nose to the ear, or e-f	2	6
The upper arm, or g-h	1	..
The forearm, or h-i	1	..

The hand to the tip of the middle finger, or i-k	1	2½
From the chin to the pubis, or d-m	5	1
From the neck to the pubis, or l-m	4	7
Length of thigh, or n-o	1	11½
Length of the shin bone, or o-p	2	1
Length of the entire foot, or q-r	1	11
Diameter of the thickest part of the abdomen, or s-t	3	2½
Greatest diameter of the head, or u-x	3	9

Paragraph 77

The stripped bone of the forearm, elbow and wrist, I find knotty, misshapen, bent and the substance almost similar to that of a rachitic child, so that this deformity seems to me to be a true bone disease.

Perhaps I could have discovered more if I had been able to examine this child when it was quite fresh.

Is this very remarkable specimen, perhaps, an example of a true so-called congenital English disease (rickets)?

OSTEOMALACIA

Thomas Cadwalader

Thomas Cadwalader was born at Philadelphia in 1708, the son of John Cadwalader, who came to Pennsylvania in 1669 with William Penn. He went to France and England at the age of nineteen to complete his medical education, studying first at Rheims and later going to London, where he spent a year dissecting with William Cheselden, the famous surgeon. After his return to Philadelphia he acquired a large practice in that city and became one of its most influential citizens. He was a friend of Benjamin Franklin, who published Cadwalader's only known publication—*An Essay on the West India*

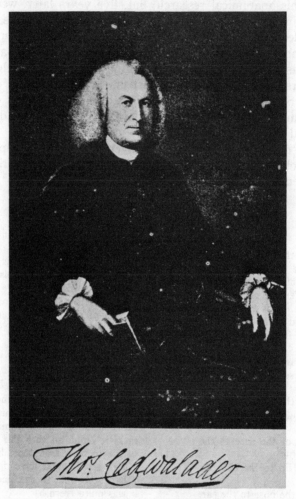

THOMAS CADWALADER (1708-1779)
A portrait by Charles Wilson Peale (1770) in the College
of Physicians, Philadelphia

Dry Gripes, to which is added an extraordinary case in physic. Philadelphia. Printed and sold by Benjamin Franklin MDCCXLV. "The West India Dry Gripes," which was studied especially by William Hillary, was later shown by Sir George Baker to be lead colic, due to the use of rum distilled through leaden pipes, and "the extraordinary case in physic" was the first description of mollities osseum, or osteomalacia.

Dr. Cadwalader was one of the founders of the Pennsylvania Hospital and one of the original members of the Philadelphia Medical Society. He died in Philadelphia in 1779.

AN EXTRAORDINARY CASE IN PHYSICK

The following Account being attended with some very uncommon Circumstances, I thought it would not be improper to make a full Enquiry into the Particulars, of which I was first informed by several Persons of Credit.

The wife of one B. S. who had been a healthy, lively Woman, and the Mother of two Children, was seized, in the Year 1738, with a *Diabetes,* and the usual Symptoms, *viz.* a frequent and copious Discharge by Urine, a gradual Wasting of the Body, a Hectic Fever, with a quick, low Pulse, Thirst, great Pains in her Shoulders, Back and Limbs, and Loss of Appetite. She continued in this Manner two Years, notwithstanding the Use of Medicines usually prescribed in such Cases, but much emaciated. She was then attacked with an *Intermitting Fever,* which soon left her; and after this the *Diabetes* gradually decreased; so that in a few Months she was entirely free from that Disorder; but the Pains in her Limbs still continued. She recovered her Appetite very well, breathed freely, and her *Hectic Fever* was very much lessened, tho' she sometimes had Exacerbations of the same. About the Beginning of Winter, 1740, she had such a Weakness and Pain in her Limbs as to confine her to Bed altogether; and in a few Months afterwards the Bones in her Legs and Arms felt somewhat soft to the Touch, and were so pliable, as to be bent into a Curve; nay, for several Months before her Death, they were as limber as a Rag, and would bend any way with less Difficulty than the muscular Parts of a healthy Person's Leg, without the Interposition of the Bones.

The 12th of *April,* 1742, she died, being then near the Age of Forty; and, having the Consent of her Friends, I had the Curiosity to examine the Body. Upon raising the *Cutis,* I found the *Membrana Adiposa* much thicker than I expected in a Person so much emaciated; the *Sternum* and Ribs, with their Cartilages, very soft; and all the cartilaginous Productions of the *Ribs* on the Left-side doubled over one another, about an Inch long, in this Form Z, but flatter. Upon rais-

ing the *Sternum,* I found the *Lungs* adhering very close to the *Pleura* on each Side, but more loose and flaccid, and much less in Size than usual. Her *Heart* was of the common Bigness, and upon viewing her *Liver,* I found it at least a third Part bigger than ordinary. Her *Spleen* was about an Inch and a Half in the longest Part, and about a Quarter of an Inch thick, and the *Intestines* were very much inflated.

She had Appearances of several *Anchyloses* formed in the small Joynts, *viz. Carpal* and *Metacarpal* Bones, &c. which had been without Motion for several Months; but upon laying them open, I found they were only like a thin Shell. The cartilaginous *Epiphyses* of the Bones were entirely dissolved, and no Part of the Heads remaining, but an Outside, not thicker than an Egg-shell. Upon making incisions in her Legs and Arms of five or six Inches long, I found the outer *Lamina* of the Bones soft, and perfectly membranous, about the Thickness of the *Peritoneum;* and containing (instead of a boney Substance) a Fluid of the Consistence of Honey when thick, and of a reddish Colour, but not at all disagreeable to the Smell. There was, however, an Appearance of Bones near the Joynts of her Legs and Arms, tho' in part dissolved; but what remained was very soft, and full of large Holes, like a Honey-comb. The Bones of the Head yielded easily to the Pressure of my Finger. It may seem surprising, that those Parts of the Bones, which are the most compact and hard, should be dissolved, while their Heads, which are more spongy and soft, had not altogether lost their Substance—She was, when in Health, five Foot high, as I was informed by her Husband; but having measured her after Death, she was no more than three Foot seven Inches in Length, tho' all her Limbs were stretched out strait.

Quaere. Whether a corrosive, *acid* State of the Fluids, might not have been the Cause of this uncommon Dissolution of the Bones? For had it been an *alcaline* Acrimony, I am of Opinion, those Fluids so long extravasated, would have arrived to a great Degree of

Putrefaction, and consequently must have been extremely offensive to the Smell, as is usual in other Cases proceeding from such a Cause.

Supposing, therefore a corrosive, *acid* State of the Fluids, to have been the proximate Cause; *Quaere,* Whether an *alcaline* Regimen, timely pursued, would not have been the most likely Method to have succeeded in this poor Woman's Case?

Henry Thomas

XXIII. A REMARKABLE CASE OF THE SOFTNESS OF THE BONES, BY MR. HENRY THOMAS, SURGEON, TO THE LONDON HOSPITAL. COMMUNICATED BY THOMAS DICKSON, M.D., F.R.S.*

James Stevenson, a shoe-maker in Wapping, aged thirty-three five feet seven inches high, enjoyed a good state of health till about the year 1766, when he was seized with violent pains in his knees and feet, and was tormented with a headache, which came on at irregular periods; these pains he supposed to be rheumatic, and had recourse to a variety of medicines, and to empirical aid, without finding any alleviation whatever of his complaints. In the month of November of the same year, he injured his left shoulder by a fall, which occasioned him considerable pain; and he was unable to move it for several months afterwards.

In November 1768, he slipped down in his shop and fancied he had sprained his right thigh; this injury confined him to his bed about a week; and he was afterwards unable to walk without the support of a person's arm and a crutch-stick. On the twenty-first of December following, as he was endeavouring to go up stairs to bed, supported by his wife, he struck the toe of his right foot upon the edge of the step and instantly cried out that his thigh was broke. He was put to bed, and an apothecary being sent for the next morning, who, paying little attention to the injured thigh, attributed the great pain he suffered to an increase of his rheumatic complaints, gave him medicines accordingly. In this situation he continued upwards for a fortnight, when Dr. Dickson, physician to the London Hospital, was called in. Upon his viewing the thigh so much complained of, he found it crooked and much shorter than the other, and therefore advised a surgeon to be sent for.

I saw him the following day, and on examination, found a fracture of the thigh-bone near its upper extremity. I effected the reduction as well as I could, by means of very little extension and had reason to suppose that the ends of the bone were in due contact, by the limb being of an equal length with the other. It was secured in this position by the usual apparatus; and I was in hopes that his pain would now cease: the event however proved different; his pain continued, though not so violent. This circumstance obliged me frequently to unbind the splints, and to reaccommodate the bandage, judging that either the puckering of the bandage, or tightness of the splints, might occasion in some measure the uneasiness which he felt. About the end of five weeks from the time I had replaced the thigh-bone, desirous of knowing how far the union was completed, I undid the whole apparatus, and requested his wife to lift up the leg, by placing one hand under the m, and the other to embrace the leg above the ancle, whilst I examined the degree of firmness where the fracture had been. In doing this, I was surprised to find the thigh-bone yield and fall in about a hand's-breadth above the knee, similar to that of a fracture, excepting that in this case, there was no sensation of grating, as is usual, where the broken bone is of a solid texture. Upon turning my head about to give his wife directions to lower the leg upon the pillow, I became more astonished, for I found the leg almost doubled in her hands; a similar separation of the *tibia* and *fibula* had taken place about a hand's breadth below the berosity, as had been just before noticed, in the *os femoris*. Both these separations were unaccompanied by any remarkable signs of additional pain to the patient.

Dr. Hunter did me the favour of assisting in the examination of the body. Upon opening the *thorax,* we found the ribs and *sternum* had lost all their solidity, being easily cut through with a common scalpel; the cartilages of the ribs were unaltered; the contents of the *thorax* and *abdomen* ap-

---

* *Med. Obs. & Inq.,* London, 1776, v, p. 259.

peared in a healthy state, and were no otherwise affected than by situation, owing to the deformity of what originally formed the bony supports of the *thorax,* the *spine,* and *pelvis.* The gallbladder however was destitute of bile, greatly contracted and contained a considerable number of very small, black, jagged stones, resembling coal-dust. We next proceeded to examine the state of every bone in the body; the result was, that we could easily pass the knife through those of the *cranium, sternum* ribs, *vertebrae, pelvis,* and

the *epiphyses* it appeared as if this cartilaginous covering was in a manner annihilated, whilst in other parts it appeared prominent and full of bumps. The *epiphyses* were equally compressible and springy to the touch as the *diaphyses* of the same bones; and though there was an apparent diminution of cartilaginous covering, yet it by no means appeared to be abraded, since what remained preserved its pearly colour and smooth polish; and it is remarkable, that though the joints of the lower extremities, in particular,

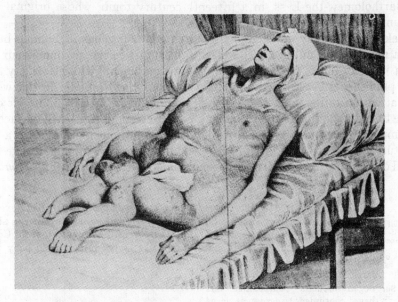

A remarkable case of the softness of the bones by Henry Thomas. From the *Medical Observations and Inquiries.* Vol. v (London, 1776)

all the cylindrical bones which formed the extremities; and the *phalanges* of the fingers were even so much altered, that they were capable of being slit through longitudinally. All these originally bony parts consisted of a mere cortical or outside osseous covering, of the thickness of rind of cheese, and of an inside flesh-coloured mass. The cartilaginous covering of the *epiphyses* of the bones of the extremities appeared to have lost much of their original thickness; in many parts of

had been destitute of motion, above six years, the *sinovia* was perfectly good, and in great quantity.

I have only to add, that the muscular parts in general, but more particularly of the lower extremities, were exceedingly pale, having lost the appearance of flesh; and it would scarcely have been possible to have traced them by dissection, from their contortion and adhesion to each other.

MYOSITIS OSSIFICANS PROGRESSIVA

John Freke

John Freke was born in London in 1688, the son of John Freke, surgeon. He was apprenticed to Mr. Richard Blundell, a well known surgeon of London and in 1726 was elected assistant-surgeon to St. Bartholomew's Hospital. Shortly afterwards he was appointed the first curator of the hospital museum, one of his chief duties consisting in arranging the calculi which were placed on exhibition when the surgeons came to collect their fees for the removal of the stones. Freke married the eldest daughter of his master, Mr. Blundell, and, in 1729, was elected surgeon to St. Bartholomew's Hospital, holding this position until 1755, when gout and infirmity necessitated his resignation. He was elected a Fellow of the Royal Society in 1729 and, in 1736, published in the Philosophical Transactions one of the earliest accounts of myositis ossificans progressiva. He died in 1756 and was buried beside his wife in the Church of St. Bartholomew-the-Less, in a fifteenth-century tomb, whose original owner was unknown.

Freke was not only one of the most prominent surgeons of London but was also a man of wide culture, well versed in natural science, a connoisseur in art and a judge of music. He carried out many experiments with electricity and in 1748 published a very interesting *Essay on the Art of Healing*. In this work he calls attention to the danger of infected lymph glands in operations for cancer of the breast and advises their removal. He also recommends early paracentesis for empyema, his method being to divide the skin and muscles with a knife, puncture the pleura with his fingers and then insert a cannula. Freke was a friend of Fielding, the novelist, and is mentioned twice in the latter's *Tom Jones*.

A Case of extraordinary Exostoses on the Back of a Boy, by Mr. John Freke, F.R.S. Surgeon to St. Barth. Hosp. No. 456. p. 369. Jan. &c. 1740

IV. April 14, 1736, there came a Boy of a healthy Look and about 14 Years of Age, to ask of us at the Hospital, what should be done to cure him of many large Swellings on his Back, which began about 3 Years since, and have continued to grow as large on many Parts as a Penny-loaf, particularly on the left Side: They arise from all the *vertebre* of the Neck, and reach down to the *Os sacrum;* they likewise arise from every Rib of his Body, and joining together in all Parts of his Back, as the Ramifications of Coral do. they make, as it were, a fixed bony Pair of Bodice.

HEBERDEN'S NODES

William Heberden

DIGITORUM NODI

What are those little hard knobs, about the size of a small pea, which are frequently seen upon the fingers, particularly a little below the top, near the joint? They have no connexion with the gout, being found in persons who never had it; they continue for life; and being hardly ever attended with pain, or disposed to become sores, are rather unsightly than inconvenient, though they must be some little hindrance to the free use of the fingers.*

* Heberden, William, *Commentaries on the History and Cure of Diseases,* Boston, Wells and Lilly, 1818, p. 119.

ACROMEGALY
Pierre Marie

Pierre Marie, one of the greatest of modern neurologists, was born in Paris in 1853. He was externe of the hospitals of Paris in 1876 and from 1878 to

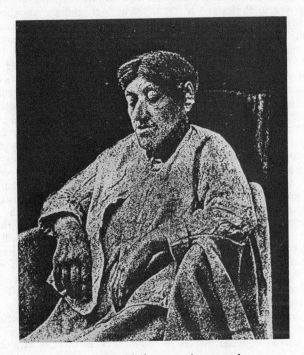

Picture of Marie's first case of acromegaly

1881 was interne, serving his last year under Bonchard. In 1883 he graduated in medicine and became the chief of Charcot's clinic at the Salpetrière and in 1889 became associate professor. Later he became the chief of a service at the Bicêtre and in 1906 was elected to the chair of pathologic anatomy, which had been previously occupied by Charot.

In 1886 he described with Charcot the form of progressive muscular atrophy since known as "atrophy of the Charcot-Marie type." In 1886 he described acromegaly, pointing out the pituitary lesion. This was not, however, the first description of acromegaly. Vicenzo Brigidi in 1877 described a case of acromegaly with autopsy in which a marked enlargement of the pituitary gland was found. Fritsche and Klebs in 1884 reported in great detail a classic case of acromegaly, and also emphasized the marked enlargement of the pituitary found at autopsy. Marie also made three other original descriptions of disease entities: hypertrophic pulmonary osteo-arthropathy, hereditary cerebellar ataxia, and rhizomelic spondylosis. One of his most important recent investigations is that upon aphasia in which he attacked the classical concept of Broca and asserts that the third left frontal convolution plays no special rôle in the function of speech. His conclusions have been confirmed by many neurologists. Pierre Marie died in 1940.

TWO CASES OF ACROMEGALY*

The two cases which are the subject of this article were observed in Professor Charcot's clinic. They present a disease which has not yet been separately described in all its features. Yet it seems to possess a special morbid entity, for among all the patients are found the same symptoms, and characters. Whether this disease is very rare, it is difficult to say, as so little has hitherto been known concerning it. We have simultaneously observed two cases, but though we have made extensive literary researches, we have been able to find on record only a very small number of examples of it.

Case I. Fusch, a woman, aged 37 single.— There was no family history of rheumatism or nervous disease. Her mother and father had died of chest disease; the rest of her relatives were healthy. The patient herself had always been strong and healthy, and had never had rheumatism or syphilis. At the age of twenty-four, following great fatigue and exposure in washing a house, her menstruation suddenly ceased. Fifteen days afterwards she took to her bed, with shivering, general weakness, and trembling in all her limbs. At the end of four or five days her menses reappeared. She remained in bed three weeks; there was no pain in the joints, but she noticed, on raising herself, a weakness of the left hand, with tingling sensations in it. At the end of some weeks the strength returned to a great extent in this hand, though not completely. From this time she went for three months without menstruating.

Having again been exposed to draughts, she was seized with headaches, and pain in the back and arms. There was no redness or swelling of the joints. She was not laid up, but noticed that there were grating sensations in the shoulders and knees. She took sitz baths and the menses reappeared, but have since not returned. She experienced a sensation of sinking at the pit of the stomach, which seemed to be empty a quarter of an hour after food, when she had a fresh desire to eat. She was treated by a doctor for

* Pierre Marie, translated by Proctor S. Hutchinson, M.R.C.S., London, New Sydenham Society, 1891

anaemia. After resting for a time, her strength came back, and she was able to recommence work, but was not so strong as formerly. She had now for seven years lived in the country and done very heavy work. In 1880 she came to Paris, being then aged thirty, and remained in a somewhat more satisfactory condition till the commencement of 1883. After this she was troubled with violent pains, sometimes over the forehead, the parietal eminences, or the temples. These pains often prevented sleep, and they had been worse lately. The patient had always had somewhat large limbs, but nothing compared to their present size. It was at the age of twenty-four, at the time the menstruation suddenly ceased, that she noticed the sudden increase in her hands. Her face at this time also underwent changes, which will be referred to later, so that when the patient returned home none of her relatives could recognize her.

Present condition. The whole feet are large, including the toes. Though the latter are increased in size, they have preserved their form, there is no true deformity, their appearance is simply that of a very big person. The nails, skin &c., show no change. The tibia is not increased in size, but there is a marked projection at the inner side of the knee, which, as there is no effusion into the joint, is due either to thickening of the patella or of the inner condyle of the femur. There is grating felt on moving the kneejoint, but not so marked as in dry arthritis, and due possibly to friction of the fibrous tissues. All the movements of the leg and foot are normal. The chest shows nothing peculiar, beyond a marked posterior curve in the dorsal region. This, though not angular, is distinctly marked. The hands are very large, but of regular form; their thickness and width are relatively greater than their length, and attention is at once attracted to them on seeing the patient. The joints of the fingers are not specially enlarged in proportion to the bones, which have certainly shared in the hypertrophy; the fingers present a somewhat flattened appearance. The width of the nails is increased. There is apparent atrophy of the interosseous muscles, which, according to the account of the patient, took place early in the disease. Movements of the fingers are well performed. On making passive movements of the shoulder-joint, very marked grating is felt. The muscular movements of the left arm and neck seem weaker than normal. The thyroid cartilage seems increased in size, but the thyroid gland is found with difficulty, and is probably less developed than normal. The tongue is enlarged. The patient is a little deaf, and the sight is also slightly defective. There are two symmetrical depressions in the parietal bones, that on the left side being less marked then on the right; it being over the latter that the patient complains of intense persistent pain. Briefly, the face presents the appearance of a lengthened ellipse, with the diameter from above downwards. The centre of this ellipse is situated on a level with the bridge of the nose, and its greatest diameter is opposite the malar prominences. The cranial vertex is of nearly the same size as the end of the chin. The lower jaw is well developed. The complexion is pale and the eyelids a little pigmented. The patient's thirst is intense, obliging her to beg tea of her friends in order to satisfy it. The quantity of urine is excessive; but no measurement of the amount has been made, and no record of analysis kept beyond the fact of there being no sugar.

FRÖHLICH'S DISEASE

Alfred Fröhlich

Alfred Fröhlich was born in 1871 in Vienna and received his M.D. from the University of Vienna in 1895. He became, after graduation, an assistant of von Basch, then worked with Frankl-Hochwart, and in 1905 became assistant of Hans Horst Meyer in the Pharmacological Institute of the University of Vienna. In 1923 he was raised to the rank of full professor. In 1901 he described dystrophia adiposogenitalis, since known as Fröhlich's disease.

A CASE OF TUMOR OF THE HYPOPHYSIS CEREBRI WITHOUT AGROMEGALY*

By Dr. Alfred Fröhlich

Gentlemen: I am taking the liberty of demonstrating a case, which I have had the opportunity of observing in the out patient department of Professor V. Frankl-Hochwart attached to the clinic of Hofrat Northnagel.

R. D., a boy of 14 years, has been under our observation since November 1899. At that time the mother stated that twice a week, sometimes at intervals of 14 days, he came home from school with a headache. He had to go to bed: two hours later vomiting, sometimes vomiting as soon as he came home. This condition has been present since April 1899. Headache on the left side, sometimes on both sides, mostly in the anterior portion of the head. He learns well, good memory, no signs of nervousness or hysteria. No former diseases, no previous trauma. Vision good. Otherwise no subjective complaints.

* *Wien klin. Rundschau*, 1901, xv, 883.

No bladder or colon disturbances. Objectively no pathological findings made out. In the history the status is described as good. Fundus normal. The eye-grounds, the mother states, were examined at that time by Professor *Königstern* and found normal. We considered the condition, because of the negative findings migraine and gave the appropriate therapeutic advice. Then we lost sight of the patient.

On the 19th of August he appeared again, this time with a series of grave symptoms. The mother relates the following: Since March 1899 the patient who was then a thin child, began to increase rapidly in weight. In January 1901, he complained of loss of vision in the left eye, but no further attention was paid to this. In July 1901 the headaches began to reappear and later increased in intensity. At the same time he complained of exhaustion. Frequently vomiting, especially after meals. Further diminution in vision in the left eye, then blindness in the left eye. Later vision in the right eye diminished.

On the 23rd of September 1901, I made the following findings: Subjective improvement for several weeks. Less headache, no dizziness. For ten days no vomiting body weight decreases 5½ kg. against 54 kg. in May 1901. Appetite and sleep good. Objectively; intelligence and speech quite normal. Head

left pupil does not react to light, but well to accommodation. Right pupil reacts promptly to light and accommodation. Eye-balls freely movable, no nystagmus, *Fundus: genuine atrophy of the left optic nerve; right normal. Left amaurosis, right 5/20* (glasses do not improve) *right temporal hemianopsis.* The visual fields of the right eye are normal in the nasal half. The nasal portion which sees is sharply separated from the blind temporal

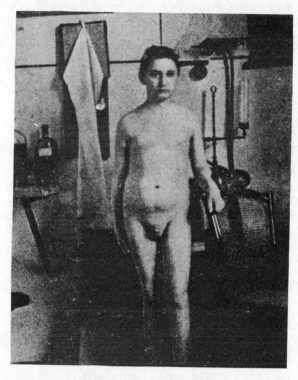

The patient in Fröhlich's article on *A Case of Tumor of the Hypophysis Cerebri without Acromegaly.* From the *Wiener Klinische Rundschau,* 1901

movements free. The left temporal fossa and *only this* painful on percussion.

No disturbances of the taste, of smell or of sensation in the face. Hearing normal. The remaining cerebral nerves normal. Motility and sensation in the extremities and on the trunk quite normal. The tendon reflexes namely the knee reflexes active. No foot clonus, no *Romberg* phenomenon. Sphincters negative. Internal organs normal. Urine free from sugar and albumin.

Ophthalmoscopic examination (Docent Dr. Kuln).—Pupils circa 4 mm. wide, equal. The

portion by a nearly vertical line of separation, which runs from the periphery to the center, surrounding it in a kind of circle. The left optic papilla is snow-white, but sharply outlined; no changes in the vessels.

In regard to the improvement during the last few weeks as well as the loss of weight, it should be mentioned that the patient has been treated with thyroid tablets since September 9.

The significance of these symptoms causes no great difficulty. All point to a process localized at the base of the skull in the optic chiasm. The onset with headache and vomiting, the long course all point to a gradually increasing encroaching process; the irregular affection of both eyes (atrophy of the left optic nerve with loss of pupillary reflexes, right temporal hemianopsis, diminution of vision in the right eye) makes certain the supposition of a new growth of the hypophysis, or to be more exact in the region of the hypophysis. . . .

* * *

Also in this case under our observation, everything points to the assumption of an encroaching process at the base of the skull in the neighborhood of the chiasms. Since however, as already mentioned, there are no signs of acromegaly, we must be content with a purely topical diagnosis. I wish however to make the attempt to proceed beyond this, and to localize the disease in a definite organ, and will therefore examine more closely the symptoms, which appear important to me. In the first place I wish to stress the *obesity* in the body of our patient.

We have an individual who is well developed and apparently well nourished. The weight of this fourteen year old boy in August of this year was 54 kg: The average weight of a boy of the same height is 39.40 kg. We must emphasize, that the first signs of this illness were vomiting and headache 2½ years ago, and that *after* the onset of these symptoms, the patient, who until that time was thin, began to rapidly gain weight. He weighs now 51 kg. He has lost 3 kilograms since the institution of thyroid therapy three weeks ago. However he still presents the picture of a well nourished boy. The fingers are thick, with *exception of the terminal phalanges*, the hands are plump. The osseous system is not involved in this increase in size. The most marked collections of fat are in the skin of the trunk especially the abdomen and in the region of the genitalia. There the masses of fat are so marked that they bulge out around the genitalia. The penis, which is otherwise normally developed, is so hidden between these masses of fat that the genitalia approach the feminine type. The testicles are palpable in the masses of fat and are infantile. There are collections of fat in the region of the nipples. There are some nodules in the breasts, no fluid can be expressed. There are no hairs in the axillae, there are only a few hairs on the genitalia.

The hairs on the skull are brittle, short scanty and since the onset of this illness continually falling out.

As a characteristic of the skin should be added that it is dry and somewhat harsh. In many places, especially on the trunk it can be lifted in thick folds with the fat underneath. In other places especially on the fingers and wrists, palpation gives the impression that the skin is increased in thickness.

* * *

From what has been described we can conclude that *with symptoms, which point to a tumor in the neighborhood of the brain stem, with the absence of acromegalic symptoms, the presence of other trophic symptoms, such as rapidly developing obesity or skin changes suggesting myxedema, points to the hypophysis as the point of origin of the tumor.*

PERSISTENT THYMUS

Felix Platter

OBSERVATION IV

SUFFOCATION FROM AN INTERNAL CONCEALED STRUMA

AROUND THE THROAT*

The son of Marcus Peresius, five months old, healthy appearance, no other preceding affection, suddenly with stridor and difficulty of respiration, is taken from our midst: from which manner of death he had already before lost two sons, desiring to know the cause, he himself requesting it, we lay bare the chest.

In the region of the throat we discover the gland in that place to have grown into quite

*Bonetus, Theophilus, *Sepulchretum*, Geneva, Cramer and Perachon, 1700, Vol. I, p. 577.

a large struma, one part with the half hanging down, spongy, filled with blood-vessels and only by the aid of membranes it adhered to the great vessels, it is filled up with material like flesh and blood. which rushing suddenly in and dilating the gland so much that it presses upon the vessels in this spot, we judge the infant to have been suffocated.

F. Platerus *Observ.* lib. 1, pag. 184.

The gland in that place, we understand as thymus, concerning which see Warthon *Adenographiae* Chapter xvi. To it he assigns four classes of vessels, arteries, veins, nerves and lymphatics, which he saw running through this organ in great numbers. According to this same authority, the function of the glands of all the body is to transport the lymph, unless this function is carried out, the lymph thickens and the gland is elevated into a tumor, by this hard mass, the trachea is compressed. This happens more easily in infants, in whom this gland is much larger than in adults. In the case cited, he ascribes the increased size to blood brought through the arteries.

III. LEAD POISONING

Lead poisoning has the most interesting history of all diseases due to chemical agents. Nikander, the Greek poet-physician, was obviously quite aware of the deleterious effects of lead, and Paul of Aegina wrote the first clear description of epidemic colic followed by paralysis. Citois, nearly one thousand years later, described the same disease as *colica Pictonum* but did not suspect its

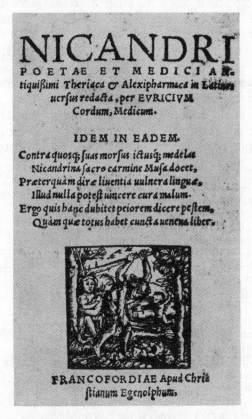

Title-page of Nikander's *Theriaca and Alexipharmaca*. From the translation by Euricius Cordus (Frankfort, 1532)

cause. Huxham's account of the Devonshire colic called attention to the prevalence of this disease in England and ascribed it to the presence of tartar in the crude cider. Tronchin clearly recognized that the colica Pictonum of Amsterdam was due to drinking water impregnated with lead, but he made the error of attributing this colic to other causes as well. It was Baker who first clearly proved, by clinical observation and by experiment, that colica Pictonum and Devonshire colic were the same disease and due to poisoning with lead. His

Essay remains a model of careful experimentation and of accurate deduction. Burton's discovery of the lead line was epochal since it pointed out a pathognomonic sign in this disease, which has been of immense value in its diagnosis.

Nikander

Nikander (or Nicander), Greek poet, physician, and grammarian, was born at Claros near Colophon in the second century before Christ. His family held the hereditary priesthood of Apollo at Colophon. Nikander wrote several poems, two of which are preserved; the longer *Theriaca,* describing the nature of venomous animals and their bites, the other *Alexipharmaca,* treating of poisons and their antidotes. Nikander was praised by Cicero, imitated by Ovid, and held in great esteem by Pliny. Plutarch, however, remarked that his verses had nothing poetical about them except the meter and that their style was bombastic and obscure.

Nikander's *Theriaca* and *Alexipharmaca* were translated into Latin by Euricius Cordus in 1532 and by Joannes Gorraeus in 1549. A French translation by the French poet, Jacques Grévin, was published in 1567. The following translation is from the Latin version of Euricius Cordus and gives a vivid picture of lead poisoning with its colic, paralysis, and ocular disturbances.

> The harmful cerussa, that most noxious thing
> Which foams like the milk in the earliest spring
> With rough force it falls and the pail beneath fills
> This fluid astringes and causes grave ills.
> The mouth it inflames and makes cold from within
> The gums dry and wrinkled, are parch'd like the skin
> The rough tongue feels harsher, the neck muscles grip
> He soon cannot swallow, foam runs from his lip
> A feeble cough tries, it in vain to expel
> He belches so much, and his belly does swell
> His sluggish eyes sway then he totters to bed
> Complains that so dizzy and heavy his head
> Phantastic forms flit now in front of his eyes
> While deep from his breast there soon issue sad cries
> Meanwhile there comes a stuporous chill
> His feeble limbs droop and all motion is still
> His strength is now spent and unless one soon aids
> The sick man descends to the Stygian shades.

Paul of Aegina

Paul of Aegina (629-690) was the most important Greek physician of the seventh century. Very little is known of his life except that he lived for a time at Alexandria and probably taught in the medical school there. He apparently enjoyed a great reputation during his lifetime and for several generations later. His works, which were mainly compilations, were early translated into Arabic and he is frequently quoted by Rhazes and other Arabian physicians.

Paul seems to have been a skillful surgeon and describes lithotomy, trephining and tonsillotomy, paracentesis, and amputation of the breast. His description of an epidemic of colic terminating in paralysis is the earliest known description of the clinical picture of lead colic.

The first Greek edition of his works was printed at Venice in 1528. Numerous Latin translations soon followed. The following translation was made from the Latin version of Johannes Guinterius von Andernach, published in Venice in 1542.

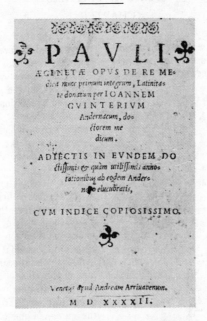

Title-page from the Latin version of Paul of Aegina's works by Johannes Guinterius von Andernach (Venice, 1542)

I consider moreover a colicky affection, which still becomes violent from a kind of collection of humors, which took its origin from regions in Italy, moreover in many other places in Roman territory whence it spread like the contagion of a pestilential plague. Wherefore in many cases it passed into epilepsy, to some there came loss of motion, with sensation unhurt, to many both, and of those who fell victims to the epilepsy, very many died. Of those indeed who were paralised, not a few recovered; for the cause which attacked them ended by crisis.*

* Paul of Aegina, *Opus de re medica. Liber tertius,* Venice, Arrivabenum, 1542, Cap. XLIII, p. 120b.

François Citois

François Citois was born at Poitiers in 1572 and received his doctor's degree at Montpellier in 1596. He practised medicine for a time in his native city but later removed to Paris, where he became personal physician to Cardinal Richelieu. His description of a maiden in Poitiers who lived for two years without taking any food, aroused a lively discussion in the medical profession.

In 1616 he published his well-known account of Poitiers colic or "colica

Pictonum," without, however, suspecting its cause. Citois returned late in life to Poitiers, where he became Dean of the Medical Faculty. He died in 1652.

The following extract is translated from Citois' *De novo et populari apud Pictones dolore colico bilioso, diatribe,* Poitiers, 1616.

A DISCUSSION OF THE NEW AND COMMON PAINFUL BILIOUS COLIC AT POITIERS*

CHAPTER I

Giants cause, when they attack with the weapons of the Gods, new and varied monsters of animals to be born throughout the entire earth. In almost the same manner at

Title-page of *De novo et populari apud Pictones dolore Colico bilioso Diatriba* by François Citois (Poitiers, 1616)

the end of the century it seized, with great audacity and daring rashness, the Princes of all Europe as well as everyone else, it was a judgment from God and his religion, (although it is certainly other than engaging in combat with God). He protected the country from wars and rebellion and he concealed this fault by a name and besides the Chris-

tian of the entire earth was afflicted with various and before now unknown kinds of diseases, I should not say monstrous.

First Lues venera appeared, the scourge of prostitutes, in the year 1494, and originating from the expedition to Naples, then throughout all Europe it spread to certain regions thereof, from which it received the name of disease now of the French, now of the Spaniards, now of the Parthenopians or the Neapolitans. . . .

Some time later, about the year 1529, which because it first invaded greater Britain, they called the English sweating sickness, many thousands of people it destroyed with so powerful poison within twenty-four hours. with prodigious fatal sweating.

A little later scurvy arose which first attacked the Danes, Norwegians and Lithuanians: now in nearly all places the sailors and navigators were attacked with rottenness of the gums, falling of the teeth, with virulent ulcers of the throat, foetid breath, with swelling of the whole body, at first of the legs and feet and livid spots on the skin which degenerated most destructively into malignant ulcers.

Most recently about the year one thousand five hundred sixty or seventy, that Plica Polonorum appeared described repeatedly by Hercules Saxonia, which blemished with its embrace and horrid tangle of hair the heads of men and women, so that it appeared like the Gorgon's head, full of lice and pus, which they neither dare cut off with scissors nor disentangle with a comb. . . .

At about the same time, or at least about the year one thousand five hundred and seventy two, with that new constellation Cassiopeia, not without the secret judgment of God, indeed observed with great admiration by all Astrologers: a new painful Colic appeared called Bilious from the most severe pains due to the bile so it is believed, and it still rages. Those whose bodies it attacks,

---

* Citois, François, *De novo et populari apud Pictones dolore Colico Bilioso Diatriba* (Poitiers, Mesnier, 1616, pi.

sink down as if struck, suddenly he changes his posture, a pallor spreads over his face, his extremities shiver, his strength languishes, his mind is disturbed, his body is troubled, constant wakefulness, fainting spells, or severe frequent stomach pains, loss of appetite, perpetual nausea, eructation, vomiting, the latter with green bile like leeks, which if it continues a most severe hiccoughing vexes the miserable sick man, an insatiable thirst, a troublesome painful urination, and more often this resembles the pain of a stone.

Their abdomens are inflamed, however without fever, more often with a slow fever, and what is most of the whole trouble, the most acute pain of the stomach, the intestines, the loins, the flanks and the groins: meanwhile in these parts once and again, it causes a very violent change: often especially in the beginning, frequent stools but not in abundant amounts, more frequently constipation with it. Soon the poison spreading itself, or at least the acrid vapor arising from the morbid material plagues, bites and nips as if with darts the arms, breasts and entire chest. Indeed in this way the thighs and os sacrum. Nor do they fail to have most severe pains in the soles of the feet, with motion unimpaired, pains in the abdomen follow and again become more severe. And after so much suffering, remarkable to relate, the patient now believing things to be going better with him, for indeed the abdominal pains in some way easing, he feels his arms and feet to be relaxed, and he stirs up that material which scattered through all his joints, he then feels his strength broken.

The motion of his elbows and hands, legs and feet is lost, sensation however is intact, but as if there were needles pricking the skin everywhere. And in many several epileptic convulsions preceded this paralysis, which sometimes carried off many, at other times few. Those attacked showed blindness for many hours, yet with a clear mind: after moreover this persists alone, and lasts for seven days or thereabouts, with no other function of the senses interfered with except vision: and then there are either no pains or they are mild and are gradually relieved, if the cause is subdued by timely and opportune remedies. In others the pain increases and epilepsy recurs with great danger to the patient.

Those indeed who survive so many and so great misfortunes, as the result of diligent treatment, are for a long time confined to their beds and the men affected recover little by little from the paralysis of all their parts below the head, and after several months with the strength restored now to their joints, they are seen moving about through the hamlets crooked and hanging down from their own weight, they can be moved only with great effort to the mouth or upper parts of the body and not down to the feet but only to the muscles of the thighs. Their gait is ridiculous rather than provoking pity, their voice noisy and rattling. Neither does the same accident happen to all, for the forms of this Monster are varied and changing, nor is there lacking any reason for it, for those who invoke at the proper time the beneficial power of a Protecting Panacea, prescribe proper remedies for the causes of the severe pains as well as for the symptoms themselves, now in the first place the pain increases with the use of purgatives, but after alternating first a course of cathartics then of anodynes, it becomes milder as well as lighter.

John Huxham

JOHN HUXHAM
TO
THE MOST EXCELLENT
DOCTOR JAMES JURIN,
Fellow of the ROYAL COLLEGE
OF
PHYSICIANS
AND OF
The ROYAL SOCIETY

SIR.

As it was owing to your particular Exhortation that I entered upon making these meteorological Observations, which I have now finished, the Public is chiefly indebted to you for any Benefit it may receive from them—From a grateful Remembrance of the many Favours I have received from you, I dedicate this little Piece to you.—Wishing you long Health and much Happiness, I am
&c &c
J. HUXHAM

November 13th
1738.

* * *

ON THE DEVONSHIRE COLIC*

On the Beginning of Autumn, 1724, a Disorder exceedingly empidemical spread itself over the Country of *Devon*, amongst the Populace especially, and those who were not very elegant and careful in their Diet. Perhaps it will not be unuseful to give a History of the Disease, and the Method of treating it, because, though it may not range with the same degree of Violence, and affect a vastly less Number of People, yet, it infests this Country more or less almost every Autumn.

This Disease began its Attack by an excessively tormenting Pain in the Stomach, and epigastric Region, with an unequal, weak Pulse, and coldish Sweats; the Tongue in the mean Time was coated with greenish or brown, Mucus, and the Breath was most offensive. An enormous Vomiting soon followed, for the most Part of exceeding green Bile, sometimes black with a great Quantity of Phlegm excessively acid and very tough; nay the foul matter brought up was oftentimes so very acrid, that, by excoriating the Throat and Oesophagus, it was tinted with Blood and created a Difficulty and Pain in Swallowing—Things continuing in this State for a day or two, the Belly became extremely bound, neither answering to the most drastic Purges or sharpest Clysters, the latter coming off without Wind or Stool, the former being soon vomited. The Vomiting abating somewhat, the Pain descended, and most grievously tortured the umbilical Region, and Small of the Back, so that you would have thought the Patient actually laboured under a nephritic Paroxysm, and the rather as a Suppression of the Urine now also comes on, and yet a perpetual Desire of that Discharge is urgent; nay very frequently there is a most troublesome Sense of a Weight in Perinaeo, as if from an incumbent Stone.— Such a Difficulty of Urine in colical Disorders *Aretæus Cappadox*, of old, hath noted *Capit. de Colic.* And *Hippocrates* in the first *Book of Epidemics*, Sect. 2d.

The Urine was high-coloured and resembled a Lixivium, depositing a large Quantity of mucous, red and sometimes a greenish Kind of Sediment—The Abdomen was for the most Part very hard, and exceedingly tense, inso-

much that the Sick were very anxious lest it should burst; on the contrary, in some, it was so greatly contracted by Spasms that there was Scarce any Belly to be observed; This however did not so very often happen as the tense swoln Belly—There was frequently a violent, fixed, burning Pain in the right Hypochondrium, where was also both Hardness and Swelling. In the Region of the Epigastrium there was often felt a great and troublesome Pulsation: Whenever Nature of her own Accord (which was very seldom) discharged any Thing from the Guts, or when solicited, or forced by Medicine, it was always in the Form of exceeding hard, small Balls, of a greenish black Colour resembling Sheep's Dung: After two or three such Stools what was brought off was somewhat softer, but green, or black and some times tinged with Blood, which created a very troublesome Tenesmus: But the Belly was soon shut up, and if purged again, though but at the Interval of a few Hours, again discharges such small and exceedingly hard Globules.

Thus was the first Stage of the Disease; but the Tragedy was not yet over, nor this the End of the Calamity, for though the terrible Griping and Pain of the Belly might have ceased a little, (an extream Tenderness of the Skin, scarce bearing the least Touch, however remaining) a most excruciating Pain now seized the whole spine of the Back, most violent between the Shoulder-Blades; then soon affecting the Arms it fixed chiefly in the Articulations, and altogether destroyed the Motion of the Hands—nor were the Legs and Thighs much less tormented, for a very sharp Pain affected them, fixed in the very Bones as it were, and resembling those of the Lues Venerea, and yet there was seldom any Redness, or swelling of the Parts.

Whilst the morbid Matter was passing from the intestines to the Limbs the Pulse beat stronger, and the Sick had feverish Heats; nay some in this State of the Disorder grew delirious, which was a Kind of limpid Urine certainly and constantly indicated; And indeed it was very remarkable, that if the Sick rendered pale Urine without a Sediment, at any Time of the Disease, they were suddenly seized either with Convulsions, or a Delirium, or a Palsy of the Hands, sometimes with, and sometimes without Pain.

When the Malady had fallen on the Limbs,

* Huxham, John, *Observations on the Air and Epidemic Diseases together with a Short Dissertation on the Devonshire Colic,* London, Henton, 1759, p. 5.

a large foetid, sour-smelling migrated the Pains, and if any Griping in the Belly remained, upon the Coming on of the Sweat it vanished. Some, dissolved as it were in a long and very profuse Sweat, totally lost the Use of their Hands, the Power of Feeling only remaining; Palsy for Pain, a miserable Exchange. However I scarce knew any one, that laboured under this Disease, seized with a Palsy in his legs—Sometimes a great many red itching Pustules, and often very burning and smarting, broke out with the Sweat all over the Body, which was of very happen Omen, as on this the rheumatic and colical Pains soon vanished.—This indeed was the most favourable issue of the Disease, but much more commonly the Rheumatism succeeded the Colic, the Colic the Rheumatism, and thus alternately tormented the miserable Patients, the Disease now being translated to the Limbs, now the Bowels.

Sometimes the tormenting Pains would cease for a few Days, and then return with equal Vehemence, especially on taking the least Cold, or drinking Beer, or Cyder—The Appearance of a Jaundice sometimes took off the Colic for a Time, but as soon as that went off the Colic immediately returned—In one, or two Cases, however, a permanent Icterus absolutely carried off the Disease, some Pains only remaining in the Limbs.

Although the colical Pains most commonly preceded the Rheumatic, yet frequently the Disease affected the Limbs first, and then by a Metastasis of the morbific matter, the Stomach and Intestines in the Manner described—I knew a certain Inn-Keeper attacked in a truly surprising Manner, for he almost intirely lost the Use of his Hands and Arms, though before a strong Man, antecedent to any other Symptoms of the Malady, nor did any come on for a Day or two, only that he seemed to be a little more languid than ordinary; however very soon after both a Vomiting and Colic seized him, and at length a rheumatic Pain tormented the paralytic Limbs.

Some, but very few, after having been long and greatly afflicted with this Disease, were seized with Epileptic-Fits and died of it; But to say the Truth, whether I consider the very great Number of Persons that laboured under it, or its Violence and Duration, I greatly wonder so few became Victims to it.

This Distemper was most violent when northerly Winds prevailed, which was likewise true of the Small-pox, that raged also at that Time.

They, who had naturally lax Bowels, suffered less by far from this epidemic Disease than they, who were more costive; this perhaps may be the Reason why Children (who are generally loose) were not so severely tormented by it as the Adult.

This epidemic Colic continued from the Autumn to the following Spring, but as the Summer advanced it totally vanished.

Théodore Tronchin

Théodore Tronchin, the physician of Voltaire and a favorite pupil of Boerhaave, was born in Geneva in 1709. He was a member of a noble Provençal Calvinist family who had fled from France after the massacre of St. Bartholomew's Day and established themselves in Switzerland. His father, one of the wealthiest bankers in Geneva, lost his fortune in the collapse of John Law's financial schemes and sent his son to Lord Bolingbroke in England. Bolingbroke was at the time in disgrace and could do but little for the youth of sixteen except to introduce him to certain scholars and advise him in his studies. Théodore Tronchin was sent to the University of Cambridge, where he was attracted so much by reading the works of Boerhaave that he proceeded to Leyden to study under this illustrious physician. After completion of his medical studies, he settled in Amsterdam, where he married the granddaughter of Jan de Wet, the "martyr of liberty." He was soon appointed president of the college of medicine and the Stadholder of the Netherlands offered him the position of his first physician. He declined, however, and returned to Geneva in 1750, where he was appointed professor of medicine.

He remained in Geneva for many years, where he enjoyed the esteem and confidence of his native city and was consulted by patients from all parts of Europe. He introduced inoculation against small pox into Holland, Switzerland, and France, and inoculated more than twenty thousand persons. He was called to Paris in 1756 to inoculate the children of the Duke of Orleans and later left Geneva to become physician to the Duke. He became the friend of Voltaire, of Jean Jacques Rousseau, and of Diderot, and attended Voltaire in his last illness. Tronchin died in Paris in 1781 at the age of seventy-three. Although he gained

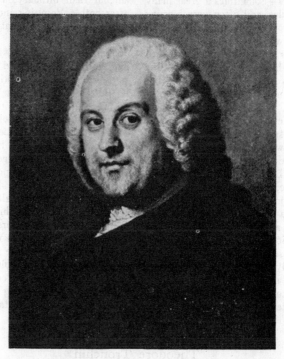

THÉODORE TRONCHIN (1709-1781)
After a pastel by Liotave

a very large income through the practice of his profession, his liberality, especially to the poor, was so great that he left his children only a very small patrimony.

Théodore Tronchin enjoyed the reputation of being a safe and conservative physician, and is well remembered for his insistence upon exercise, plain food, and fresh air as the most important requisites for the preservation of health. His best-known works are his edition of the works of Baillou and his essay *De colica pictonum*, published in Geneva in 1757. In this essay he showed that the "colica pictonum" in Amsterdam was caused by water passing over leaden roofs into cisterns where it was kept for drinking purposes. Tronchin's essay was published ten years before the "inquiry" of Sir George Baker.

CHAPTER X
SECOND REMOTE CAUSE. POISONS*

Fernel relates that an Empiric gave to an arthritic, a pound and a half of powdered lead in soup in the place of sugar; within the space of fifteen days on the twelfth day he was attacked by a severe dysentery, accompanied by fever with the most severe cramps not only of the stomah but in the intestines also; there was great weakness of this, moreover there was injury of the mouth so that indeed the softest contact by no means could be borne, and there was such belching that everything seemed to be changed into flatus: the dysentery healed, heaviness of the stomach, of the abdomen and pain of the loins, lasting twenty days, with the most disturbing sense of internal burning, and just as many nights he was sleepless, the intestine did not respond to the action of either cathartics or clystes; all the evacuated faeces were constantly foul with a lead color. Meanwhile the entire body was disfigured with jaundice and all these ills were caused less by the weight than by the hidden malignity of the lead.

The remote causes best described by Fernel

* * *

The potters who fashion earthern vessels with leaden glass are subject to the same kind of pain. Besides practical observations prove, that Lead Medicaments, which Quacks employ in treating Gonorrhoea leave behind an unconquerable stricture of the intestine with frightful griping.

A man of thirty years in the calcination of red lead inhaled Saturnine vapors, with a mild taste; the next day there was an intolerable pain about the umbilicus with a persistant constriction of the intestine. Then followed nausea, vomiting, disturbing pains of the heart and cold sweating: the day after, the pain affected his left hand slightly with loss of motion.

Observation 1

A youth suffering from Gonorrhoea, from unwise use of the tinctura antiphthisica, a prescription with Sugar of Lead as a base, fell into a most obstinate constriction of the intestine with paralysis of both hands.

Observation 2

* Tronchin, T., *De Colica Pictonum*, Geneva, Cramer, 1757, p. 24.

I saw a youth likewise suffering from Gonorrhoea, who from shame went to a Quack, and for twenty-one days took daily two powders of Sugar of Lead, after constriction of the bowels, suffered from painful and atrocious colic, and frequent convulsions, moreover was feeble in all his extremities. I have both of these confessed parties.

Observation 3

And I saw a Matron, twelve years ago, who suffering from a slight hemoptysis, make use internally for a long time of Sugar of Lead, although small doses yet frequently repeated (who was) pale, bloated, weak, trembling, moreover lax in her hands.

Observation 4

Indeed such and so many pestilential poisons are hidden among metallic poisons, the diggers of red lead daily prove who are subject to dyspnoea, phthisis, cachexia, tremors of the limbs, painful colics, paralysis, and although their lungs are mostly affected, the effluvia of red lead admitted into the vital parts, attacks the cerebrum and nerves, so that tremors, stupor and worst paralyses arise. Nor is it a wonder that for this thing they blame red lead. For bad, so dry, since with the mine powder stirred up, and penetrating the trachea, there appears in the lungs a malady which is called Asthma, as soon as the saliva is swallowed there is a painful colic, and often a fatal paralyisis. No wonder it is said that in the mines there are women who have married seven men all of who suffered a premature death from the poisonous fumes. Agricola saw such widows in the mines of the Carpathian Mountains. Indeed the animals infected by this same poison commonly become bloated, soon lose their motion, and moreover die when unconscious. The diggers in mines are daily seen to suffer in climbing the rounds of the ladders from the pits where the poison is concentrated, falling backwards in the pits, because of inertia of the hands and flaccidity of the feet.

Worst in miners

Thus the potters applying burnt and calcined lead to glass vases while they grind the lead, smear the vases with liquid lead, before they are placed in the furnace, whose poison is dissolved or scattered in the water, they take up through the nostrils, mouth and whole body, tremors appear in the hands and soon they are paralysed.

* * *

No less fortunate are those who drink water impregnated with lead. Houses roofed with lead sheets, where rain-water only is drunk, collected in cisterns, or preserved in

T. TRONCHIN,

IN ACADEMIA GENEVENSI MED. PROF. COLLEGII MEDICI AMSTE-LODAMENSIS OLIM INSPECTORIS, ACAD. REG. SCIENT. BEROLIN. &c.

D E

COLICA PICTONUM.

Vidi in arte peritissimos huncce morbum non intellexisse. Spigel.

G E N E V Æ,

Apud F R A T R E S C R A M E R.

MDCCLVII.

Title-page of *De colica pictonum* by Théodore Tronchin (Geneva, 1757)

leaden vessels, produces commonly this very bad and frequent disease: and this is the reason why the painful colic formerly rare, now rages in Amsterdam. Formerly the houses were roofed with tiles but today with lead, formerly declining from above, now flat. At the close of Autumn the shed leaves flying about, indeed you have known it as a city of trees, they are carried on the roofs by the wind, macerated there by the stagnant water, they imbue this with acid, by which soluble lead is changed into Cerussa, from there it is carried off by the rain-water into a Cistern, thus gradually the water is infected. It is no wonder that in other places where lead is lacking, and trees are absent, painful colics are less frequent. Thus is explained why if no continued breezes be upon the shed leaves, if the lead is protected by wood, the water is more healthy.

(margin: And in lead work-shops)

(margin: Water with impregnated cerussa)

The observations deserve belief: I have seen the malady rage in whole families. Eleven in one house at one time down in bed, convulsed with horrible torments, with their extremities flaccid; the roof changed, the water renewed, they recover.

Wines, adulterated with sugar of lead or litharge produced the same effect, in the first place Rhine and Moselle, by this artifice there is a more sparkling color, a milder flavor, certainly they were very harmful, because they are adulterated more secretly and more pleasantly.

(margin: Wines adulterated with litharge or cerussa)

Sir George Baker

George Baker was the son of the Vicar of Modbury in Devonshire, where he was born in 1722. He was educated at Eton and at King's College, Cambridge, and received his M.D. degree in 1756. He first began practice at Stamford in Devonshire but removed to London in 1761. He rapidly acquired a large practice, became physician to the royal household, and was nine times president of the Royal College of Physicians. He was created a baronet in 1776 and died in 1809, in his eighty-eighth year.

Baker was noted among his colleagues not only as a brilliant physician but as a profound and elegant scholar, and one who knew all that had been said or written on medical subjects from the most remote antiquity. In 1767 he read his famous *Inquiry concerning the cause of the Endemial Colic of Devonshire* before the Royal College of Physicians and in this paper proved that the Devonshire colic was not caused by cider but by lead in the cider. Baker noted that the colic was very common in Devon but very rare in Hereford and found the farmers in Devon used lead-lined cider presses. He extracted lead from the cider of Devon but found none in cider made in Hereford. Baker's essay created

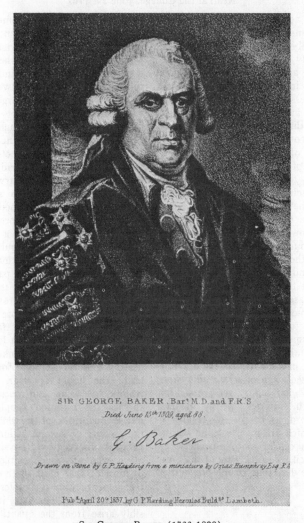

SIR GEORGE BAKER, Bar.^t M.D. and F.R.S

Died June 15th 1809, aged 88.

G. Baker

Drawn on Stone by G. P. Harding from a miniature by Ozias Humphrey Esq. R.A.

Pub.^d April 20th 1837 by G. P. Harding Hercules Build.^{gs} Lambeth.

SIR GEORGE BAKER (1722-1809)
From G. P. Harding's drawing on stone of the miniature
by Ozias Humphrey, Esq., R.A.

a storm. He was fiercely attacked by his old neighbors in Devonshire and de-nounced from the pulpit as a faithless son of Devon. His enemies asserted that the lead he found in the cider came from shot employed to clean the bottles, and that the colic was due to the humours of the body. The farmers, however, re-moved the lead from their cider presses and Devonshire colic disappeared.

XII. AN INQUIRY CONCERNING THE CAUSE OF THE ENDEMIAL COLIC OF DEVONSHIRE

By George Baker, M.D., Fellow of the College of Physicians, and of the Royal Society, and Physician to Her Majesty's Household*

Read at the College, June 29, 1767

A very small acquaintance with the writings of physicians is sufficient to convince us, that much labour and ingenuity has been most unprofitably bestowed on the investigation of remote and obscure causes; while those, which are immediate and obvious, and which must necessarily be admitted, as soon as discovered, have been too frequently overlooked and disregarded. Such a spirit of refinement in theory has, in several instances, been the parent of dangerous errors in practice: men are apt to be as partial to their own conceits, as to their own offspring: and those opinions seldom fail to govern at the bed-side, which have been the result of much contemplation in the closet. It is with true pleasure I acknowledge, that this spirit is a fault, not so much to be imputed to the present, as to the last age. We have now learned not to indulge ourselves in visionary speculations, but to attend closely to nature. We observe diseases in themselves; and trace the powers of medicines in their effects on the human body; and experiment is the great *basis* of our reasoning. In many cases indeed, from our very limited knowledge, we are still obliged to allow, in some degree, the doctrine of the empiric sect, *non interesse quid morbum faciat, sed quid tollat;* yet are we far from being such empirics, in the modern sense of the word, as to pay no regard to those causes, which are manifest and within our reach; such causes more especially, as lead us directly either to the cure of diseases, or, what is more desirable, to the prevention of them.

* * *

In some letters which I have lately received from Dr. Wall, of Worcester, the following facts are asserted. "The counties of Hereford, Gloucester, and Worcester, are not, so far as I know, subject to the colic of Poitou, or any other endemic illness, unless it may be the rheumatism: which I think, the inhabitants of Herefordshire are more

* The following extracts from Baker's essay are taken from the *Med. Tr. Coll. Phy.,* London, 1772, I, pp. 175-177, 202-204, 217-218, 221-226.

liable to, than those of some other counties. There is no lead, which can give occasion to that colic, used in any part of the *apparatus* for grinding or pressing the apples, or fermenting the liquor. Once indeed, in a plentiful year of apples, I knew a farmer, who, wanting casks, filled a large leaden cistern with new cyder, and kept it there, till he could procure hogsheads sufficient to contain the liquor. The consequence was, that all, who drank of it, were affected by it as lead-workers usually are. We had eleven of them, at one time, in our infirmary.

"I have lately had two or three patients in that distemper, occasioned by their having drunk cyder made in a press covered over with lead. But this fact of a cyder-press covered with lead, is a singular, and perhaps the only instance of the kind in this part of England. It happened in a part of the county of Worcester, adjoining to Warwickshire, where very few apples grow; and the bed of the press being therefore cracked by disuse, the sagacity of the farmer contrived this covering, to prevent a loss of his liquor. In general, the cyder-drinkers with us are healthy and robust; but for the most part lean. The liquor is clear, and passes off readily by urine and perspiration; which enables the common people to drink immense quantities of it when at labour, to the amount of several gallons a day. I have heard it observed by a physician, late of this place, who was much employed in the cure of lunatics, that more of those unhappy people come to him from Herefordshire, than any other place. The fact, if true, may possibly arise from the quantity drunk, rather than the quality."

* * *

I Determined therefore to make use of the first opportunity, which might occur, to satisfy myself by experiment, whether or no there might be in fact any solution of lead discovered in the cyder of Devonshire. Happening to be, in the month of October 1766, at Exeter, I procured some of the expressed juice of apples, as it flowed from a cyder-press, lined with lead, in the parish of

Alphington. On this I made and repeated several experiments, by means of the *atramentum sympatheticum,* or *liquor vini probatorius;* and of the volatile tincture of sulphur. The experiments satisfied me, that the Must did contain a solution of lead. The same experiments were made on some cyder, made in the parish of Alphington, of the preceding year. This likewise showed evident signs of lead contained in it; but in less proportion than in the Must.

* * *

EXPERIMENT I

A small quantity of Devonshire cyder being exposed upon clean paper to the fumes of the volatile tincture of sulphur, became immediately of a darkish colour. And we could only imitate this colour by exposing a dilute solution of *saccharum Saturni* to the same fumes. A small quantity of Herefordshire cyder, exposed in like manner to the same fumes, exhibited no such appearance, until a few drops of a solution of *saccharum Saturni* were added to it.

OBSERVATION I

FROM this experiment we are to understand, that the acid, before united with the lead in the cyder, and the volatile alkali in the tincture of sulphur, mutually attracted each other; and that it was the precipitate of the lead, united with the sulphur, which produced the dark colour above-mentioned.

EXPERIMENT II

A small quantity of *hepar sulphuris* (prepared by digesting together in a sand-heat one ounce of orpiment, and two ounces of quick-lime, with twelve ounces of water, in a close vessel) being added to some Devonshire cyder, in a few minutes occasioned a darkish colour in the body of the liquor; and the whole become very opaque. No such change was produced in the cyder of the county of Herefordshire until a few drops of a solution of *saccharum Saturni* were infused; when the same appearance likewise was perceived.

OBSERVATION II

THE reasoning made use of in the former observation, is applicable here. The decomposition of the *saccharum Saturni* and of the *hepar sulphuris* was affected by the same laws of elective attraction.

EXPERIMENT III

To a small quantity of Devonshire cyder a few drops of *hepar sulphuris* (Prepared by boiling equal parts of fixed vegetable alkali and sulphur together in water) were added; and a precipitation of a very dark colour was produced.

WHEN Herefordshire cyder was treated in the same manner, the precipitate of a dilute solution of *saccharum Saturni*, that a precipitate of the same colour with the former could be obtained.

OBSERVATION III

THERE is some nicety required in making this experiment. The *hepar sulphuris* is not to be added in any large quantity; for, as all the lead is precipitated upon the first addition, it is easy to perceive the several successive shades of colour in the precipitate, until all the lead is separated; and then the precipitate, upon a further addition of *hepar sulphuris,* assumes the whiteness of the precipitate obtained from the Herefordshire cyder, which entitles it to the appellation of *lac sulphuris.* If a large quantity of *hepar sulphuris* be at once added, the whiteness of the too copious precipitate is such, as to render the dark colour of what is first precipitated imperceptible.

EXPERIMENT IV

SOME Devonshire cyder was examined by means of the volatile tincture of sulphur, as in experiment III: and a very dark colour precipitate was obtained. A similar precipitate could not be obtained from Herefordshire cyder, until a weak solution of *saccharum Saturni* had been added to it.

SOME of the Must (taken from the press in the parish of Alphington) treated in the same manner, produced precipitates of a deeper dark colour. This sufficiently shews, that the solution of lead in the Must, was stronger than that in the cyder.

IT is a matter of no consequence, whether the lead, the existence of which is proved, was applied to the cyder in its state of Must, or in that of a vinous liquor. However, as the Must afforded more considerable signs of impregnation than the cyder, it should seem probable, that the lead was incorporated with the Must; and that, as the acid, during the fermentation, is in a great measure converted into alcohol, a proportional quantity of lead would necessarily be precipitated.

THE same experiments were afterwards tried on several other specimens of Devonshire and of Herefordshire cyder, from the cask as well as the bottle. The result of them was constantly and uniformly the same as has been described, except only in three or four instances. Three bottles of different kinds of the former shewed no signs of having been impregnated with lead; and one of the latter, which I very lately examined, gave a darkish precipitate.

IT has been proposed by several authors, to detect such adulterations of wines by means of the vitriolic, or of the muriatic acid; which, by uniting with the lead, will make it precipitate. But it is ascertained, by the experiment of Professor Gaubius, that trials, made with the acids, are less conclusive than those which have been described.

Henry Burton

ON A REMARKABLE EFFECT UPON THE HUMAN GUMS PRODUCED BY THE ABSORPTION OF LEAD*

By Henry Burton, M.D., Fellow of the Royal College of Physicians, and Physician to St. Thomas's Hospital

Read January 14, 1840

No branch of medicine is perhaps of greater importance than that which contemplates the means employed in the prevention and cure of diseases. But notwithstanding a vast number of observations have been made with a view of ascertaining the medicinal efficacy of various substances, and many well-regulated experiments instituted, yet the sum of the information resulting from these inquiries is small in comparison with the labour bestowed in collecting it, and our knowledge of the virtues of medicines still continues very imperfect. Nevertheless, the histories of cinchona, iodine, mercury and antimony, offer proofs of the benefit which has been often experienced from the discovery of new medicines and afford a reasonable expectation that additional improvements in the treatment of disease will emanate from future discoveries.

The opinions however of therapeutists differ very widely in respect to the virtues of the same medicine, and it was whilst endeavouring to confirm or refute the statements published with reference to the action of lead on men, that I noticed an interesting phenomenon which, so far as I can ascertain, has not been hitherto recorded: and, as I believe it will prove useful in the treatment of disease, I hope the following reference to it will deserve the favourable consideration

of the Royal Medical and Chirurgical Society.

Medical authors have stated that a salivation is occasionally produced by the action of lead introduced in a very comminuted form into the human body. Dr. R. Warren, in an essay read before the Royal College of Physicians in 1768, gives (Med. Trans. vol. ii, p. 87.) an account of "Four persons out of thirty two, who were attacked by lead colic, and fell into salivations for several hours every day, and said their pain was abated by the spitting." Dr. Christian also, speaking of the action and symptoms of lead on man, (Treatise on Poisons, 1829 and 1836), says, "The saliva is increased in quantity and bluish in colour."

Dr. A. T. Thomson likewise states, (vol. ii. Therapeutics, p. 64) "The saliva assumes a bluish colour." But these very eminent authorities have not, I believe, noticed the peculiar discolouration on the gums, produced by lead, which is the chief object of this paper to describe. My attention was first directed to the phenomenon in the year 1834, when a patient under the treatment of my friend and late colleague, at St. Thomas's Hospital, Dr. Roots, was said to have been salivated by the internal use of acetate of lead; and from that time I have been accustomed to examine the mouths of patients admitted into my wards, who have been exposed to the action of lead in the course of

* Med. Chir. Tr., London, 1840, XXIII, p. 63.

their usual avocations; and those also who had swallowed the acetate of lead medicinally. The result of this investigation has proved highly interesting. It has led to the belief that a salivation in the ordinary sense of the word does not occur in one case out of thirty-six cases of lead colic, the number examined in my wards; nor in one case out of fourteen cases of pulmonary disease, which were treated by me with acetate of lead; but in the total number of fifty patients who were examined whilst under the influence of lead, a peculiar discolouration was observed on their gums, which I could not discern on the gums of several hundred patients, who were not under the influence of lead, and which I believe cannot be produced by any other internal remedy.

I believe the sign will enable physicians to establish with increased facility a precise diagnosis in derangements of health, depending on the unsuspected presence of lead; and also to obviate, in many cases, the infliction of lead colic, during the treatment of other diseases by saturnine preparations.

The discolouration was carefully observed on fifty patients, and although it varied a little in point of intensity as well as extent, yet the following description will apply with sufficient accuracy to the majority of cases in which it was remarked. The other phenomena referrible to the state of the mouth, noticed on these patients, were neither peculiar, nor invariably present. The edges of the gums attached to the necks of two or more teeth of either jaw, were distinctly bordered by a narrow leaden-blue line, about the one-twentieth part of an inch in width, whilst the substance of the gum apparently retained its ordinary colour and condition, so far as could be determined by comparing the gums of these patients with those of other patients of the same class in the hospital: there was no invariable tumefaction, softening or tenderness about them; neither was there any peculiar foetor in the breath; nor increased salivary discharge to be observed on any of the fifty patients; and on thirteen out of fourteen patients, who were treated in the hospital with acetate of lead, and carefully watched during its employment, the substance of the gums, the smell of the breath, as well as the quantity and colour of the saliva, pre-

served the same characters, after the appearance of the blue line, as they respectively possessed before the saturnine preparation was administered; but on the fourteenth patient, who died from haemoptysis, the gums, which were, previously to the use of lead, tumid and soft, became contracted and firm, after the blue line had appeared.

With reference to the state induced by lead, it should be remembered, on making an examination of the mouth, that the gums and breath of patients who frequent hospitals (and by whom the practice of cleansing the teeth is habitually neglected), very often present an unhealthy aspect, independent of constitutional disease arising from lead; and amongst the fifty patients who were examined under the influence of this metal, as well as others not under its influence, the gums of many were either ulcerated, tumid, or partially detached from the teeth by incrustations; but even on the patients with ulcerated gums, the peculiar leaden-blue border line was distinctly visible. I do not remember to have seen one example of the bleeding tumefied gum, peculiar to confirmed scorbutus, produced by the internal use of lead; nor do I think it consistent with experience or reasonable, to suppose that a powerful and very useful astringent in haemorrhages should simultaneously check haemoptysis, and produce bleeding and tumid gums. The colour also of the scorbutic gum differs from the blue colour produced by lead, and there is likewise a peculiar foetor in the breath of scorbutic patients with bleeding gums, which did not exist in the fifty patients above alluded to.

Neither is the state of the gums and salivary glands induced by mercurial preparations, similar to that produced by those of lead; for in fourteen cases of pulmonary disease treated with the acetate of lead, no pain, heat, redness or tumefaction of the gums, characteristic of the action of mercurials, were observed; nor was there any increased flow of saliva, nor looseness of the teeth, notwithstanding the blue line was evident on the gums of all the fourteen patients. On the contrary, the blue line was obliterated on some patients with lead colic, to whom calomel was administered in quantity sufficient to affect the system.

IV. DISEASES OF THE CIRCULATORY SYSTEM

The history of diseases of the circulatory system forms one of the most interesting chapters in medical history. A few less well-known facts may be pointed out. Heart-block, commonly known as the Adams-Stokes syndrome, was described by three observers before Adams. Aortic insufficiency was first clearly described by Cowper, and the collapsing pulse of this condition was noted by Vieussens more than a century before Corrigan. Mitral stenosis was first clearly described and pictured by Vieussens, the presystolic thrill was first noted by Corvisart, and the pre-systolic rumble first heard by Laënnec. Pericarditis was noted by many physicians in the routine of carrying out autopsies but it remained for Rotch and the Broadbents to paint its characteristic physical findings. Angina pectoris was noted by the Earl of Clarendon, its clinical picture clearly portrayed by Heberden, and the sclerosis of the coronary arteries described by Fothergill. The autopsy of a distinguished victim of angina pectoris, John Hunter, is included. The history of coronary occlusion is one in which American physicians have played a dominating rôle.

Aneurysms were described with increasing frequency after the advent of syphilis, but it remained for Corvisart to describe the physical signs of aneurysm of the aorta, and for Oliver to call attention to the pathognomonic tracheal tug. Apoplexy after the appearance of Wepfer's book was no longer an unsolved mystery and Raynaud's disease and erythromelalgia are now readily diagnosed. thanks to the observations of Maurice Raynaud and of Weir Mitchell. Buerger's painstaking studies of thrombo-angeitis obliterans belong to the group of notable modern contributions to clinical medicine and their importance is shown in the increasing frequency with which this disease is recognized.

––––––

HEART-BLOCK
Marcus Gerbezius

Marcus Gerbezius or Verbez was a physician in Laibach, who published a large number of observations in the transactions of the Leopold Academy of Natural Sciences. He was also the author of a work in which he stressed the importance of weather and climate upon the origin and development of disease. He was perhaps the first to note and record the slow pulse of heart-block. He died in 1718.

The following account of heart-block is translated from the *Appendix ad Ephemeridum Academiae Caesaro-Leopoldino-Carolinae Naturae Curiosum in Germania,* Nuremberg, 1719, Centuriae VII et VIII, p. 23.

––––––

I recall moreover in the Augsburg hall years before an infant dead of epilepsy, and after the anatomical section in my presence the subject to have had a brain most similarly constituted.

Others ill, who came to me for treatment

elsewhere in the course of the years, I treated happily by a Method, and remedies noted in my medical Chronicologia: for example under fevers, arthritides, colics, hemoptysis &c. More unusual moreover I observed this in two patients about the pulse: truly that one of them a melancholy hypochondriac indeed had commonly when well a pulse so slow, that before a subsequent pulse followed the preceding one, three pulsations would have certainly passed in another healthy person; who moreover after the passing of August fell into a malignant fever, had on the contrary a frequent pulse, and through all the different ills of varying kinds, such as I had never observed. Therefore afterwards at the commencement of the disease and until now I had predicted a bad termination of the illness. Such remarkable

departure from nature, from the healthy state did not seem possible, and only the worst fate was predicted. The man at other times was robust, exact in his movements, but is now slow, often seized with dizziness, and from time to time subject to slight epileptic attacks.

Another man, likewise robust fell into a similar fever, in the tenth day continually had a pulse and urine quite regular and natural, so that on the contrary a bad prognosis had been given, some of the symptoms continued, he had a very intense loss of strength, dryness of the tongue, disturbed slumber, delirium, subsultus tendinum &c, but only a little inconsequential fever; he was believed to have been in special danger: yet on the 13 day of the disease succumbed with supervening convulsions.

Giovanni Battista Morgagni

Giovanni Battista Morgagni was born at Forlin near Bologna in 1682 and studied philosophy and medicine at Bologna, where he graduated in 1701. He taught for a time in the University, later settling in his native town. He was very successful in practice but soon gave it up and accepted the chair of theoretical medicine at Padua. Morgagni began his career at Padua when he was thirty-one years of age and taught there until his death, sixty years later. Three years after he removed to Padua, he was appointed to the chair of anatomy, a famous chair, whose previous occupants were Vesalius, Fallopius, Casserius, and Spigelius. He was exceedingly popular, both as a teacher and as a man, and a favorite with both his students and colleagues.

In 1761, when he was eighty years of age, he published his famous *De sedibus et causis morborum,* a book which founded the science of pathological anatomy. Here Morgagni remarks, "Those who have dissected or inspected many bodies, have at least learned to doubt; when others, who are ignorant of anatomy and do not take the trouble to attend to it, are in no doubt at all." Morgagni died in 1771, at the age of ninety.

In this monumental work, Morgagni describes cerebral gummata, mitral disease, aneurysms, acute yellow atrophy of the liver, tuberculosis of the kidneys, and gives the first clear account of heart-block. The following account of heart-block is taken from the translation of his *De Sedibus,* The Seats and Causes of Disease, by Benjamin Alexander.

LETTER THE NINTH
WHICH TREATS OF EPILEPSY*

7. To which, therefore, that I may return.

* Morgagni, J. B., *The Seats and Causes of Diseases,* translated by Benjamin Alexander, M.D., London, Millar and Cadell, 1769, 1, p. 192.

I will just skim over, in as few words as I shall be able, those many things which I have observ'd, for a long time, in my fellow-citizen Anastasio Poggi, a grave and worthy priest. He was in his sixty-eighth year, of a habit moderately fat, and of a florid complexion, when he was first seiz'd with the epilepsy, which left behind it the greatest slowness of pulse, and in like manner a coldness of the body. But this coldness of the body was overcome within seven hours, nor did it return any more, though the disorder often return'd; but the slowness of the pulse still remain'd. The first epilepsy had suc-

in the cure of this refactory disorder, less than the patient himself, made no scruple to pronounce, that it arose from the irritation of the hypochondria. And, indeed, as you have it also in this section of the Sepulchretum,[m] there is extant in Galen a history of a certain grammarian, "who having abstain'd too long from food, became epileptic, from no other cause than bile." And examples are very common of adults,[n] not

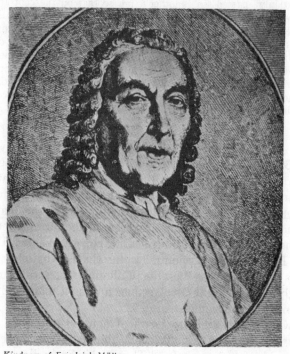

Kindness of Friedrich Müller

GIOVANNI BATTISTA MORGAGNI (1682-1771)
Etching by Angelica Kauffman

ceeded to a pain of the right hypochondrium, which was resolv'd by bilious dejections: the other paroxysms, which were slighter, generally succeeded to the sensation of a kind of smoke, ascending up to the head from the hypochondria, the fullness of which parts was continually troublesome to the patient, and was scarcely encreas'd from the ingesta, but especially from liquids. And this being the state of the case, and as the pain of the head, and all the marks of it being affected of itself, were absent, the senior physicians, who had not wish'd for me to be their companion

only of children,[o] who have been troubl'd with epilepsies, from worms, harbour'd in the intestines. And to this purpose also is that observation of the Spigellius,[p] on a whelp thus kill'd by worms; not very unlike to which, is that formerly written by me to Vallisneri, and by him publish'd.[q] And you know that this disorder often arises, also,

[m] Sect. 12 in schol. ad obs. 19.
[n] *Ibid*. schol. ad obs. 41.
[o] Obd. ead. § 2 & schol. ad obs. 15. in additam
[p] *Ibid*. obs. 41. § I.
[q] Consideraz. in. alla. gener. de' Vermi.

from other viscera of the belly being diseas'd, which the section, that I have already quoted, confirms.[r]

But although that kind of cure was applied to my fellow-citizen Poggi, with my assent, which was proper to open, cleanse, and relax, the hypochondria, yet, nevertheless, the accessions still return'd frequently; so that we now began to fear, lest the head itself had also contracted the injury, especially as, upon a very quick turn of the head, the epileptic insults recurr'd, and left a sense of weight with stupidness in the head; and frequently some blood came, together with the mucus, from the nose. Wherefore, as in the beginning, they had already drawn blood once and again from the arm, nor had omitted to give such things as are generally of use to the head, I persuaded them to let blood be taken away from those veins, which lie about the anus also; and that several things should be given internally, which are recommended as extremely proper against this disease, by the most excellent physicians. These remedies, however, were of no advantage; but the bleeding, whether it reliev'd the head, or rather those viscera which are serv'd with blood by the vena portarum, was so far of advantage, that for a short time the paroxysms were quiet. When, therefore, they return'd again more frequently, it was of use to make the patient sit up, sometimes to rub the lower limbs, and sometimes to tie them alternately with bandages thrown round about, and sometimes to fix cupping-glasses without scarification, and presently to vex the patient by taking them off; for thus he seem'd to have a longer intermission from his paroxysms. And I was even assur'd that when they sometimes attack'd him much more often, the spirit of sal ammoniac, applied to the nostrils, had driven them away as they were coming on; or, even when they were already, in a manner, begun, had suppress'd them, although the patient was entirely without the power of smelling. They were, for the most part, very short, but by no means slight. For distortions of the eyes, agitations of the limbs, and a suspension of all the senses, always accompanied the attack: oftentimes there was a strangulation, and that sometimes joined together with a stertor; and even, now and then, an involun-

tary afflux of urine attended. But he was exceedingly bad that day on which the solstice happen'd, and in like manner, that on which the eclipse of the sun happen'd.

And though you may suppose this might be by chance, yet you cannot suppose it merely accidental, that when the quantity of urine was either naturally or artificially encreas'd,[s] the epileptic paroxysms not only became not slighter, but were even very frequently very much exasperated. For we were oblig'd to have regard to this excretion sometimes, when a sudden difficulty of breathing rous'd the patient, as he was beginning to sleep, and compell'd him to sit up; which symptom, doubtless, gave us some suspicion of a dropsy of the thorax; and the more so, because the patient told us, that his right leg had, for a long time past, been accustom'd to swell a little with water, and that even then, which, when he told us, we examin'd into, the swelling was ascending up the thigh. But it was easy to encrease the quantity of urine, by obvious and innocent remedies, and therefore to diminish the tumour, and the suspicion, which was afterwards entirely remov'd; but not so the force of the attacks, which, from the encreas'd afflux of urine, and that of itself, sometimes opaque, and blackish, was so far from being weaken'd or diminish'd, that even on the contrary, as I said above, they grew stronger and stronger. When these things, and others, which for the sake of my promis'd brevity I pass over, were of no effect against the inroads of this disease, and even such as had been sometimes useful to retard or suppress them, as I said above, were now of no advantage, as they did not continue to afford these effects; there was one thing, however, which was constantly of service; I mean opium, given at the beginning of the night, in the quantity of half a grain. For the frequency and force of the insults, and added to these also, obstinate watchings so weaken'd the patient in other respects, that we were under a necessity of gaining a truce by some means or other. And by this means, good nights, and easy sleeps, were procur'd to the patient; and so far was his head from being made heavy, or dull, by the use of this medicine, that even the heaviness and dullness, left behind by the daily attacks, were by this means taken away; which

---

[r] Obs. 39. cum schol.

[s] Vid. infra, n. II.

otherwise, that is, when the use of the opium was intermitted, continu'd, while the former restlessness and watchings also oppress'd him. And, indeed, after he had pass'd a night of that kind, which was far more troublesome than the rest, when to the greatest rarity of the pulse, which I mention'd in the beginning, an inequality had suddenly been added, so that very often they were perceiv'd to be much more rare, then not more so, than usual, and presently much rarer again; which symptom made us the more uneasy, because the disease, at that time, was wont, first of all, entirely to obscure the pulse, and then immediately to begin its attack; and when we had tried all the remedies, recommended to dissolve, and promote, the circulation of the blood, in vain; upon giving the opium again, the quiet nights again return'd and diminish'd that inequality of the pulse; and, by the continu'd use of opium every night, it was entirely remov'd, and even the former rarity was diminish'd.

But, perhaps, you will suspect, whether the rarity of the pulse be, in fact, a very uncommon symptom, to remain after an epilepsy, in hypochondriac patients, when you shall have compar'd this observation of mine with that of the celebrated Gerbezius,[*] which describes the pulse of a strong hypochondriac man, "who was now and then subject to slight epileptic paroxysms," even when he was in health, "as being so very slow, that before the subsequent pulsations followed that which went before, three pulsations would certainly have pass'd in another healthy person." But to return to my subject; after

* Eph. N.C. Cent. 7. in Append.

that no fit had now return'd for thirteen days, and the use of opium was intermitted, the first night indeed was not bad; but the following ones, by reason of the continual watching, and restlessness, and at length by reason of that difficulty of breathing, which I spoke of above, were exceedingly troublesome; so that we were oblig'd to have recourse again to the opium, in order to procure quiet nights. which nothing but opium would procure. And, to comprehend all in a few words; that the attacks of the disease, from being very frequent, as they had happen'd every day. in the month of June, had been so far reduc'd in their number, that but one happen'd in July, one in August, nor more in September. and after that none in the two next months at least, and upwards, till I departed to teach medicine publicly, we judg'd was owing to the use of opium, given opportunely, sometimes every night, sometimes every other night, and at length at intervals of many nights. For by that medicine we were able to appease the tumultuary motions, which arose, and frequently by a very manifest sensation, from the hypochondria, to the thorax, and head; and by this means to procure a truce, both for nature and art: and this gave us sufficient time to cleanse and confirm the hypochondriac viscera, which we had determined to do, in the beginning, but in vain attempted, among those first continual tumults. with which the patient was harass'd: and from these viscera alone, and not from water being redundant in the brain, that these sudden commotions arose, this history. or I am much deceiv'd indeed, evidently shews.

Thomas Spens

Thomas Spens was born in Edinburgh in 1769, the son of Dr. Nathaniel Spens, a distinguished physician of that city. He was elected a Fellow of the Royal College of Physicians at the early age of twenty-five and was successively Librarian, President and, for the last thirty-three years of his life, Treasurer. He died in Edinburgh in 1842.

Spens' published papers were six in number. One of these papers, published in 1793, contained the first account of heart-block written by a British physician. This account precedes that of Adams by forty-eight years and Stokes' account by fifty-three years. Spens' case, however, was published thirty-two years after Morgagni's celebrated case of "epilepsy with a slow pulse."

SECT. II
MEDICAL OBSERVATIONS*
I
HISTORY OF A CASE IN WHICH THERE TOOK PLACE A REMARKABLE SLOWNESS OF THE PULSE. COMMUNICATED TO DR. DUNCAN, BY DR. THOMAS SPENS, PHYSICIAN IN EDINBURGH

On the 16th of May 1792, about 9 o'clock in the evening, I was sent for to see T. R. a man in the 54th year of his age, a common labouring mechanic. After having heard from him, some account of his complaints, I was much surprised, upon examining the state of his pulse, to find, that it beat only twenty-four strokes in a minute. These strokes, however, as far as I could judge, were at perfectly equal intervals, and of the natural strength of the pulse of a man in good health.

He informed me, that, about 3 o'clock in the afternoon, he had been suddenly taken ill while standing on the street; that he had fallen to the ground senseless; and that, according to the accounts given him, by those who were present, he had continued in that state for about five minutes. His face was slightly cut, in two different places, by the fall; but his head did not seem to be in any way materially injured. From the time of this first attack, till I saw him, he had been affected with three other fits, nearly of a similar nature. These, however, were attended with some convulsive motions of his limbs, and with screaming during the fit. When I saw him, he was somewhat drowsy, but perfectly recollected and distinct, and his voice was as strong as when he enjoyed a state of perfect health; nor had he, at that time, any other complaint.

He imputed these attacks, to having been intoxicated the night before, with strong ale and whisky; and to his having drunk in the forenoon, when very thirsty, a large quantity of cold water. In the morning, he had two natural stools; but, besides being uncommonly thirsty during the former part of the day, he was frequently affected with sickness at stomach, and had vomited up his dinner soon after it was taken.

Upon visiting him, in the morning of the 17th, I found that he had been attacked with several fits during the night, which were of

* *Medical Commentaries*, Edinburgh, 1793, VII, 463.

considerably longer duration, and more violent than the former ones: he was attacked with one of them, while drinking some infusion of camomile to assist vomiting. Upon examining his pulse, I found that it beat only twenty-three strokes in the minute; nor was any change produced upon it, by his drinking a tea-cupful of wine, and a glassful of whisky, which I directed for him; and, an hour after, I found it in precisely the same state as before. He was now directed to take some spirit of Hartshorn; but, by mistake, it was given him very little diluted, and produced much uneasiness in his throat and mouth. From this cause, I found him in great distress at one o'clock; but it seemed to have produced no change on the state of his pulse, which at this time beat twenty-four strokes in a minute, and was of the same strength and regularity as before. Washing his mouth with vinegar and water, gave him almost immediate relief; and, at nine in the evening, I found that he had continued free from any return of fits or of faintness, since five in the morning. At this time, I gave him thirty drops of Spiritus Ammoniae aromaticus, in about two ounces of water, which he found very agreeable. But he had hardly swallowed it, when he felt himself faint, and cried out that one of his fits was coming on: but, upon taking a tea-cupful of wine, which I directed for him, this uneasiness went off. His pulse still continued in the same state as before. During the course of the day, he had frequently sat up in bed, without feeling any uneasy faintness, or threatening of fit.

When I visited him in the morning of the 18th, I was informed that he had slept a good deal during the night, but had been frequently faint. He had, however, eaten an egg and some bread as breakfast. He had no headache, vertigo, or pain in any part of his body; but his pulse beat only twenty-six strokes in the minute. About mid-day, he got up and put on his clothes. He had a natural stool, and afterwards walked out to his workshop. Upon his return, finding himself very well, and inclined to eat, he sat down to dinner; but, upon taking some broth, he almost instantly felt faint, and had the same most distressing sensation as if one of his former fits were coming on. The same circumstances took place twice afterwards, on his attempting to swallow something solid. About eight in the evening, wishing again to try what would be the effect of swallowing, while I was present, he took a bit of newly toasted bread. But he had no sooner smelt it, than he felt some of the sensations of a beginning fit; and, as soon as he had tasted it, he almost instantly cried out, and fell back senseless, with smart convulsions of all his muscles. He apparently recovered, however, in a few seconds; but hardly any pulse could be felt for a good many seconds.

On the morning of the 19th, I learnt that he had been very faint almost the whole night, and that he had been attacked with frequent fits, attended with violent convulsions; and every thing he attempted to take, seemed to have had the effect of inducing a fit. He now felt, at their commencement, a violent pain which darted through his head; but when free from the fit, he was perfectly recollected and distinct. When I numbered his pulse, I found that it beat only ten strokes in the minute, though it still continued equally strong and regular as before. I ordered him to take a glassful of whisky, after which he remained for an hour pretty quiet and easy; and his pulse rose again to twenty-four strokes on the minute. But at three in the afternoon, I found that his pulse was only nine in the minute; and it was neither so strong, nor so regular as before. He was now in great distress from constant sickness and faintness; but perfectly sensible and recollected. At seven in the evening, I found his pulse still nine in the minute, but much weaker. He continued sensible, but unable to speak. He was not, however, affected with any more returns of the convulsions. During the whole of the following night, the people who attended him, observed that he never moved his right hand or leg; and he expired on the 20th, about nine in the morning.

During the continuance of this patient's disease, recourse was had, on different occasions, to trials of cordials, stimulants, and opiates. But none of them seemed to produce any obvious change on the state of his complaints.

The day after his death, the body was opened by Mr. Fyfe, and, upon the most careful examination, no morbid appearance, of any consequence, could be discovered, either in the thorax or abdomen. Upon examining the head, about two ounces of a watery fluid were found in the ventricles of the brain; and a gelatinous appearance was observable in some parts of the pia mater. But nothing of this kind could be discovered about the thalami nervorum opticorum, as is often observed in cases of hydrocephalus. A small ossification was discovered on the back part of the dura mater; but no other morbid appearance could be detected.

What may have been the state of this patient's pulse prior to the attack on the 16th, I know not. But I was informed by Mr. Latta, surgeon in Edinburgh, who had attended him when he laboured under a fever two years before, that, during the course of that disease, his pulse was often above 120 in the minute; and that when the fever left him, it returned to the natural standard of between 60 and 70 in the minute.

How far the different symptoms, which occurred in this case, particularly the slowness of the pulse, were to be attributed to the effusion of water in the ventricles of the brain, may perhaps be a question. A slow pulse, at least at a particular period of the disease, is well known to be one of the most remarkable symptoms in hydrocephalus; and the water found in the ventricles of the brain, was the only cause detected on dissection, to which this symptom could be attributed. If, however, we suppose water in the ventricles of the brain to have been here the sole cause of disease, we must of necessity conclude, that hydrocephalus may not only exist, but even prove fatal, though the greater part of those symptoms, which are commonly considered as marking that affection, be totally absent.

Robert Adams

Robert Adams was born in 1791 in Dublin, entered the University there in 1810 and received successively the degrees of B.A., M.A., and M.D., obtaining the doctor's degree in 1842. While still a medical student, he became the apprentice of William Hartigan, a leading surgeon of Dublin. After graduation he was appointed to the staff of the Jervis Street Hospital and later to that of the Richmond Hospital. He founded, with two colleagues, the Peter Street School of Medicine but later withdrew and established another school in connection with Richmond Hospital. In 1861, Adams was appointed Surgeon to the Queen and Regius Professor of Surgery in the University of Dublin. He died in 1875 at the age of eighty-four.

Robert Adams was highly respected for his medical ability, for the soundness of his views and for his innate honesty. He is now best remembered for his classic account of essential heart-block, which appeared in 1826.

CASES OF DISEASES OF THE HEART ACCOMPANIED WITH PATHOLOGICAL OBSERVATIONS*

By Robert Adams, A.B., Member of the Royal College of Surgeons in Ireland, and one of the Surgeons to the Jarvis Street Infirmary, &c.

An officer in the revenue, aged 68 years, of a full habit of body, had a long time been incapable of any exertion, as he was subject to oppression of his breathing and continued cough. In May 1819, in conjunction with his ordinary medical attendant, Mr. Duggan, I saw this gentleman: he was just then recovering from the effects of an apoplectic attack, which had suddenly seized him three days before. He was well enough to be about his house, and even to go out. But he was appressed by stupor, having a constant disposition to sleep, and still a very troublesome cough. What most attracted my attention was, the irregularity of his breathing, and remarkable slowness of pulse, which generally ranged at the rate of 30 in a minute. Mr. Duggan informed me that he had been in almost continual attendance on this gentleman for the last seven years; and that during that period he had seen him, he is quite

*Dublin Hosp. Rep., 1827, iv, p. 396.

certain, in not less than twenty apoplectic attacks. Before each of them he was observed, for a day or two, heavy and lethargic, with loss of memory. He would then fall down in a state of complete insensibility and was on several occasions hurt by the fall. When they attacked him, his pulse would become even slower than usual; his breathing loudly stertorous. He was bled without loss of time and the most active purgative medicines were exhibited. As a preventive measure, a large issue was inserted in the neck and a spare regimen was directed for him. He recovered from these attacks without any paralysis. Oedema of the feet and ankles came on early in December; his cough became more urgent, and his breathing more oppressed; his faculties too became weaker.

November 4, 1819, he was suddenly seized with an apoplectic attack, which in two hours carried him off, before the arrival of his medical attendant.

Sir William Burnett

William Burnett was born at Montrose in 1779 and educated at the Grammar school in his native town. He began the study of medicine at Edinburgh, but studied only a short time and entered the navy as a surgeon's mate. He was present at the battles of the Nile and of Trafalgar, and for his services was created a K.C.B. and awarded four war medals. In 1810, he became physician and inspector of hospitals for the Mediterranean fleet and, in 1814, became the medical inspector of the Russian fleet. After service with the Russian fleet, he settled in Chichester as a physician. In 1829, he again entered the naval service and subsequently became physician general to the navy.

William Burnett became a member of the Royal College of Physicians in 1825 and a fellow in 1836. He was knighted in 1831, and in 1835 was appointed physician to the king. On his retirement from active life, he returned to Chichester, where he died in 1861.

CASE OF EPILEPSY, ATTENDED WITH REMARKABLE SLOWNESS OF THE PULSE*

By William Burnett, M.D., Member of the Royal College of Physicians; Physician in Ordinary to His Royal Highness The Duke of Clarence; and Honorary Fellow of the Imperial Medico-Chirurgical Academy of St. Petersburg, &c.

Communicated by Dr. James Johnson. Read April 13th, 1824

An officer of the navy, aged about forty-six, who had served much at sea in different climates, experienced about sixteen years ago, a single attack of epilepsy, from which time, till about four years preceding the present period, there was no recurrence of the disease; he then, however, had another attack while in bed, and in consequence, fell upon the floor. From this time till August, 1820, he enjoyed good health, but, on the 23rd of that month, I was requested to visit him, and though on this occasion I had no opportunity of seeing him during any of the paroxysms, I had every reason to conclude, from the symptoms mentioned, that the disease under which he laboured was epilepsy, which, by moderate bloodletting, both local and general, purgatives, and light tonics, together with small doses of the pil. hydrargyri, I soon succeeded in checking. He remained quite free from complaint till the end of January, 1821, and appeared to have regained his usual health. Indeed on the day preceding his attack on this occasion, I met him while on my road to visit a patient in the country, driving his chaise, and looking remarkably well.

On the 27th of January, I was again requested to visit this patient, and found him labouring under all his former symptoms, having suffered many paroxysms. Indeed, they were now so frequent that, in the space of half an hour, while I was with him, he had four or five attacks. During the paroxysms he exhibited all the usual symptoms of epilepsy; yet these were of very short duration, some times lasting only a few minutes, and never being followed by a disposition to

sleep. They were commonly preceded by nausea, and a sensation as if something arose in the stomach, and proceeded upwards to the head. Occasionally the nausea proved very troublesome, and was accompanied by vomiting even when the fits did not come on. The same plan of cure was pursued as on the former occasion, with the addition of the tinct. valerianae ammoniata. A seton was inserted in the nape of the neck; great attention was paid to the regulation of his diet and the state of his bowels and the disease soon ceased.

About the latter end of April or beginning of May, I was again called upon to visit him, and found the paroxysms had been slighter, and not so frequent, but he complained of great uneasiness and distention about the epigastrium, which some purgatives he had previously taken had failed to remove. He also complained of dyspnoea, which frequently made it necessary for him to sit up in bed; and on examining his pulse, I found it to beat about thirty-six to the minute, but it was regular and small. On the following morning the pulse was only beating twenty in the minute, but, in the evening, it got up to 32, and from this time till the 6th of May, it varied from 28 to 56, but was generally under the latter number, though without any return of the paroxysm.

* * *

The foregoing case exhibits a train of symptoms which I have never before dealt with in epilepsy; and the only instances I am acquainted with in any degree resemble that which is here detailed, are related by the celebrated Morgagni.

The first he mentions is recorded in Book

* *Med. Chir. Trans.*, London, 1827, XIII, 202-211.

1. Letter ix. Article 7, in which he gives the case of a "worthy priest, of a moderately fat habit, and florid complexion, who in his sixty-eighth year was attacked by epilepsy, which left behind it the greatest slowness of pulse, and, in like manner, a coldness of the body." The latter however was soon overcome, though the disease often returned, but the slowness of the pulse still remained. The first attack of epilepsy was succeeded by a pain in the right hypochondrium, which was resolved by bilious dejections; the other paroxysms, which were slighter, generally succeeded to a sensation of something like smoke arising in the hypochondria and ascending to the head. A sense of fulness about the hypochondria was troublesome to the patient, and increased by ingesta, especially fluids. As the disease advanced, he was subject to sudden attacks of dyspnoea, which, as in the case I have related, compelled him to sit up in bed. Morgagni does not mention the minimum of the pulse in this instance, but from a quotation he has introduced from Gerbezius, I should conceive it was not below 24 in the minute.

The other case mentioned by Morgagni is in the Letter lxiv. Article 5., which exhibited an equal slowness of pulse, and was considered to have arisen from the same cause, viz. disorder of the chylopoietic viscera. This case terminated fatally, and, on examination, many pints of water were found in the thorax; adhesions of the lungs to the pleura costalis, and a collection of puriform fluid in the superior lobe of the left side. The spleen was larger than usual, and several of the other viscera shewed slight marks of disease.

The case of this gentleman was one in which, on several accounts, I felt greatly interested; and it is but right to add, that I considered the disease to have arisen from the same cause as Morgagni assigns in these cases, before I consulted his invaluable works. Whether I was justified in doing so, is at present a matter of opinion. I may mention, however, that I have lately had occasion to treat a young lady who had been long and painfully subject to the most severe attacks of this disease; and by pursuing a plan of treatment calculated to improve the digestive functions, she has been now for nearly two years in the enjoyment of the best health: nor is this a solitary instance.

Welbreck Street, April 6th, 1824.

William Stokes

William Stokes, whose name is indelibly linked with two well-known syndromes—Stokes-Adams disease and Cheyne-Stokes respiration—was born in Dublin in 1804. The Stokes family, although of English origin, had been transplanted to Ireland for five generations and had occupied prominent positions in Irish public life. Whitley Stokes, the father of William Stokes, was Regius Professor of Medicine at Dublin, a gifted physician, a highly cultivated gentleman and a devoted Irish patriot. William Stokes began the study of medicine at the Meath Hospital in Dublin, proceeding later to Glasgow and finally to Edinburgh, where he obtained his degree in 1825. While still a medical student he published in 1825 a small *Treatise on the Use of the Stethoscope,* the first systematic treatise on the subject in the English language. After graduation, Stokes returned to Dublin and in 1826 was elected physician to the Meath Hospital. Here he became a colleague of Robert James Graves, who was, in Stokes' opinion, the most remarkable man in the medical profession of Ireland. Stokes and Graves became devoted friends and worked for years at the Meath Hospital, initiating and carrying out a system of clinical instructions that brought world-wide fame to the Dublin School of Medicine. In 1842 Stokes became Regius Professor of Medicine at Dublin in succession to his father.

In 1837 Stokes published his *Diseases of the Chest,* which added to his rapidly growing reputation and was soon translated into German. In this work,

Stokes notes that physical signs reveal mechanical conditions which may proceed from different causes. In 1854 Stokes' *Diseases of the Heart and the Aorta* was published. This work was also received with great acclaim and immediately recognized as the authoritative work on this subject. It was immediately translated into German and, a few years later, Italian and French translations were published. In 1861, Edinburgh, Stokes' alma mater, conferred the degree of

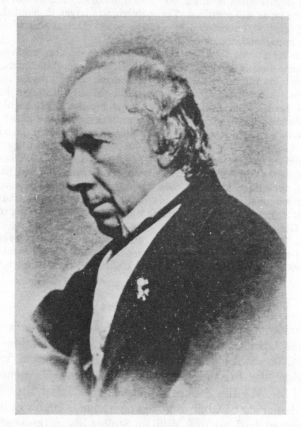

WILLIAM STOKES (1804-1878)
From a photograph—Kindness of Dr. George Blumer.

LL.D. upon him, in 1865 Oxford gave him the degree of D.C.L. and, in 1874, Cambridge presented him the degree of LL.D. Stokes, in 1876, was decorated by the German Emperor William I with the order of "Pour le Mérite," the crowning honor of Stokes' life. He died in 1878.

Stokes was a keen observer, possessed an unusual sense of humor, and was intensely interested in his fellow men of every age, occupation, condition, and station in life. He was intensely interested in prevention of disease long before preventive medicine had attracted much attention. Stokes once remarked, "My father left me but one legacy, the blessed gift of rising early." He often rose at four or five and worked steadily at writing until eight, when he had breakfast and began his professional duties. Stokes' account of Stokes-Adams disease was published in 1846 and his description of Cheyne-Stokes respiration appears in his *Diseases of the Heart and the Aorta*. This latter work also contains an account of paroxysmal tachycardia antedating the observations of both Cotton and Bouveret.

ART. III.—OBSERVATIONS ON SOME CASES OF PERMANENTLY LOW PULSE*

By William Stokes, M.D., Physician to the Meath Hospital, &c.

In the fourth volume of the *Dublin Hospital Reports*, Mr. Adams has recorded a case of permanently slow pulse, in which the patient suffered from repeated cerebral attacks of an apoplectic nature, though not followed by paralysis. The attention of subsequent writers on diseases of the heart, has not been sufficiently directed to this case, which is an example of a very curious, and, there is reason to believe, special combination of symptoms. The following cases will still further elucidate a subject on which there is but little information extant:—

CASE I.—*Repeated pseudo-apoplectic attacks, not followed by paralysis: slow pulse, with valvular murmur.*

Edmund Butler, aged sixty-eight, was admitted to the Meath Hospital, February 9, 1846. He stated that his health had been robust, until about three years ago, at which time he was suddenly seized with a fainting fit, in which he would have fallen if he had not been supported. This occurred several times during the day, and always left him without any unpleasant effects. Since that time, he has never been free from these attacks for any considerable length of time, and has had, at least, fifty such seizures. The fits are very uncertain as to the period of their invasion, and very irregular as to their intensity, some being much milder and of shorter duration than others. They are induced by any circumstances tending to impede or oppress the heart's action, such as sudden exertion, distended stomach, or constipated bowels. There is little warning given of the approaching attack. He feels, he says, a lump first in the stomach, which passes up through the right side of the neck into the head, where it seems to explode and pass away with a loud noise resembling thunder, by which he is stupified. This is often accompanied by a fluttering sensation about the heart. He never was convulsed or frothed at

the mouth during the fit, but has occasionally injured his tongue. The duration of the attack is seldom more than four or five minutes, and sometimes less; but during that time he is perfectly insensible. He never suffered unpleasant effects after the fits, nor had anything like paralysis. His last fit occurred about one month before admission. He has never heard it remarked that there was anything peculiar about his heart or pulse. At first he found that spirits was the best restorative or prophylactic, but latterly he has not used them, being "afraid to die with spirits in his belly."

On admission, he was haggard and emaciated, but seemed the wreck of what was once a fine, robust man. He lay generally in a half drowsy state, but when spoken to was perfectly lively and intelligent.

What he sought admission into the hospital for was an injury he had sustained, by a fall, on the left shoulder; this, however, was of no consequence, and he soon recovered under the use of an anodyne liniment.

He makes no complain of his general health; his appetite is good, and he sleeps well, bowels regular, and, in fact, all the functions are in good order. He has, however, some cough, attended with a slight mucous expectoration. His intellectual powers are perfect. He complains of a feeling of chilliness over the body, and is never warm except when close to the fire. This has long been the case; and he says that each day he gets a periodical chill, generally in the afternoon, which is followed by increased heat of the surface, but without sweating.

On percussion, the chest is universally resonant. The respiratory murmur loud, and combined, more especially posteriorly, with large mucous râles. The impulse of the heart is extremely slow, and of a dull, prolonged, heaving character, giving the idea of feeble, as well as of slow, action. The first sound is accompanied by a soft *bruit de soufflet*, which is prolonged until the commencement

* *Dublin Quart. Jour. Med. Sc.*, 1846, ii, p. 73.

of the second sound, and is heard very distinctly up along the sternum and even into the carotid arteries. The second sound is also imperfect, though very slightly so; the imperfection being much more evident after some beats than after others. Pulse twenty-eight in the minute, of a prolonged. sluggish character: the arteries pulsate vividly all over the body, but no *bruit* is audible in them. They appear to be in a state of permanent distention; the temporal arteries ramifying under the scalp, just as they are seen in a well injected subject. All the other cavities and viscera appear to be in a perfectly healthy state. Urine, neither acid nor alkaline; of a light colour, clear; specific gravity 1010; and does not afford a precipitate with nitric acid. He was ordered four ounces of wine, and a liniment for the shoulder.

February 17th. The pulse was varied from twenty-eight to thirty in the minute. The cardiac murmurs continue unchanged; that with the first sound is plainly audible over the upper part of the thorax, but most evident along the course of the aorta.

21st. Pulse thirty. Cough quite gone. Has been complaining of a feeling of the "lump in the stomach" for several days and was once threatened with the approach of a fit during the night; it passed off, however, without becoming a true attack.

23rd. An oedematous swelling has appeared behind the left ear, extending up the side of the head, slightly tender on pressure; no redness; has had no shiverings; tongue clean, bowels free. Pulse up to 36.

March 3rd. On the 24th of February the oedema had left the left side, and made its appearance on the right, from which it was dispersed on the following day by the application of poultices. The pulse fell to the usual range.

His aspect and general health are greatly improved since his admission. He gets up every day, and is much stronger. The shoulder is almost quite well. The pulse has continued at 28 or 30. He says he has had two threatenings of fits since his admission, both occurring in bed, *and both warded off by a peculiar manoeuvre; as soon as he perceives symptoms of the approaching attack, he directly turns on his hands and knees, keeping his head low, and by this means, he says, he often averts what otherwise would end in an attack.*

4th. He has mentioned for the first time today. that he is much troubled with irritability of the bladder, so that he is obliged to rise very often during the night to pass water. His urine was examined and found to be healthy. Specific gravity 1015. He has been subject to this for the last twelve months, and it probably depends on the disease of the prostate so common in old men.

We remarked today that on listening attentively to the heart's action, we perceived that there were occasional semi-beats between the regular contractions, very weak, unattended with impulse, and corresponding to a similar state of the pulse, which thus probably amounts to about 36 in the minute, the evident beats being only 28, so that there must be about eight of these semi-beats in the minute;—but these signs are very indistinct.

14th. Health improving; has had no fit; no cough. Both morbid sounds are loudest over the sigmoid valves and thence along the aorta. No semi-beats audible. Pulse 29; not quite as prolonged as before.

18th. He complains to-day of palpitation, and a feeling of uneasiness about the heart; the impulse is increased and is found to consist of two distinct pulsations. The bruit, with the first sound, is somewhat louder than before. On listening attentively, there are heard occasional abortive attempts at a contraction, probably about four in the minute. They do not destroy the regular intervals between the stronger sounds, but are heard, as it were, filling up the interval. We could not recognize a corresponding state of the pulse, which counted 32 in the minute.

After this, little change was observed. His health continued improved; he had no fit, or threatening of one; and he appeared anxious to leave hospital, in order to go to work again. The pulse continued about the same standard, and regular; I believe it never exceeded 36 in the minute since his admission into the hospital. The physical signs remained unchanged, as was observed the day before he left the hospital. An examination of the lungs revealed no morbid sign, the bronchial râles heard at the time of admission, having quite disappeared.

He left the hospital in March, intending to go for sometime into the country before he resumed work. He was advised to be careful not to overexert himself; and never to allow himself to be bled when threatened with one of his fits.

Within the present month (June) this patient has been again admitted to the hospital. The cardiac phenomena remain as before, but a new symptom has appeared, namely, a very remarkable pulsation in the right jugular vein. This is most evident when the patient is lying down. The number of the reflex pulsations is difficult to be established, but they are more than double the number of the manifest ventricular contractions. About every third pulsation is very strong and sudden, and may be seen at a distance; the remaining waves are much less distinct, and some very minor ones can be also perceived. These may possibly correspond with those imperfect contractions which have been already noticed in the heart. The appearance of this patient's neck is very singular, and the pulsation of the veins is of a kind which we have never before witnessed.

He has had scarcely any of the cardiac attacks since he was discharged; he refers the premonitory sensations to the right supraclavicular region, but states that he has often experienced them without any loss of consciousness following.

AORTIC INSUFFICIENCY
William Cowper

William Cowper was born in Petersfield, Sussex, in 1666, the youngest son of Richard Cowper. He began the study of medicine as an apprentice to William Bignall, a surgeon of London, and in 1691 was admitted to the Barber Surgeons' Company. He immediately began to practise in London, devoting himself especially to the study of anatomy. In 1694 he published an account of the muscular system of the body under the title of *Myotomia Reformata*. Two years later he was elected a Fellow of the Royal Society and in 1698 published *Anatomy of Humane Bodies*. The publication of this work aroused the ire of Godfrey Bidloo, the great Dutch anatomist who called Cowper a "highwayman" and accused him of having published a pirated edition of his *Anatomia Corporis Humani*. Cowper retorted that the plates of Bidloo's Anatomy were originally drawn for Swammerdam and that he, Cowper, had as much right to them as Bidloo. Some two hundred years later Dr. Hewitt of the Royal College of Surgeons discovered that on the frontispiece of Cowper's Anatomy a circle of thin paper bearing Cowper's name had been pasted over the name of Bidloo with the title of Bidloo's Anatomy in Dutch. This discovery apparently bears out Bidloo's contention that Cowper's Anatomy was really a piece of scientific piracy.

In spite of this controversy Cowper seems to have maintained his professional standing in London and was the teacher of the immortal Cheselden. In 1702 Cowper described the urethral glands since known by his name, although Mery had previously discovered them in 1684. In 1705 Cowper contributed an interesting paper to the *Philosophical Transaction of the Royal Society* describing "Ossifications or Petrifactions in the Coats of the Arteries, particularly in the Valves of the Great Artery," in which he clearly described the lesions of aortic insufficiency.

Cowper died in 1709 at the age of forty-three and is buried at Bishops Sutton in Hampshire.

III. OF OSSIFICATIONS OR PETRIFACTIONS IN THE COATS OF ARTERIES, PARTICULARLY IN THE VALVES OF THE GREAT ARTERY, BY WILLIAM COWPER, SURGEON, AND F.R.S.*

How far Anatomical Enquiries inform in the true causes of Diseases, which have been ascribed to the want of Spirits in some, and Radical Moisture in Aged People, etc. may be in some measure seen by two Observa-

sened to more than a third part of its natural size; insomuch that a part of the Trunk of the Artery cut Transversel very much resembled a bit of the stem of a Tobacco-pipe, its sides were so thick and its Bore conse-

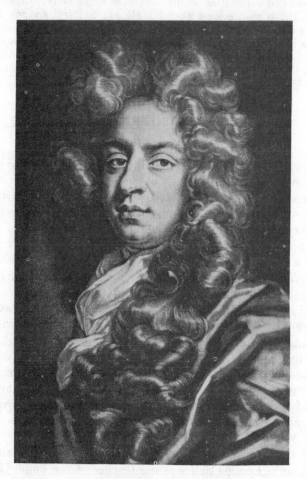

WILLIAM COWPER (1666-1709)
From a portrait by Closterman

tions, among others, publisht in the *Transactions* No. 280: The first there mentioned, page 1195, is of a young Gentlewoman, in whom the *Parietes*, or Membranes, that compose the Trunks of the Arteries of the Arm near the *Axilla*, being very much thickened, so that the *Diameter* of its Bore was les-

quently so much lessened: The other was of the Trunks of the Arteries of the Leg, pag. *ib.* that were Obstructed by Petrifactions or Ossifications, in a person about the 67th year of his Age. Since which I have met with several of the like Instances in people of years, particularly in the Leg of an old Gentlewoman, whose Toes and Foot were Sphacelated, the Arteries of whose Leg I

* *Phil. Tr. Roy. Soc.*, London, 1706, XXIV, 1970.

have still by me, and have sent them herewith Injected as much as they could be, with Red Wax; in which the Ossifications diminishing their Channels in some places, and totally obstructing them in others, is made very evident. (See the Preparation in the *Repository* of the *Royal Society*.)

The Dissections of Morbid Bodies not only instruct us in the Seats and Causes of Diseases, but very often inform us in the true Use of parts, as will appear by the following Instances.

The Ossification or Petrification in the Great Artery, at is rise from the Heart, has been so commonly found, that some think it is constant; how it may be in some Animals I cannot be certain, but in Humane Bodies I am well assured whenever it happens it is a Disease, and does in some measure incommode those parts in the due execution of their office, as the following Cases will evidence: But that this Paper may be of some use, I shall set down the Symptoms before Death, which may help our Conjectures when the like offers again. A spare man about 30, who languisht with an Ulcer in the Thigh, attended with a *Caries*, or Rottenness of that Bone at its Articulation with the *Tibia* and *Patella* call'd the Knee, where all those Bones were affected, at length fell into a true *Phthisis*, and coughed up no small quantity of *Pus*; some months before his Death I frequently saw him, when he would often offer me his Wrist, to feel his unequal Pulse, which was wont to amuse him; the Artery there missing sometimes one, sometimes two strokes in 6 or 7: At first he told me he observed it mist but one in ten but at length those stops became more frequent, especially on any agitation of the Body or Mind: tho a *Polypus* in any of the Great Vessels about the Heart may induce that Symptom, yet the continuance of it so long before Death, shews it owing to some other Cause, as appear'd on opening the Heart and Great Artery of this person. A A A D G. Fig. 1st.

You will not be surprized I send the Figures printed from Copper Plates, when I tell you they are designed, among others (I am now about) to explain the Muscles, in another Edition of my *Myotomia Reformata*, this Fig. the 1st being one of those that represent the muscular Structure of the Heart; the rest I have added to explain the Petrifaction of the Valves of the *Aorta* in the following instance.

A A. The Trunk of the Great Artery opened and display'd.

a a a. The three Semilunary Valves of the *Aorta*, which hinder the Blood from returning to the Heart, after it is expell'd thence by its *Systole* or Contraction; these Valves in this case were somewhat thicker, and not so plyable as naturally, and did not so adequately apply to each other, as is exprest Fig. 4. aaa. Whence it hapned sometimes, that the Blood of the Great Artery (A A A. Fig. 1.) would recoil, and interrupt the Heart in its *Systole*. But this stubbornness of these Valves was owing to a Bony or stony body, markt b. Fig. 1st, which appear'd much plainer when the Valves were dry, a is represented in the Figure beneath markt with an x: a a. the two Valves pinn'd out and dry'd, b the Petrifaction or stony Body at their junction. In this instance I observ'd the Left Ventricle of the Heart, exprest at G G. D D. e e. f f. Fig. 1st, to be a little dilated from its natural size, but was not by two parts in three so big as the Left Ventricle of the Heart of one I dissected in the Presence of Dr. *Sloane*. The Symptoms, some years before the Death of this person, who was about 40 years of Age, were extraordinary Shortness of Breath, especially on any fatigue, with an intermission of one stroke in three of the Pulse; his posture of sitting up was more Eligible than any other, he complain'd of great faintness, and now and then pain about the Heart; the extreme parts often cold, which towards his Death increased more and more on him; his Legs and Arms being Gangreen'd some hours before; insomuch that the Corps was very offensive in opening, so 'twas done within 24 hours after he expired, in the month *November*.

Upon opening the Chest, the Heart, particularly its Left Ventricle, was found larger than that of an ordinary Ox, and fill'd with Coagulated Blood. The Valves of the Great Artery a A. Fig. 1. were Petrify'd, insomuch that they could not approach each other, as exprest Fig. 2. and 4. But an Orifice, represented at Fig. 5, remain'd always open by the Petrifactions b b, Fig. 3. and a a, Fig. 5, which had clogg'd these Valves, and hindered their application to each other, as in a Natural state is represented in Fig. 2 and 4, a a a.

The explication of the Symptoms in both these Cases is obvious enough; for tho the Person first instanced did not dye of the same disease with the last mentioned, yet the

Symptoms in his Illness plainly shewed what must follow, from the disorders of these *Valves,* as they are rendred more or less useless: For as their Offise is to prevent the return of the Blood into the Heart, in its *Diastole,* by exactly shutting up the passage these Valves) cannot contract to prepare the passage for the Blood of the Left Ventricle, when to be expelled into the *Aorta.* Hence the Intermissions of the Pulse in the first instance may be accounted for. In the latter instance. these Valves were wholly useless.

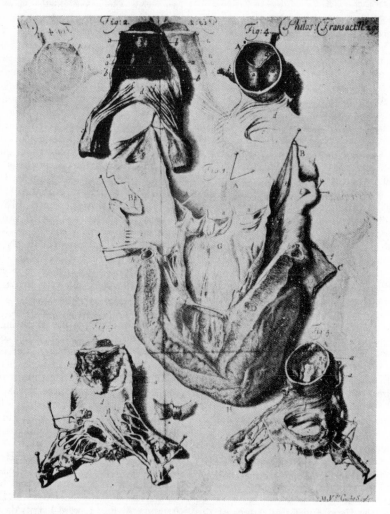

Figures 1, 2, 3, 4, and 5 showing ossification in the coats of arteries. From Chapter XXIV of the *Philosophical Transactions of the Royal Society* (London), 1706. Engraver M. Vander Gucht

of the *Aorta* (as the Flaps in Water Engines) so if by any accident they are hinder'd from doing their duty, as they were by the Petrifactions mentioned, the consequences must be, not only a regurgitation of Blood into the Heart, but they baulk its impulsive force, when the Muscular Fibres (which are in the Circulation became more difficult, as appear'd by the refrigeration of the extreme parts, Gangreens, etc. In both these cases the Left Ventricle of the Heart was dilated proportionably to the ill constitution of these Valves, which clearly shews these Valves give that assistance to the Heart in its Office that it cannot be without, and that it gradually suffers according to their indisposition.

Before these Papers were sent to the Press, I had an opportunity of observing a like Instance of that first mention'd in this latter part of them. It was an Elderly Gentleman, about 72, who had sometimes Intermissions in his Pulse several years before his death, in whom I found divers Petrifications in the Mitral and Semilunar Valves of the Left Ventricle of the Heart.

If my time would give leave, I might here add some Anatomical remarks on the Structure and Mechanism of this noble Organ, particularly of the Use of that Transverse Tendon exprest at f f. Fig. 1. and the Progress and Insertions of the Tendon f. Fig. 3, arising from the *Carneae Columnae* e e, which do not all terminate in the lower Margin of the Mitral Valve d, Fig. 2 and 3, but pass to the upper and middle part of that Valve, whilst others terminate in the Basis of the Heart, with the Muscular structure of the Semilunar Valves; but these I must reserve for another place.

THE EXPLANATION OF THE FIGURES

FIG. 1

The Left Ventricle of the Heart open'd, etc.

AAA. The inside of the *Aorta* slit open to the Left Ventricle.

BB. The Bulbous Trunk of the *Vena Pulmonalis* divided through, and pinn'd aside to shew.

a a a. The Three Semilunar Valves of the *Aorta*, which hinder the Blood from returning to the Heart.

b. A small Stony Body at the conjunction of two of the Semilunary Valves, exprest at the * below this Figure.

a a. Parts of the two Valves dryed.

b. The Petrifcation, as it appears in the dryed Valves.

C. Part of the lower Trunk of the *Vena Cava*, cut off immediately above the Liver.

c c c. The Left Auricle open'd and pinn'd out.

CC. The sides of the Left Ventricle divided and drawn aside, to show its inside d d e e f f G G.

d d. The Mitral Valves of the Left Ventricle of the Heart or *Arteria Pulmonica* divided and turn'd aside.

e e. The *Carneae Columnae*, whence spring

the Tendons fasten'd to the Valves, d d, exprest Fig. 3. d f.

f f. A Transverse Cord or Tendon, by which the *Columnae Carneae* are drawn nearer each other in the *Systole*, or contraction of the Heart, when the Blood is expell'd into the *Aorta*; whereby the Tendons (express'd f f Fig. 3 and 5) draw the Mitral Valve laterally; by which means its Orifice g f Fig. *ibid*, is not only closed to prevent the return of the Blood by the *Vena Pulmonalis*, but at the same time it opens a passage for the Blood of the *Arteria Magna*, by withdrawing the Mitral Valve, d. Fig. 2. from the Orifice of the *Aorta*, a a a g. Tho this Artifice in Nature may be indifferently explain'd by these Figures; yet I have design'd some others, that I think will make it more intelligible in another place.

GG. The Internal Surface of the Left Ventricle where it is somewhat smoother as it leads to the *Aorta*.

g g. The Trunk of the Coronary Vein divided when filled with Wax.

h h. The Coronary Artery in like manner divided.

i. One of the Trunks of the *Vena Pulmonalis*.

k k k. The three Orifices of the Trunks of the *Vena Pulmonalis*, as they open into the Bulbous Trunk, express'd at B B.

H. The Cone of the Heart.

FIG. 2

A. Part of the *Aorta* next the Heart.

a a a. The three Semilunary Valves, as they appear next the heart in a Natural State, when the Heart is in *Diastole*, and the Blood hinder'd by these Valves from returning to its Left Ventricle.

b b. Part of the Basis of the Heart cut off.

e e. The two *Columnae Carnae* of the left Ventricle.

d. The Mitral Valve.

f f. The Tendons Springing from the *Carneae Columnae*, and inserted into the upper and middle parts of the Valve, as well as to its lower Margin; which is better exprest in the following Figure.

g. The Orifice of the *Aorta* compleatly clos'd by the application of these three Valves to each other.

FIG. 3

Shows the same parts exprest in the preceding Figure, as they appear'd when the Valves of the *Aorta* were Petrified: The same Letters also directing to the parts already explain'd, except a.

a. Part of one of the Valves which was not cover'd with the Petrifaction.

b b b. The Petrifcations on the rest of the Valves.

† A small Petrifaction on the Mitral Valve.

h h h. Some of the Transverse Tendons which draw the *Carneae Columnae* to each other, when the Heart is in *Systole*, for the more effectual closing the Orifice of the Mitral Valve, exprest here at g.

FIGS. 4 AND 5

Show the same parts represented in the two preceding Figures, as they appear view'd towards the Heart, when dry'd and display'd.

AA. The Trunk of the *Aorta*.

a a a. Fig. 4. The Semilunary Valves in a Natural State, when the Blood in the Arteries presses them close to each other.

b b b b. The Trunks of the two Coronary Arteries cut off.

a a Fig. 5. The Semilunary Valves Petrify'd.

c. The Orfice of the Mitral Valve next the *Vena Pulmonalis*.

d d d. The Internal Surface of the Mitral Valve leading into the Left Ventricle.

e e e. The *Columnae Carneae*.

f f. Their Tendons.

g g. The Transverse Tendons which draw the Fleshy Columns to each other when the Heart is in *Systole*.

Raymond Vieussens

Raymond Vieussens was born in 1641, in a small village in Rouergue, the son of a Lieutenant-Colonel. The father having bequeathed nothing to his son, he was left to make his own way in the world on his own resources. He entered the University of Montpellier as a student of philosophy and then became a student of medicine, showing a great interest in anatomy and devoting a great deal of time to dissections. At the age of thirty, Vieussens became physician to the Hospital of Saint Eloy. In 1685, Vieussens published his *Neurographia universalis*, a description of the brain, spinal cord, and nerves. This book received instant recognition and brought great fame to its author, who was immediately elected a member of the Academy of Sciences and a foreign member of the Royal Society of London. In 1688 he went to Paris as a Physician to Mlle. de Montpensier, and was granted a stipend by Louis XIV. After the death of the princess, he returned to Montpellier where he lived until his death in 1715.

There has been much difference of opinion in regard to the merits of Vieussens' principal work, his *Neurographia universalis*. Many of his contemporaries were very lukewarm in their praise of his work and many later writers share this disdain. Laying aside the controversial questions, no one will begrudge him unstinted praise for his clear and vivid portrayal of a case of mitral stenosis and a case of aortic insufficiency, both with autopsies. His patient with mitral stenosis had "lips the color of lead" and a pulse "very small, feeble, and absolutely uneven" (pulsis irregularis perpetuus?), while his patient suffering from aortic insufficiency was pale, had a pulse "very full, very fast, hard, uneven and so strong that the arteries of both arms struck the ends of my fingers like a cord which had been tightly stretched and then violently shaken." These striking descriptions are in his *Traité nouveau de la structure et des causes du mouvement naturel du cœur*, Toulouse, 1715.

The valves of the aorta sometimes become osseous

* I know that many Anatomists have found in some animals, & indeed in some men, the trunk of the aorta bony; but I have never read nor heard tell that they had recognized any alterations in the natural texture of the sigmoid valves: however I have found them, once, only partly

subject to epilepsy for a long time, was seized twenty years ago, by a paroxysm of this disease, so violent that he almost fell into apoplexy: as he was very poor, they carried him into the Hospital Saint Eloy of Montpellier, where he was promptly delivered of his paroxysm of epilepsy by remedies which were ordered for him by M. Verny, a

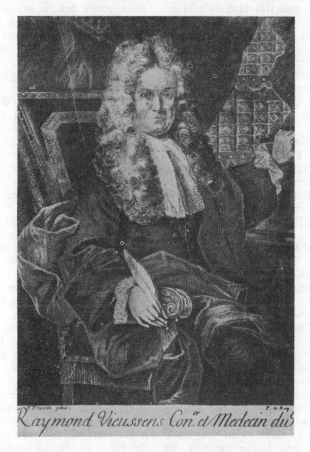

Raymond Vieussens Con.er et Medecin du

Frontispiece of *Œuvres Françoises* de M. Vieussens
(Toulouse, 1715)

osseous, as will appear from the observation which I shall report as soon as I have finished the history of the following illness.

History of the disease of Jean Chifort

Jean Chifort, native of Mouguyo, in Languedoc, Diocese of Montpellier, age thirty-five years, of a melancholy temperament, &

* Vieussens, Raymond, *Traité nouveau de la structure et des causes du mouvement naturel du cœur*, Toulouse, Guillemette, 1715, p. 107.

wise and experienced Physician, so that they believed him, if not entirely cured, at least out of danger; but this did not hinder me from studying his condition in making my rounds, according to my custom to the patients of this hospital. After having remarked the sunkenness of his eyes, the puffiness, & the pallor of his face, I examined his pulse, which appeared to be very full, very fast, very hard, unequal, & so strong that the artery of first one & then the other arm, struck the ends of my fingers just as a cord would have done which was very tightly drawn & violently shaken. The pulse of this patient, the like of which I had never seen and do not hope to again, persuaded me that he was suffering from a violent palpitation of the Heart. I was not deceived, for having questioned him upon this fact, he told me that for a long time he had not been able to sleep comfortably, neither on one nor on the other side, nor indeed upon his back, if his head were not very high, because the strong beating of his heart prevented it; & he added that when he reclined on one or the other side, & particularly on the left side, it seemed to him as if one struck on his ribs with a hammer.

When I had examined with care the pulse of this patient, I said to M. Verny, & to several Students of Medicine who accompanied us, that there was a polyp in the right auricle of the Heart, & that there was not any in the ventricles, because it seemed to me, on account of the freedom of his respiration, & because of the fullness & height of his pulse, that the blood passed freely from the right to the left; something that never happens, when there is a polyp of any size in one or the other ventricles. I added that besides the polyp, there was something else extraordinary which I did not understand, in some part of his heart, which would soon cause the death of the patient.

My prognosis proved correct; for the patient died in three days: I opened his body, I found a polyp in the right auricle; the left ventricle was extraordinarily dilated; the walls of the trunk of the aorta appeared to me very thick, very hard, & like cartilage; the semilunar valves are markedly

Description of what was observed in the Heart of Jean Chifort when one opened his body

stretched & cut off at their tips: all these cuts which bore some resemblance to the teeth of a saw, were in fact osseous. The walls of the trunk of the aorta had become very thick, hard, & like cartilage, the lymph which the blood of the canals of the Heart, to which they were very closely attached, furnished for nourishment, had no longer a free flow; it was no longer present, at least abundantly enough, in the tissue of the walls of all the branches of the arteries, of which I have spoken; this is why they became dry little by little, & lost enough of their natural suppleness to have the appearance of fingers stretched from one trunk to the other like cords. Since the lymph designed for the nourishment of the aorta could not pass through the walls of the trunk, it turned towards the base of the semilunar valves, & was pushed in such a large quantity into their tissue, that it diminished their natural suppleness, & fixed itself at their ends in the manner which will be described, & hardens in the gashes which are formed like plaster or stone; so that the great tension of these valves allowed the left ventricle to pass the blood which the right furnished it into the aorta only by their very violent contractions, & as they had been cut off the ends could never approach each other closely enough to prevent any opening between them; that is why whenever the aorta contracted, it sent back into the left ventricle a part of the blood which it had just received. It was then the irregularity in the flow of the blood, caused by the tension & the bony gashes of the sigmoid valves of the aorta, which caused the palpitation of the Heart and the throbbing of this artery, which was produced by very strong beats.

The semivalves of the aorta had become osseous & why

The explanation of the cause of palpitation of the heart

Giovanni Battista Morgagni*

BOOK II. OF DISEASES OF THE THORAX. LETTER XXIII. ARTICLE 9

8. A woman, a little younger than that last describ'd, complain'd, in the same hospital, of a palpitation of the heart sometimes, but always of a difficulty in her breath,

*Morgagni, J. B., *The Seats and Causes of Disease,* translated by Benjamin Alexander, M.D., London, Millar and Cadell, 1769, i, p. 684.

which she could not draw but with her neck erect; and still more of so great a streightness and anxiety at her heart, that very often she seem'd just at the point of death. Some suppos'd her to labour under a dropsy of the pericardium. Her pulse never was intermitting; but her veins were large. She died at the time that the genital parts of a woman were wanted to finish the public demonstrations of the year 1731, a little before the middle of March.

The Thorax and belly being open'd some quantity of water was found in both cavities; but there was no dropsy of the pericardium. The valves of the aorta were indurated, and one of them even bony. The trunk of the artery itself shew'd, up and down in its internal surface, either something bony, or something verging to the nature of a bone; so that the part of the artery which went through the belly, and which I dissected after demonstration of the genital parts, was the same state. Nor did I find it bony only at the side of the interior mesenteric artery, and in other places, but even at the very division of it into the iliacs: and in several places it was unequal, and here and there of a whitish colour, as it generally is when it begins to become bony.

9. It certainly cannot be denied, that the aorta, in the state I have describ'd it, must resist the blood, as it is driven by the heart, and, for that reason, be able to create a palpitation, a difficulty of breathing, and that sense of streightness with which the woman was tormented. But at the same time it is necessary to declare, why, out of so great a number of persons in whom there was an aorta of this kind, as I have already written to you, and shall write hereafter, many of them, certainly, did not labour under these disorders at all, or, at least, not so vehemently. And in order to do this, other circumstances, without doubt, must be added to the disorder of the aorta, which did exist in this woman and did not exist in the others; as, for instance, a different fault in the organs, or a different constitution of the blood, different quantity, and other things of a similar kind besides, that we may not seem to be always bringing in the more exquisite side of the nerves, and convulsions. So in an observation of Vedrisius, already pointed out[m] after a violent palpitation of the heart; and a very great asthma, the aorta was found to be internally bony near the heart; but the heart itself was found to be of a stupendous magnitude, hard, and tumid. So in another person, who having been long afflicted with various disorders, had

been, in the beginning of them, very much subject to a palpitation of the heart. the celebrated Plancus[n] not only found the aorta in many places become bony, but also both the coronaries of the heart, and the heart itself very large, particularly its right auricle, which was the largest and strongest of all: and from hence you may easily perceive, that, in consequence of this one disorder, the heart might be more vehemently irritated by the blood being more strongly impell'd into the subjected ventricle; and may we the less wonder, if in the observation of Grassius the younger, spoken of already in this work,[o] it shall perhaps appear, that nothing else could be the cause of the palpitation, but the right auricle being enlarg'd to the double of its usual capacity. Finally, not to detain you too long, in a woman of an illustrious family, whose palpitation of the heart was so great, and so constant, as to be heard by those who stood near her, and be discern'd by those who were at some distance. the celebrated Cohausen[p] not only saw the aorta entirely callous; but he even saw in the heart itself, not to mention the lungs. scirrhi, and the blood viscid and mucous.

Wherefore, in the woman, also spoken of by me, besides the aorta being here and there bony, or inclining to a bony state, the valves of it are also to be attended to. For as one of these was bony, and the others indurated, so being of consequence, less yielding to the blood, they might encrease the obstacles to its exit, and, on the other hand not sufficiently prevent its return, when, soon after, repuls'd by the contraction of the great artery; so that, as some portion of it return'd into the left ventricle of the heart, when this ventricle ought to receive the blood that was coming in from the lungs, it would necessarily happen, that the returning portion, as well as the portion which had not been extruded just before, must occupy some part of that space, which, from the design of nature, was entirely due to the blood that was coming in from the lungs. Which circumstance, finally, could not but overload both the lungs and the heart and compel the latter to throw out, every now and then, with a great impetus, the blood that stagnated in it.

[m] Epist. 18 n. 4.

[n] Epist. de Monstr.
[o] Epist. 18 N. 4.
[p] Commerc. Litter. A. 1743. Hebd 21 n. 4.

Thomas Hodgkin

ON RETROVERSION OF THE VALVES OF THE AORTA*

By Thomas Hodgkin, M.D.

Read before the Hunterian Society, Feb. 21, 1827

9, New Broad Street, 6-2, 1827

My Dear Friend:

Thou wilt probably recollect having pointed out to me, a few months ago, a particular state of the valves of the aorta, which, by admitting of their falling back towards the ventricle, unfits them for the performance of their function.

Though the derangement of the thoracic viscera had for some years been a peculiar object of my attention, the lesion in question was new to me and it seems to have equally escaped the observation of those pathologists to whom we are the most· indebted for the knowledge which we possess respecting the disease of the heart. Corvisart, Laënnec, Bertin, Rostan, Bouilland and Andral, have none of them made any allusion to it. Since the first specimen was pointed out to me by thyself, I have had the good fortune to meet with two or three additional cases. In the deficiency of a better description, the following sketch may be found to possess some interest. If thou thinkest so, it is quite at thy service.

To avoid circumlocution,· and in defect of a better name, I shall designate by the term retroversion of the valves that diseased state which allows of their dropping in towards the ventricle, instead of effectually closing the vessel against a reflux of the blood.

The valves in which this derangement has taken place, have their loose edge considerably stretched and lengthened: hence, when raised and applied to the side of the vessel, instead of forming a straight or rather concave line, they form a curved one, with its convexity upwards. In some instances there is a manifest laceration of the edge. The structure of the valves is more or less thickened, and the appearance of the corpora Arantii is nearly lost. The point where the lip of the valve is connected with the side of the vessel seems to be the principal seat of mischief. It is at or near this spot that the laceration before mentioned, when present, is met with; and almost always the

portion of the artery to which the valve is attached is thickened and drawn downwards, assuming the appearance of a fleshy column, and evincing that a considerable degree of traction has been exerted upon it. In no instance which I have met with are the three proportions of the valve all equally deranged. Those which correspond with the origins of the coronary arteries are either principally or solely affected. A more or less diseased state of the artery has, almost without exception, concurred with retroversion of the valves. In some instances there has been merely a little unequal thickening, with disposition of earthly deposit; in others this derangement has been much more considerable, and accompanied with dilatation of the artery.

Having described the morbid appearance, I proceed to offer a few remarks on its nature and causes, and shall afterwards give one or two examples, with the hope that, when followed up by further investigation, the symptoms and the lesion may be so connected as to render its diagnosis tolerably easy.

The mere inspection of the parts would at once induce one to attribute the derangement to a mechanical cause. In what other manner can the laceration of the edge of the valve, or the elongation of the part of the artery to which it is attached, be accounted for? That such causes do at times act on this part, we have abundant proof, in the occasional sudden production of aneurism of the aorta from violent straining, forcible retention of the breath &c. A force calculated to effect the dilatation of the first part of the aorta, if exerted through the medium of a fluid, as e.g. the blood, must, from its pressing equally on all sides, have also a tendency to send the valves backwards towards the heart. Though I am not aware that such an injury has hitherto been noticed by any author, as occurring in the aortic valves, examples are not wanting or partial ruptures having taken place in other parts of the heart, as a consequence of urgent straining. Corvisart has given three cases in which the

* *London Gaz.*, 1828-29, III, p. 433.

carnae columnae, the tendons of the valves, were ruptured from this cause; and Laënnec and Bertin have each added another.* A previously diseased state of the structure of the artery is probably an important condition as a predisposing cause; and its dilatation may also contribute to induce retroversion of the valves, precisely as Bichat explains the imperfect action of the valves of the veins.

The specimen No. 1422, in the collection at Guy's Hospital, the one in which retroversion of the valves was first observed by thyself, exhibits this derangement in a well-marked manner. It is now some years since it was taken from the subject, and I am not in possession of any of the symptoms which distinguished the case, except that the patient was anasarcous and had enlarged heart.

The next example occurred in a stout and vigorous man, about thirty years of age. He was admitted into Guy's Hospital on the 29th of March last, having severe affection *of the chest, under which he had been laboring for some time.* Blood had already been taken from him, but without relief, and after his admission, the operation was again repeated, with no abatement of the urgency of his symptoms. He had great dyspnoea, with anxiety and palpitation. He died on the second of April.

I had scarcely seen this patient during life, and had not myself examined him with the stethoscope. The impulse communicated to the ear by the cylinder was reported to be remarkably strong, but I do not know that any *bruit de scie* was noticed.*

* Since this letter was written, I have noticed the following remark in Dr. Baillie's *Morbid Anatomy:* "There is a preparation in Mr. Hunter's Museum shewing one of the semilunar valves thickened and ruptured to a considerable extent. It is very rare that such an occurrence happens, and in this instance the rupture was so large, that I conceived it must have proved almost immediately fatal."

* Some months after this letter was written, I received further particulars respecting this case from my friend J. H. Pickford, of the Guards. He examined this patient's chest about an hour and a half before death, and inserted the following remarks in his note-book:

"Right side.—Anteriorly and superiorly on the

This examination having been made so short a time before death, it ought to afford no surprise that the impulse of the heart was not proportioned to the thickening of its parietes discovered after death. The great extent over which the sound was heard ought, in all probability, to be attributed to the indurated state of the lungs. The *bruit de scie* not having been noticed in two or three other cases of retroversion of the valves, may have been an accidental symptom of short duration. May it not have been produced by the partial coagulation of the blood, which there are various reasons for supposing to commence before death?

On examination, the aortic valves were found in the state which I have already described, and which an inspection of the preparation, No. 1423, will render perfectly intelligible. The heart itself was of large size, its cavities dilated and its parietes thickened. There was a little fluid in the pericardium. The left side of the chest bore marks of recent pleuritic inflammation. A considerable portion of the lung was hepatized, and a small spot had suffered from pulmonic apoplexy. The right lung, though denser than natural, and containing much serosanguinolent fluid, was far more permeable to air than the left. The abdomen contained about two gallons of clear, bright, yellow serum. The other appearances noted in this cavity were unimportant, and foreign to the subject before us.

right side, the sound of the breathing gave an idea that the air was injected with great force, and had very great difficulty in insinuating itself into the substance of the lungs, as though they were compressed. The respiration became gradually less audible inferiorly, until it was quite lost.

"Left side.—Precisely similar results were obtained on the left side, except that the respiration was not audible below the third or fourth rib.

"Heart.—The impulse of the heart was not particularly feeble, but was considerably diffused; the sound very general over the whole of the left side, and nearly the whole of the right side of the chest, with the exception of the superior part. Each contraction appeared lengthened, accompanied with a purring, thrilling, or sawing kind of noise."

James Hope

James Hope, whose studies on the heart did much to clear up many points in diagnosis, was born in Stockfort, Cheshire, in 1801 and while yet a youth in school, showed great talent and industry. He wished to study law, but was urged by his father to study medicine. He had always felt a strong dislike for the medical profession and finally agreed to study medicine on the condition that he be allowed to practise in London. He began the study of medicine in Edinburgh in 1820 and found it at first most distasteful. He disliked anatomy especially and he always dissected with gloves and forceps. After spending five years at Edinburgh, Hope went to London for a year in surgery at St.

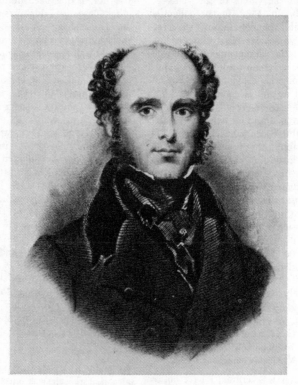

JAMES HOPE (1801-1841)
From the biography—*Memoir of the late James Hope,
M.D.*—written by Mrs. Hope and published
in London in 1848

Bartholomew's Hospital and then proceeded to Paris, where he decided to remain a year. His knowledge of French was very imperfect but he devoted twelve hours daily to practice in French conversation and at the end of one month was able to speak the language fluently. He became a clinical clerk to Dr. Chomel and delighted his chief with his skill in drawing pictures of pathological specimens. After a year in Paris and a tour of Switzerland and Italy he returned to London.

Hope began his active career with the advantage of a good medical education, but with the disadvantage of not possessing a degree from an English university and of not having membership in the Royal College of Physicians. He became a pupil and a governor in St. George's Hospital, where he became noted for his regular attendance and constant application. There was a strong prejudice at St. George's against auscultation so Hope was to take a leading rôle in proving the great value of Laënnec's discovery. He made many observations on the physical signs of aneurysms, of diseases of the heart, and upon the mechanism of the production of the heart sounds. The latter experiments were carried out upon an ass, stunned by a blow on the head and kept alive by artificial respiration. To obtain recognition among his colleagues Hope decided to publish his clinical pathological observations. He set to work and wrote with such application that in one year he had completed his work on the heart. This work, *Diseases of the Heart and Great Vessels,* appeared in 1831 and had an immediate success. It was translated into German, passed through several American editions, and spread its author's reputation far and wide. In 1834 he was appointed assistant physician to St. George's Hospital and in 1839 became physician to the same hospital. Six months after his appointment to St. George's Hospital he was attacked with pleurisy and died two years later of pulmonary tuberculosis at the early age of forty.

Hope achieved great success at a comparatively early age. He was greatly esteemed by his colleagues, not only for his intellectual acumen, but for his moral qualities as well. A short time before his death he stated that he owed his great success to a faithful observance of the advice given him by his father, just before entering practice. "1st, Never keep a patient ill longer than you can possibly help. 2ndy. Never take a fee to which you do not feel yourself entitled. And 3rdy, Always pray for your patients."

The biography of Hope written by his wife (*Memoir of the late James Hope, M.D.,* by Mrs. Hope, London, 1848) is a very intimate and interesting account of the life of this unusually gifted and admirable physician.

THE PULSE IN REGURGITATION THROUGH THE AORTIC VALVES*

Under this head must be included regurgitation out of the aorta into the right ventricle (Mitchell), or into the pulmonary artery (Evans). Aortic regurgitation produces a pre-eminently *jerking* pulse, a high degree of the pulse of unfilled arteries, as seen in anaemia from any cause. The diastole or beat of the artery is short and quick, as if the blood were smartly jerked or shot under the finger, the vessel during the intervals feeling unusually empty. This is the most remarkable, appreciable, and constant pulse produced by disease of the heart. In the immense majority of cases, the practitioner may conjecture the disease by this sign alone. It differs from the jerking pulse of anaemia, in being more marked, and in not necessarily being frequent, as the anaemic

A Treatise on the Diseases of the Heart, by J. Hope, London, Churchill, 1839, p. 379.

pulse is, when its jerk is distinct. It may be absent, or scarcely appreciable, if the regurgitation be very slight; and it may be neutralised by free mitral regurgitation (Payne) or great contraction, in consequence of the enfeebling effects of these lesions on the pulse.

* * *

I described this pulse (which had not previously been noticed by any writer on diseases of the heart), in several parts of the first edition of the present work in 1831; especially at p. 434; but having up to that time noticed it solely in cases of aortic regurgitation combined with inflammation of the heart or adhesion of the pericardium, I was in doubt as to its cause, and ascribed it more to the latter affections than to the regurgitations, propounding, however, the question in reference to the case of Copas, written in 1829, whether it was not due to the regurgitation. This question I soon afterwards resolved in the affirmative by discovering the pulse in question in cases of regurgitation alone. Dr. Corrigan, who wrote in 1832 or 1833 on permanent patency of the aortic valves as a supposed new disease, has so completely overlooked this pulse as even to state the reverse: "It rises without any jerk under the finger" (Dublin Jour. vol x, p. 186). M. Donné subsequently wrote a thesis on aortic regurgitation, which I have not been able to procure: but as M. Bouillaud, who quotes him, does not anywhere allude to the jerking pulse, I presume that it was overlooked by M. Donné also.

SIGNS OF DISEASE OF THE AORTIC VALVES*

When there is regurgitation through the permanently open aortic valves, a murmur accompanies the second sound, and its source may be known, by the following circumstances:—1. It is louder and more superficial opposite to and above the aortic valves than above the apex of the heart, by which it is distinguished from a murmur in the auricular valves with the second sound. 2. It is louder along the course of the ascending aorta than along that of the pulmonary artery, and down the tract of the left ventricle than down that of the right; by which circumstances its seat is known to be in the aortic, and not in the pulmonic valves. This inference is strongly corroborated by the state of the pulse, which, when the aortic regurgitation is at all considerable, is singularly and pre-eminently jerking—the pulse of unfilled arteries. 3. It is distinguished from a systolic murmur in the aortic orfice by its accompanying the second sound; by its being more audible (though with a gradual diminution), down the course of the ventricle, than a systolic murmur; by its being prolonged through the whole interval of repose, and even through accidental intermissions of the ventricular contraction (case of W. Esq.); and by the weakness of the refluent current always imparting to it the softness of the bellows-murmur, an inferior degree of loudness, and a lower key, like whispering the word awe during inspiration. It often becomes musical.

Purring tremor, though necessarily produced by an inconsiderable, salient, or rugged contraction of the aortic valves, can rarely be felt, because the sternum is interposed; but when the heart is displaced from beneath the sternum, as by hydrothorax, empyaema, emphysema, tumors, consolidation and contraction of one lung and hypertrophy of the other (case of Mitchell). I have never known it accompany aortic regurgitation. Probably the refluent current is too feeble to render it perceptible through the walls of the chest. Aortic regurgitation, however, by unfilling the arteries, eminently favours the production of tremor from contraction of the aortic valves, during the ventricular systole (see p. 142).

Irregularity of the pulse is not necessarily or usually produced by contraction of the aortic valves, unless extreme (e.g. case of Hedgley); nor are the size and strength of the pulse materially diminished by the moderate contraction. Aortic regurgitation produces the eminently jerking pulse; and this does whether the regurgitation be into the left ventricle, or through a false opening into the pulmonary artery or mouth of the right ventricle (Mitchell and Evans).

* J. Hope, A Treatise on the Diseases of the Heart, London, Churchill, 1839, p. 383.

Sir Dominic John Corrigan

Dominic John Corrigan, whose description of the "Corrigan Pulse" has assured him of immortality in medical history, was born in Dublin, in 1802, the son of a prosperous merchant. Unlike Graves and Stokes, the other two most famous men of the Dublin School, Corrigan was not the descendant of transplanted Anglo-Scotch colonists, but was of simon-pure Irish ancestry. He was educated first at the Catholic College of Maynooth and later studied medicine in Dublin and Edinburgh, taking his degree at the latter university in 1825. He was much interested in the new science of pathology and devoted himself, on settling in Dublin, to original pathological investigations. He early obtained an appointment as physician to the Jervis Street Hospital, where his service consisted of only six medical beds. However, by carefully choosing his patients and studying them with great care and attention, he made here his great reputation as a physician, pathologist, and teacher.

In 1832, while physician to the Jervis Street Hospital, he published a

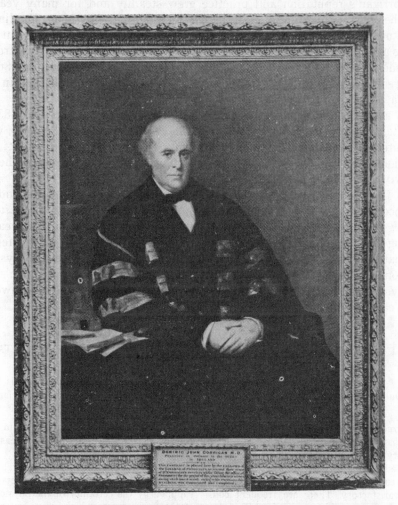

SIR DOMINIC JOHN CORRIGAN (1802-1880)
The portrait by W. Catterson Smith which hangs in the Royal College of
Physicians, Dublin

paper in the *Edinburgh Medical and Surgical Journal* on the "Permanent Patency of the Mouth of the Aorta or Inadequacy of the Aortic Valves," in which he described the typical pulse of aortic insufficiency, the excessive pulsation and the sudden expansion and equally sudden collapse of the arteries. This article contained three neat illustrations showing the morbid appearance of the valves.

Corrigan's great ability was not at first appreciated by his colleagues and when he was first proposed for membership in the Irish College of Physicians, he was blackballed. Later, however, they atoned for their mistake in judgment and not only elected him to membership, but made him their president for five successive terms and had a statue made of him upon his retirement from the presidency.

Corrigan's reputation and practice grew steadily and for many years he was the most popular and most highly remunerated physician Dublin had ever known, his practice exceeding 9000 pounds per annum in fees. In 1847 he was appointed Honorary Physician in ordinary to Queen Victoria in Ireland, an honor never bestowed before upon a Roman Catholic, and in 1866 he was created a baronet. In 1870 he was elected to Parliament. He died in 1880 from a paralytic stroke.

In addition to his paper on aortic insufficiency, he published in 1837 an important paper, *On Aortitis, as One of the Causes of Angina Pectoris,* which antedated by seventy years the well-known views of Sir Clifford Allbutt upon the etiology of this disease. Corrigan's epochal papers were written at the ages of thirty and thirty-five respectively.

In Corrigan's early professional career, when patients were few and fees only occasional, he was much heartened, he tells us, by reading *The Lives of British Physicians, from Linacre to Gooch.* He referred to it in later years as proving that "there is but one road to excellence and success in our profession, and that is by steady, sturdy and hard labour; and you will at least always have this consolation in your dreariest hours of labour, that no proud man's contumely, no insolence of office, nor spurns that patient merit of the unworthy takes, can bar your way."

ART. I.—ON PERMANENT PATENCY OF THE MOUTH OF THE AORTA, OR INADEQUACY OF THE AORTIC VALVES*

By D. J. Corrigan, M.D., one of the Physicians to the Charitable Infirmary, Jervis Street, Dublin; Lecturer on the Theory and Practice of Medicine; Consulting Physician to St. Patrick's College. Maynooth (With Engravings.)

General Symptoms.—On the general symptoms that accompany this disease. little is necessary to be said. Like most of those connected with affections of the respiratory and circulatory organs, they are uncertain and unsatisfactory There are frequent convulsive fits of coughing, more or less dyspnoea. sense of straitness and oppression across the chest, palpitations after exercise, sounds of rushing in the ears, and inability to lie down. Neither one nor all of these symptoms are essential to the disease. They may all arise from varied affections of the lungs, heart, liver or nervous system. They neither tell us the seat of the disease, nor the extent of the danger.

Signs.—What is deficient in general symptoms from their obscurity, is, however, amply supplied by the certainty of the physical and stethoscopic signs, which may be referred to the three following indications. *1st,* Visible pulsation of the arteries of the head and superior extremities. *2nd, Bruit de Soufflet* in the ascending aorta, in the carotids, and subclavians. *3rd, Bruit de Soufflet* and *frémissement,* or a peculiar rushing thrill felt by the finger, in the carotids and subclavians. In conjunction with these may be reckoned the pulse, which is invariably full. When a

* Edinb. Med. & Surg. Jour., 1832, XXXVII, 225.

patient affected by the disease is stripped, the arterial trunks of the head, neck and superior extremities immediately catch the eye by their singular pulsation. At each diastole the subclavian, carotid, temporal brachial and in some cases even the palmar arteries, are suddenly thrown from their bed, bounding up under the skin. The pulsations of these arteries may be observed in a healthy person through a considerable portion of the tract, and become still more marked after exercise or exertion; but in the disease now under consideration, the degree to which vessels are thrown out is excessive. Though a moment before unmarked, they are at each pulsation thrown out on the surface in the strongest relief. From its singular and striking appearance, the name of *visible pulsation* is given to this beating of the arteries. It is accompanied with *bruit de soufflet* in the ascending aorta, carotids, and subclavians; and in the carotids and subclavians, where they can be examined by the finger, there is left *frémissement,* or the peculiar rushing thrill, accompanying with *bruit de soufflet* each diastole of these vessels. These three signs are so intimately connected with the pathological causes of the disease, and arise so directly from the mechanical inadequacy of the valves, that they afford unerring indications of the nature of the disease. In order to understand their value, it is necessary to consider their connection with the cause by which they are produced. The visible pulsation of the arteries of the neck, etc. may first be examined.

In the perfect state of the mechanism at the mouth of the aorta, the semilunar valves, immediately after each contraction of the ventricle, are thrown back across the mouth of the aorta by the pressure of the blood beyond them, and when adequate to their function of closing the mouth of this vessel, they retain in the aorta the blood sent in from the ventricle, thus keeping the aorta and larger vessels distended. These vessels consequently preserve nearly the same bulk during their systole and diastole. But when the semilunar valves, from any of the causes enumerated, became incapable of closing the mouth of the aorta, then after each contraction of the ventricle, a portion of the blood just sent into the aorta, greater or less, according to the degree of the inadequacy of

the valves, turns back into the ventricle. Hence the ascending aorta and arteries arising from it, pouring back a portion of their contained blood, become, after each contraction of the ventricle, flaccid or lessened in their diameter. While they are in this state, the ventricle again contracts and impels quickly into these vessels a quantity of blood, which suddenly and greatly dilates them. The *diastole* of these vessels is thus marked by so sudden and so great an increase of size as to present the visible pulsation which constitutes one of the signs of the disease.

That this visible pulsation of the arteries is owing to the mechanichal cause here assigned is made evident by several circumstances. It is most distinct in the arteries of the head and neck, which empty themselves most easily into the aorta, and of course into the ventricle. In the arteries of the lower extremities, of even larger size than those which present it about the head and neck, it is not seen to any comparative degree, and most generally not at all while the patient is standing or sitting. It is much more marked in the arteries of the head and neck in the erect than in the horizontal posture; and a patient suffering under the disease himself, first pointed out a circumstance which is convincing of its being produced as asserted. He would increase the pulsation of the brachial and palmar arteries in a most striking degree by merely elevating his arms to a perpendicular position above his head. He thus enabled the brachial and palmar arteries to empty themselves more easily back upon the aorta. They became more flaccid, and then, on the next contraction of the ventricle, their diastole became comparatively greater, and their visible pulsation of course more marked. The same effect could be produced in the arteries of the lower extremities by lying down and elevating the legs on an inclined plane. The strength of the heart has little to do in producing this singular pulsation, for it is never observed in an equal degree, and most generally not at all, in the arteries of the lower extremities.

If it be asked, is the explanation here adduced of the cause of this visible pulsation sufficient to account for its appearance in the brachial and radial arteries, since the blood to return back from these vessels into the arch of the aorta should flow upward when the patient holds his arms in the ordinary position, flexed or hanging by his side? The following reply may be made. When the subclavians are pouring back their blood into the arch of the aorta and ventricle, the elasticity of the brachial arteries, acting upon the blood just urged into them, forces it back along with the retrograde current of the subclavians, no obstacle meeting it in that direction. The brachial arteries thus partially empty themselves, and become in their systole of a lessened diameter like the carotids and subclavians, but in less degree. The next jet of blood from the ventricles dilates them, and as in the subclavians, produces in them a visible pulsation: and if they be assisted in returning their blood by elevating the arms to a perpendicular position, their pulsation becomes, as has been already observed, much more strongly marked. The arteries of the lower extremities are not similarly circumscribed. The arteries of the upper extremities are assisted in emptying themselves back towards the heart, by the retrograde current in the subclavians and ascending aorta; but on the blood contained in the arteries of the lower extremities, the tall column of blood in the descending aorta is pressing, and prevents any return; or if it be supposed that of the large mass of blood in the descending aorta, a small portion flows back into the arch, it can produce little change in the contents of the iliacs and femorals; and moreover, whether the column of blood in the aorta be lessened or not in diameter, the pressure on the contained blood of the iliacs and femorals will remain the same, and keep these vessels distended. If we, however, as already observed, alter the relation of the several arteries to the arch of the aorta, so as to facilitate the reflux of their contained blood, for instance from the radial arteries, by raising the arms to a perpendicular line above the head, from the iliacs and femorals, by placing the patient in a recumbent posture, and raising the legs upwards on an inclined plane, the visible pulsation becomes more marked in these respective arteries.

The *bruit de soufflet*, which is heard in the ascending aorta, carotids, and subclavians, with the accompanying *frémissement* in the latter arteries, is next to be considered. The *bruit de soufflet* characterizing this disease, is heard, as already observed, in the ascending aorta, its arch, and in the carotids and suh-clavians. It can be followed upwards from the fourth rib along the course of the aorta, increasing in loudness as it ascends, until it is heard of great intensity at the upper part of the sternum, where the arch of the aorta most nearly approaches this bone, and then branching to the right and left, it can be traced into the carotids and subclavians of both sides; and in these trunks it assumes a harshness that it did not passess in the aorta. This *bruit de soufflet* is synchronous with the visible pulsation, with the diastole of the arteries. It is of no consequence whether the ascending aorta and its large branches be sound or be diseased; the *bruit de soufflet* is as loud in the one case as in the other. To account for the presence of this sign, and why it extends so far from the seat of the disease and along sound vessels, it is necessary to refer to a paper published in the Lancet of 1829, Vol. ii, p. 1. Continued observations from the date of that paper to the present, have confirmed the view then taken of the cause of that singular sound; of its being dependent purely on a physical cause, on a mechanical change in the manner of the blood's flowing.

In that paper is related an experiment, which it may be well to recapitulate here. A flexible tube, such as a piece of small intestine, or a portion of artery, is connected by one end with a tube which has a current of water of considerable force running through it. While the piece of intestine or artery is kept fully distended by the supply of water from the tube, no sound is produced by the motion of the fluid; but if the flexible tube, while the fluid is moving through it, be pressed upon in any part, so that the quantity of fluid passing through the contracted part is no longer sufficient to keep the further portion of the tube tense, then, beyond the contracted part, where the tube is less tense, or in some degree flaccid, a distinct, and, according to the velocity or force of the current, a loud *bruit de soufflet* is heard; and, at the same time, if the finger be gently laid upon the part of the tube where the *bruit de soufflet* is heard, a slight trembling of the tube is perceived, evidently arising from the vibrations into which the current within is throwing its sides. If, in place of constricting any one part of the flexible tube, the whole tract of tube be allowed to become partially flaccid, by diminishing the supply of fluid, and the fluid be then allowed to rush along the tube by jets, at each jet the tube is suddenly distended, resembling the visible pulsation described above; and with each diastole of the tube, there is a sudden and loud *bruit de soufflet;* and, synchronous with the *bruit de soufflet,* there is *frémissement* felt by the finger.

Both the sound heard and the sensation felt by the finger in this experiment may be explained by the principles which regulate the motion of the fluids. It may be remarked, that it is a property of fluid in motion, that, when discharging itself from the orfice of a tube into open space, or into a vessel of wider capacity not fully distended, its particles move in lines from the orfice, like so many *radii* tending to leave vacuums between them. When the flexible tube, artery, or intestine, therefore, is kept fully distended, the fluid moves forward as a mass, there is no tendency in its particles to separate from one another,—they all press equally,—there is no vibratory motion of the sides of the tube, and consequently no sound, no *frémissement* or trembling. But if the tube be not kept fully distended, then the fluid propelled through it rushes along as a current; and its particles tending to leave vacuums between them, throw the sides of the tube into vibrations, which can be very distinctly felt by the finger, and which give to the ear the peculiar sound *bruit de soufflet,* and to the touch *frémissement.*

These principles may be applied to the state of the ascending aorta and its branches in the instances before us. When the aortic valves are fully adequate to their function of perfectly closing the mouth of the aorta, and thus preventing any regurgitation of the blood, the aorta and its branches are kept fully distended, the blood is at each contraction of the ventricle propelled forward *en masse,* and there is no trembling, or vibratory motion of the sides of the aorta, carotids, and subclavians, and, as in the flexible tube when fully distended, no sound is emitted. But when the valves, becoming inadequate to their office, permit some of the blood contained in the ascending aorta, carotids, and subclavians, to return into the left ventricle after each contraction, then the aorta and these trunks become, like the flexible tube in the second part of the experiment, partially flaccid; and at the next contraction of the ventricle, the blood propelled into them is sent along as a rushing current, which throws the sides of these arteries into vibrations, and these vibrations give to the ear *bruit de soufflet,* and to the finger *frémissement.* These two signs may be traced to a varying distance from the mouth of the aorta, and also along the carotids, and to the outer third of the subclavians, and sometimes in the brachial arteries, as far as the bend in the arms, the distance to which they are heard being determined by the limit to which the current-like motion of the blood producing them is extended. In these cases in which the deficiency of the valves is considerable, allowing a full stream of blood to rush back into the ventricle, there is heard in the ascending aorta a double *bruit;* the first accompanying the *diastole* of the artery, the second immediately succeeding; and, in listening to the two sounds constituting this double *bruit de soufflet,* the impression made distinctly on the ear is, that the first sound is from a rushing of it back into the ventricle. It is impossible for those who have not heard this double *bruit* to conceive the distinctness with which the impression described is made on the ear. A patient in one instance heard this double sound distinctly in his own person, and referred it to its cause, a rushing of blood *from* and *to* the heart. The *bruit de soufflet* and *frémissement* are not perceived in the arteries of the lower extremities, when the patient is in a sitting or standing posture. The pressure of the blood in the abdominal aorta is sufficient in these postures to keep the vessels arising from it fully distended; and thus no vibratory motion of their parieties being permitted, there is no bellows sound, nor *frémissement* or rushing thrill.

Austin Flint

Austin Flint's name has been handed down to posterity linked with the names of Laënnec, Skoda, and Piorry. And rightly so, for he was one of that small band of pioneers who appreciated the great discovery of Laënnec and enriched it by his own studies.

Austin Flint was born at Petersham, Massachusetts, October 20, 1812. At Harvard Medical School, he was fortunate in having as teachers Jacob Bigelow and James Jackson. Jackson at that time, although about to retire, had taken up Laënnec's discovery in earnest and was rarely seen without his

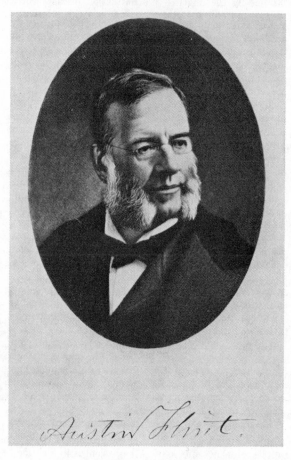

AUSTIN FLINT (1812-1886)
From William B. Atkinson's *Physicians and Surgeons of the United States*, Charles Robson, Philadelphia, 1878

stethoscope. Jackson's influence was a powerful stimulus to young Flint. Flint, unlike many of his colleagues, did not study in Europe. He advised young students not to go to Paris, then the medical Mecca, using, among other arguments, that there was much vice there and that the French language was difficult to learn. Flint, during the course of his professional life, practised and lectured in no less than six widely separated localities, among them New York City, Buffalo, Louisville, and New Orleans. In 1833, he began to record his medical experiences and continued to do so for more than half a century, leaving records covering 16,922 folio pages of manuscript written in the author's own hand.

Flint is perhaps best remembered in connection with what we still term "Flint's murmur," which he observed in a patient in 1860. This discovery was first published in 1862 and an extract of this article follows. It will be seen that what Flint calls a direct mitral murmur is a murmur which he describes elsewhere in the same article as "a presystolic murmur"; this name expresses its proper relation to the heart sounds, and it is the only murmur which does occur in that particular relation. He says furthermore, "The mitral direct murmur . . . always continues up to the first sound, and instead of losing any of its intensity, it becomes more intense, and appears to be abruptly arrested, in its greatest intensity when the first sound occurs." Flint's explanation of this murmur follows his description. It is a matter of interest that Vaquez in his "Maladies du Coeur," after reviewing the various theories regarding the production of this murmur, finds the original theory of Flint the most plausible.

Austin Flint died in 1886. No man has had greater influence upon the medicine of this country.

ART. II.—ON CARDIAC MURMURS

By Austin Flint, M.D., Prof. of the Principles and Practice of Medicine in the Bellevue Hospital Medical College, N.Y., and in the Long Island College Hospital*

So much for the reality of the mitral direct murmur and the means of discriminating it from other murmurs. It remains to consider another important practical point, viz., the pathological import of this murmur. As already stated, it is developed in connection with a contracted mitral orfice, and, so far as my experience goes, especially in connection with contraction caused by adherence of the mitral curtains, forming the *buttonhole slit;* the murmur, then, being due, not to the passage of blood over a roughened surface, but to the vibration of the curtains. And the sound, as thus produced, is peculiar, resembling the sound which may be produced, in an analogous manner, by causing the lips to vibrate with an expiratory puff. The murmur, however, may be produced with the flowing of the current of blood over a roughened surface, without contraction of the aperture. This is undoubtedly rare. As a rule, the force of the mitral direct current is not sufficient to develop a murmur unless there be mitral contraction. Is this murmur ever produced without any mitral lesions? One would *a priori* suppose the answer of this question to be in the negative. Clinical observation, however, shows that the question

is to be answered in the affirmative. I have met with two cases in which a well-marked mitral direct murmur existed, and after death in one of the cases no mitral lesions were found; in the other case, the lesion was insignificant. I will proceed to give an account of these cases, and then endeavor to explain the occurrence of the murmur.

Case 1.[1] In May, 1860, I examined a patient, aged 56, who had had repeated attacks of palpitation, sense of suffocation, with expectoration of bloody mucus and a feeling of impending dissolution, but without pain, the paroxysms resembling angina, except the absence of pain. In the intervals between these attacks he was free from palpitation, did not suffer from want of breath on active exercise, and considered himself in good health. He had never had rheumatism. On examination of the chest, the heart was found to be enlarged, the enlargement being evidently by hypertrophy. At the apex was a pre-systolic blubbering murmur, which I then supposed to be characteristic of the button-hole contraction of mitral orifice. At the base of the heart was an aortic regurgitant murmur, which was diffused over nearly the whole praecordia. There was no systolic mur-

* *Am. J. M. Sc.,* 1862, XLIV, N.S., 29.

[1] Private Records, vol. x, p. 713.

mur at the base or apex. Three days after this examination the patient was attacked with another paroxysm, and died in a few moments after the attack, sitting in his chair. The heart was enlarged, weighing 16½ oz., the walls of the left ventricle measuring 4/5ths of an inch. The aorta was atheromatous, and dilated so as to render the valvular segments evidently insufficient. The mitral valve presented nothing abnormal, save a few small vegetations at the base of the curtains, as seen from the auricular aspect of the orifice.

In this case, it is assumed that the mitral direct murmur, which was loud and of the blubbering character, was not due to the minute vegetations which were found after death. There was no mitral contraction. The mitral valve was unimpaired, so that the murmur could not have been due to mitral regurgitation.

Case 2.[2] In February, 1861, I was requested to determine the murmur in a case at the Charity Hospital, New Orleans. I found an aortic direct and an aortic regurgitant murmur, both murmurs being well marked. There was also a distinct pre-systolic murmur within the apex, having the blubbering character. On the examination after death, the aorta was dilated and roughened with atheroma and calcareous deposit. The aortic segments were contracted, and evidently insufficient. The mitral curtains presented no lesions; the mitral orifice was neither contracted nor dilated, and the valve was evidently sufficient. The heart was considerably enlarged, weighing 17½ oz., and the walls of the left ventricle were an inch in thickness.

In the second, as in the first of the foregoing cases, it is evident that a mitral systolic murmur was not mistaken for a mitral direct murmur, for in both cases, the condition of mitral systolic murmur were not present. In both cases the mitral direct murmur was loud and had that character of sound which I suppose to be due to vibration of the mitral curtains. In both cases, it will be oserved, an aortic regurgitant murmur existed, and aortic insufficiency was found to exist post mortem. How is the occurrence of the mitral direct murmur in these cases to be explained? I shall give an explanation which is to my mind satisfactory.

The explanation involves a point connected

[2] *Ibid.,* vol. XI, p. 241.

with the physiological action of the auricular valves. Experiments show that when the ventricles are filled with a liquid, the valvular curtains are floated away from the ventricular sides, approximating to each other and tending to closure of the auricular orifice. In fact, as first shown by Drs. Baumgarten and Hamernik, of Germany, a forcible injection of liquid into the left ventricle through the auricular opening will cause a complete closure of this opening by the coaptation of the mitral curtains, so that these authors contend that the natural closure of the auricular orifices is effected, not by the contraction of the ventricles, but by the forcible current of blood propelled into the ventricles by the auricles. However this may be, that the mitral curtains are floated out and brought into apposition to each other by simply distending the ventricular cavity with liquid, is a fact sufficiently established and easily verified. Now in cases of considerable aortic insufficiency, the left ventricle is rapidly filled with blood flowing back from the aorta as well as from the auricle, before the auricular contraction takes place. The distention of the ventricle is such that the mitral curtains are brought into coaptation, and when the auricular contraction takes place the mitral direct current passing between the curtains throws them into vibration and gives rise to the characteristic blubbering murmur. The physical condition is in effect analogous to contraction of the mitral orifice from an adhesion of the curtains at their sides, the latter condition, as clinical observation abundantly proves, giving rise to a mitral direct murmur of a similar character.

A mitral direct murmur, then, may exist without mitral contraction and without any mitral lesions, provided there be aortic lesions involving considerable aortic regurgitation. This murmur by no means accompanies aortic regurgitation lesions as a rule; we meet with an aortic regurgitant murmur frequently when not accompanied by the mitral direct murmur. The circumstances which may be required to develop, functionally, the latter murmur, in addition to the amount of aortic regurgitation, remain to be ascertained. Probably enlargement of the left ventricle is one condition. The practical conclusion to be drawn from the two cases which have been given is, that a mitral direct murmur in a case presenting an aortic regurgitant murmur and cardiac enlargement, is not positive proof of the existence of mitral contraction or of any mitral lesions. The coexistence of a murmur denoting mitral regurgitation, in such a case, should be considered as rendering it probable that the mitral direct murmur is due to contraction or other lesions, and not functional.

Heinrich Quincke

ɪʏ. OBSERVATIONS ON CAPILLARY AND VENOUS PULSE

By Dr. H. Quincke,* Assistant in the Medical Clinic, Berlin

It is a well known principal in physiology that the pulsation in the arterial system which originates in the heart, extends to the smallest arteries, and that the blood stream in the capillaries, is not in the same manner influenced by the heart beat. This view is based largely on microscopical observation of the capillary stream in the mesentery of different animals, in the swim bladder of the frog, and the web of the bat. Only when the flow of blood in the veins is diminished or when there is a very marked lowering of the arterial pressure and slowness of the heart beat, such as take place during the death of an animal, does one notice a pulsatile movement of the blood in the capillaries.

There is only a single such observation of Lebert (*Handbuch der praktischen Medizen* I. p. 725), who saw in a case of aneurysm of the aorta, systolic reddening and diastolic paling of the cheeks, that is, a true capillary pulse.

Claude Bernard noticed a transmission of the pulse to the vessels of the submaxillary gland through the capillaries, clear in the draining veins when, after cutting of the sympathetic, stimulation of the lingual branch, produced dilatation of the arteries.

As far as man is concerned, there are only a few observations made on the venous pulse by King, which were referred to briefly by Stokes in his Diseases of the Heart. The original article is in Guy's Hospital Reports, IV, XII, which, unfortunately, are not accessible.

However, there are certain places in the human body which, under normal conditions, but more clearly still in abnormal states, show a transmission of the pulse wave clear out to the capillaries and then into the veins: such areas are—the finger nails, the hand, forearm and foot.

As far as the capillary pulse is concerned, so can one see it best on his own finger nail, or better, on that of another, in the area be-

* *Berl. Klin. Wchnschr.*, 1868, v, 357.

tween the whitish, blood-poor area and the red injected part of the capillary system of the nail-bed; in the majority of persons examined, there is, with each heart-beat, a forward and backward movement of the margin between the red and white part, and he can convince himself that the increase of the redness follows a moment later than the apex beat and is still clearly systolic and rather rapid, while the backward movement of the edge of the redness seems to take place more slowly. That is, a lingering in the wave which can be seen by the eye, just as palpation and the sphygmograph show it in the pulse waves of the radial artery.

But the finger nails of everyone do not show this white zone; with general full-bloodedness, strong and frequent heart action and high blood-pressure, in warm air the nails are not evenly reddened. Under these conditions, a clear zone on the nails can be produced by an even pressure, or, better still, by holding the hands up in the air; with the latter manipulation we have at the same time, the advantage that the blood-pressure in the vessels of the arms falls, and the increased pressure (with uniform cardiac action) which the blood has with every heart-beat is greater than the average pressure which shows when the hand is not raised.

Similar conditions, which are produced by elevating the hands, increase of anemic area of the nails and reduction of arterial pressure, occur generally in anemic persons: therefore in such the capillary pulse is usually clearer and also visible without elevating the arm: however, the activity of the heart must not be diminished, and for this reason it is clearest in mild chlorosis and not in convalescents from severe diseases.

Powerful and sudden heart contractions are favorable for observing the capillary pulse, while hypertension and tachycardia are unfavorable. The clearness of the capillary pulse in fever and excitement depends upon the predominance of these factors.

A large and rapidly falling pulse is seen especially in aortic insufficiency, and for this reason the capillary pulse is especially clear in this condition. Even in a horizontal position of the hand we see a very clear and rapid appearance and disappearance of the margin between the red and white zone and also with an uniform coloration of the nail and lightninglike and evanescent reddening, so that the manner of the appearance and disappearance of the capillary pulse is, for the eye, a characteristic sign of active visibility of the capillary pulse in health, and in addition the transparency of the nails and the proper degree of elasticity of the arteries must be considered.

It is, in general, impossible to state upon which finger nail the phenomenon is clearest, but usually, it seems to me, the index finger is best. The white zone is present usually in the third portion of the finger nail, reckoning from the nail root, and the pulsation is somewhat clearer upon the upper portion, at other times, in the lower portion.

Up to the present time I have not observed the capillary pulse in the toe nail: the cause being probably the weakening of the pulse wave in the long artery and the marked hardness and thickness of the nails.

Of importance in the production of the capillary pulse in the nail-bed, is the observation of Kölliker, that the average diameter of the capillaries is 0.005-0.008, while elsewhere in the body it is only .002-.006.

I have succeeded only a few times recently in observing a transmission of the pulse wave through the capillaries into the veins in individuals without valvular lesions. The first object of observation was my own hand. I saw, several times, after the veins on the back of my hand were dilated markedly from heat, a weak but undoubted post systolic pulsation.

Much clearer was the venous pulse in a fifty year old woman, who came to the hospital because of cholelithiasis. She had never suffered from palpitation of the heart, the heart tones were clear: there was perhaps a slight hypertrophy of the left ventricle, but this could not be established without certainty, because of the unusually rigid thorax. The palpable arteries were somewhat rigid, the pulse full, rather resistant, the pulse waves not particularly short but rapidly falling away. Here was seen an extraordinary clear pulse in the distended and prominent veins of the very thin, relaxed skin of the back of the hand, as well as in the anastamoses in the middle of the forearm, the pulse following the radial pulse and even more evidently after the counted pulse. The capillary pulse in the nails was here, also, very striking.

A third case of venous pulse which I observed quite recently was in a strong young man who, in diving into water, struck his head on the bottom and suffered a paralysis of all the spinal nerves emerging below the fourth cervical vertebra (the autopsy showed a fracture of the vertebra, with destruction of the cervical cord). In the veins of the back of the hand extending to the middle of the forearm, a post systolic pulsation could be clearly seen. Here we were dealing most probably with a paralysis of vasomotor nerves, which, together with the high temperature, produced a dilation of the vessels causing the venous pulse. Here, there is an analogy with the pulse produced in Bernard's experiment of the salivary glands.

Besides these three cases there were also cases of the aortic insufficiency, in which the forceful and rapid pulse wave was propagated to the veins, indeed I noted this recently in four cases I had an opportunity of examining. To be sure, not always with the same clearness, for here, as in the production of the capillary pulse, certain conditions are necessary: the skin must be very thin and relaxed (especially not edematous), the veins must be filled to a certain degree and not under tension, also elevation of the arms or obstruction of the veins can cause the venous pulse in the hand to disappear.

In several of these cases of venous pulse, the centripetal direction of the waves can be clearly demonstrated by comparison of the veins on the back of the hand. Peripherally from the compressed area the pulse continues, centrally it disappears, then reappears when the compression is withdrawn. Compression of the brachial artery (without obstruction of the venous flow) abolishes regularly the venous pulse on the back of the hand.

Aside from the hand and forearm, the venous pulse was observed only once elsewhere, and on the back of the feet. This was the first case of venous pulse a tergo and was observed in the medical clinic of Dr. Riess. It was found in a fifteen year old girl, poorly developed and highly chlorotic, who suffered possibly from heart disease, which, as often, in the patient, could not be diagnosed with certainty: there was a loud systolic murmur heard all over the heart, loudest over the pulmonary artery and aorta: also there was a moderate hypertrophy of both ventricles. There was probably a communication between the aorta and pulmonary artery. The arterial pulse was soft, somewhat rapid, often whining when the arm was raised. In the remarkably stretched-out venous network of the pale, paper-thin skin on the backs of both hands and foot, there was a full, even palpable pulse, which disappeared completely with the gradual disappearance of the chlorosis and the improvement in her nutrition.

Lately I had an opportunity of observing the capillary pulse in still another place besides the finger nails, namely in the retina, and it was in one of the two cases of aortic insufficiency already mentioned, in a man who is still under my observation. In addition to a remarkably strong arterial pulse in the retina, which extends far beyond the papilla, he showed in both eyes, on ophthalmoscopic examination when standing, an uniform reddening and diastolic pallor of the papilla, which was due to an alternating strong and weak filling of the capillary net: The color change was seen most clearly in the middle, bordering on the physiological cupping, whereas in the finger nails, the border between red and less red moved with the pulse. The capillary pulse could not be seen beyond the border of the papilla, even if present, since here the color changes, because of the dark background of the chorois was not so sharp. Moreover, neither of the eyes showed any other abnormality as a basis for the pulsations.

The diastolic pulse of the central vein of the retina, which is often present normally, was seen here with great intensity; since the origin of this pulsation has not yet been entirely explained, and is probably not due to propagation through the capillaries, this pulse will not be considered further here.

From the above observation, it is seen that the pulse wave which originates in the left heart, is not so general as supposed and disappears in the small arteries. Under proper conditions, only partly pathological, at times on the limits of the normal, the wave is propagated through the capillaries, even into the veins; and it is also probable that the capillary pulse can be observed in other places than those mentioned; for example, in organs filled with blood, such as the spleen and kidneys. The hands are a good place for observing it, partly because of the superficial position of the capillary and nervous network and also because the peripheral portions have a side blood supply and relatively broad arteries: the marked change in volume when hot or cold, shows how remarkably good the blood supply is.

I wish to express my best thanks to Geheimrath Frerichs for his liberality in turning over the material in his clinic for these observations.

Paul-Louis Duroziez

Paul-Louis Duroziez was born at Paris in 1826 and received his doctor's degree in 1853. While still a medical student he won the Corvisart Prize for a dissertation on the therapeutic properties and physiological action of digitalis. In 1856, he became chief of the clinic at the Charité and in 1870 served as an army surgeon in the Franco-Prussian War. In 1882, he was elected president of the Society of Medicine and in 1895 was made Chevalier of the Legion of Honor. Duroziez died in 1897 at the age of seventy-one.

Duroziez was never professor at the medical school and never had a service in any of the great hospitals of Paris. "Although he had no hospital service of his own, the doors of all the hospitals were open to him." He was a general practitioner, a remarkably keen observer, a simple and gentle man who sought no honor or preferment but whose name was honored throughout the medical world. His *Traité Clinique des Maladies du Cœur,* which appeared in 1891, received universal acclaim, and for it he received the Itard Prize of the Academy of Medicine and the Montjou Prize of the Institut de France.

Duroziez is remembered for his description of pure mitral stenosis, "Duroziez's disease," the presystolic rumble, and reduplication of the second heart sound, but especially for his description of the double femoral murmur, "Duroziez's sign," in aortic insufficiency. The following selection is the summary of his article which describes in detail a series of patients in whom this sign was either present or absent.

CONCERNING THE DOUBLE INTERMITTENT CRURAL SOUFFLE AS A SIGN OF AORTIC INSUFFICIENCY*

By Dr. P. Duroziez, former chief of the clinic of the faculty at the Charité Hospital
(Service of Professor Bouillaud)

CONCLUSIONS

1. The double intermittent crural murmur noted by many authors in aortic insufficiency has never, at least in my knowledge, been given as a constant sign of this lesion.

2. Most commonly it is not present and it is necessary to produce it by means of compression.

3. In aortic insufficiency, the blood carried by the left ventricle almost to the extremities, flows back from the extremities towards the heart, repulsed by the arteries of the periphery and forced by the left ventricle.

4. The finger, pressing the artery about 2 cm. above the stethoscope produces the first sound; 2 cm. below the instrument, the second murmur is produced.

5. The secondary murmurs which can be produced by lesions of the pericardium, by stenosis of the myocardial orifices, by stenosis of the right auriculo-ventriculo orifices, by insufficiency of the pulmonary artery, can be separated from the murmur of aortic in-

*Arch. Gén. de Méd., 1861, Avril, 417.

sufficiency by aid of the double crural murmur, which does not exist except in this last lesion.

6. If aortic insufficiency is combined with one or more of the lesions indicated below, and when a diagnosis of it becomes on this account very difficult, the crural sign will aid a great deal, indeed will make certain the diagnosis.

7. The crural sign distinguishes perhaps less well between the lesions of the aortic orifice and lesions of the aorta. The double murmur can appear in certain aneurysms without insufficiency at autopsy.

8. The temporary insufficiency can be demonstrated by an intermittent murmur.

9. The continuous murmur can pass through the arteries when it is never heard in aortic insufficiency with a double constant intermittent crural murmur.

10. The double crural intermittent murmur is present in typhoid fever, chlorosis and lead toxication, etc., but transitory; it is soon replaced by a constant murmur.

MITRAL STENOSIS

Raymond Vieussens

CHAPTER XVI

CONCERNING THE STRUCTURE OF THE INTERNAL SURFACE OF THE LEFT VENTRICLE OF THE HEART*

The left ventricle of the Heart has, like the right, two large openings in its base, of which one should be regarded as its mouth,

*Vieussens, Raymond, Traité nouveau de la structure et des causes du mouvement naturel du cœur, Toulouse, Guillemette, 1715, p. 101.

& the other as the mouth of the aorta. After having opened this ventricle, we find in its cavity, as in that of the right ventricle, a membranous substance, very thin, supplied at the base with many small round ligaments, tendinous, which are united one

Description of the triglossal valves & the columnae carneae of the left ventricular heart and their functions

with the other & which are inserted on the superior part of the three unequal eminences to which one has given the name of columnae carneae. (See second figure of the tenth plate.) Although this membranous body is not divided at its apex, the first anatomists who described it, seeing that the tendinous ligaments were inserted at the summit of the three columnae carneae, did not fail to divide them into three valves which they called triglossal (mitral). These valves are very closely united at the top of the internal surface of the tendon which occupies the superior part of the mouth of the left ventricle, & is nourished by the lymph, drawn from the blood which the muscular ducts carry, which are very numerous in this tendon, they prevent the blood carried by the blood-vessels of the lung into the cavity of the ventricle from entering these vessels: & consequently this blood is obliged to enter into the aorta while the Heart contracts. I will not waste time in explaining the manner in which they carry out the function which I have just attributed to them, because it is very easy to understand this from what I have said in the preceding Chapter, in explaining here the function of the mitral valves of the left ventricle.

I will say in passing, that the lymph which nourishes the mitral valves of the left ventricle, is sometimes found so filled with earthy saline particles that they become bony, as it will appear from the very rare observation I am going to report, after having finished the history of the disease, which has given me occasion to report it. Master Thomas d'Assis, apothecary, native of the place of Florensac in Gascony, Diocese of Auch, age thirty years or therabouts, with a sanguine, melancholy temperament, had dysentery at Paris in the month of August of the year 1705. He was cured of it by the use of ipecac; but soon afterwards his legs commenced to swell up, respiration became very difficult, & he had a slow fever. As the remedies which were ordered for him brought no relief to his trouble, he believed that his native air would help in the re-establishment of his health.

The triglossal valves of the left ventricle sometimes become bony

History of the malady of Thomas d'Assis, apothecary

Buoyed up by this pleasant hope, he departed from Paris for his home in the beginning of the month of October & arrived at Montpellier & finding himself without money, he asked to be taken to the Hospital Saint Eloi. As soon as he had been admitted, he asked me through one of his friends to come to see him; after which he told me that which I have just recorded, I examined his condition; he was lying on his bed, his head quite high; his respiration seemed to me very difficult, his Heart was working with a very violent palpitation; his pulse appeared very small, feeble & quite unequal, his lips were the color of lead and his eyes sunken; & his legs & his hips were swollen; & rather cold than hot. After I had examined with attention all of the symptoms above reported & had sought for every cause, I said to M. Deidier, my son-in-law, the very worthy Professor of Medicine, with whom I consulted in regard to this patient, that I did not doubt but that he had a hydrops of the chest, of which he would certainly die in a few days; I added that the violence of the palpitation of the Heart, & the circumstances which accompanied it, persuaded me that there was some change which I did not understand in the tissue of some part of this organ, which had produced the disease of this young man: My diagnosis and my prognosis were true, as will appear from what follows.

The patient died the fifteenth of November of the same year; I opened his body on the morrow, in the presence of M. Diedier, & of several Students of Medicine: the sternum having been separated from the ribs and thrown back above, we saw that the entire cavity of the chest was filled with a yellow serous fluid; the lungs were extraordinarily large & soft, because all of its tissue was soaked with an aqueous lymph; the posterior portion of the left side appeared to us to be inflamed. After having recognized the condition of the lung, I removed the Heart with the trunks of the blood-vessels from the cavity of the chest, in order to examine all of their parts; its size was so extraordinary, that it approached that of a beef's Heart: the coronary veins & all of their branches were very much dilated;

All the unusual things observed in the Heart of Thomas d'Assis the cavity of the right ventricle & the right auricle were very large. (See figure on the twelfth plate.)

When I had opened the right ventricle to study its excessive dilatation, I examined with a great deal of attention the tissue of internal surfaces, & in examining it, I noticed in the first place, that the size of the columnae carneae & the trabeculae carneae, which formed the sides of the fossa, surpassed a great deal their natural size. I observed in the second place that the usual openings of this ventricle had been so markedly dilated, that they had become very evident, & that the membrane which covered them, had been so distended, that it allowed the blood which came from it to pass freely: the sheaves of the canals, which form the sides of the fossa of the right auricle, had become extraordinarily large: The usual openings of this auricle had become markedly dilated, as well as the pores of the delicate membrane which covered it: so that pressing in the valves on the walls of the right ventricle or those on the right auricle, the blood ran from the holes of their interior surface, which I have called the usual openings. There is no reason to doubt that these openings such as I have described are in the Heart of all men.

I did not find any sinus on the internal margin of the anterior part of the roof of the right auricle, but I discovered here a large number of common openings which was sufficient in the absence of this

The venous sinus the right auricle

sinus. I remarked again that a portion of the vena cava where these two trunks appear was markedly dilated, & that more of

its surface had become so large that blood was easily brought forth when I pressed with the fingers. One could estimate the excessive dilatation of that part of the vena cava, of which I have just spoken, by that of the fossa, on which one could see the Isthmal vein, of which the trunk & the branches had become excessively large. Although the tissues of the walls of the arteries were very thin, & consequently less supple than that of the walls of the veins, the trunk of the pulmonary artery could not have dilated very much, and stretched also very much the sigmoid valves. (See figure of the twelfth plate.)

Great as was the dilation of the part of the vena cava where the two trunks join; it

was not however as remarkable as that of the pulmonary vein, which one can see in the first figure of the thirteenth plate. In proportion as the trunk of this vein was excessively dilated, the common openings became larger, & the left auricle was also dilated in such a manner that finally the fossa disappeared, if you will except a few of those at the tip. In examining the extraordinary dilatation of the body of the pulmonary vein, & of its common openings, I perceived that the mouth of the left ventricle appeared very small, and that it had an oval oblong shape; & in searching for the cause of such a surprising fact, I discovered that the mitral valves of this ventricle were really bony, & realized that as they became hardened, they would become thickened and rough enough to cause a marked narrowing of the lumen, & give a picture such as is represented in the figures of the plate indicated below.

After having examined well the trunk of the pulmonary vein, I opened the left ventricle, & I discovered here first that which I have just pointed

The branches of the columnae carneae of the left ventricle had some of them become very small without losing their natural color; others had taken on the form of tendinous pale ligaments & why?

out: namely, that the substance of the mitral valves has become bony, & that it had very markedly diminished, & indeed changed the natural appearance of its lumen: I observed in the second place that the bundles of the columnae carneae which formed the sides of the fossae of this ventricle, had lost, some of them, much of their natural size, because they did not receive as much blood as they had been accustomed to receive before the mitral valves were changed into a bony substance, & others not receiving any at all, had become pale, & had taken the form

of small tendinous ligaments very little like those of the mitral valve. (See the second figure of the thirteenth plate.)

The lumen of the left ventricle being markedly narrowed, & its margin having lost all of its natural suppleness, blood could no more enter freely & as abundantly as it should have into the cavity of this ventricle: so that in the beginning the circulation was impaired, it commenced to dilate extraordinarily the pulmonary vein, because the blood remained too long & accumulated in too large an amount. The blood had no longer commenced to make too long a stay in the trunk of this vein, than it retarded the course of that in all the blood-vessels of the lungs: so that the branches of the pulmonary artery and pulmonary vein extending throughout all the tissue of this organ, were always too full of blood, & consequently so dilated that they compressed the vesicles, interfered with the free entrance of air or prevented it from leaving freely; that is why the patient always breathed with a great deal of difficulty. As the blood thickened considerably in the lung because of its stay in the blood vessels, its serous portion separated little by little & fell into the cavity of the chest.

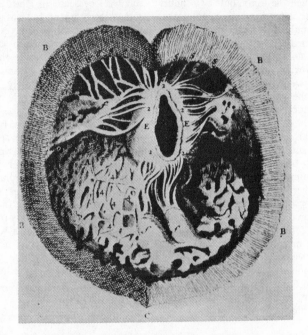

An illustration of mitral stenosis from Vieussen's *Traité nouveau de la structure et des causes du mouvement naturel du cœur* (Toulouse, 1715)

Explanation of the second figure of the thirteenth plate.

A.A.	The left ventricle of the Heart of Thomas D'Assis.		internal surface.
BBBB.	The thickness of its walls.	44444	Several small bundles of the trabeculae carneae of the right & inferior part of the cavity of the left ventricle, changed into small tendinous bodies.
C.	The apex of the Heart.		
D.	The opening of the left ventricle.		
E.E.	Mitral valves changed into an osseus substance.		
ffff	Four trabeculae carneae attached to the internal surface.	555555&c	Several other small bundles of trabeculae carneae of the superior part of the same cavity, also changed into small tendinous bodies.
22222	The tendinous ligaments by which the trabeculae are attached to the		

Giovanni Battista Morgagni[*]
BOOK I. OF DISEASES OF THE HEAD. LETTER III

Peter Fasolati, an engraver, at Padua, in

the sixty-second year of his age, yet still of a full habit, and liable to no indispositon, died at the very same season as Tita[(m)] and

* Morgagni, J. B., *The Seats and Causes of Disease*, translated by Benjamin Alexander, M.D., London, Millar and Cadell, 1769 I, p. 59.

[m] Vide supra n. 11.

even the very day after him in the following manner. He had gone through no labour, had not been troubled with care and anxiety, as he had been us'd at other times, and made no complaint of any thing. He had even supp'd heartily, for he always us'd to eat freely; and desir'd to go to bed more early than usual, which he did: but two hours afterwards, his wife happening to wake, found him not only dead but even cold, and stretch'd out in the same manner he had lay'd himself when he went to bed.

The day following, when the integuments of the cranium were cut into, and while the upper part of the skull was saw'd through, and taken off, much blood was dicharg'd. Yet there was none at all extravasated within the skull; none in the substance of the cerebrum, or cerebellum, and both these parts seem'd to the touch to be perfectly natural: there was, I say, nothing ruptur'd, nothing injur'd in any part. There was some water in the lateral ventricles almost limpid, but in small quantity, and some also seem'd to flow from the sides of the cerebellum, which was found, as I have said, or might it not come from the tube of the vertebrae? But such a quantity of fluid blood distended all the vessels in and about the brain, that I do not remember to have seen the like before: even some small vessels, which us'd to be scarcely per-

ceptible, were extremely large and turgid.*
I ordered, however, that the thorax should be open'd also. The left lobe of the lungs was strongly connected to the ribs, but both of them were found. The colour of the fat, in the mediastinum, was brown; which I attributed to the blood remaining in the smallest vessels. In the pericardium was some bloody water, but not much. The heart was large, and its proper vessels and auricles turgid with blood, which came forth very black and grumous, while the heart was cut off from its larger vessels, that I might examine it the more closely, out of the body. The blood was also black and grumous, in the ventricles of the heart, yet not in very great quantity. The right valvula mitralis was white; and in like manner some of the semilunar valves; the former were much harder than usual, and the latter a little so; but in both mitral and semilunar, the membranous nature had degenerated almost into the nature of a ligament. In the middle and posterior surface of the heart, a kind of little membrane protruded, of a white colour, and look'd like the remains of a hydatid. On the right auricle externally, also, were some white spots. But the aorta and other vessels, as far as I could see, were according to their natural appearances.

* Vid. etiam Epist. 60, n. 12.

Jean Nicholas Corvisart

Jean Nicholas Corvisart, the translator of Auenbrugger's *Inventum Novum* and the teacher of Laënnec, was born in 1755 in the small village of Dricourt in Champagne. Although his relationships to Auenbrugger and Laënnec have immortalized his name, he was a great man in his own right and one of the engaging and outstanding figures in medical history.

Originally intended for the bar he entered the College of Saint Barbe at the age of thirteen. He was a rather lazy and mischievous pupil, much devoted to outdoor sports, and showed no signs of future greatness. While a student of law he visited the medical clinics at Paris and was so fascinated by what he saw that he determined to study medicine. This decision so infuriated his father that he drove him from the paternal roof. Having neither pecuniary means nor influence he obtained a position as a male nurse at the Hôtel-Dieu, where he received board and lodging and was given an opportunity to study medicine. He soon became a great favorite with his teachers and graduated in 1782, the youngest and first in his class.

In 1788 he became physician to the Charité Hospital and when the medical school of Paris was created in 1795, was chosen to fill the chair of medicine. Later he became personal physician to Bonaparte, the First Consul, and when

Napoleon became Emperor, Corvisart was appointed chief physician to the Emperor and to the Court. Napoleon subsequently created him a Baron of the Empire and an Officer of the Legion of Honor.

Napoleon was much attached to Corvisart and had the greatest confidence in his medical ability. He was fond of discussing medical questions with his physician and often chatted with him while he was taking his morning bath. The three men whom Napoleon respected most for their honesty and frankness were Corvisart, Larrey, and Percy, all of whom were physicians. Corvisart's

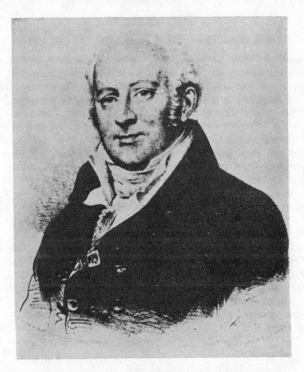

JEAN NICHOLAS CORVISART (1755-1821)
From the portrait by Charles Bazin. Etching by Delpech

frankness later led him to his estrangement from the Emperor for he opposed the Emperor's marriage to Marie Louise, and later advised Marie Louise not to follow Napoleon during the latter's exile at Elba.

In 1806, Corvisart published his *Essai sur les maladies et les lésions organique du cœur et des gros vaisseaux*. In this work he emphasized cardiac symptomatology and pointed out the differentiation between cardiac and pulmonary disease. Here we find the signs of aneurism clearly defined and the first description of the pre-systolic thrill of mitral stenosis.

Corvisart had unusual powers of observation. Upon viewing a portrait one day Corvisart remarked: "If the painter has been exact, the original of this portrait died of a disease of the heart." An investigation revealed that Corvisart's diagnosis was correct.

In 1808, Corvisart translated Auenbrugger's *Inventum Novum* into French and made known to the medical world the important discovery of percussion by the Viennese physician. With a fine sense of integrity he wrote in the preface, "I could have raised myself to the rank of an author by revamping the work of Auenbrugger and publishing a work on percussion. But by that I would sacrifice the name of Auenbrugger to my own vanity, that I do not wish to do: It belongs to him, it is his beautiful and rightful discovery (*Inventum novum,* as he justly says) which I wish to bring to life."

ARTICLE III*

THE SIGNS CHARACTERISTIC OF STENOSIS OF THE ORIFICES

The cartilaginous, or bony hardening of the auriculo-ventricular orifices, of the mitral and tricuspid valves, of the semilunar pulmonary valves, the vegetations which grow on the valves, either ventricular or arterial, all have as a principal effect, the production of a more or less complete narrowing of the affected orifices. When these stenoses exist, the circulation is impeded and its phenomena strikingly altered. By examining the disturbances of the circulation the physician can discover in a patient the signs, I would say, are positive, of this type of affection. In order to indicate with precision these signs, it is important to establish the distinctions between the different affections of which I have spoken. First, those which produce obliteration of the orifice—incomplete but permanent and always constant. Second, those which do not produce this narrowing except at certain times.

* * *

It is necessary then, to have the agreement of a large number of symptoms to make a diagnosis of the stenoses of the right orifices, it is necessary that we have a face of a color like ecchymoses, that we have a very marked enlargement of the veins and particularly those of the liver; that the volume of this organ be increased; that breathlessness be marked and of long standing. All the signs in a word, which could indicate an affection of the right cavities, dilated because of a narrowing of the orifices and these things to be the characteristics of the pulse which in

* Corvisart, J. N., *Essai sur les maladies et les lésions organiques du cœur,* Paris, Migneret, 1806, p 231.

this case is less irregular than that in narrowing of the right orifices, but less regular, however, than in the natural state. The obscurity which surrounds the signs of the narrowing of the right orifice, does not entirely disappear, when we try to recognize the imperfect obliteration of the left auriculo-ventricular orifice. Moreover, besides the general signs of heart disease, which are constantly found in this latter condition, as well as in the former, because there is almost always an aneurysmal complication, there are certain signs which allow us to recognize the affection in question.

Among these there is a certain thrill (bruissement) difficult to describe, perceptible when the hand is applied to the precordial region, a thrill which comes without doubt, from the difficulty which the blood finds in passing through an orifice which is not large enough for the quantity of blood which it is supposed to let pass. This same thrill is also recognizable, but is much less marked, by the hand, which studies the phenomena of the pulse. This characteristic is not the only one, by which the pulse shows the existence of a narrowing of the left orifice; it is more irregular in the case of narrowing of the right orifice, but less irregular than when the aortic orifice is changed. Moreover, it shows that neither the force, the hardness, nor the fullness, because the quantity of blood, which the left ventricle puts out is proportional to that which it receives from the left auricle, which does not empty completely, because the action of the ventricle is not so vigorous since it is only feebly stimulated by the small quantity of blood.

R.-T.-H. Laënnec

ARTICLE II*

SIGNS OF CARTILAGENOUS OR BONY HARDENING OF THE VALVES

The signs of ossification of the mitral valve differ little from those which indicate this condition in the semi-lunar valves. The principal sign of ossification of the mitral valve, according to M. Corvisart is "a thrill (bruissement) particularly difficult to describe, felt by the hand when applied to the precordial region."

This thrill is none other than the purring thrill (frémissement cataire) of which we have already spoken. This sign is met with indeed very often when ossification of the mitral valves or of the aortic valves is present in a marked degree: but as we have already said, it can be present however when the valves are entirely healthy, and it is absent nearly always when the osseous or cartilagenous induration is not sufficiently advanced to markedly obstruct the lumen.

A blowing murmur (bruit de soufflet) accompanies much more constantly ossification of the valves; it accompanies the contraction of the left auricle when the mitral valve is affected and it accompanies the contraction of the ventricle when the induration affects the aortic valves. But this phenomenon is also absent when the lesion is slight, and as it is moreover very common in hearts which are quite normal, we can conclude nothing from this sign in a case in question unless it is found linked with other findings necessary to confirm the diagnosis: thus when the blowing murmur, the file sound and the rasp sound persist in the left auricle continuously or intermittently for several months; when it is present only there, when it persists during quiet moments and after a long rest, when it diminishes scarcely at all after bleeding or when disappearing under these conditions it leaves behind a roughness in the sound produced by the contraction of the auricle; when especially the purring thrill is also present, we can then state that there is a stenosis of the left auriculo-ventricular orifice, a stenosis which is more commonly due to ossification of the mitral valve than to any other cause. If the same phenomena occurs under the same circumstances in the

*Traité de l'Auscultation médiate . . . par R.-T.-H. Laënnec, II Edition Paris, Chaudé, 1826, Vol. II, p. 579.

left ventricle, we can state that there is a stenosis of the aortic orifice.

* * *

Also, a slight degree of cartilagenous, stony or calcareous induration of the valves may exist a long time without any perceptible change in the health or indeed in the action of the heart, and, with hygienic measures and bleedings, at the proper times, we can often prolong for a long time the lives of patients who show all the signs of a marked stenosis of the cardiac orifices. The following observation will present the proof of this.

Observation XLVI, Louis Ponsard, sixteen years old, a gardener, of a height a little below the average, of a strong constitution, muscular and well developed, and somewhat fat, and having all the appearance of splendid health. entered the Neckar Hospital the 11th day of February, 1819, complaining of oppression and palpitation of the heart. These symptoms have been present for two years; they commenced suddenly one day when the patient was occupied in carrying some soil on a wheelbarrow. He was forcibly stopped in the midst of his work by a violent beating of the heart, accompanied by oppression. spitting of blood and nasal hemorrhage, coming on without any preceding discomfort. These symptoms quieted down under rest; but they reappeared each time the patient attempted to take the slightest bit of exercise. He then changed his trade and went into a paper factory. The occupation which they gave him was still too fatiguing and his symptoms became more frequent. The day after he entered into the hospital he presented the following symptoms:

Respiration was good throughout all parts of the chest, which was also resonant throughout; the hand, applied to the region of the heart, felt its beats with considerable force and received also the sensation which we have described under the term of "purring thrill" (frémissement cataire). This thrill was not continuous, but came at regular intervals of equal length, without intermissions. It was not synchronous with the pulse beat, it appeared rather to alternate with the beat.

This sensation was not solely one of touch; it seemed also that the sense of hearing was concerned in it, although nothing was heard when the hand was withdrawn. The cylinder (stethoscope) applied between the cartilages of the fifth and seventh ribs on the left side, allowed one to hear the contraction of the heart in the following manner; the contraction of the auricle was extremely prolonged, took place with a dull bruit, very strong and quite like the sound produced by a file rubbing on wood. This bruit was accompanied by a purring, heard by the ear, and which was evidently the same as that felt by the hand. At the end of the contraction one heard a loud bruit, accompanying the impulse and synchronous with the pulse; the contraction of the ventricular was too short by three-quarters. This bruit was somewhat harsh and rough.

Along the lower portion of the sternum, the contractions of the heart were of an entirely different character. The impulse of the left ventricle was very strong; its contracting being accompanied besides, by a very marked sound; it also was of long duration; that is to say, twice as long as that of the auricle. The sound of the auricle was a little dull, but there was nothing analogous to the thrill observed over the left ventricle.

The heart could be heard, but feebly, below the two clavicles and over the two sides of the chest, especially to the right. Over the entire sternum and on the left side, as well as under the left clavicle, contraction of the heart showed the same rhythm as at the end of the sternum. On the left side, on the contrary, one heard the rumble of the left auricle described above, very well, but feebler than in the left precordial region.

After these signs I made the following diagnosis: *Ossification of the mitral valve; slight hypertrophy of the left ventricle, perhaps slight ossification of the aortic valves; marked hypertrophy of the right ventricle.*

The pulse was strong and very regular. The face had no other color than that which youth and health gives it; his tongue was clean, his appetite was very good, stools and urine normal. He had never had any edema of the extremities, but his slumbers were constantly disturbed by terrifying dreams and the patient could not carry out any arduous exercise, nor could he walk very rapidly without feeling strong palpitations and feeling himself threatened with suffocation.

Four bleedings, at intervals of several days, relieved the patient very much. After the first bleeding his pulse became weak rather than strong and this characteristic has not changed since. Immediately after each bleeding the purring thrill ceased to be felt by the hand and the rumble of the auricle instead of being like the noise of a file, became like the sound of a bellows, when one holds the valve open with his finger. Even after the bleeding the impulse of the right ventricle was always very strong.

After a month's rest in the hospital the patient was very well, from his point of view, and demanded his release. He returned several times to consult me and I had him bled from time to time. In 1822 he came to consult me anew. He had given up his trade as a gardener and had become the domestic of a priest, who only let him do work which was not fatiguing. Since this time he suffers little. The same symptoms are present, but are much less pronounced.

Réné-Joseph-Hyacinthe Bertin

Réné-Joseph-Hyacinthe Bertin, the eldest son of E. J. Bertin the famous anatomist, was born in 1767 at Johard, a small village near Rennes. He studied medicine at Paris and at Montpellier, taking his degree at Montpellier in 1791. The following year he became army surgeon and in 1798 was sent to England as health officer to the French prisoners at Plymouth. His observations while in England were published in 1808. In 1808 he took part in the campaigns in Prussia and in Poland and upon his return to Paris, was appointed physician-in-chief to the Cochin Hospital and the Hospital for Venereal Diseases. In 1822 he became professor of hygiene as successor to Hallé. He died in 1828.

Bertin's studies on the pathology of the heart were very important and the conception of "eccentric" and "concentric" hypertrophy of the heart dates from his observations. His most important publication was his *Traité des Maladies du cœur et des gros vaisseaux,* Paris, 1824.

SECTION III

OF THE SYMPTOMS AND DIAGNOSIS OF INDURATION, AND VEGETATIONS OF THE VALVES OF THE HEART*

* * *

It is certain that the characters of the pulse indicated by Corvisart, the rushing murmur of the precordial region, are exceedingly valuable symptoms which ought not to be neglected. The same is true of the defect of harmony, the species of contradiction, if we may be allowed the expression, which exists between the pulsations of the heart and those of the pulse, in the affections of which we are speaking. We have, now and then, been able to suspect a contraction of the orifices of the heart by means of this symptom; that is, by observing the very strong pulsations of the heart coinciding with the extreme smallness of the pulse. But we must acknowledge that this symptom is met with in different diseases from those which at present occupy us. There is a method of exploration for ascertaining the contraction of the several orifices of the heart, which no other can supply: we refer to auscultation, either *immediate* or *mediate.* The symptoms which this mode of exploration furnishes, already pointed out by M. Laënnec, are the following: 1st, When the disease affects the auriculo-ventricular orifice, we hear, during the contraction of the auricles, which continues longer than in the natural state, a very distinct sound, which resembles the sound of a blow given by a file on wood, or that of a bellows quickly pressed. 2nd. When the contraction is situated about the arterial orifices (ventriculo-pulmonary and aortic) the sound of rubbing, to be presently described, is the same; but it is coequal with the contractions of the ventricles, and of the pulse. 3d. If the left orifices are contracted, the pathognomonic sound will be heard more especially

in the region of the cartilages of the fifth, sixth and seventh ribs: Whereas, if the contraction occupies the right orifices, the same sound will be more particularly heard at the inferior part of the sternum. 4th. The bellows-sound appears to coincide with the cartilaginous, or fibro-cartilaginous induration, and with the contraction produced by vegetations; that of the *file,* on the contrary, announces rather the contraction produced by open induration.

We have so frequently had occasion to confirm the absolute certainty of these symptoms, they have enabled us to ascertain the contractions of the orifices of the heart with so great facility that we do not fear to repeat, that the diagnosis of this disease may be established in the most positive manner. We allow, only, that some cases now and then occur, in which it is somewhat embarrassing to designate with precision which is the orifice constricted: but, on supposing that this cannot be determined, the inconvenience would be of no consequence. The only thing truly important is to know whether any orifice be contracted. Now, it is always possible to arrive at this certainty, by means of the symptom which has been so frequently indicated. It has never failed us, it has never deceived us. We have reported six cases in which the autopsy has demonstrated its exactness. We might augment the number, if it appeared necessary; and this would be of much consequence, if the contractions of the orifices of the heart were a rare disease.*

* It sometimes happens, that we hear a bellows-sound in the precordial region, without there being contraction of the orifices; but then this sound only takes place at intervals; and this circumstance is sufficient not to confound it with that produced by the contraction, which is heard continuously.

The intermittance, inequality and irregularity

* *Treatise on the Disease of the Heart and Great Vessels,* by R. J. Bertin, translated from the French, by Charles W. Chauncy, M.D., Philadelphia, 1833, p. 224.

Nothing appears to us more easy to be conceived, than the mechanism of the sound which accompanies the constriction of the orifices of the heart. The blood being obliged to pass from the cavity of the auricles or the ventricles, across a very narrow opening,

of the pulsations of the heart, are observed, more particularly, in the cases of lesions and contractions of its orifices. It would be superfluous to offer, in this place, any cases relative to this subject; but we would request the reader to consult the article relative to it, in the work of M. Laënnec.—*Traité de P. Auscult. Méd.*, tom. II, p. 230 *et suivantes*.

must necessarily produce more or less friction; and it is precisely this friction which produces the murmur, or jarring thrill of which we have spoken. In the same manner we may explain the vibratory tremor, which is heard in the precordial region, and which M. Laënnec has justly designated by the term purring tremor (frémissement cataire), because it so nearly resembles the sound produced by cats when the hand is drawn kindly over their back, in which they respond to such caresses by the peculiar *râle* which every one may have observed.

James Hope
SIGNS OF DISEASE OF THE MITRAL VALVE†

When the valve is permanently open, admitting of regurgitation, the first sound is intended with a murmur. It may be rough (rasping), or smooth (bellows-murmur) according to the nature of the contraction (the force of the circulation and the character of the blood), &c. (p. 107). Its key is low—more or less like whispering *who* (p. 110); yet it sounds louder and *near* if explored about the apex of the heart, and a little to the sternal side of the nipple. It may thus be easily distinguished from a direct semilunar murmur, which, in this low situation, always sounds feeble and *distant*. The murmur in some cases completely drowns the natural first sound on the left side; in others, the sound can be distinguished at the commencement of the murmur.

I have found perceptible purring tremor to be produced more frequently by regurgitation through the mitral valve than by any other valvular lesion—especially when the ventricle was hypertrophous and dilated, by which the refluent current was rendered stronger.

If the regurgitation be considerable, but not otherwise, the pulse is more or less small, weak, intermitten, irregular and unequal (p. 359); and this, even though the impulse of the heart be violent.

When the mitral valve is considerably contracted, a murmur (best heard in the same situation as the murmur from regurgitation

and distinguishable in the same way from semilunar murmurs) attends the ventricular diastole and second sound. From the weakness, however, of the diastolic current out of the auricle, the murmur is always very feeble, soft like the bellows-sound, and usually on a rather low key than a whispered *who* (p. 110). I have found this murmur absent unless the contraction of the valve was considerable; for the blood had still sufficient room to pass with tranquility; and I have also found it absent when the contraction was *great*—when, for instance, the aperture admitted one finger only, or merely a quill, provided the current was preternaturally weakened by softening, by extreme dilatation of the heart, or by both (cases of Anderson and Mrs. ——I——N). In such cases, however, the mitral disease would not be overlooked, as there is almost invariably a murmur from regurgitation. On the whole, this murmur is exceedingly rare, though Laënnec and authors in general have supposed quite the contrary, from mistaking it for the murmur of aortic regurgitation (see p. 103).

I have never known purring tremor accompany a diastolic mitral murmur, the current being too feeble to produce it.

When the contraction of the mitral valve is great, the pulse (whether there be regurgitation or not) is more or less small, weak, intermittent, irregular and unequal, in consequence of the supply of blood to the left ventricle being insufficient and irregular (p. 359). I have known the same to be occasioned by a polypus choking up the left auricle.

† Hope, J., *A Treatise on the Diseases of the Heart*, London, Churchill, 1839, p. 387.

Sulpice-Antoine Fauvel

Sulpice-Antoine Fauvel was born in Paris in 1813 and took his doctor's degree in Paris in 1840. His graduation thesis was on capillary bronchitis and a few years afterwards he published articles on scurvy, on typhoid fever, and on "the stethoscopic signs of left auricular ventricular stenosis." These articles attracted much attention and aided him in securing the post of chief-of-clinic at the Hôtel-Dieu. He was there in 1847, seeing a brilliant future shaping itself before him, when at the creation of an institution for health officers in the Levant, because of the discussion regarding the plague, he was called to occupy one of the most important posts, that of Constantinople.

In 1848 Fauvel was made a member of the Imperial Council of State of the Ottoman Empire, and in 1849 professor at the school of medicine in Constantinople, and in 1856 he founded the *Gazette Médicale d'Orient*. He was most active and energetic in both administration and research and in addition to the introduction of many reforms in sanitation, published important papers on the epidemiology of plague, cholera, typhus, and scurvy. He remained in Turkey for nineteen years and returned to Paris in 1866 when he was appointed General Inspector of Health Service of France. He died in 1884.

Fauvel was one of the greatest of modern sanitarians. His best-known publications are in the field of epidemiology, but one of his earliest medical articles is one of the first clear discussions of the auscultatory signs in mitral stenosis.

COMMUNICATION CONCERNING THE STETHOSCOPIC SIGNS OF NARROWING OF THE LEFT AURICULO-VENTRICULAR ORIFICE OF THE HEART*

By A. Fauvel, chief of clinic of the Faculty of medicine at the Hôtel-Dieu,
member of the Medical Society of Observation

It is generally held today that one can, by certain characteristics of the abnormal sounds of the heart, state with precision the type and the location of the lesion with which the organ is affected. According to this statement, the progress of auscultation has been tremendous during recent times, and the discovery of Laënnec has been perfected in an unexpected manner. Among the causes which have produced this result, physiological experiments take the first rank. Thus, an appreciation of the order in which the movements of the heart take place, and their relationship to the normal heart sounds have been the basis of all the theories. Then came the researches of M. Bouilland, the discovery of insufficiency of the valves by Doctor Corrigan, and finally the localization of the abnormal bruits, the importance of which in the determination of the orifice involved, has been shown, almost simultaneously by Messrs. Hope in England, Barth and Rogers in France, and Skoda in Vienna.

Arch. gén. d. med., Paris, 1843, 4 sér., I, 1.

Many times I have been able to demonstrate the fact already pointed out by M. Gendrin, that, in certain cases, the abnormal bruit precedes the shock of the heart: but I did not then attach any great importance to it.

This year, my attention was particularly attracted by a patient in whom this phenomenon existed with certain remarkable characteristics. It was a man of 25, who presented all the signs of an organic affection of the heart, because of which he had been dismissed from military service. He entered the Hôtel-Dieu the 16th day of June, because of an acute articular rheumatism of moderate intensity. In the precordial region, besides a forceful impulse and a considerable area of dullness, one heard an *intense rasping murmur (bruit de râpe), preceding the first sound, finishing with it,* having its maximum intensity at the apex of the heart and to the left. The patient was dismissed cured of his rheumatism the fifteenth of July.

Soon chance favored me to such an extent

that, in a very short space of time, four new cases have just come one after the other, to fix my attention and anew because of a repetition of the same stethoscopic signs.

Three of these individuals succumbed to different affections, and I was not permitted to ascertain, by autopsy, whether the nature of the lesions coincided with the pathological signs noted during life. The importance of these observations requires that I report them here. I shall content myself with extracting from these observations that which is relative to the subject.

OBSERVATION I—AURICULO-VENTRICULAR STENOSIS WITHOUT INSUFFICIENCY

A woman named Logrogue, aged 50 years, grocer, was admitted to the Hôtel-Dieu, Saint-Bernard hall, the 19th of September 1842.

This woman showed the signs of a chronic cerebral affection, characterized by a hemiplegia of the right side. The state of her intelligence did not make it possible to obtain information concerning her previous health. We learned only that she was subject to palpitations.

On admission it was noted that besides the complications resulting from a cerebral lesion, there was an elevation coinciding with the forceful heave in the precordial region. Percussion showed a dullness of about eight to ten centimeters.

On auscultation there was made out a rasping murmur *quite loud, having its maximum intensity at the level of the fifth rib, to the left of the nipple. This abnormal sound began during the silence which follows the second normal sound, and finishes at the moment when one hears the first sound, the abnormal sound becomes faint as one passes to the right or towards the base of the heart.* The beats show some intermittence. The pulse was small, irregular. There was no edema of the extremities.

The patient died the 29th of September, following a progression of the cerebral affection. Every day, until death, we confirmed the existence of the same phenomena in the heart.

Autopsy showed a *stenosis of the left auriculo-ventricular orifice allowing scarcely the introduction of the tip of the fore-finger.* The narrowing was due to a yellowish deposit of a fibro-cartilagenous consistence placed in the substance of the mitral valve, and to warty-like concretions adherent to its auricular service. The *chorda tendinae* and the free margin of the valve had retained their suppleness and their normal length, in such a manner that there was no insufficiency. The walls of the ventricle were a little hypertrophied, without notable increase in size of the cavity. The other orifices were normal.

In the left hemisphere of the brain we found some cysticerus cysts located principally in the substance of the convolutions, and in addition a considerable amount of red softening towards the posterior portion of the middle lobe.

This observation, in which I regret the absence of certain anatomical details, is important, since it shows that in a marked stenosis of the auriculo-ventricular orifice there is present an abnormal sound, of such nature that it commences shortly after the middle of the long silence, and finishes at the instant when the first sound was heard. This fact has all the more value, since it was not possible to explain it by any lesion than a stenosis.

* * *

In conclusion, I conclude from the facts presented in this communication, that an abnormal pre-systolic[1] murmur, localized towards the apex of the heart, in the present state of the science, is the most probable stethoscopic sign of a stenosis of the left auriculo-ventricular orifice. I do not say the certain sign: for the small number of cases upon which this conclusion is based, does not allow us to regard this conclusion as other than provisional, and requiring confirmation by new observations.

[1] An expression which I have borrowed from M. Gendrin, although giving it an entirely different signification.

Graham Steell

Graham Steell was born in Edinburgh, in 1851, the youngest son of Sir John Steell, the sculptor. He was educated at Edinburgh Academy and the

University of Edinburgh. After serving as house physician at Edinburgh and resident at fever hospitals in London and Leeds, he removed to Manchester where he was elected to the staff of the Manchester Royal Infirmary and appointed to the chair of clinical medicine at Victoria University.

He soon made a reputation as an excellent teacher and published two widely used books on cardiac diseases and on pulmonary diseases. He presently acquired a large consulting practice and his interest in cardiac disease led to a close friendship with James Mackenzie, who spent many afternoons in Steell's wards in Manchester.

Graham Steell retired in 1911 and died on January 10, 1942, at the advanced age of ninety-one. "Old students of Steell will ever associate him with his habit of changing into the old frock coat which Sister Reid kept for his entry into the ward, the absolute quiet which had to prevail during his lengthy round, the little cough which first introduced us to the Bromptom lozenge." Steell, who had been champion boxer at the University, developed pulmonary tuberculosis shortly after beginning practice, but soon recovered. His best remembered contribution is his description of the pulmonary diastolic murmur, since known as the Graham Steell murmur.

THE MURMUR OF HIGH-PRESSURE IN THE PULMONARY ARTERY

By Graham Steell, M.D., Assistant Physician to the Manchester Royal Infirmary*

There has been long question among physiologists of a safety-valve action of the tricuspid valves. Few clinicists will deny that, in disease, a similar occurrence takes place on the left side of the heart, the mitral valves becoming incompetent when the left ventricle is embarrassed under the effort which it is called upon to make. The muscle-element in the valve apparatus of the auriculo-ventricular orifices must be borne in mind in this relation, for it is by interference with muscle-action that incompetence of the valves is secured and relief temporarily afforded in both cases. It is, therefore, the important part played by the heart-muscles in the establishment and maintenance of closure of both the tricuspid and mitral valves which renders possible the sudden production of their incompetence under special circumstances. In the case of the mitral valves, the causes which demand regurgitation in the way indicated have been, as a rule, long at work, and the accomplishment of regurgitation has been preceded by a series of changes. The valve-apparatus of the great arteries of the heart, unlike that of the auriculo-ventricular orifices, is independent of muscle-action, so that an analogous safety-valve action, in its

case, appears to be out of the question. In health I believe it to be so, and, at the same time, I do not hesitate to express my disbelief in the rupture of a sound valve. In disease it is otherwise, and the clinical study of arterial high tension, aortic dilatation, and final incompetence of the valves, forces me to the admission that the arterial valves, like the auriculo-ventricular, do, under the strain of extreme tension long continued, permit the regurgitation through them. Thus there occurs an action analogous to a safety-valve one, although the name is less appropriate, since there is no threatened asystole to be obviated in their case, as there is in that of the mitral valves, inasmuch as the recoil or systole, of the elastic arteries is not a vital action. It is not my purpose here to discuss aortic regurgitation arising from dilatation, and to trace its origin directly and apart from induced disease of the valves, to high arterial tension. I wish to plead for the admission among the recognized ausculatory signs of disease of *a murmur due to pulmonary regurgitation occurring independently of disease or deformity of the valves, and as the result of long-continued excess of blood pressure in the pulmonary artery.*

In cases of mitral obstruction there is

* *Med. Chron.*, 1888, IX, 182-188.

occasionally heard over the pulmonary area (the sternal extremity of the third left costal cartilage), and below this region, for the distance of an inch or two along the left border of the sternum, and rarely over the lowest part of the bone itself, a soft blowing diastolic murmur immediately following, or, more exactly, running off from the accentuated second sound, while the usual indications of aortic regurgitation afforded by the pulse, etc., are absent. The maximum intensity of the murmur may be regarded as situated at the sternal end of the third and fourth intercostal spaces. When the second sound is reduplicated, the murmur proceeds from its latter part. That such a murmur as I have described does exist, there can, I think, be no doubt. Let me quote, with regard to it, the testimony of my revered master, Dr. G. W. Balfour, though he gives a very different explanation of the murmur from that which I advocate. Speaking of the rare occurrence of pulmonary incompetence from disease of the valves he says:† "I mention it just now mainly for the purpose of warning you against being led into mistaking an auricular diastolic murmur for a pulmonary diastolic one. I have already pointed out that mitral stenosis is not infrequently associated with a diastolic murmur apart and distinct from its own peculiar presystolic murmur. Now and then this diastolic murmur of auricular origin has its position of maximum intensity at the sternal end of the fourth rib, a position in which it might readily be mistaken for a pulmonary diastolic murmur, and possibly has been so mistaken." In another place, he speaks of the position of maximum intensity being "frequently in the pulmonary area."* I must here remark, that the murmur, which I have described, is altogether different from the obstructive diastolic murmur of mitral stenosis, which is essentially an apex murmur, and, moreover, is wanting in the soft blowing quality of the pulmonary regurgitant murmur. The mitral murmur too, runs off from the first part of a reduplicate second sound, the pulmonary from the last part.

* * *

The murmur of high-pressure in the pulmonary artery is not peculiar to mitral steno-sis, although it is most commonly met with, as a consequence of this lesion. Any long-continued obstruction in the pulmonary circulation may produce it. The plumonary valves, like the aortic, do not readily become incompetent, apart from the structural change. Probably no amount of blood-pressure in the pulmonary artery will render them so suddenly, as, at least, theoretically, the mitral valves may be rendered incompetent. Changes in the vessel, with widening of its channel, and, eventually, of its orifice, long precede the occurrence of incompetence of its valves. The pulmonary murmur of high-pressure is probably never persistent at first, and one of its most remarkable features is, as a rule, its variableness in intensity. On some days it will be distinctly heard, on others it will be indistinct, or even inaudible; while extreme accentuation of the pulmonary second sound is always present, the closure of the pulmonary semilunar valves being generally perceptible to the hand placed over the pulmonary area, as a sharp thud. This non-persistence of the murmur, in the earlier stages, at any rate, is only what the study of dilatation of the aorta and the consequent regurgitation would lead us to expect. Indeed, so common is a soft, blowing murmur, after an accentuated aortic second sound, that extreme accentuation should make us listen, with special care, for a murmur, and even though it be absent on the first occasion the search should not be abandoned. My belief, is, that when the aortic second sound is extremely accentuated, regurgitation, to some extent, will probably occur sooner or later. Its supervention in aneurism of the first part of the arch of the aorta is a familiar fact. Post mortem, enlargement of the left ventricle, in these cases, may be a better indication of regurgitation having occurred during life than the usual test of filling the cut aorta with water, a proceeding which cannot imitate the action of the forcible blood-currents in the living body. An accentuated second sound is no way incompatible with a certain amount of incompetence of the semilunar valves; on the contrary, an accentuated second sound, associated with a regurgitant murmur, is clinically common.

Writing in 1881,† after describing the regurgitant murmur of aortic dilatation, I

† *Clinical Lectures on Diseases of the Heart and Aorta*, p. 218.
* Note p. 119.

† *The Physical Signs of Cardiac Disease*, Edinburgh, Maclachlan and Stewart, 1881.

referred to the murmur which is the subject of this paper, as follows: "I am inclined to believe that a murmur of similar mechanism occurs on the right side of the heart, when there is much obstruction to the pulmonary circulation, with a dilated pulmonary artery." My subsequent experience has only served to confirm the opinion thus cautiously expressed more than seven years ago, though my faith has from time to time been shaken by a case presenting a murmur which I had at first imagined to be an example, but which, on further investigation, proved to be of aortic origin.

PULMONARY STENOSIS

James Hope

SIGNS OF DISEASE OF THE PULMONIC VALVES*

The signs of contraction of the pulmonic valves are the same as those of the aortic, (p. 365) with this difference; that, from the vessel being nearer the surface the murmur with the first sound seems *closer* to the ear, and is on a higher key, ranging from the sound of a whispered *r* towards that of *s*. I have, however, known it fall below *r* when the circulation was feeble and slow, and the obstruction slight. It may be known that the murmur is not seated in the aorta, by its being inaudible, or comparatively feeble, two inches up that vessel; whereas, at a corresponding height up the pulmonary artery, it is distinct: also, by its being louder down the tract of the right ventricle than down that of the left (Bowden). It may be known that the murmur does not proceed from regurgitation through the auricular valves, by its being distinct along the course of the pulmonary artery, where auricular murmurs are either wholly inaudible, or very feeble and remote.

When a murmur in the pulmonary artery is considerably louder between the second and third left ribs, close to the sternum, than opposite to the valves, and is there attended with impulse and purring tremor, dilatation of the pulmonary artery may be suspected (see *Dilatation of Pulmonary Artery*). In one instance I have known a murmur to be pro-duced by complete ossification of the pulmonary artery penetrating deeply into the lungs (case of Lady R.).

When there is regurgitation through the pulmonic valves, a murmur accompanies the second sound. Its nature and diagnosis are the same, (the necessary inversions being made,) as in the case of aortic regurgitation, (p. 366,) except that the pulse is not jerking (case of Rogers. A tremor attended).

I presume that purring tremor with the first sound may be occasioned by contraction of the pulmonic orifice, though I have not met with an instance verified after death: but I have met with three in which the tremor attended dilatation of the pulmonary artery (Weatherly, Bowden, and Miss L. P.——r). A purring tremor occasioned by the pulmonic valves would be more readily felt than one occasioned by the aortic valves, because it would probably be transmitted as far as the space between the second and third ribs, (where it is out of the cover of the sternum,) provided the patient lay in the horizontal position, and inclined to the left side.

Disease of the pulmonic valves is so rare, that it ought never to be suspected unless the signs described are perfectly well marked, or unless there be patescence of the foramen ovale, or some other communication between the two sides of the heart,—states which experience has proved to be generally accompanied with contraction of the orifice in question.

* Hope, J., *A Treatise on the Diseases of the Heart*, London, Churchill, 1839, p. 385.

AORTIC STENOSIS
James Hope
SIGNS OF DISEASE OF THE AORTIC VALVES*

One of the murmurs above alluded to is heard during the ventricular contraction (i.e., with the first sound) on the sternum, opposite to the lower margin of the third rib, and thence for about two inches or more upwards, along the course of the ascending aorta towards the right; and it is louder in these situations than below the level of the valves. Its pitch or key is usually that of a whispered *r*, from being superficial, and it accordingly conveys the idea of being pretty near to the ear. When a murmur of this kind is considerably louder along the tract of the ascending aorta than opposite to its valves, and is, at the same time, usually near-sounding and superficial—in other words, on

a higher key than a whispered *r*, it proceeds from disease of the ascending aorta itself. As the murmur from this cause is audible in the situation of the valves, it might lead to the supposition that they also were diseased, and it is sometimes very difficult to ascertain positively that they are not. That a murmur is seated in the aorta, and not in the pulmonary artery, may be known by its being inaudible or very indistinct high up the course of the pulmonary artery, while it is distinct high up that of the aorta. That a murmur is seated in the aorta or its valves, and not in the auricular valves, may be known by its sounding loud and *near* above the aortic valves, where an auricular murmur, if audible at all, sounds feeble, *remote,* and on a low key, like a whispered *who.*

* Hope, J., A Treatise on the Disease of the Heart, London, John Churchill, 1839, p. 383.

William Stokes
EXTREME OSSIFIC DISEASE OF THE AORTIC ORIFICE†

Strong action of the left ventricle; extremely loud and musical murmur at the extent of the arterial tree; the heart's action of the arterial tree; the heart's action generally regular.—I have witnessed two or three cases of this combination. The phenomena arise from extensive ossific diease of the aortic opening, which is rendered not only rigid, but singularly irregular, from the deposit of great quantities of earthly matter in the form of intersecting and irregular plates, stretching downwards into the ventricle, as well as into the aorta, for an inch above the sinuses. In one of these cases the appearance of the opening might be aptly compared to that of the mouth of a shark in minature; all traces of the valves had disappeared.

In these cases every superficial artery emitted a most distinct musical tone at each pulsation: the radial artery at the wrist, the palmar arteries, the ramifications of the temporal arteries, the anterior tibial, and the branches on the dorsum of the foot, all

† Stokes, William, The Diseases of the Heart and the Aorta, Dublin, Hodges and Smith, 1854, p. 139.

exhibited the same phenomenon. In two cases the sounds were distinctly audible to the patients, who were conscious of their existence at almost every point of the body. With one patient the perception of these sounds was the principal cause of his suffering, for his general health long continued excellent, and the heart's action was but little excited. This gentleman once observed to me, *that his entire body was one humming-top.* The loudness of the tone varied with the force of the heart. When I first saw him the sounds were audible at the distance of at least three feet; but when the force of the heart had been reduced by local treatment, the use of sedatives, and by removing all causes of bodily and mental excitement, the loudness of the sound at the aortic orifice was so much reduced as to render it inaudible, unless by applying the ear. Even under these circumstances the musical sound of the small arteries still continued, though not to such a degree as to cause annoyance to the patient. Dissection in this case showed but little disease in the aorta from about two inches above the orifice; the descending aorta and the arch were healthy; the left ventricle was hypertrophied and dilated; the general arterial system exhibited no disease.

Under such circumstances we may safely make the diagnosis of extensive and irregular ossification of the aortic orifice, with contraction, if the pulse be small and hard and without contraction, if its ordinary volume be preserved.

To these cases, presenting physical signs sufficiently constant and well-marked to justify such a diagnosis of the condition of the valves as will be safe or practically useful, we may add the case of varicose aneurism, of which a description will be found in the section devoted to that subject.

But the practitioner must be prepared to meet with many cases which he will be unable to refer satisfactorily to any of these forms; for the complications of heart disease are so numerous and varied that, as we have said before, it becomes impossible to determine the exact nature of every case that may come before us. Fortunately it is unnecessary to do so, for if we can be certain that organic disease really exists, the treatment, as has been before remarked, will depend less on the nature of the valvular affection than on the vital and anatomical state of the heart itself.

Among the causes which concur to produce such varied phenomena in heart disease, the following may be enumerated:

1. The existence of valvular disease in more than one situation.
2. The changes incident to the advance of disease.
3. Alterations in the muscular structure of the heart.
4. Variation in the action of the heart.
5. Intercurrent attacks of endocarditis or of pericarditis.
6. Variations in the condition of the blood itself, causing the appearance and disappearance of anaemia, in addition to the organic murmurs.

To this catalogue other causes might be added; but the practical physician knowing these things, will not feel that the difficulties of the subject reflect disgrace upon his art, when he considers that the great end of medicine is the proper treatment of the patient, rather than the exhibition of unnecessary refinement in diagnosis.

IRRITABLE HEART

Jacob M. Da Costa

Jacob Mendes Da Costa was born on the Island of St. Thomas, West Indies in 1833. His family was originally of Spanish and Portuguese extraction, his father being a gentleman of wealth and culture, descended from an English branch of the family. His parents left St. Thomas when he was only four years of age and lived for many years in Europe. Later young Da Costa was sent to a gymnasium at Dresden where he devoted his time mainly to the study of the classics and modern languages. He learned to speak both French and German with great fluency and also acquired a good knowledge of Spanish, Portuguese, Italian and Dutch.

Da Costa entered Jefferson Medical College of Philadelphia in 1849 and graduated three years later at the early age of nineteen. After graduation he spent eighteen months in Paris and Vienna. In Paris, he became a favorite pupil of Trousseau and in Vienna, a pupil and close friend of Hyrtl. In 1853 he returned to Philadelphia where he began the practice of medicine and gave instruction in physical diagnosis to students and graduates in medicine. His *Medical Diagnosis* appeared in 1864 and immediately attracted the attention of the medical profession. It passed through nine editions during the life of its author and was translated into German, Russian and Italian.

In 1866, Dr. Da Costa was appointed lecturer in clinical medicine at Jefferson Medical College. Dr. W. W. Keen, speaking of this appointment, remarked that the Philadelphia clinics "until Da Costa, in the session of 1866-67, took hold of them, were about as inane and useless as one could imagine." In 1872, Da Costa was elected Professor of the Theory and Practice of Medicine, holding this chair until his resignation in 1891. He died in 1900.

Da Costa's skill in diagnosis became proverbial, almost legendary. As a lecturer, he was simple, clear and concise. His public clinics were events in the

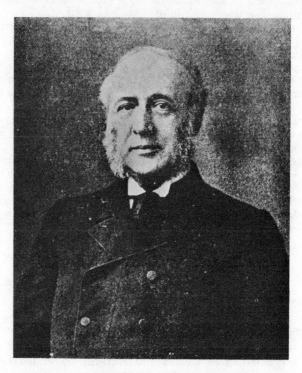

JACOB M. DA COSTA (1833-1900)
From Memoir of Da Costa by J. C. Wilson, 1902.

medical life of Philadelphia. A lifelong student and lover of the classics, their influence was apparent in his writings and public addresses. "He disliked, in writing, all compound words, as well as interjections, of which he never made use. A purist in language, he loved all that was pure and best in literature. Slang was most repugnant to him. A coarse expression gave him positive pain." (Clarke)

During the Civil War, Da Costa served at a military hospital in Philadelphia. Here he gathered much of the material for his study of the "Irritable Heart" which was mentioned in his *Medical Diagnosis* but was more fully described in his paper of 1871. This cardiac disorder which Da Costa described in soldiers during the American Civil War was later encountered in the first World War and is again very prevalent in the present conflagration.

ON IRRITABLE HEART; A CLINICAL STUDY OF A FORM OF FUNCTIONAL CARDIAC DISORDER AND ITS CONSEQUENCES*

In this paper I propose to consider a form of cardiac malady common among soldiers, but the study of which is equally interesting to the civil practitioner, on account of its intimate bearing on some obscure or doubtful points of pathology. Much of what I am about to say I could duplicate from the experience of private practice; yet I prefer to let this inquiry remain as it was originally conducted on soldiers during our late war. The observations here collected were made on a series of upwards of three hundred cases. That so large a number were examined is thus explained. Shortly after the establishment of military hospitals in our large cities, I was appointed visiting physician to one in Philadelphia, and there I noticed cases of a peculiar form of functional disorder of the heart, to which I gave the name of irritable heart—a name by which the disorder soon became known both within and without the walls of the hospital.

* * *

Palpitation.—Both the severity and frequency of the palpitations differed considerably in individual cases. In some, the attacks lasted several hours, and were attended with increased pain in the cardiac region, and under the left shoulder. They were often accompanied by a great deal of distress, and were really painful. They occurred at all times of the day and night, varying in frequency from one to five or six attacks, or more, in the twenty-four hours. Yet there were cases that did not have them for days at a time. The seizures were, of course, most readily excited by exertion, and might be then so violent that the patient would fall to the ground insensible. This happened to some on the march, or field of battle; or they fell in the ranks, and were taken prisoner. But attacks also occurred when the patient was quietly in bed, disturbing his rest, or waking him up; and some reported that they were worse at night, and early morning. They were very variously, sometimes whimsically, described.

* * *

Cardiac Pain.—Pain was an almost constant symptom. I cannot recall a single well-

* *Am. J. M. S.,* 1871, LXI, p. 17.

marked instance of the complaint in which it was wholly absent; and often it was the first sign of disorder noticed by the patient. It was generally described as occurring in paroxysms, and as sharp and lancinating; a few likened it to a burning sensation, or spoke of it as tearing, or as burning at times, and at others cutting; or as a "dull sullen" pain, becoming at times acute. In some cases no other pain happened than what occurred in these sharp attacks, or a mere feeling of uneasiness in the region of the heart existed; but in the large majority there was a substratum, as it were, of discomfort, or of dull heavy pain. In exceptional cases the pain was altogether of this character. Unwonted exercise or exertion would generally produce an attack of sharp pain, and a fit of palpitation was very apt to do the same; but the acute pain also happened without any unusual disturbance of cardiac action, and was, in truth, in rare instances, noticed to be decreased by exercise, or to be most severe when the patient was free from palpitation. Deep breathing was stated to make the pain severe, when it was otherwise but slight; cough produced a kindred result.

* * *

Pulse.—The pulse was mostly noted to be very rapid, varying from 100 to 140. In character it was small, and easily compressible; it might or might not exhibit the abrupt or jerking character, which, as we shall presently see, is one of the chief peculiarities of the cardiac impluse. and this might have a certain amount of force which the pulse would lack. In some cases it was under 90, and was then apt to be fuller; these were, for the most part, the cases passing into cardiac hypertrophy. The pulse exhibits under any circumstances great variations; and especially in a case following an injury to the spine from a falling tree it changed about between 76 to 120, little influenced by any remedy employed. Slight irregularities in the succession of its beats, and, indeed, in the general rhythm, are very common. The pulse is always greatly and rapidly influenced by position.

* * *

Respiration.—Shortness of breath, or rather oppression on exertion, was constantly complained of, and was a prominent symptom during attacks of palpitation. When the heart was acting in its usual way, a certain amount of embarrassment in breathing was also commonly spoken of, and was at times so severe that the patient was obliged to sit up in bed. Yet, notwithstanding all the signs of dyspnoea, it was astonishing that the respiration was so little hurried.

* * *

Nervous Disorders.—These manifested themselves chiefly by headache, giddiness, disturbed sleep; and were symptoms which, though common, were not so constant as those already described. The headache was not apt to be persistent, but to occur in spells, and was generally of a dull, heavy character. It was more particularly noticed after severe attacks of palpitation; and might be associated with giddiness, and with increased heat and redness of face.

Dizziness was often complained of. It was increased by stooping; by exercise; and sometimes preceded the attacks of palpitation. In one instance, the vertigo was so severe that the man fell from his horse.

* * *

Digestive Disorders.—These were very frequent. All kinds of indigestions, great abdominal distension, and diarrhoea were symptoms constantly encountered. But they were symptoms having reference rather to the causation of the cardiac trouble than due to this; and we shall examine their bearing further on.

* * *

Physical signs.—In describing the physical signs I shall first bring those together which are the most usual.

The *impulse* is almost always extended, yet not correspondingly forcible; rather, it is quick, and abrupt or jerky. When the hand is applied to the praecordial region, it may note the quick impulse happening in a regular manner, or it takes cognizance of the irregularity of rhythm of the irritable organ. Further, it may at times perceive the two sounds of the heart; feel them as it were. On listening to the heart, the first sound is found to be lacking in volume, feeble or short and valvular, and just like the second sound.

* * *

Murmurs obscuring or replacing the cardiac sounds are not as a rule present; yet they are met with, and particularly is that form of murmur, systolic, chiefly above the apex, and not connected with venous hum or other signs of anaemia, which I have described as significant of functional valvular disorder. It has all the peculiarities there dwelt upon; in truth, it was a study of the cases now under analysis that first familiarized me with it; and until I found out its meaning I was often much puzzled to know whether I was dealing with a case of organic valvular trouble or not. The inconstancy of the blowing sound is of much value; in cases of perverted rhythm it may only be heard with the first beat succeeding the intermission.

Course of the Disorder.—Having discussed the symptoms and physical signs, it will be useful to inquire into the course of the malady. This mostly either gradually subsides, or it passes by degrees into cardiac enlargement.

When the disorder yields the heart becomes less and less irritable, exercise no longer affects it so much, the cardiac pain and soreness disappear, and finally the patient is again able to bear fatigue and undergo exertion; or in other instances, he is well as long as he is not too active, but his heart is always liable to be more disturbed by undue exertion or by excitement than the heart of a healthy person is.

* * *

In bringing this inquiry to an end, I may be permitted to point out what I believe to be its chief interest and value. To the medical officer it may be of service as investigating a form of cardiac disorder which every severe or protracted campaign is sure to develop. And from a military point of view, further, it enforces the lessons, how important it is not to send back soldiers just convalescent from fevers or other acute maladies, too soon to active work; it suggests that their equipments be such as will not unnecessarily constrict, and thus retard or prevent recovery; that recruits, especially very young ones, be as far as practicable exercised and trained in marches and accustomed to fatigue before they are called upon to undergo the wear and tear of actual warfare; and it exhibits some of the dangers incident to the rapid and incessant manoeuvring of troops. True, on a movement executed on the double-quick may depend the tissue of a battle, a forced march may determine the fate of a nation; and the time can never come when purely physical considerations can forbid, either one or the other, or dictate how often they may be ordered. But every commander should be made aware that in so using his men he is rendering some unfit for further duty, impairing others, and thus be led to count the cost of the frequent use of such active movements as carefully as he would the holding of a particular part of a line or the assault on another.

PULSUS ALTERNANS

Ludwig Traube

Ludwig Traube was born in Ratibor in 1818 and studied medicine at the universities of Breslau, Vienna, and Berlin. He was a fellow-student of duBois-Reymond, Virchow, and Helmholtz and in Vienna was much inspired by the lectures and demonstrations of Rokitansky and Skoda. Rokitansky and Skoda gave him the incentive to pursue anatomico-pathological studies, which remained throughout his life one of his major interests. In 1848, Traube became a Privatdozent in Berlin and the following year became assistant in Schönlein's clinic, a position he held for ten years. He refused during the next few years calls to Heidelberg, Breslau, Zürich, and Bonn, remaining an instructor in Berlin until 1872, when he became full professor. He died in 1876.

Traube is best remembered as the first physician who systematically utilized thermometry at the bed-side and hastened the introduction of the clinical thermometer into medicine. He was a most successful practicing physician and for twenty years was regarded as the leading consultant of Berlin. As a teacher, he was endowed with a rare gift of clarity in expression and his lectures and demonstrations were unusually interesting. His greatest abilities lay in the field of experimental medicine and his experimental work covers a wide field. His early work on blood-pressure and upon the physiological effects of digitalis were noteworthy contributions to scientific medicine. In 1846 Traube's first work, his Contributions to Experimental Pathology and Physiology, appeared. Twenty-five years later he revised this work for publication but found no occasion to change any of the conclusions he had drawn in the first edition.

Traube made many important contributions to the field of cardiac and circulatory diseases. He was the first to note and study that now well-known phenomenon—the pulsus alternans.

A CASE OF PULSUS BIGEMINUS WITH REMARKS ON ENLARGEMENT OF THE LIVER IN VALVULAR DISEASE AND CONCERNING ACUTE STROPHY OF THE LIVER*

By Prof. Dr. L. Traube

In my experiments on animals years ago, I became acquainted with a kind of pulse, which I called Pulsus bigeminus. The observations upon it which are somewhat scattered, may be found in my collected *Beiträge zur Pathologie und Physiologie*.

The essential feature of the Pulsus bigemi-

* *Berl. Klin. Wchnschr.*, 1872, IX, p. 185.

nus is that after every two pulses which originate in the aorta, there follows a longer
pause. It is differentiated from the Pulsus
dicroticus by the fact that in the latter there
is only one contraction of the heart for every
two beats of the pulse, while in the Pulsus
bigeminus there are two contractions of the
heart, which follow each other closely and

*of the cardiac portion of the nervous control,
which is still active.*

If this conclusion is correct, we can
obviously conclude from the appearance of
the Pulsus bigeminus in patients that there
is a paralysis of spinal nervous control and
the prognosis under such conditions would
be bad.

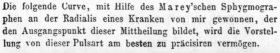

Die folgende Curve, mit Hilfe des M a r e y'schen Sphygmogra-
phen an der Radialis eines Kranken von mir gewonnen, der
den Ausgangspunkt dieser Mittheilung bildet, wird die Vorstel-
lung von dieser Pulsart am besten zu präcisiren vermögen.

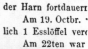

der Harn fortdauerr
    Am 19. Octbr. ·
lich 1 Esslöffel vere
    Am 22ten war

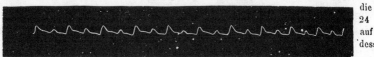

die
24
auf
des:

Ich theile die Krankengeschichte ausführlich mit, weil sie
mir in mehrfacher Beziehung interessant erscheint.
Beobachtung.

derselben erhält de
2 stündlich 1 Esslöff
    Ich selbst unte

Curve of pulsus alternans from Traube's article on *A case of pulsus bigeminus*
in the *Berliner Klinische Wochenschrift*, 1872

are separated from the preceding and succeeding contractions by a long pause. For
every two beats of the Pulsus dicroticus
there are, as in the normal pulse only two
heart sounds, while in the Pulsus bigeminus
there are four heart sounds audible. An accurate illustration of the Pulsus bigeminus is
found on Table 9 under C in the first volume
of my *Beiträge*. Here it was in an animal
who had been curarized and poisoned with
potassium cyanide, in whom, shortly after
being poisoned, the vagi were cut in the neck.
We see the Pulsus bigeminus appear shortly
after cutting the second vagus, after the
pressure and pulse rate were increased from
the effects of the operation.

I concluded from these facts, *that for the
appearance of the Pulsus bigeminus two conditions are necessary.*

1) *The heart must be released from the
influence of the spinal part of its nervous
control and also*

2) *There must be some agent circulating
in the blood, which increases the irritability*

Up to the present time I have succeeded
in three or four cases in demonstrating the
Pulsus bigeminus in men: in two of these
death followed shortly after its appearance.

The following case, which came under my
observation towards the end of last year,
shows us a variation of the Pulsus bigeminus;
I designate it with the name of *Pulsus
alternans*. It has in common with the Pulsus
bigeminus the fact that the normal rhythm
is not replaced with an arrhythmia but by a
new strange rhythm in which two consecutive
pulses are in close relationship to each other:
it has to do with a succession of high and
low pulses, in such a manner that a low pulse
follows regularly a high pulse and this low
pulse is separated from the following high
pulse by a shorter pause than that between
it and the preceding high pulse. The following curve taken by me with the aid of
Marey's sphygmograph from the radial
artery, which forms the beginning joint of
this communication, gives us a more exact
conception of this type of pulse.

GALLOP RHYTHM
Pierre-Carl Potain

Pierre-Carl Potain was born in Paris in 1825, the descendant of a line of
physicians who had practiced medicine and surgery from time immemorial.

His father however did not complete his medical studies but became postmaster at Saint-Germain. Potain received most of his early education from his father and mother and began the study of medicine at the wish of his father. He became an interne of the hospitals of Paris in 1848 and in 1849 was at the Salpêtrière where he contracted cholera during the epidemic but fortunately recovered. In 1856 he became chief of the clinic of Bouillaud and in 1861 was appointed professeur agrégé at Paris and gradually fulfilled the prophecy of Trousseau that he would become the first clinician of Paris. In the Franco-

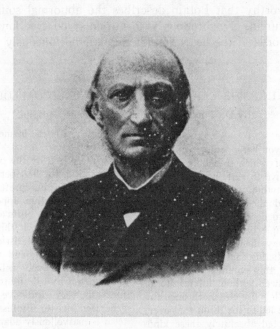

PIERRE-CARL POTAIN (1825-1901)
from Bulletin de l'Académie de Médecine 1927 XCVIII 569

Prussian war of 1870, he was asked to take charge of an ambulance service, but declined and served as an infantryman, taking part in several battles. In 1882 he became physician to the Charité Hospital, where he was active until he reached the age of retirement in 1900. He died in 1901.

Potain fulfilled Trousseau's prophecy because of his sterling worth, integrity, and ability, and not because of any physical charm. "Certainly," as his pupil Vaquez wrote in his eulogy of Potain, "nature did not put herself out for him. A large thin body, somewhat bent, of lean appearance; a tall figure, ascetic, symmetrical, furrowed with deep wrinkles and framed with sparse whiskers; a prominent nose hanging over thin lips; a bony skull, as if hammered out, surrounded by a crown of scanty greying hair falling down his neck."

Potain was a great clinician and a remarkably keen observer. He believed firmly in the union of clinical medicine and physiology and kept constantly in the closest touch with the physiologists, namely, François-Frank and Malassez.

Potain made many important clinical discoveries especially in diseases of the heart, devised a sphygyomanometer which was used for many years and an aspiration apparatus which is still universally employed. Potain wrote but little, but lavished great pains upon everything that came from his pen. One article, commenced in 1864, was not published until 1893. He wrote two works, one his *Leçons cliniques* edited by Vaquez, and another on *Blood Pressure*. Both of these works were written with the most meticulous care and bear the impress of a profound thinker and clinician.

It is noteworthy that Potain describes the abnormal sound of the gallop rhythm as occurring synchronous with auricular contraction, a fact recently verified by records of the heart sounds taken simultaneously with the electrocardiogram.

CONCERNING THE CARDIAC RHYTHM CALLED GALLOP RHYTHM*

By Dr. Potain, physician of the Necker Hospital

Gentlemen:

I presented to you here, some years ago, a communication of which I should perhaps remind you, relative to certain modifications of the cardiac rhythm, which I propose to call "normal reduplications of the heart sounds." It had to do then with clearing up the field of multiple bruits, the significance of which had always been very obscure, because of the conflicting facts, included up to that time, under this common designation. Now, it has not been without interest to attempt to see a little more clearly through this obscurity; since it led to the result that every semiologist neglected absolutely these kinds of anomalies as unimportant, while others thought they found in them a certain sign of heart disease. In studying the normal reduplications, a special variety of multiple bruits, I have attempted first to rid the subject of that which one might call its nonessentials. And indeed, you have been able to see, at that time, how the bruits of which I speak, resulting from transitory changes and which one hears occasionally at the beginning of a pericarditis. In the second group, that of anapests, we find first the constant reduplication of the first sound, which one observes in some cases of organic disease of the heart, without knowing until now either its mechanism or its pathological significance; than finaliy, the special anomaly which I wish to discuss with you today, and which I shall

*Bull. et mém. Soc. med. d. hóp. de Paris, 1876, XII, p. 137. Presented . . . at the meeting of July 23, 1875.

designate with the name of *gallop rhythm (bruit de galop).*

Characterized by the presence of a double sound during the first period, both these *anapests,* or if you prefer, these two last anomalies of rhythm, appear likely to be confused and to only form one, but that which I propose to study at this time presents certain special characteristics, which render it absolutely distinct, and upon which I shall insist at once you will understand then, gentlemen, why I desire to reserve exclusively for it, the very expressive term created by my venerated master Professor Bouillaud. This term is marvellously adapted to the sound it designates, and it will be especially useful in distinguishing a very particular group of findings and quite worthy, as you are going to see of a special designation. Besides, it is this variety itself which M. Bouillaud had us formally hear, in applying to it this name of gallop rhythm which the respiratory movements superimpose upon the pressure of the blood contained in the heart and in the large vessels, their pathological importance is nil; so that they have nothing to do with heart disease, and that it is important solely to distinguish them, so that we can not confuse them any more with the truly pathological forms of multiple bruits.

* * *

. . . There remains a certain number of true multiple bruits and truly pathological; among which these are some which have already acquired a certain diagnostic value, while others are still awaiting their interpretation. One can divide them into two groups; one in which the multiplication of sounds takes place during the second period of the heart, the *dactyls,* if you will; the other those where it belongs to the first period, the *anapests.*

In the first group is the reduplication of the second sound which announces the mitral rhythm, considered today, especially since the excellent communication of my colleague and friend Dr. Duroziez, as characteristic of stenosis of the left auriculo-ventricular orifice: it is the drum sound (*bruit de rappel*) of M. Bouillaud: then besides the forms of double sounds the second period as yet well differentiated, which one sees, as I attempted to show previously, with a generalized adhesive pericarditis.

* * *

I

The formation of this rhythm of which I wish to speak, is as follows. We distinguish here three sounds, namely: the two normal sounds and an additional sound. The normal sounds show most frequently their normal characteristics, without any modification. The first especially maintains its normal relationship to the apex heart and to the arterial pulse. As to the abnormal sound, it is placed immediately before it, preceding it some times by a very short time; always notably larger however, than that which separates the two parts of a reduplicated sound; in general and almost always much shorter than the short silence. The sound is dull, much more so than the normal sound. It is a shock, a perceptible elevation, it is scarcely a sound. If one applies the ear to the chest, it affects the tactile sensation more perhaps than the auditory sense. And if one attempts to hear it with a flexible stethoscope, it lacks only a little, almost always, of disappearing completely. The place where one perceives it best is a little below the apex of the heart, somewhat towards the right, but sometimes one can distinguish it throughout the entire precordial region.

* * *

II

Now what does this bruit signify and what diagnostic value does it have? As I said a moment ago, it usually exists with a simple hypertrophy of the heart. Is it the simple result of hypertrophy and should we see in it only one of the characteristic symptoms of this affection? Evidently not because we do not need it, by any means, in all cases of cardiac hypertrophy; it can appear or disappear in certain patients, independent of the hypertrophy itself; finally I diagnosed it positively in a case where the autopsy showed no trace of an appreciable hypertrophy.

This abnormal sound, so peculiar, so distinct from all others has no special significance, no particular diagnostic value? It has one, in which I believe: strange always, at first glance. It can be, if I am not mistaken, the indication of a renal affection.

* * *

V

Does the abnormal sound result from an early systole of the right ventricle or rather from a premature closure of the tricuspid valve and is the rhythm with which we are concerned nothing but a reduplication of the first sound? This is the opinion adopted and defended lately, in England, by Doctor Sibson. I believe this absolutely erroneous and for the following reasons. In the first place, the abnormal sound has, in no way, the timbre or usual characteristics of a valvular sound. In the second place, it is not loudest, as it should be, in the region of the right cardiac cavities. In the third place, finally (and this is the unanswerable argument which makes unnecessary all other reasons), I have heard, in certain patients, successively and in the same cardiac revolution, the "bruit de galop" itself and a reduplication of the first sound. I mean that after the dull sound which constitutes the first part of the gallop rhythm, one noted clearly a doubled first sound, a reduplicated clicking of the usual type. And this, I have demonstrated to the pupils on my service, in a way I do not believe I could have been in this case, the victim of an illusion. Now, if the tricuspid produced, by its closure, the dull sound of the gallop, it evidently could not click a second time to produce a reduplication. And as it is accepted by everyone that the reduplication of the first sound depends upon the clicking of the mitral and tricuspid valves, the gallop sound must have a different cause.

We see that it is impossible to refer the abnormal gallop sound to any of the movements which take place at the beginning of the ventricular systole. If, on the other hand, one observes it with care, if one seeks to specify the place which it occupies in the cardiac revolution, one can rapidly convince himself that it is during presystole: or, if you prefer, during the moment when the auricle, in contracting, finishes and completes the ventricular diastole; the moment immediately followed by the beginning of the ventricular systole and of the first sound.

* * *

VIII

We summarize now gentlemen if you permit, the result of this work. That can be done in a few words.

We find in the heart in patients suffering from interstitial nephritis, a special sound which is the bruit designated by Professor Bouillaud with the name "Gallop rhythm" (*bruit de galop*).

This sound results from the abruptness with which the dilation of the ventricle takes place during the pre-systole period, a period which corresponds to the contraction of the auricle. It appears to be an indirect consequence of the excessive arterial tension which interstitial nephritis produces habitually by a mechanism of which we have a glimpse but which still remains to be determined in a thoroughly accurate manner. It can start us on the way to a diagnosis of the renal disease, and reveal it before any other symptom has attraction to it. It can, consequently, be of service in diagnosis and prognosis, and therefore give useful indications for treatment.

AURICULAR FIBRILLATION

Heinrich Ewald Hering

Heinrich Ewald Hering was born in 1866 in Vienna, the son of the well-known physiologist, Ewald Hering, who was later professor in Leipzig. Ewald Hering became in 1895 Privatdocent at the German University of Prague, five years later was promoted to the rank of extraordinary professor and in 1902 he became professor of general and experimental pathology. In 1913, he was chosen rector of the University of Prague and shortly afterwards accepted a call as professor of pathological physiology in the University of Cologne. In 1935, he became emeritus professor.

Hering's scientific investigations have been mostly in the field of the physiology and pathology of the circulatory system. Among his early investigations were those upon the irregularities of the pulse, especially of the type which he named pulsus irregularis perpetrus. His best known work, however was the discovery and demonstration of the importance of the carotid sinus in the maintenance of blood pressure and his investigations on the carotid sinus syndrome.

* * *

ANALYSIS OF THE PULSUS IRREGULARIS PERPETUUS

By Prof. H. E. Hering*

The pulsus irregularis perpetuus has not yet been analysed and it seems at first glance to be quite difficult to get any firm basis for

analysis in the confusion of short and long cycles, small and large pulses. We find however, after a certain reflection and with the aid of previous experimental results that we

Prag. Med. Wchnschr., 1903, xxviii, 377.

can today carry out very well such an analysis.

From the theoretical standpoint a cardiac arrhythmia can consist of two different types, and result either from (A), an *abnormal behavior of the stimulus,* or (B), an *abnormal*

tain symptoms the corresponding conclusions.

In the following pages it will be shown that we can separate these different kinds from each other on the basis of *clinical* observations, that we now also have a basis for differentiating at least to a certain degree one

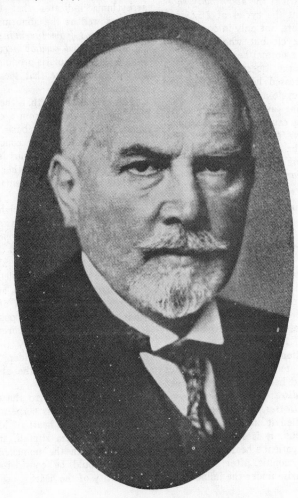

HEINRICH EWALD HERING (1866-   )
Courtesy of Münchener Medizinische Wochenschrift

behavior of the irritability of the heart or certain of its parts or (C), when both (A plus B) are present.

We can distinguish these different types quite well experimentally: it is a question however whether we can do this on the basis of *clinical* observation, since the human heart in general can not be subjected to direct investigation and we can only draw from cer-

of the possibilities under type A, which will be discussed later.

In the analysis of an irregular pulse, that is, an irregular heart action whose nature on the basis of previous observations is not well understood, I proceed as follows.

By means of a pulse curve taken with great exactness or a curve of the cardial impulse taken during apnoea, the frequency of the beat per minute is determined. From this curve one sees at the same time the different durations of the irregular cycles.

* * *

The most important feature for analysis of the Pulsus irregularis is the *abnormally short* cycles. We see that the cycles of 2.5/5 sec. are abnormally short, not only in comparison to an estimated cycle but when compared with the cycle of a normal heart.

There is now the question to answer, how can the increased heart rate and the abnormally short cycle arise? Certainly only by some accelerating cause.

The accelerating cause can only be a *prematurely appearing powerful stimulus,* and this stimulus can be either an *extra stimulus* or a stimulus *arising prematurely at the place of normal formation.*

* * *

Since we have until now no basis for explaining the long cycles which appear sporadically, by a sporadic decrease in irritability, so there remains as a cure of the abnormally short, *as well as for the abnormally long cycle only an abnormal behaviour of the stimuli,* and we now seek to determine for the former as well as for the latter, whether they are produced by extra stimuli or through premature or delayed formation of normal stimuli.

In this connection some further *clinical* facts should be mentioned. The Pulsus irregularis analysed here, which is observed in *valvular heart diseases, coronary sclerosis* and *myocardial diseases,* is *lasting* and for that reason, I called it in the title Pulsus irregularis perpetuus; it is furthermore the *same* whether the patient's heart beats *faster* or *slower,* as for example, after giving digitalis: it does not arise under the influence of

respiration, it is then not a Pulsus irregularis respiratius.

All these facts indicate that the Pulsus irregularis perpetuus has its origin from some cause within the heart, and is of *cardiac origin.* The fact that there is no respiratory arrhythmia indicates that the abnormally short as well as the abnormally long cycles *do not result from the indirect influence of the extra-cardial cardiac nerves.* Since there is no Pulsus irregularis produced by the extra-cardial nerves save that seen in respiratory disturbances.

The circumstance that the Pulsus irregularis takes its origin from a cause within the heart, leads us on the basis of our present knowledge to a further conclusion that the Pulsus irregularis perpetuus is very probably of *Myogenic* origin, whether it is produced by extra stimuli or by premature or delayed normal stimuli.

When we now ask, which of these two latter causes is probably responsible, we answer *extra stimuli.* The appearance of extra stimuli explains to us not only the abnormally short but also the abnormally long cycles, and indeed the complete picture of the Pulsus irregularis perpetuus, and we also have evidence for the presence of extra stimuli, while in favor of the other possible cause—an irregular production of normal stimuli—we can at present not only produce no evidence, but must consider it improbable, especially in view of the abnormally short cycles.

Our analysis leads to the conclusion that the Pulsus irregularis perpetuus is due to an irregularity of the heart of Myogenic origin, produced by extra stimuli, and therefore in agreement with the nomenclature proposed by me, should be considered a moerethic irregularity of the heart.

Sir James Mackenzie

Few man have had their lives so intimately interwoven with the history of any phrase of medicine as had Sir James Mackenzie with the history of heart disease. James Mackenzie, a Highlander of ancient stock, was born on the farm of Pickstonhill in the parish of Scone, in the year 1853. He went first to the village school and later, at the age of twelve, was sent to the ancient grammar school of Perth for three years. His experience at Perth was a very unhappy one and he left school to enter an apothecary's shop where he remained until he was twenty years of age. The following year he entered the University of Edinburgh, graduating in medicine in 1878. He served a year in the Edin-

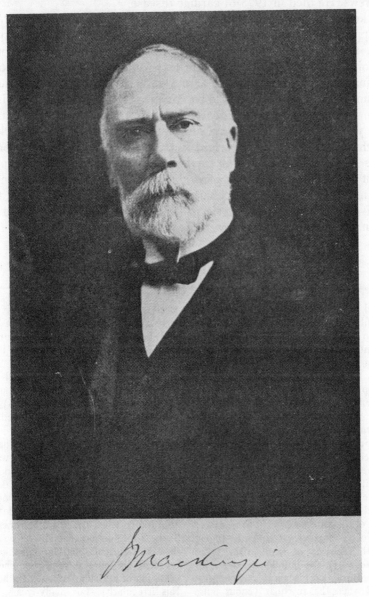

SIR JAMES MACKENZIE (1853-1925)
Photograph by Emery Walker

burgh Royal Infirmary and then settled down to practice in Burnley, a town in Lancashire. He remained here for over twenty-five years. In 1907 he removed to London, and there he rapidly achieved a great reputation. He became Sir James Mackenzie and soon had one of the largest consulting practices in the metropolis. In 1918 he left a consulting practice "worth rather more than 8000 pounds a year" and returned to general practice in the Scottish town of St. Andrews. He died in 1925 of cardiac disease.

Mackenzie's name is associated particularly with his *Study of the Pulse* which appeared in 1902 and his *Diseases of the Heart* which was published in 1909. The first book, which is a remarkably keen analysis of the pulse and which pointed out already the different types of irregularity and the means of diagnosing them, did not have at first a wide sale but it made Mackenzie's name known throughout the world to students of cardiac disease. His second book, however, not only made his reputation but brought him patients and in a single year increased his income nearly ten fold. Mackenzie's work on the heart, which was the most important in the generation and revolutionized all concepts of cardiac disease, was carried out not in a magnificent university clinic but in the rounds of a busy general practice. The story of this remarkable physician is told in a singularly charming and interesting fashion by R. Macnair Wilson in *The Beloved Physician*—a book whose perusal should be obligatory in the curriculum of every medical school.

CHAPTER XXX
AURICULAR FIBRILLATION*

Personal experiences in the recognition of auricular fibrillation.—My attention was first directed to this condition as a separate and definite entity about 1890. I had been endeavouring to discriminate between the different forms of irregular heart action, and it occurred to me to employ the jugular pulse as an aid. By this means I was able to separate the great majority of irregularities into definite groups, according to the mechanism of their production, as revealed by simultaneous records of the jugular and radial pulses. There was one group which showed a distinct difference from all others, by the presence of the ventricular form of the venous pulse. I was at a loss to understand the nature of the heart's action in these cases; and as I found them very frequently among people with a history of rheumatism, I determined to watch the individual cases with rheumatic hearts, to see when this irregularity arose, and when the auricular venous pulse changed to the ventricular. The individual recorded as Case 48 came under my care in 1880, suffering from an attack of rheumatic fever. I examined her at intervals until her death in 1898. Up to 1897 her heart was regular, except for occasional ventricular

extra-systoles. Her jugular and liver pulses were always of the auricular form (Fig. 119 and 120). There was a well-marked presystolic murmur. She became very ill in 1897, with a rapid and irregular heart. When the heart slowed down after a partial recovery, I found that the jugular and liver pulses were of the ventricular form (Fig. 121), that the presystolic murmur had disappeared, and that the heart was irregular; in other words, all evidences of auricular activity had disappeared. From this date onwards, I was able to confirm these observations, and add to them other cases which showed waves due to the auricle, in jugular and apex tracings before the heart becomes irregular, and their disappearance when the heart becomes regular. Thus, I established that all the positive evidences of auricular activity, capable of being revealed by clinical methods, showed the cessation of auricular action with the onset of this irregularity. For many years, I speculated as to the causes of auricular fibrillation. As the auricle was found distended and thin-walled at the post-mortem examination, I came to the conclusion that the disappearance of the signs of auricular systole was due to the auricle having become distended, atrophied, and paralysed. This view I put forward in a book on the pulse, which I pub-

* Mackenzie, James, *Diseases of the Heart*, III Ed., London, Oxford, 1913, p. 212.

lished in 1902. Shortly after this was published, I had a series of cases, some of which I had watched for years, and at the post-mortem examinations the auricles were not thinned, but were hypertrophied. With this fact before me, I saw that my previous explanation could not be correct; for the fact that the auricles were hypertrophied indicated that they must have contracted during the years that I had watched them, and when there had been an absence of all signs of auricular activity. As it was clear that the auricles could not have contracted during the normal period—that is to say, immediately before ventricular systole—the only alternative I could see was that they contracted during ventricular systole. As, in the meantime, I had studied several hundreds of cases and had seen this condition start under a variety of circumstances, particularly in individuals with frequent extra-systoles, I put forward the view that ventricles and auricles contracted together, and assumed that the stimulus for contraction arose in some place that affected auricles and ventricles simultaneously. As at this time I could not conceive of any other possibility to explain the facts, I suggested that the stimulus for contraction arose in the auriculo-ventricular node; and I called the condition 'nodal rhythm,' under which name the clinical aspects of auricular fibrillation are described in the two editions of this book, the first being published in 1908.

With the advent of the electrocardiograph, we obtained a more accurate method of recognizing the contractions of the chambers of the heart. When electrocardiograms were taken of the cases that I had called nodal rhythm, my clinical observations were verified, inasmuch as no evidence of the normal auricular systole was found. In cases where the heart periodically became disorderly in its rhythm, and where I was able to demonstrate that the auricular form of venous pulse was present with the regular heart action, and the ventricular form during the period of irregular action, the electrocardiograms also showed evidence of auricular contraction during the normal period of the heart's action, and a disappearance of the normal auricular activity during the period of irregular action, fully confirming the observations I had made on nodal rhythm.

The attention of other observers had also

been arrested by some of the clinical features of this condition. Thus Hering, in 1903, separated from among other irregularities the irregularity peculiar to auricular-fibrillation, and called it the *pulsus irregularis perpetuus*. He was mainly concerned with the physiological aspect of the subject, and did not recognize the full clinical picture, with the disappearance of all signs of auricular activity. Many other observers had noted the 'positive' venous pulse, and in attributing it merely to tricuspid incompetence they had failed to appreciate its real meaning, and so missed the significance of its appearance.

Although the disappearance of the auricular contraction was the feature that puzzled me in these cases, I realized that my explanation of it, as being due to synchronous contraction of auricles and ventricles, was far from being established; and I endeavoured to interest others in the subject, who might investigate the matter by experimental methods, and find out, if possible, what the auricle was doing. Cushny was the first to suggest that auricular fibrillation might be a factor of clinical importance; and in 1906 he and Edmonds drew attention to the resemblance of the radial tracings in a case of paroxysmal irregularity in the human subject to the tracings from a dog, in which they produced experimental fibrillation of the auricles. On reading this communication, I was struck with the idea; and on a visit Professor Cushny paid to me in Burnley in 1906, he discussed with me the probability of auricular fibrillation being the cause of the irregular heart action in certain cases of 'nodal rhythm' and he agreed that certain small waves, which I had recognized in the jugular pulse of one case (Fig. 122), were due to the fibrillation of the auricle.

I published in 1907, tracings with this explanation, but I failed to appreciate the real significance of what auricular fibrillation was; I thought it only a passing event; and I practically gave up the idea that it was at the bottom of these cases that went on for years. Lewis had been pursuing an inquiry clinically and by experiment into the nature of cardiac irregularities and had produced experimental fibrillation in the dog. In 1909 he took graphic records of the venous and arterial pulses. With the onset of fibrillation, he found that the arterial pulse became irregular, and the venous pulse changed from the auricular to the ventricular form. Pursuing his investigations further, Lewis was able to detect in the electrocardiogram of experimentally produced fibrillation, certain oscillations during ventricular diastole, which were induced by the fibrillating auricle. Examining more critically the electrocardiograms of typical cases of nodal rhythm which I sent to him, he found these oscillations also present and demonstrated their correspondence with the small fibrillation waves I had noted in the jugular pulse.

When Lewis placed these facts before me,

I had no hesitation in abandoning my views, and accepting the fact that these cases owed their abnormal actions to auricular fibrillation; and I now recognize that the reason those evidences of auricular activity, to which I have been referred, disappear, is because the auricle ceases to act as a contracting chamber.

Rothberger and Winterberg had independently, in 1909, drawn attention to the fact that in *pulsus irregularis perpetuus* the electrocardiogram corresponded to that of auricular fibrillation experimentally produced.

* * *

CHAPTER XX

PARALYSIS OF THE AURICLE AND THE VENTRICULAR FORM OF THE VENOUS PULSE*

§178. Paralysis of the auricle.—This increase of the ventricular wave and diminution and disappearance of the auricular wave implies the paralysis of the auricle. The auricular appendage is usually described as being the last part of the heart to cease contracting,—the *ultimum moriens*,—so that the notion of a patient continuing to live with an auricle incapable of contracting is a somewhat novel idea in cardiac symptomatology, and it seems necessary to devote a little study to the condition.

I have already demonstrated, in Figs. 183 to 186, how in one patient the steadily advancing failure of the heart was accompanied by the diminution in size and final disappearance of the auricular wave, with the increase in size and final persistence of the ventricular wave. At the *post-mortem* examination one could easily surmise that the greatly distended, thin-walled sac of an auricle was incapable of exercising any pressure on its contents. In quite a number of cases I have noted the same steady progress of events, and occasionally I have had the opportunity to watch the restoration of the auricle to temporary activity. All who are familiar with cases of heart failure consequent on mitral disease recognise periods of extreme failure when the heart's dulness increases. Sometimes it happens that a presystolic murmur that was present entirely disappears during the time of temporary failure, and returns with increased vigour of the heart. The explanation usually given for this is that the distended

right side had pushed the left ventricle away from the chest wall, so that the sound was no longer capable of being heard, that during this period of heart failure in some cases the auricle has become so enormously distended that it ceases to contract, but that with restoration of compensation it again regains its power of activity. In Fig. 211 there is a tracing taken from a patient suffering from extreme heart failure. It will be noticed that there is no sign of an auricular wave, the venous pulse wave being synchronous with the arterial outflow from the ventricles. (E). Gradually this patient's strength improved, the area of cardiac dulness diminished, and the venous pulse then presented a distinct though relatively small wave, a, due to the contraction of the auricle (Fig. 212). The improvement continued, and the last tracing I took (Fig. 213) shows a still larger auricular wave. Figs. 214 and 215 show the same thing. This patient had symptoms of extreme heart failure, during which Fig. 214 was obtained. When he had much improved the tracing Fig. 215 was taken, which shows a well marked auricular wave. Here I have not the slightest doubt there was a temporary paralysis of the auricle, and very likely with recurring attacks of heart failure the auricular wave would entirely disappear. In another patient, whom I first saw in May 1892, there was a faint venous pulse of the auricular type (Fig. 216). After an attack of heart failure in July of that year the venous pulse was ventricular in form, with the occasional small beat due to the auricle, a (Fig. 217). The following year this small wave had ceased to appear, and up to the time of her death in 1900 the venous pulse was invariably of the ventricular form only.

EXTRA-SYSTOLES

James Mackenzie

§81. *The dropped beat.**—In many cases the finger fails to recognize the small pulse beat due to an early occurring systole. In such cases it is usual to assume that either the heart has missed a beat, or that it has sent on a wave too small to be recognized. What usually happens is that the ventricle has made a premature systole, but the force has been so small that it has not been able to overcome the pressure in the aorta and open the aortic valves, or that having done so, the wave of blood sent forth has not been of sufficient strength to be felt by the finger. The duration of the period including the long pause and the preceding beat will often be found to correspond accurately to two cardiac cycles, as represented by two beats of the pulse. In the tracing, Fig. 79, there are two dropped beats, the radial pulse showing no

* Mackenzie, James, *The Study of the Pulse,* Edinburg, Pentland, 1902, p. 95.

sign whatever of a beat when examined by the finger. In the tracing there is a slight prolongation of the dicrotic wave at the irregular period, which may be assumed to be due to a minute premature beat occurring at that period. If the apex tracing taken at the same time be examined, it will be found that the ventricle did make a contraction at that period (s′). If the heart be auscultated there will be heard the two short, sharp sounds, as already described, occurring at the beginning of the long pause, and caused by the rapid premature systole of the ventricle. When the apex beat is absent the presence of these sounds will often reveal the true nature of the delay on the pulse. Occasionally, however, it happens that the ventricular systole has not sufficient strength to raise the aortic valves, and then only the faint, muffled sound may be detected corresponding to the first sound. Sometimes even this may be absent.

PAROXYSMAL TACHYCARDIA†

William Stokes

A remarkable case, illustrative of what has been said, occurred in Dublin some years ago. The patient, a lady of great intelligence, was for some years the subject of long-continued attacks of violent and extraordinary palpitations during which the action of the heart became greatly excited, extremely irregular, and attended by a loud bellows murmur, approaching to the *bruit de rape*. During these attacks she was visited by several experienced physicians, who all concurred in the opinion that some extreme and singular disease of the valves existed. After having been the subject of this disease for several years she consulted me. The paroxysm was then in its decline, after having lasted for some weeks, but the action of the heart was irregular, with a loud and

† Stokes, William, *The Diseases of the Heart and the Aorta,* Dublin, Hodges and Smith, 1854, p. 161.

somewhat metallic murmur apparently attending the first sound. She mentioned her anxiety that I should not make up my mind as to the nature of her case until I saw her a second time, which she arranged should be in the course of about ten days, observing that her physicians had not had fair play, inasmuch as they had only examined her heart during the continuance of its excitement. The patient was perfectly persuaded that she laboured under a fatal organic disease. I saw her again in about ten days; the heart's action was perfectly tranquil, the pulse natural, and every trace of murmur had disappeared. Several years afterwards I saw this lady; she was then in perfect health, and mentioned, with a good deal of self-complacence, that she had not only puzzled all her physicians, but had discovered her own cure, and this was in the use of an emetic at the commencement of each attack, a practice to which she had been led by the occurrence of accidental vomiting from the effect of some medicine which had been administered. She then determined to take an emetic of mustard or ipecacuanha on the supervention of each attack. The paroxysms became less and less severe, and finally disappeared. When I last saw her she was able to take active exercise, and the action and sounds of the heart were natural.

A case, probably of a similar nature, was that of a young man who was brought to the hospital suffering from extraordinary excitement of the heart, the action of which was so violent that the most severe form of carditis was believed to exist. The patient was treated with extreme but erroneous activity; he was repeatedly and largely bled, mercury was freely exhibited, and all other means of subduing local inflammation resorted to; yet not the slightest impression seemed to be made on the disease; and as his strength was much exhausted, while the action of the heart continued with terrific violence, the gentleman under whose care he was placed suspended treatment, the death of the patient being daily expected. A draught, containing ether, laudanum, and other ingredients, having been taken, was followed by full vomiting, after which the action of the heart became regular and tranquil; the murmur disappeared, and convalescence was rapid and complete.

Richard Payne Cotton

Richard Payne Cotton was born in Kensington in 1820 and received his medical education at St. George's Hospital and at Paris. He served for many years on the staff of the Hospital for Consumption and Diseases of the Chest at Brompton and retired from this position in 1875. He had a very large practice in London and was most highly esteemed by his colleagues and patients. He obtained in 1852 the Fothergillian Gold Medal for his prize essay on consumption and published a small manual on *Phthisis and the Stethoscope* which was very popular and which appeared in several editions. He died in 1877. While Cotton is best remembered by his colleagues for his publications on tuberculosis, posterity will probably remember him best for his description of paroxysmal tachycardia.

NOTES AND OBSERVATIONS UPON A CASE OF UNUSUALLY RAPID ACTION OF THE HEART (232 PER MINUTE)*

By RICHARD PAYNE COTTON, M.D., F.R.C.P. Lond.,
Physician to the Hospital for Consumption, etc., Brompton

About three years back, I was consulted by a tradesman—a tailor, aged 42—on account of shortness of breathing, with a sense of general distress, which had lasted several days. It was the first attack of the kind he had had. The pulse was too rapid to be counted; the respirations were forty; and the *pulsations of the heart two hundred and thirty, in a minute*. Dr. Peplow saw the case several times with me. In about three weeks from the commencement of this attack, the patient entirely recovered; the action of the heart becoming *suddenly* in every respect natural, and the pulse eighty in the minute.

About fourteen months from this period,

a similar attack occurred; but it was less severe, and of short duration, the heart never exceeding one hundred and sixty in a minute. Six months subsequently there was a return of the symptoms, on which occasion the patient was attended by Mr. R. W. Dunn. And within the last winter, two slight attacks have occurred, lasting, however, only a few hours.

All these seizures differed from each other, and from the one I am about to give more in detail, chiefly in their duration—the general symptoms having been, on each occasion, remarkably alike.

The last attack commenced four weeks ago. It was preceded, as before, by loss of appetite, acidity, and disordered stomach, with constipation; the rapid action of the

* *Brit. M. J.*, 1867, I, 629.

heart following immediately upon a sensation of faintness and short breathing.

When called to see the patient, I found him anxious, but not otherwise seriously distressed; his breathing was short, hurried, and irregular, varying from thirty to forty in a minute. The pulse was too rapid to be depended on; but the beating of the heart was distinct, regular, free from murmur, and *two hundred and thirty-two per minute*. Immediately over the semilunar valves both sounds could be clearly distinguished, scarcely differing from each other, and closely resembling the peculiar "tic-tac" beats of the foetal heart; but in every other part of the cardiac region a single and abrupt sound only could be heard. No valvular murmur could anywhere be detected, neither was there any visible pulsation in any of the larger arteries; but the jugular veins, as well as the larger veins at the head of the arms, could be distinctly seen to pulsate.

The case being of so remarkable, and, as I believe, unique a character, I was anxious that my friend and colleague, Dr. J. Burdon Sanderson, should examine the patient by the aid of his sphygmograph. We met accordingly in consultation, Dr. Sanderson succeeding in getting an accurate tracing of the radial pulse. Figure 1 represents this tracing, which Dr. Sanderson informs me, marks the number of the pulsations at exactly *two hundred and twenty per minute*.

It will be observed that the pulse was singularly uniform and regular in its beat, varying from the natural pulse principally in its extreme feebleness and great rapidity. The usefulness of the sphygmograph was thus sensibly illustrated; since, without it, the pulse, from its extreme rapidity, was so difficult to count, that it appeared *previously*, both to Dr. Sanderson and myself, neither to be synchronous with the action of the heart, nor at all regular.

The treatment consisted at first in the use of antacids and stimulants, together with aperients: during the action of which, a considerable quantity of tapeworm was expelled. After a short time, the tincture of digitalis was given in doses of from ten to fifteen minims three times a day; and it was during the use of this medicine that the heart returned to its healthy condition. Whether such occurrence was a *post* or a *proper hoc*, I cannot pretend to determine, but it is worthy of remark that, during the patient's first two attacks, a similar condition obtained, the recollection of which induced me, on this occasion, to try the digitalis again. Two or three days before the heart returned to its natural pulsation, a considerable amount of hemoptysis occurred, the bases of both lungs being at the same time dull on percussion, and having the respiratory murmur very feeble. With this single exception of slight pulmonary congestion, there was no change in the general condition of the patient during the whole attack, until the heart regained its healthy condition, which as on every previous occasion happened very *suddenly*, being immediately preceded by a sense of faintness, which from former experience, the patient himself recognized as a forerunner of his recovery.

A few days after this, Dr. Sanderson and I had a second consultation; when we found the respiration natural, the heart perfectly healthy, the pulse regular, and rather below seventy in a minute.

The only remaining symptoms were slight oedema of the legs, which had come on as the heart quieted; and which was less easy to account for, a slight pulsation in the right jugular vein, upon which I shall make an observation presently.

This case thus briefly, but as I hope, sufficiently described, is interesting in many ways. It shows very clearly that mere functional rapidity of the heart's action, that is to say, rapidity unconnected with valvular diseases or alternation in heart structure, is not necessarily a dangerous condition. Notwithstanding its immense rapidity in this case —a rapidity perhaps seldom, if ever, surpassed, the patient could at no time be said to have been in danger. From the very commencement to the close of the attack, he was calm, and even cheerful, and suffered surprisingly little either bodily or mentally.

The interesting question remains—upon what did the heart's rapid action depend?

It appears to me that such extreme rapid action of the heart, when free from organic or inflammatory disease, and when unconnected with displacement, must arise from one of two causes. Either the heart itself is so extremely sensitive that it contracts upon the healthy blood before its cavities have had sufficient time to become properly filled with this fluid; or the blood itself is of so abnormal and irritating a character as to excite such premature contraction. The first condition may be occasionally seen in certain diseases of the nerve-centres, but more frequently in simple nervous and hysterical palpitation; the second, in palpitation arising in the course of an attack of gout, or acid dyspepsia.

In the case before us, either of the two conditions may have existed. The presence of the tapeworm may have produced a reflex irritation of the heart itself; or the acidity and dyspepsia under which the patient invariably suffered at the period of his attacks may, by giving rise to an abnormal condition of the blood, have provoked the heart to its rapid and premature contraction; and it is even possible that these two conditions may have coexisted. I will not, however, insist upon such an explanation: but, in the absence of even the slightest indication of brain or spinal affection, or indeed, of any unusual amount of general nervous sensibility in our patient, I am at a loss for any other.

One of the still remaining symptoms to which I have referred, viz, the pulsation of the right jugular vein, noticed both by Dr. Sanderson and myself, is not easy of explanation. It is a natural conclusion from such a condition, that the tricuspid valve must allow of regurgitation. During the previous extreme rapidity of the heart, insufficiency of this valve, and the consequent venous pulsation is easy to understand; but after the heart had returned to its healthy state, why the valve should still remain incompetent, or, remaining incompetent, should not have given rise to a regurgitant murmur, is not so easy of comprehension. If regurgitation really existed, as the venous pulsation would indicate, the case is still further interesting, as an addition to the evidence which most of us must have had, that valvular regurgitation is not necessarily productive of valvular murmur.

* * *

ADDITIONAL NOTES ON UNUSUALLY RAPID ACTION OF THE HEART*
By RICHARD PAYNE COTTON, M.D.
Senior Physician to the Hospital for Consumption, Brompton

In the *British Medical Journal* of June 1st, 1867, I related a case, illustrated by sphygmographic drawings by Dr. Sanderson, in which the pulse reached 232 per minute. It was the first of the kind which had been published. In the *Journal* of June 22 of the same year is a letter addressed to me by Sir Thomas Watson, Bart, in which he describes a similar case which had fallen under his notice several years previously, and where the pulse reached 216 in the minute. Dr. James Edmunds also describes a like case (*Journal*, June 15th, 1867). A short time afterwards, four other cases were recorded—one by Dr. J. D. Brown (*Journal*, July 20th, 1867). Two by Dr. R. L. Bowles (*Journal*, June 20th, 1867); and one under the care of Dr. Broadbent at St Mary's Hospital, (*Journal*, August 3rd, 1867).

As this closes the number of cases hitherto placed on record, and the condition is, as Sir Thomas Watson justly remarked, "a very rare form of disorder," I have thought it right to be worth while to add the following case, which has lately fallen under my observation.

* *Brit. M. J.*, 1869, II, 4.

A few months ago, I was requested by Dr. Langhorne, of 227 Brompton Road, to meet him in consultation upon a case of excessive palpitation of the heart. We found the patient—a gentleman aged about 35, and leading ordinarily a very active and anxious life —suffering with severe dyspnoea and general depression, accompanied by marked symptoms of gastric derangement and slight muscular rheumatism. It was impossible to count the pulse, the beats being far too quick, feeble, and apparently irregular; but on placing the stethoscope upon the heart, we could distinctly count 200 pulsations in the minute —each pulsation being regular and uniform, and consisting of but one sound, and that quite free from murmur. The patient stated that his palpitation and distress had come on simultaneously two days before; and that he had had several previous attacks, but of a milder form.

Remembering the treatment of my former case, I suggested the free use of stimulants, with ammonia, potassa, and digitalis; and in the course of two days, the heart returned *suddenly* to its normal action, and at the same moment the patient to his ordinary condition—whether as a sequel or consequence of the treatment, a *post* or a *propter*, I cannot say.

I have very recently seen the same gentleman in perfect health, his heart beating quite naturally, and not exceeding 80 in the minute. He told me, however, that, since the attack which I have described, he has had several other similar in kind, but less severe; and that on each occasion the heart returned *suddenly* to its proper action.

Of the seven cases now recorded, in four instances the excessive action of the heart terminated *abruptly* and *suddenly;* the patients having been able to tell the exact moment of its occurrence. In the remaining three cases, the same may or may not have obtained; the circumstance either having escaped observation, or not having been stated. This forms an interesting feature in the dis-order, and is well worthy of notice in any similar cases which may occur.

I feel much hesitation even in suggesting an explanation of the strange phenomena exhibited in the cases I have related. In my former paper, I ventured upon the supposition that they were due either to an obscure and abnormal irritating state of the blood, or to an extreme and inexplicable sensitiveness, but having the common effect of causing the heart to contract upon its contents long before its cavities have had time to become filled to their normal extent. It remains, however, to reconcile with this, or, indeed, any other view of the matter, the *sudden* return of the heart to its healthy action. I confess that I am unable to understand this, but There are more things in heaven and earth Than are dreamt of in our philosophy.

Leon Bouveret

Leon Bouveret was born in 1850 at St. Julien-sur-Reyssouze, a small hamlet in the department of l'Ain, where his father was a country doctor. Leon Bouveret began the study of medicine at Lyon, then proceeded to Paris, where he became interne des hopitaux in 1873, receiving his doctor's degree in 1878. That year he returned to Lyon and in Lyon he spent the rest of his professional life. In 1880 he became professor agrégé at the University of Lyon but, in spite of his great merit and obvious ability, he never became a full professor. He died in 1929.

Bouveret left a very devoted group of disciples, who, as students, had followed him on his hospital rounds. "If indeed," wrote Lyonnet, "the young physicians have lost a great deal not to have heard his teaching, they have lost still more not to have known that Bouveret was not only a learned man, but an admirable man of rectitude, dignity, of independence and of devotion." Bouveret soon enjoyed a large practice and in Lyon and in that part of France was considered "the great consultant."

Bouveret's scientific achievements were of great excellence. He wrote articles or monographs on perspiration, cholera, typhoid fever, empyema, and aerophagia. His most ambitious work was his *Traité des maladies de l'estomac,* but the work by which he is best remembered is his article on paroxysmal tachycardia, since called by many French physicians *la maladie de Bouveret.*

CONCERNING ESSENTIAL PAROXYSMAL TACHYCARDIA

By L. Bouveret,* agrégé, physician to the hospital of Lyons

During the year 1885, I observed in my service at the hospital a man of fifty-five,

Rev. de méd. 1889, IX, 753.

attacked by a singular affection of the heart. A violent attack of palpitation had ceased suddenly, a few days before the admission of the patient. Since a certain time, similar attacks had often appeared, always without any appreciable cause. It was nearly impossible to feel the pulse at the radial artery. At the heart one could count more than 200 beats to the minute. These beats were moreover regular. The heart sounds, very short but very clear, were not accompanied by any murmur. What was still more unusual, at least during the first few days, was that the patient did not seem to suffer very much from this extreme acceleration of the cardiac rhythm. He was a little pale, he did not voluntarily leave his bed, but he did not present any of the serious trouble which ordinarily develops during the heart failure in valvular cardiopathies. His dyspnoea was always moderate, and this relative calmness of respiration presented a striking contrast to the extreme disturbance of the heart.

I was inclined to think that we were dealing, not with an organic lesion of the heart, but with a disturbance of the cardiac innervation. The hypothesis of a paralytic condition of the pneumogastric nerve seemed probable and I attributed this paralysis either to some bulbar lesion or to a deep tumor of the mediastinum compressing the pneumogastric nerve. But it soon became necessary to abandon this hypothesis. One day the extreme acceleration of the heart-beats ceased suddenly, and the pulse returned to a normal rate. It was equal, regular and beat 60 to 70 times per minute. The patient remained several days longer on my service, then he was able to leave the hospital and take up his old occupation. A careful examination, repeated after the termination of the attack, did not show signs of any lesion whatsoever of the heart, of the great vessels, of the lungs, of the mediastinum or of the nerve centers. The sudden and lasting disappearance of the tachycardia, moreover, was difficult to reconcile with the hypothesis of a permanent lesion of the nerve centers of the pneumogastric nerve. I lost sight of the patient and this observation remained incomplete. The interpretation of this case appeared very obscure to me. Certainly this violent attack of tachycardia, lasting several days during which the pulse almost disappeared at the radial artery, was not an ordinary attack of palpitation. On the other hand the patient showed neither exophthalmos nor enlargement of the thyroid, and besides, in

Basedow's Disease, the tachycardia is not present to such a degree.

I have recently, at the end of the year 1888 and at the beginning of the year 1889, encountered two new cases of this singular form of tachycardia, and I can relate the complete history of these two last patients. The three observations are quite similar. There are no differences between them from the point of view of their duration and of the seriousness of the secondary disturbances, caused by the weakness of the heart. Also, I have been able to find in the foreign literature several similar observations, one of which at least is accompanied by an autopsy.

The analysis of all these observations allows us to conclude that we are dealing with a certain neurosis of the heart, with a distinct species in the group of tachycardias. I propose to give this affection the name of *essential paroxysmal tachycardia (tachycardie essentielle paroxystique)*. I employ the term essential in the absence of a better expression; I wish to say that the symptoms observed point much more to a functional disturbance of the motor innervation of the heart than to any permanent lesion of the heart, of the cardiac nerves or of the nerve centers. As to the term paroxysmal, it expresses very clearly the fundamental characteristic of this form of tachycardia; it continues by attacks more or less long, in the intervals between, the function of the heart returns completely to the normal state.

I. *Personal observations.*—These two observations are complete and suffice to give a very exact idea of essential paroxysmal tachycardia.

In the first case, the affection has lasted more than fifteen years. The patient was fifty years of age. He was an intelligent man, well informed, very capable of observing himself, and who was able to give me numerous details of the attacks previous to the one of which I myself was a witness. In the beginning, the attacks were infrequent and of short duration; after some years they became more frequent and of longer duration, without it being possible to advance any cause to explain the irregular recurrences of the tachycardia.

The cause of the affection itself remains obscure enough. The patient shows no symptoms of a disease of the nerve centers. He is neither hysterical nor neurasthenic. There is no exophthalmos and the thyroid gland is not hypertrophied. The heart, examined frequently in the interval between attacks, is quite healthy, without a trace of hypertrophy or dilation, without any indication of a valvular lesion. The kidneys are also normal; in the interval between attacks, albuminuria, increased arterial tension and polyuria are entirely absent. There is no appreciable dyspeptic trouble, no intestinal disturbances and the stomach is not dilated. The liver is also normal; the patient has never suffered from hepatic colic or congestion of the liver. Besides, a true attack of essential paroxysmal tachycardia is a very different thing from an attack of reflex palpitation of gastric, intestinal or hepatic origin. The patient, it is true, for several years has used to excess coffee and tobacco; but during the past year, he has given up their use, and it was precisely during this period that he suffered from the most violent attacks.

In the history of the first patient, there have been long attacks and short attacks. The former lasted more than four or five days, the latter only a few hours, twenty-four hours most frequently. The distinction is important between these two types of paroxysms. If the tachycardia is of short duration, scarcely anything else is observed during the attack than an extreme acceleration of the heart beats. If the tachycardia persists longer than four or five days, then there appear disturbances of the pulmonary circulation and indeed of the systemic circulation.

Each paroxysm begins and ends suddenly, in a few seconds. These sudden transitions from normal rhythm to a tachycardial rhythm and vice versa are accompanied sometimes by peculiar sensations in the head or in the precordial region. During the attack, the patient often feels a painful sensation of thoracic constriction with a little numbness of the left arm, but this pain has only a slight resemblance with that which is characteristic of angina pectoris. The acceleration of the heart-beats is very extreme: in one attack 300 beats were counted, and I myself counted 220 and 230 to the minute. The attack ended, the patient was depressed for several days, especially after a severe attack, then his strength returned and he

soon was able to take up his occupation.

The second observation shows us a very long and severe attack, accompanied by alarming disturbances of the pulmonary and of the systemic circulation, and which, after a duration of about three weeks, terminated in a fatal collapse. An autopsy was not obtained but the clinical history is sufficient to allow us to discard the hypothesis of a lesion of the heart, of the cardiac nerves or of the nerve centers. In the midst of the paroxysm, the heart became weak and we found signs of a considerable dilation of the cardiac cavities. The cardiac dullness was so markedly enlarged, that, if the hand had not felt so clearly, from the apex to the base, the forceful beats, one could have believed that a pericardial effusion was present. The acceleration of the heart was extreme; one could count 200 and 220 beats to the minute. There was moreover a moment of respite in the course of this long paroxysm; for thirty-six hours, the pulse, up to that time almost imperceptible, reappeared at the radial artery, where one could count from 60 to 70 pulsations to the minute, quite forceful, equal, regular. Then the tachycardia reappeared with the same intensity and without a new interruption until the death of the patient.

The enfeeblement of the heart at first showed its harmful influence upon the pulmonary circulation. A wheezy and frequent cough, viscid expectoration then bloody, true hemoptysis, a dyspnoea more and more marked, such were the signs of a rapidly advancing pulmonary congestion, complicated by a pleurisy on the right and probably also by true hemorrhagic infarctions of the lung. The cyanosis of the face, the delirium, the congestion of the jugulars, the swelling of the liver and of the spleen, the marked diminution of urinary secretion and the albuminuria were evidences of grave disturbances of the systemic circulation, of the increasing congestion of the venous system and of the progressive fall of the arterial tension. Death was caused by cardiac weakness, but there was here a cardiac failure of a very peculiar kind, whose course is extremely rapid and whose primary cause is not a lesion of the valves or of the muscular fibres, but in a grave disturbance of the motor innervation of the heart.

PERICARDITIS
Guillaume Baillou
CONSULTATION CIX
CONCERNING PALPITATION OF THE HEART*

At one time in the heart itself is the cause of the affection, & then it is more dangerous: at another time it is from the neighboring parts, at another time from more remote parts, as from the uterus, from a malignant ulcer of the tibia. A tubercle in the heart, likewise an abscess can be the cause of the affection, too much blood producing an obstruction, too much heat, the heart impregnated with wriggling worms suddenly released. Just as moreover women who are wont to be afflicted with the affections of old age when they have become pregnant they are liberated and miraculously released indeed they are attacked again on the birth of fetus, thus, too, haughy pregnant women can be attacked by an illness, such as palpitations

& epilepsies, intense pain in the teeth and heaviness of the head. Besides these mentioned causes, inflammation, water contained in the sac of the heart, likewise if the sac contain within either a fluid putrid and smelling badly, or stones, it causes throbbing. Also a poisoned condition, a heavy exhalation or vapor either from the arteries or from the body of the heart, or from the lungs, or from the spleen or some other part, either brought from near or far: a severe spasm, a sore on the kidneys and back, particularly if the great arteries moving press on the spine, as vapor is raised up from the inflamed putrid fuel, there is a conducting (drawing together) of pestilential air and breath: adhesions of the pericardium to the body of the heart itself, which was observed in two dropsical patients.

* Ballonius, Gulielmus, *Consiliorum medicinalium libri* ii, Venice, Jeremia, 1735, ii, 388.

Richard Lower

Richard Lower was born in 1631 at Tremere near Bodmin, Cornwall, the second son of Humphrey Lower. He was educated at Westminster School and at Christ Church College, Oxford, receiving his B.A. in 1653, his M.A. in 1655, and his M.D. in 1665. He remained at Oxford after receiving his arts degrees and assisted Thomas Willis in his researches on the anatomy of the nervous system. He followed Willis to London in 1666, was elected a fellow of the Royal Society the following year and in 1675 became a fellow of the Royal College of Physicians. After the death of Willis in 1675, he was, according to his friend and patient Anthony à Wood, "esteemed the most noted Physician in *Westminster* and *London,* and no Mans name was more cried up at Court than his, he being then also Fellow of the *Coll. of Physicians.* At length upon the breaking out of the Popish Plot in 1678 (about which time he left the *Royal Society,* and thereupon their Experiments did in some manner decay) he closed with the Whiggs, supposing that Party would carry all before them: But being mistaken, he thereby lost much of his Practice at and near the Court, and so consequently his Credit." This quotation is from Anthony à Wood, who was one of his patients and good friends. He died in London in 1691, and was buried in the parish church of St. Tudy in Cornwall where he had been baptized 59 years before. He died in London in 1690 and was buried in the parish church of St. Tudy near Bodmin.

Lower was an excellent anatomist and an able physiologist. Willis praised him highly in his *Anatomy of the Brain* and gives him credit for most of the anatomical researches. His name remains in the anatomy of the heart from the tubercle of Lower, named in his honor. His researches in physiology were even more important. In 1665 he performed the first direct blood transfusion from one dog to another. The idea of blood transfusion had been previously suggested by Andreas Libavius in 1615 and, about 1640, according to Anthony à Wood, Francis Potter "entertained the notion of curing diseases by transfusion of Blood out of one Man into another: the hint whereof came into his

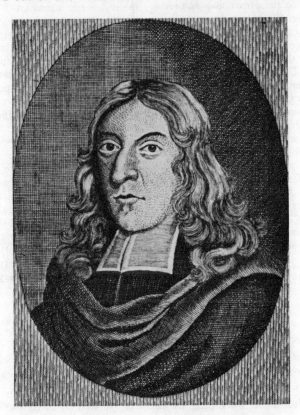

RICHARD LOWER (1631-1691)
A portrait of Lower at the age of fifty-five years

Head from *Ovid's* Story of *Medea* and *Jason*. Which matter he communicating to the *Royal Society* about the time of its first erection was entred into their Books." In 1669 Lower injected dark venous blood into the lungs of an animal and, noting that it immediately became bright red in color, concluded that it had absorbed air from the lungs. Lower's *Tractatus de corde,* which was first published in 1669, describes the heart as a muscle and contains illustrations of the unrolled muscular fibers which resemble very much those shown in anatomical papers which have appeared recently. In his *Tractatus de corde*, he described his transfusion experiments and also a case of adhesive pericarditis with autopsy. The following translation of the account of the case of adhesive pericarditis was made from the edition of 1728, published at Leyden.

3. With regard to this, the covering of the Heart, let it be said, it cannot have its function described by one term, for it serves to keep the Heart moist and to protect it from external injuries, thus injury can come to it not through one manner alone, for when too much water accumulates in it, injury of the Heart results and when water is lacking, it adheres closely to the Heart and moreover it may adhere on all sides to it; since it is also attached to the diaphragm it is inevitable that the motion of the Heart is combined & united with it; that this must be regarded as a great impediment and inconvenience to both, I show above, and it will appear more completely from this history.*

A married woman of the city of *London*, age 30 years, formerly healthy enough & lively, for the last three years of her life was very dejected, & melancholy, panting from any movement whatever, with a small & intermitting pulse, besides she complained continually of pain with a marked heaviness attacking the praecordium; & indeed of repeated swooning, & shortness of breath from any quick movement whatever of the body, & she became especially liable to coldness of

* Richard Lower, *Tractatus de corde,* Leyden. Verbek, 1728, p. 109.

the extremities, in which state she at last received aid from no medicine and, gradually with loss of strength, died.

On opening the body, no lesions in general were visible in the viscera of the lower abdomen, but when the other parts were examined, we detected an affection of the Heart, to which fault we ascribed the source of all the ills: for on opening the Thorax the lungs were healthy enough, however, the pericardium of the whole Heart was everywhere closely adherent, so that with the finger it was scarcely possible to separate it from the Heart: further, this membrane was not as it should be, thin & transparent, but thick, opaque & as if transformed into callus; hence with no space for the free movement of the Heart, & nothing by which it was moistened, if water had been present, it is no wonder that she complained immediately of all these ills. Besides, since the diaphragm is always attached to the pericardium in man, where the Heart itself also happens to be united, it can not be but that the Heart in every inspiration is drawn down with it, and so much so that the movements of it are so much slowed, & of necessity are suppressed; whence the intermission itself of the pulse followed so constantly every inspiration.

Albrecht von Haller

Albrecht von Haller, "the greatest systematist after Galen and one of the most imposing figures in all medical history" (Garrison) was born at Berne in 1708. He was a very precocious youth, writing Latin verses at the age of ten and composing scientific treatises at the age of fourteen. He began the study of medicine at Tübingen at the age of fifteen and the following year disproved the contention of his teacher, Professor Coschwitz, that the lingual vein was the salivary duct.

The rough student life of Tübingen displeased him very much and the inefficient medical teaching even more, so he proceeded to Leyden. After graduation at Leyden, where he had as teachers the great Boerhaave and the anatomist Albinus, he proceeded to Paris, where he studied anatomy with Winslow, and then to London, where he became the friend and pupil of Douglas. He returned to Berne in 1729 and entered the practice of medicine, became the librarian of the city library and began to teach anatomy. His fame as an anatomist and botanist led to his appointment as professor of anatomy, surgery and botany in the newly founded University of Göttingen.

Haller remained at Göttingen for seventeen years, living a life of the greatest activity. He founded a botanical garden, built an anatomical theatre, established the first physiological laboratory in Germany and found time to write some thirteen thousand scientific papers. Although professor of surgery, he could never bring himself to perform a surgical operation on a patient, in spite of the fact that he was most skillful in animal experimentation, and the master physiologist of his age.

At the age of forty-five he returned to his Swiss home and lived in Berne until his death in 1777, withstanding numerous inducements to return to Göttingen and to accept calls at Berlin and Halle.

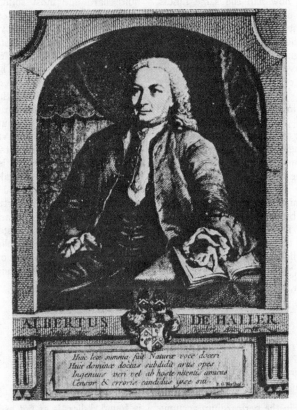

ALBRECHT VON HALLER (1708-1777)
A portrait by E. J. Handemann. Engraved by P. F. Tardieu

Haller was eminent as a botanist, anatomist, and physiologist. His most classic research was his demonstration that irritability is a specific property of muscle and sensibility of nerves. This work was based upon 567 separate experiments—190 of them being performed by his own hand. Haller also wrote historic novels and poems, these productions occupying an honorable place in the history of German literature, in spite of the derision with which Goethe greeted some of his verse.

The following observation from his *Opuscula pathologica* discusses a patient with palpitation of the heart, in whom an autopsy revealed adhesive pericarditis, aortic insufficiency, and mitral disease.

OBSERVATION NO. 52
STONE IN THE HEART*

But in the first place, the following unusual disease is worthy of discussion and from it a most excellent young person died not long since. The mother of the boy, I found on medical examination eight years ago to be suffering from palpitations of the heart, the youth now had the same illness. He himself, this day on which he died, was without the pulse, which you feel in the wrist. I found however, that the carotids were beating strongly. Chilling, then drenched with sweat, I gave unwillingly a bad prognosis. Shortly after his death we opened the body.

The pericardium was everywhere attached to the heart, the pleura to the lungs and all over the surface of the pericardium there were white patches, some hard, others filled with a whitish material like pus. Through these patches the heart was united to the pericardium. The inferior part of the right ventricle was semi strong, it was adherent to the pericardium by means of a mass of tophaceous calculi formed of fine sand. The fold between the two membranes of the aortic valves was calloused and partly stony. In

* Haller, Albrecht von, *Opuscula Pathologica,* Lausanne, Trottner, 1755, p. 135.

the valves of the aorta, between the membranes, there was a strange material, indeed the tendons which held these valves were found fleshy and spotted with bony scales. But a peculiar condition was present in the valves of the pulmonary vein. These were quite hard and most solid, so full of calcareous material that they everywhere grated on cutting the fibers. Moreover the pulmonary sinus was composed of a stony material.

Neither the heart nor great vessels exceeded the usual size. The patient's age, twenty years, increases the rarity of the disease. The heart of this youth was not stopped up; neither was the aperture large enough, it lacked alternate rest without which no heart can exist. Now the left ventricle received with difficulty blood from its sinus and sent it by its own contraction through the rigid opening of the bony mitral valves into the sinus. Also the blood could return from the aorta through the rigid aortic valves into the heart. Hence when the heart was constantly goaded, it palpitated constantly & when it could not send sufficient blood to the brain, it was the cause of a kind of stupor, such as follows from a loss of blood, from venesection & from wounds.

Leopold Auenbrugger
HYDROPS OF THE PERICARDIUM†
§LXVl

When the fluid in the pericardium accumulates in such a manner, that it can disturb the action of the heart, it is called hydrops of the pericardium; two species of which are observed, for it is either watery or purulent.

THE SIGN OF HYDROPS OF THE PERICARDIUM

Nearly all the signs accompany hydrops of the pericardium, which in general are described for hydrops of the chest.

However I have observed the following specific signs.

The note in the region of the heart, described elsewhere in III numbers 2 and 3,

† Auenbrugger, Leopold, *Inventum novum,* Vienna, Trattner, 1761, p. 86.

is found duller, is as flat as if you percussed a piece of meat.

In the epigastrium there is a swelling, which by its resistance you distinguish easily from a stomach distended by wind.

The patients sleep sitting up and with the head inclined forward.

They awake a second time suddenly, as soon as they feel the weight of the head falling down in front.

For this reason they complain to those about, of a disquieting propensity to slumber.

It happens then that fainting attacks (which recur more frequently because of inequality in the regularity and size of the pulse) afflict the unhappy patients, who in all positions in which they remain, suffer extreme anguish.

A few days before death, the neck in many is swollen: and their eyes become very red like those weeping.

With these signs apoplexy supervening, ends their life in an instant, or fainting terminates it.

The same signs indeed coincide entirely with those, which purulent enclosed cavities present.

The fluid contained in a purulent hydrops of the pericardium is wont to appear like whey. Since it is indeed purulent, it cleaves like fringes to the heart.

V. Collin

SOUND ANALOGOUS TO THE CREAKING OF NEW LEATHER*

We have only once observed the sound analogous to the creaking of new leather. It occurred in a patient who died of chronic pericarditis. This sound continued for the first six days of the disease, but disappeared as soon as the local symptoms indicated a slight liquid effusion into the pericardium. M. Devilliers, intern pupil at the Hospital of St. Antoine, observed it at the same time in a patient whose symptoms indicated pericarditis. He was not aware that the phenomenon had been already observed in this disease,

and did not avail himself of it in his diagnosis. The patient left the hospital after a rather long stay. He still showed the same sound and had not shown any improvement from the treatment which had been administered to him. It is regrettable that if this patient had died it would have been impossible to verify the diagnosis by autopsy. Perhaps this bruit may be a constant symptom of pericarditis before the appearance of effusion into the serous envelope of the heart, a very fleeting symptom in the cases where the disease terminates in a few days, of a longer duration when it is chronic.

* Collin, V., *Les diverses Methodes d'Exploration de la Poitrine,* Paris, Didot le Jeune, 1823, p. 44.

Thomas Morgan Rotch

Thomas Morgan Rotch was born at Philadelphia in 1849 and, graduating from Harvard in 1870, he received the degree of M.D. from the Harvard Medical School in 1874. He then spent two years abroad, principally at Berlin, Vienna, and Heidelberg, returned to Boston in 1876. At the time he began practice in Boston, there was no physician in New England devoting himself to the treatment of children's diseases and pediatrics was not even taught at the Harvard Medical School. Rotch was interested in the diseases of children from the first days of his practice and, through his initiative, a department of pediatrics was developed at Harvard and the Infants Hospital was founded— the first institution of its kind in America. In 1888, Harvard University established a chair for the diseases of children, of which Rotch was the first occupant.

Rotch played a very important rôle in the development of pediatrics, not only at Harvard, but all over the United States as well. He made pediatrics a vital subject in medical education and was a man of the highest ideals and of untiring energy and perseverance. He introduced the percentage method of feeding in pediatrics, founded the first milk laboratory in Boston and wrote an important treatise on pediatrics. In 1878, he described a sign, since known as Rotch's sign—dullness between the fifth and sixth right costal cartilage, seen particularly in pericardial effusion. Rotch's death in 1914 was a great loss to American pediatrics and to American medicine.

ABSENCE OF RESONANCE IN THE FIFTH RIGHT INTERCOSTAL SPACE DIAGNOSTIC OF PERICARDIAL EFFUSION*

By T. M. Rotch, M.D.

* * *

Perhaps it will be well to describe here shortly the case where I was enabled to determine the first signs of effusion in an adult, by the introduction of from seventy to eighty cubic centimeters of fluid, which is from twenty to thirty cubic centimeters less than the smallest amount laid down by authors as being possible to make a diagnosis by.

April 22, 1878. Subject, a female of medium size, who had died of cancer of the rectum: percussion of lungs and heart normal; resonance in fifth right intercostal space well marked. Dr. Maurice Richardson managed the cocoa-butter apparatus for me, keeping his eye on the graduated scale and his hand on the clamp; the trocar was introduced, and I proceeded to percuss lightly the fifth right interspace about one and one-half to two centimetres from the edge of the sternum, until decided flatness was found and verified by Dr. Richardson, who then immediately applied the clamp, when we found on our scale that when the flatness first appeared seventy to eighty cubic centimetres of fluid had been introduced, we then found that no vertical increase of flatness had taken place, and that the curved line bounding the area of flatness corresponded to that in Diagram III., the percussion flatness extending in the fifth interspace to about four centimetres from the edge of the sternum.

Next we will consider the large effusion, where the pericardium is pretty well filled from top to bottom.

May 10, 1878, with the assistance of Professor Bowditch, injected the Pericardium of an infant about two weeks old, until percussion showed that the praecordial flatness had extended to the nipple on the right, and beyond the nipple to the left, in an area corresponding to the front of the thorax as high as the fourth ribs, when it approached the sternum to within about one and a half centimetres, and then perhaps upward to the sternal notch.

* * *

In conclusion I shall describe as briefly as possible the extremely small number of clini-

cal observations which I have been able to make during the past winter.

The first was a woman who died at the Channing Home. Flatness on percussion was found in the fifth right intercostal space to the distance of five centimetres from the edge of the sternum. There was no increase of vertical flatness. The autopsy showed the pericardium to be distended with about one hundred and twenty cubic centimetres of fluid.

The second case is especially interesting as showing the difficulty which may be met with in the differential diagnosis between enlarged heart and effusion without the aid of our *fifth right intercostal space*. This case, a boy six years of age, is best spoken of in connection with another, a girl eleven years of age, who was under observation at the same time, through the kindness of Dr. Davenport, of the Children's Hospital. In both patients the same rational signs were presented, such as orthopnoea, praecordial pain, etc. In both cases the attack followed acute articular rheumatism. In both cases the force of the heart's impulse was of about the same intensity, and appeared to be a little to the left and below the left nipple. The vertical flatness was not increased in either case; the area of flatness to the left of the sternum was identical in both cases. In the boy, however, flatness was found in the fifth right intercostal space, while in the girl it did not extend beyond the left edge of the sternum. In the boy a loud undoubted pericardial friction sound developed at the base of the sternum; in the girl a decided murmur developed at the apex of the heart. These two last symptoms are spoken of to show the strong probability of the correctness of the diagnosis that the boy was a case of pericarditis, and that the girl was a case of endocarditis with enlarged heart, though of course this could only be proved by autopsy, and the cases must merely be taken for what they are worth; but, when we remember that the friction sound might have been absent, and that apparently endocardial murmurs may occur when no disease of the heart itself but merely a pericardial effusion is

* *Boston M. & S. J.*, 1878, XCIX, 423.

present, we again have to appeal to our *fifth right interspace* for diagnosis.

My third and last case was a patient seen at the City Hospital whom through the kindness of Dr. Doe, I was allowed to examine thoroughly. In this patient the area of percussion flatness, verified by Dr. Doe, exactly corresponded to that marked out in Diagram III., and I made my diagnosis simply by the flatness in the *fifth right interspace*. The case was especially interesting from the fact that it illustrated Gerhard's observation of the change of the area of flat-ness in effusion on change of position of the patient. When the patient was in the position of orthopnoea we obtained the fifth interspace flatness; when she was horizontal this flatness disappeared, leaving the normal resonance of the lung.

As additional proof that this was a case of pericardial effusion, an undoubted pericardial friction sound, testified to by several of the physicians at the hospital, developed, and according to Professor Traube it is exceedingly rare to mistake this sound for a pleural friction sound.

Sir William H. Broadbent

William Henry Broadbent was born at Huddersfield, Yorkshire, England, in 1835, and was educated at Huddersfield College which he left at the age of sixteen to embark in business. Commercial life, however, had no appeal for him and he proceeded to Manchester, where he studied at Owens College, and later entered the Royal School of Medicine in that city. While a student of medicine, he was apprenticed to a surgeon in Manchester and had to visit patients, dispense medicines, and make long rounds at night on foot. He was a brilliant student and although working under great handicaps, won medals in botany, materia medica, midwifery, medicine, surgery, anatomy, physiology and chemistry. He passed the examination of the Royal College of Physicians in 1857 and applied for the post of house surgeon at the Manchester Infirmary, but was unsuccessful. He was keenly disappointed at this failure and went to Paris for eight months, where he worked under Trousseau and Ricord and acquired a remarkable proficiency in the French language. He returned to London in 1858 and received his M.B. degree at the University of London.

Broadbent then obtained a position as Obstetric Officer at St. Mary's Hospital and the following year, became Medical Officer. He was connected with St. Mary's Hospital and its medical school for nearly forty years and exercised a powerful and beneficent influence upon the institution. He became a Fellow of the Royal Society in 1896 and received honorary degrees from Edinburgh, St. Andrews, Leeds, and Toronto. He was created a baronet in 1893. He died in 1907.

Sir William Broadbent was a great clinician, a man of high ideals, strong feelings, and quick impulses. He came to London with slender financial resources, with no professional or social connections, and, by hard work and great tenacity of purpose, became one of its leading consultants. His investigations of the nervous system were striking in their originality and thoroughness, and his book on *The Pulse* and his *Heart Disease* remain classics.

Broadbent's name is familiar to medical students the world over, from Broadbent's sign, first published by his son Walter Broadbent in 1895. Sir William Broadbent, in a paper published in 1898, discusses a case in which he had observed this sign twenty years earlier.

ADHERENT PERICARDIUM*

By Sir William Broadbent, Bart., M.D., F.R.S.

* * *

Other evidences of fixation of the heart are imperfect descent of the apex-beat during inspiration and inadequate shifting of the cardiac impulse when the patient lies first on one the apex-beat and of its maximum impulse may be observed even when the heart is dilated and hypertrophied in consequence of valvular disease. Distinct evidence of free

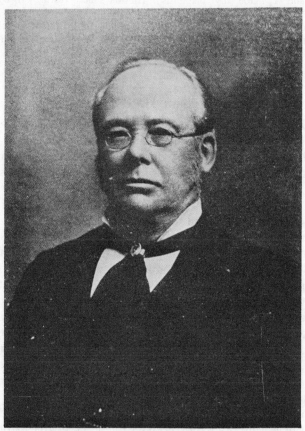

Courtesy of the "Lancet"
SIR WILLIAM H. BROADBENT (1835-1907)
Photograph by Elliot and Fry

side and then on the other, more particularly when he turns upon his right side. As a rule, in normal conditions the apex, when its beat is recognisable, disappears from the fifth space and is felt in the sixth on a deep breath being taken and held, and moves for an inch or so towards the middle line, descending also somewhat when the patient lies over on the right side. Similar shifting of

mobility obtained in this way would exclude pericardial adhesions, and a marked failure to respond to the test would raise a strong presumption of its existence. But nothing must be accepted as absolute in clinical investigation, and the exercise of judgment will be called for in estimating the significance and value of the results obtained. For example, whether the pericardium is adherent or not a deep inspiration may bring the lung over the heart and the apex-beat may be al-

* *Trans. Med. Soc. London,* 1898, XXI, 109.

together obliterated; its disappearance from the fifth or other space, therefore, is not conclusive of mobility. Again, when the patient is turned over on his right side a transference of the seat of maximum impulse may simply mean that another part of the heart has been brought in contact with the chest wall and not that the apex has shifted. Not unfrequently, however, from one cause or another, no apex-beat or impulse of any kind can be felt, so that palpation affords no assistance whatever and percussion cannot be relied upon to furnish the kind of evidence required to distinguish between fixation and mobility of the heart.

Indications may be furnished by dilatation and hypertrophy, which may sometimes be quite conclusive when there is no valvular disease. The dulness in a characteristic case usually begins in the third space, and the apex-beat will be at the nipple level or even higher and outside the mamma. It will probably not shift with a deep breath, but it may be obscured. The transverse position of the heart and the fixation of the apex above its normal point of contact with the chest wall I formerly looked upon as a consequence of effusion which had carried the apex upwards and left it adherent there. I am now convinced that the cause is not effusion but dilation. There may be conspicuous falling in the fourth and fifth spaces, and although this may be due to atmospheric pressure when the heart is very greatly enlarged from any cause it may be a true retraction or tugging. Diastolic tugging may sometimes be felt when the hand is applied over the region of the apex; there is not merely a subsidence of the push but a sharp shock as if the chest wall were dragged upon from within, which is quite different from what is felt even after the most powerful thrust which is given by the dilated and hyperthrophied heart of aortic regurgitation.

A systolic tug of the left false ribs posteriorly communicated by the diaphragm may be conspicuous. The recoil from the drag may be so distinct as to look and feel to the hand like pulsation, and in the first case in which I observed it, now more than 20 years since—a case of left empyema—it was taken for pulsation, and it was supposed that a pulsating tumor of some kind underlay the empyema. A *post-mortem* examination showed that the cause was adherent pericardium. I have often seen this tugging since, and in some cases it can be made to affect the right false ribs by causing the patient in the sitting position to lean over to the left so far as to throw the drag of the heart upon the right half of the diaphragm. It must be added that this indication is not infallible, as the tugging has been observed when the heart was hypertrophied without adhesions.

Walter Broadbent

AN UNPUBLISHED PHYSICAL SIGN*

By Walter Broadbent, M.B., Cantab.,
House Physician at the Brompton Hospital for Consumption

By the kind permission of the physicians at the Brompton Hospital I am permitted to publish the notes of four cases now under their care in the wards, in each of which there is visible retraction, synchronous with the cardiac systole, of the left back in the region of the eleventh and twelfth ribs, and in three of which there is also systolic retraction of less degree in the same region of the right back. In all these cases there is a definite history of pericarditis, and in three of them there are other conditions strongly suggesting an adherent pericardium. The only means of causing this retraction on both sides seems to be the diaphragm, which, if pulled upon, would have more effect on the floating eleventh and twelfth ribs than on the more fixed ones. In cases of large heart with adherent pericardium there is a considerable area of the ventricles closely adherent to the central tendon of the diaphragm, and the powerful contraction of the hypertrophied heart must give a decided tug to this structure. That it should effect the ribs more often on the left side would be expected from the adhesion being mainly to the left of the middle line; the liver also; which is often large in these cases, may restrain the movement on the right.

* *Lancet*, 1895, II, 200.

CASE I—A youth aged eighteen years had rheumatic fever in 1890 and pericarditis in 1893. He is pale and thin, with carotid pulsation very marked in the neck. He also shows capillary pulsation. His pulse (80) is regular in force and frequency. The artery is large and visible for two inches up the arm. The wave is sudden, large bisferiens, and almost completely collapsing. The chest bulges on the left side from the second rib downwards. The apex beat is a very powerful thrust in the sixth space four inches and a half below and one inch and a half outside the nipple. There is systolic retraction of the third and fourth left spaces, and also of the epigastric region, and pulsation in the fifth and sixth left spaces. The apex beat does not change its position on his taking a deep breath, and moves barely half an inch when he lies on one side or the other. In the left back, between the posterior axillary and scapula angle lines, retraction, synchronous with the cardiac systole, is seen and felt in the tenth and eleventh spaces, and over the twelfth rib and just below it. In the right back, systolic retraction of almost equal intensity is present over precisely the same area. The cardiac dulness is bounded above by a line from the midsternum opposite the fourth cartilage to the nipple; and in the sixth space extends from the right of the sternum to two inches outside the vertical nipple line. Deep inspiration only slightly decreases this area. The heart sounds are as follows: at the apex there is a blowing systolic murmur almost entirely replacing the first sound, and a long low murmur filling the diastole. Both murmurs are heard round to the back. In the tricuspid area there are a good first sound, a blowing systolic murmur, a second sound, and a blowing diastolic murmur. At the pulmonary cartilage a rough systolic murmur, slightly accentuated second sound, and a blowing diastolic murmur are audible. At the aortic cartilage there are a rough vibratory systolic murmur, a second sound, and a loud blowing diastolic murmur. In the neck there is heard a very loud vibratory systolic murmur, but no second sound. The liver is only just felt below the margin of the ribs. Respiration is almost entirely costal and the epigastric region recedes on inspiration. There is slight dulness at the left base, and some rhonchi and crepitations are heard over the lower part of both lungs, especially the left.

CASE 2.—A girl aged eighteen had pericarditis with rheumatic fever in 1893. She is a thin, anaemic girl with slightly flushed cheeks. Her pulse (116) is regular in force and frequency. The artery is of fair size, just felt between the beats; the wave is large and short, and very easily compressible. There is very little praecordial bulging. The apex beat is in the fifth space, an inch and a half below and half on inch external to the nipple; the sixth rib is also lifted. A presystolic thrill is felt, followed by a short powerful impulse. Slight pulsation is also visible in the second, third and fourth spaces on the left side, and to the right of the sternum in the fourth and fifth spaces. In the epigastrium there is very slight systolic retraction. The apex beat does not alter its position on her taking a deep breath, and only moves very slightly on her turning to either side. In the left back there is seen retraction, during the cardiac systole, of the tenth space and eleventh and twelfth ribs with the region just below. In the right back there is a similar retraction of the twelfth rib with the space above and below. Cardiac dulness begins in the third space from the midsternum to the left vertical nipple line, and in the fourth space extends from half an inch to the right of the sternum to half an inch outside the left nipple line; in the fifth space it extends from three-quarters of an inch to the right of the sternum to one inch outside the nipple line. Deep inspiration does not decrease the cardiac dulness. The sounds heard are at the apex, a short soft rumbling presystolic murmur leading up to a very loud banging first sound, and a whistling systolic murmur; no second sound is audible. The first sound and the systolic murmur are conducted round to the back. In the tricuspid area there are heard a first sound, a blowing and slightly whistling systolic murmur, and a second sound. At the pulmonary cartilage there was a first sound, a soft systolic murmur, and an accentuated and reduplicated second sound. At the aortic cartilage a loud first sound and second sound are audible. The liver is felt two fingers breadth below the costal margin. The abdomen moves very poorly in respiration even for a girl, and the epigastrium sinks in on inspiration. In the lungs there is tuberculous infiltration of the right upper lobe, with some excavation. There is also slight want of resonance at the left base, with diminished breath sounds.

CASE 3.—This is a young man aged twenty-one years. In 1888 and 1890 he had rheumatic fever, and in 1892 pericarditis and left-sided pleurisy. He is fairly healthy-looking, being only short of breath on exertion. His pulse (108) is regular in force and frequency. The artery is rather large and just visible at the wrist, being nearly empty between the beats; the wave is short and large and is easily compressible. There is some praecordial prominence below the third rib on the left side. The apex beat is in the sixth space, four inches below and half an inch external to the nipple. There is a powerful thrust in the fifth and sixth spaces, with a shock at the end of systole; pulsation is also seen in the third and fourth spaces. There is slight systolic retraction of the epigastric region, but pulsation is felt on deep palpation. The apex beat appears in the seventh space when he takes a deep breath, and moves half an inch internally on his lying on the right side, and one inch and a half externally on lying on the left side. In the left back systolic retraction is seen from the tenth space to just below the twelfth rib, between the posterior axillary and scapula angle lines. On the right side, the tip of the twelfth rib is seen to be drawn in during the cardiac systole. The cardiac dulness is in the third space two inches to the left of the sternum, in the fourth space from the mid-sternum to the left nipple, and in the fifth and sixth spaces from the right margin of the sternum to one inch and a half outside the vertical nipple line. This area is considerably decreased on deep inspiration. At the apex there are heard a short, loud, banging first sound and a harsh, systolic murmur, but no second sound. The first sound and murmur are conducted through the axilla to the back. Over the tricuspid area a loud first sound, a blowing systolic murmur, and a sharp second sound are audible. At the pulmonary cartilage there are heard a first sound, a systolic murmur, and slightly accentuated and reduplicated second sound. At the aortic cartilage, a short first sound, a soft systolic murmur, and a fair second sound are audible. The liver is not enlarged. Respiratory movement is absent in the epigastric region and very poor in the lower abdomen. In the lungs there is diminished resonance at both bases, and the breath sounds are weak at the right base, but good at the left base.

CASE 4.—A girl aged seventeen years had rheumatic fever and pericarditis in 1890, and rheumatic fever again in 1892. She is delicate looking, small for her age; she becomes short of breath on the slightest exertion. Her pulse (92) is regular in force and frequency; the artery is small, and not felt between the beats; the wave is short and small and is very easily compressible. There is very marked bulging of the left chest below the second rib, and of the lower sternum; the apex beat is in the sixth space two inches below and one inch outside the nipple; it is a powerful thrust. Its position does not alter on deep inspiration or on her turning on to either side. There is systolic retraction in the third and fourth left spaces, also in the epigastric region, and in the fifth and sixth right spaces for one and a half inches from the sternum. There is well marked pulsation in the fifth and sixth left spaces, and the ribs are lifted. In the left back, there is slight systolic retraction of the eleventh and twelfth ribs and the region just below. There is no retraction in the right back. The cardiac dulness is in the second space for an inch, in the third space from the mid-sternum to the nipple line, in the fourth space from one inch to the right of the sternum to one inch outside the left nipple, and in the fifth and sixth spaces from one and a half inches to the right of the sternum to one inch outside the left nipple. On deep inspiration the dulness disappears from the second space, but the rest of the area remains. At the apex are heard a short loud first sound, a loud, rough systolic murmur, and an indistinct reduplicated second sound. The systolic murmur is conducted round to the back. Over the tricuspid area, a first sound, a blowing systolic murmur, and a slightly reduplicated second sound are audible. At the pulmonary cartilage there are heard a first sound, a rough systolic murmur, and an accentuated and reduplicated second sound. At the aortic cartilage a first sound, a soft systolic murmur, and a second sound are heard. The liver extends nearly three fingers' breadth below the costal margin. The epigastrium is a little drawn in during inspiration, and the rest of the abdomen moves only very slightly in respiration. The lungs are normal, with good resonance and good breath sounds at both bases.

Of these cases the first is one of aortic disease of rheumatic origin, and the others of mitral regurgitation, with a variable amount of stenosis. In Cases 1, 2 and 4 there is evidence of adhesion of the pericardium to the chest wall as well, but in Case 3 the heart moves freely under the ribs, and the lung expands well over it, so that the sign is much more important, as being the only clear evidence that the pericardium is adherent. This sign has long been pointed out by Sir William Broadbent in the wards of St. Mary's Hos-

pital, but, so far as I have heard, has not had sufficient importance attached to it elsewhere. Adherent pericardium has frequently such a serious influence on the course of valvular disease, that any aid towards the diagnosis seems worthy of attention.

Brook-street, Grosvenor-square, **W.**

ANGINA PECTORIS
The Earl of Clarendon

One of the early accounts of angina pectoris is found in the *Life of Edward Earl of Clarendon* which describes the death of his father.

Edward Hyde was born in 1609 and graduated from Oxford in 1626. He entered Parliament and became allied with the Royal party. After the defeat of the Royalists, he retired to the Continent where he remained during Cromwell's rule. After the Restoration, Hyde returned to London with Charles II and was appointed Lord High Chancellor. In 1661 he was created Earl of Clarendon and a short time before he received his honor, his daughter Anne was married secretly to James, Duke of York, brother of Charles II. Two of Anne's daughters, Mary and Anne, subsequently became queens of England. Clarendon was later treated with base ingratitude by his sovereign, was banished from England, and spent the remainder of his life in exile. He died at Rouen in 1674.

While Clarendon had certain definite limitations as a statesman he occupies an important place in English literature as a writer and historian. His *History of Rebellion* is his best known work.

The following extract is from *The life of Edward Earl of Clarendon, Lord High Chancellor of England and Chancellor of the University of Oxford containing An Account of the Chancellor's Life from his Birth to the Restoration in 1660*. Oxford (1759), p. 9.

His Father had long suffered under an Indisposition (even before the Time his Son could remember) which gave him rather frequent Pains, than Sickness; and gave him Cause to be terrified with the Expectation of the Stone, without being exercised with the present Sense of it; but from the Time He was sixty Years of Age, it increased very much, and four or five Years before his Death, with Circumstances scarce heard of before, and the Causes whereof are not yet understood by any Physician; He was very often, both in the Day and the Night, forced to make Water, seldom in any Quantity, because He could not retain it long enough, and in the Close of that Work, without any

sharp Pain in those Parts, He was still and constantly seized on by so sharp a Pain in the left Arm, for Half a Quarter of an Hour, or near so much, that the Torment made him as pale (whereas He was otherwise of a very sanguine Complexion) as if He were dead; and He used to say, "that He had passed the Pangs of Death, and He should die in one of those Fits;" as soon as it was over, which was quickly, He was the chearfullest Man living; eat well such Things as He could fancy, walked, slept, digested, conversed with such a Promptness and Vivacity upon all Arguments (for He was *omnifariam doctus*), as hath been seldom known in a Man of his Age: But He had the Image of Death so constantly before him in those continual Torments, that for many Years before his Death, He always parted with his Son, as to see him no more; and at Parting still shewed him his Will, discoursing very particularly and very chearfully of all Things He would have performed after his Death.

lay; and He obliged his Son to accompany him thither before his Return to *London;* and He came to *Salisbury* on the *Friday* before *Michaelmass* Day in the Year 1632, and lodged in his own House that Night; the next Day He was so wholly taken up in receiving Visits from his many Friends, being

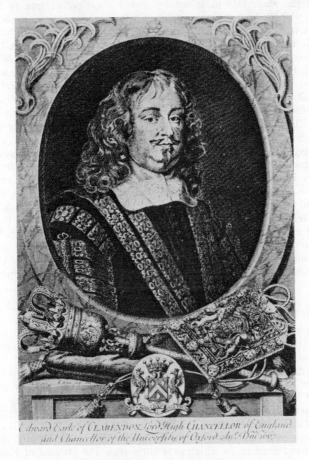

THE EARL OF CLARENDON
Frontispiece to *The Life of Edward Earl of Clarendon* (Oxford 1759). Drawn by P. Lely. Etched by R. White

He had for some time resolved to leave the Country, and to spend the Remainder of his Time in *Salisbury,* where He had caused a House to be provided for him, both for the Neighbourhood of the Cathedral Church, where He could perform his Devotions every Day, and for the Conversation of many of his Family who lived there, and not far from it; and especially that He might be buried there, where many of his Family and Friends

a Person wonderfully reverenced in those Parts, that he walked very little out of his House. The next Morning, being *Sunday,* He rose very early, and went to two or three Churches, and when He returned, which was by eight of the Clock, He told his Wife and his Son, "that He had been to look out a "Place to be buried in, but found none "against which he no some Exception, the "Cathedral only excepted, where He had "made Choice of a Place near a Kinsman of "his own Name, and had shewed it to the "Sexton, whim He had sent for to that Pur- "pose; and wished them to see him buried "there;" and this with as much Composed- ness of Mind as if it had made no impression on him; then went to the Cathedral to Ser- mon, and spent the whole Day in as chear- ful conversation with his Friends (saving only the frequent Interruptions his Infirmity gave him once in two or three Hours, sometimes more, sometimes less) as the Man in the most confirmed Health could do. *Monday* was *Michaelmass* Day, when in the Morning He went to visit his Brother Sir *Laurence Hyde,* who was then making a Journey in the Service of the King, and from him went to the Church to a Sermon, where He found himself a little pressed as He used to be. and therefore thought fit to make what Haste He could to his House, and was no sooner come thither into a lower Room, than having made Water, and the Pain in his Arm seizing upon him, He fell down dead, without the least Motion of any Limb: The Suddenness of it made it apprehended to be an Apoplexy, but there being nothing like Convulsions, or the least Distortion or Alteration in the Visage, it is not like to be from that Cause, nor could the Physicians make any reasonable Guess from whence that mortal Blow pro- ceeded. He wanted about six Weeks of at- taining the Age of seventy, and was the greatest instance of the Felicity of a Country Life that was seen in that Age; having en- joyed a competent, and to him a plentiful Fortune, a very great Reputation of Piety and Virtue, and his Death being attended with universal Lamentation. It cannot be ex- pressed with what Agony his Son bore this Loss, having as He was used to say, "not only lost the best Father, but the best Friend and the best Companion He ever had or could have;" and He was never so well pleased, as when He had fit Occasions given him to mention his Father, whom He did in Truth believe to be the wisest Man He had ever known, and He was often heard to say, in the Time when his Condition was at highest, "that though God Almighty had been very propitious to him, in raising him to great Honours and Preferments, He did not value any Honour He had so much, as the being the Son of such a Father and Mother, for whose Sakes principally He though God had conferred those Blessings upon him."

William Heberden

"Was born in London in the year 1710, and received the early part of his education in that city. At the close of the year 1724 he was sent to St. John's College in Cambridge, and six years after was elected a Fellow. From that time he directed his attention to the study of medicine, which he pursued partly at Cambridge and partly in London. Having taken his degree of Doctor of Physic he practised in the University for about ten years, and during that time read every year a course of lectures on the Materia Medica. In the year 1746 he became a Fellow of the Royal College of Physicians, and two years after- wards, leaving Cambridge, he settled in London and was elected into the Royal Society. He very soon got into great business, which he followed with unremitting attention above thirty years, till it seemed prudent to withdraw a little from the fatigues of his profession. He therefore purchased a house at Windsor, to which he used ever afterwards to retire during some of the summer months; but returned to London in the winter, and still continued to visit the sick for many years.

In 1766 he recommended to the College of Physicians the first design of the Medi- cal Transactions, in which he proposed to collect together such observations as might have occurred to any of their body, and were likely to illustrate the history or cure of diseases. The plan was soon adopted, and three volumes have successively been laid before the public. In 1778 the Royal Society of Medicine in Paris chose him into the number of their Asso- ciates. Besides the observations contained in the present volume, Doctor Heberden was the author of several papers in the Medical Transactions, and of some in the Philosophical Transactions of the Royal Society. He declined all professional business several years be- fore his death, which was mercifully postponed till the year 1801. when he was advancing to the age of ninety-one.

From his early youth he had always entertained a deep sense of religion, a consummate love of virtue, an ardent thirst after knowledge, and an earnest desire to promote the welfare and happiness of mankind. By these qualities, accompanied with great sweetness of manners, he acquired the love and esteem of all good men, in a degree which perhaps very few have experienced; and after passing an active life with the uniform testimony of good conscience, he became an eminent example of its influence, in the cheerfulness and serenity of his latest age."

The above biography of William Heberden was written by his son, William Heberden the younger, and appears in his *Commentaries on the History and Cure of Diseases*, which was composed in the Latin language and trans-

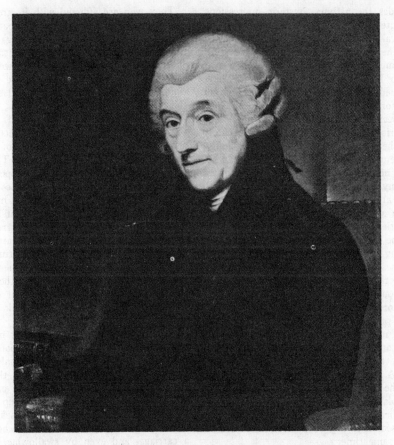

WILLIAM HEBERDEN (1710-1801)
Reproduced from a portrait by Sir William Beechey, R.A., through the courtesy of the Royal College of Physicians, London

lated by his son into English. Heberden was one of the best Latin and Hebrew scholars of his time and was a man of wide learning and culture. Dr. Johnson, in his last illness, being asked what physician he had summoned, answered, "Dr. Heberden, *ultimus Romanorum,* the last of our learned physicians."

Heberden's *Commentaries* and its English translation, ran through numerous editions and contained his original descriptions of angina pectoris and chicken pox. The descriptions of these two diseases found in this book are from the Boston edition of 1818. His descriptions of angina pectoris was published first in 1768, in the *Medical Transactions of the College of Physicians,* and his account of chicken pox in the same publication for the year 1767. Angina pectoris had been observed before but it was Heberden's account that led to its recognition by the profession as a distinct disease entity.

CHAPTER 70

PECTORIS DOLOR*

Besides the asthma, hysteric oppressions, the acute darting pains, in pleurisies, and the chronical ones in consumptions, the breast is often the seat of pains, which are distressing, sometimes even from their vehemence, oftener from their duration as they have continued to tease the patient for six, for eight, for nine, and for fourteen years. There have been several examples of their returning periodically every night, or alternately with a head-ach. They have been called gouty, and rheumatic and spasmodic. There has appeared no reason to judge that they proceed from any cause of much importance to health (being attended with no fever,) or that they lead to any dangerous consequences; and if the patient were not uneasy with what he feels, he needs never to be so on account of anything which he has to fear.

If these pains should return at night and disturb the sleep, small doses of opium have been found serviceable, and may be used alone, or joined with an opening medicine, with a preparation of antimony, or with the fetid gums. Externally, a small perpetual blister applied to the breast has been successful, and so has an issue made in the thigh. A large cumin plaster has been worn over the seat of the pain with advantage. The volatile, or saponaceous liniment, may be rubbed in over the part affected. Bathing in the sea, or in any cold water, may be used at the same time.

But there is a disorder of the breast marked with strong and peculiar symptoms, considerable for the kind of danger belonging to it, and not extremely rare, which deserves to be mentioned more at length. The seat of it, and sense of strangling, and anxiety with which it is attended, may make it not improperly be called angina pectoris.

*William Heberden, *Commentaries on the History and Cure of Diseases,* Boston, Wells and Lilly, 1818, p. 292.

They who are afflicted with it, are seized while they are walking, (more especially if it be up hill, and soon after eating) with a painful and most disagreeable sensation in the breast, which seems as if it would extinguish life, if it were to increase or continue; but the moment they stand still, all this uneasiness vanishes.

In all other respects, the patients are, at the beginning of this disorder, perfectly well, and in particular have no shortness of breath, from which it is totally different. The pain is sometimes situated in the upper part, sometimes in the middle, sometimes at the bottom of the os sterni, and often more inclined to the left than to the right side. It likewise very frequently extends from the breast to the middle of the left arm. The pulse is, at least sometimes, not disturbed by this pain, as I have had opportunities of observing by feeling the pulse during the paroxysm. Males are most liable to that disease, especially such as have passed their fiftieth year.

After it has continued a year or more, it will not cease so instantaneously upon standing still; and it will come on not only when the persons are walking, but when they are lying down, especially if they lie on their left side, and oblige them to rise up out of their beds. In some inveterate cases it has been brought on by the motion of a horse, or a carriage, and even by swallowing, coughing, going to stool, or speaking, or any disturbance of the mind.

Such is the most usual appearance of this disease; but some varieties may be met with. Some have been seized while they were standing still or sitting; also upon first waking out of sleep: and the pain sometimes reaches to the right arm, as well as to the left, and even down to the hands, but this is uncommon: in a very few instances the arm has at the same time been numbed and swelled. In one of two persons the pain has lasted some hours, or even days; but this has happened when the complaint has been of long standing, and thoroughly rooted in the constitution: once only the very first attack continued the whole night.

I have seen nearly a hundred people under this disorder, of which number there have been three women, and one boy twelve years old. All the rest were men near, or past the fiftieth year of their age.

Persons who have persevered in walking till the pain has returned four or five times, have then sometimes vomited.

A man in the sixtieth year of his life began to feel, while he was walking, an uneasy sensation in his left arm. He never perceived it while he was traveling in a carriage. After it had continued ten years, it would come upon two or three times a week at night, while he was in bed, and then he was obliged to sit up for an hour or two before it would abate so much as to suffer him to lie down. In all other respects he was very healthy, and had always been a remarkably strong man. The breast was never affected. This disorder, its seat excepted, perfectly resembled the angina pectoris, gradually increasing in the same manner, and being both excited and relieved by all the same causes. He died suddenly without a groan at the age of seventy-five.

The termination of the angina pectoris is remarkable. For, if no accidents intervene, but the disease go on to its height, the patients all suddenly fall down, and perish almost immediately. Of which indeed their frequent faintness, and sensations as if all the powers of life were failing, afford no obscure intimation.

The angina pectoris, as far as I have been able to investigate, belongs to the class of spasmodic, not inflammatory complaints, For,

In the 1st place, the access and the recess of the fit is sudden.

2dly, There are long intervals of perfect health.

3dly, Wine, and spirituous liquors, and opium afford considerable relief.

4thly, It is increased by disturbance of the mind.

5thly, It continues many years without any other injury to the health.

6thly, In the beginning it is not brought on by riding on horseback, or in a carriage, as is usual in diseases arising from scirrhus or inflammation.

7thly, During the fit the pulse is not quickened.

Lastly, Its attacks are often after the first sleep, which is a circumstance common to many spasmodic disorders.

Yet it is not to be denied that I have met with one or two patients, who have told me they now and then spit up matter and blood, and that it seemed to them to come from the seat of the disease. In another, who fell down dead without any notice, there immediately arose such as offensive smell, as made all who were present judged that some foul abscess had just then broken.

On opening the body of one who died suddenly of the disease, a very skillful anatomist could discover no fault in the heart, in the valves, in the arteries, or neighboring veins, excepting some small rudiments of ossification in the aorta. The brain was likewise every where sound. In this person, as it has happened to others who have died by the same disease, the blood continued fluid two or three days after death, not dividing itself into crassamentum and serum, but thick, like cream. Hence when a vein has been opened a little before death, or perhaps soon after, the blood has continued to ooze out as long as the body remained unburied.

With respect to the treatment of this complaint, I have little or nothing to advance: Nor indeed is it to be expected we should have made much progress in the cure of a disease, which has hitherto hardly had a place or a name in medical books.* Quiet and warmth, the spirituous liquors, help restore patients who are nearly exhausted, and to dispel the effects of a fit when it does not soon go off. Opium taken at bed-time will prevent

---

* Coelius Aurelianus, as far as I know, is the only ancient writer who has noticed this complaint, and he but slightly: "Erasistratus memorat paralyseos genus, et *paradoxon* appellat, quo ambulantes repente sistunture, ut ambulare non possint, et tum rursum ambulare sinuntur." *Chron.* lib. ii. c. 1-M. Saussure in his *Voyage dans les Alpes* says, that at the height of 13 or 1400 toises above the sea, a peculiar tiredness often comes upon those who are ascending such high hills, so that it is impossible to proceed four steps further; and if it were attempted, such strong universal palpitations would come on, as could not fail to end in swooning. Upon resting three minutes, even without sitting down, this tiredness passes, and the power of going on is perfectly restored. The climbing of steep hills, which are not so high above the sea, does not occasion this peculiar fatigue. Vol. 1. p. 482.

the attacks at night. I knew one who set himself a task of sawing wood for half an hour every day, and was nearly cured. In one also the disorder ceased of itself. Bleeding, vomiting, and purging, appear to me to be improper.

* * *

John Fothergill

XXII. FARTHER ACCOUNT OF THE ANGINA PECTORIS†

By J. Fothergill, M.D., F.R.S.

Since my former paper on this subject was delivered to the Society, I have had another opportunity of being informed by dissection of some circumstances relative to this disease, which are here submitted to your consideration.

H. R. Esq. aged sixty-three, a gentleman rather inclined to corpulency, but active, and of a very irritable habit, middling stature, and fresh complexion, employed in affairs that often required attention and confinement, writing especially, complained to me three or four years before his death, that he often found a difficulty, or rather an incapacity, to walk up a moderate ascent, especially if he attempted to do it hastily. I soon perceived that this obscure disease, which had hitherto for the most part baffled all my endeavours to remove it, was taking place. I advised great temperance and moderation in diet, in drinking, and application to ride frequently, pass his summers in the country, to shun everything that would agitate his spirits, or depress them, a gentle laxative medicine and stomach bitter to be continued for a fortnight, and occasionally to be repeated, promoted his general health; and his own care contributed greatly to prevent the increase of this malady. In the summer of 1774, he spent a few weeks at Buxton, where he bathed, and drank the water, and returned to town in better health than he had enjoyed for some years before. Being much disposed to flatulency, he now and then took a warm cardiac draught, which he found relieved him, and pretty often some aloetic pills, to prevent constiveness, but pursued no other plan of medicine, contenting himself with observing, and with some degree of attention, the general regulations I had prescribed to him; and though it did not appear that much ground was hereby gained, the same constriction returning if he attempted

† *Med. Obs. & Inq.*, London, 1776, v, 252.

any exercise beyond a certain point, which his own experience had taught him, yet he perceived no increase of the disease. He occasionally consulted me, but rather with a view to be confirmed in the plan proposed to him, than with a hope of obtaining effectual relief, as he was very apprehensive that he laboured under the disease which Dr. Heberden had so fully described.

On the 13th of March 1775; in the evening, in a sudden and violent transport of anger, he fell down and expired immediately. His family were prevailed upon to allow the body to be opened, which was done the next day, by that very skilful and accurate anatomist, John Hunter, F.R.S. whose account is as follows:

THE APPEARANCES UPON OPENING THE BODY OF H. R. ESQ.

"The blood had settled very generally on the skin, appearing in dark purple spots.

"In opening the chest, I found the cartilages of the ribs very much ossified.

"In the cavity of the chest I found a full quart of bloody serum.

"The lungs were to all appearances sound.

"The heart to external appearance was also sound; but upon examination, I found that its substance was paler than common, more of a ligamentous consistence, and in many parts of the left ventricle is was become almost white and hard, having just the appearance of a beginning ossification.

"The *valvulæ mitrales* had a vast number of such appearances in them, and were less pliant than in a natural state; but it did not appear to be unfit for use.

"The semilunar valves of the aorta were thicker than common, but very readily filled the area of the artery.

"The aorta had several small ossifications on it, and several white parts, which are generally the beginnings of ossifications, and which were similar to those found in the heart and *valves*.

"The two coronary arteries, from their origin to many of their ramifications upon the heart, were become one piece of bone."

John Hunter*

These symptoms increased in violence at every return, and the attack which was the most violent came on one morning about the end of April, and lasted above two hours; it began as the others had done, but having continued about an hour, the pain became excruciating at the apex of the heart; the throat was so sore as not to allow of an attempt to swallow anything and the left arm could not bear to be touched, the least pressure upon it giving pain, the sensation at the apex of the heart was that of burning or scorching, which by its violence, quite exhausted him and he sunk into a swoon or doze, which lasted about ten minutes, after which he started up, without the least recollection of what had passed, or of his preceding illness. I was with him during the whole of this attack, and never saw anything equal to the agonies he suffered; and when he fainted away, I thought him dead, as the pain did not seem to abate, but to carry him off, having first completely exhausted him.

He then fell asleep for half an hour and awoke with confusion in his head, and a faint recollection of something like a delirium; this went off in a few days.

The affections above described were, in the beginning, readily brought on by exercise, and he even conceived that if he had continued at rest, they would not have come on; but they at last seized him when laying in bed, and in his sleep, so as to awaken him, affections of the mind also brought them on; but cool thinking or reasoning did not appear to have that effect. While these complaints were upon him, his face was pale, and he had a contracted appearance, making him look thinner than ordinary; and after they went off his colour returned, and his face recovered its natural appearance.

* * *

In the autumn of 1790, and in the spring and autumn of 1791, he had more severe

* "Life of John Hunter," by Everard Home, in John Hunter's *Treatise on the Blood, Inflammation and gun-shot Wounds,* Philadelphia, Bradford, 1796.

attacks than during the other periods of the year, but of not more than a few hours duration: in the beginning of October 1792, one, at which I was present, was so violent that I thought he would have died. On October the 16th, 1793, when in his usual state of health, he went to St. George's Hospital, and meeting with some things which irritated his mind, and not being perfectly master of the circumstances, he withheld his sentiments, in which state of restraint he went into the next room, and turning round to Dr. Robertson, one of the physicians of the hospital, he gave a deep groan, and dropt down dead.

It is a curious circumstance that, the first attack of these complaints was produced by an affection of the mind, and every future return of any consequence arose from the same cause; and although bodily exercise, or distention of the stomach, brought on slighter affections, it still required the mind to be affected to render them severe; and as his mind was irritated by trifles, these produced the most violent effects on the disease. His coachman being beyond his times, or a servant not attending to his directions, brought on the spasms, while a real misfortune produced no effect.

At the time of his death he was in the 65th year of his age, the same age at which his brother, the late Dr. Hunter, died.

Upon inspecting the body after death, the following were the appearances; the skin in several places was mottled, particularly on the sides and neck, which arose from the blood not having been completely coagulated, but remaining nearly fluid.

The contents of the abdomen were in a natural state, but the coats of the stomach and intestines were unusually loaded with blood, giving them a fleshy appearance, and a dark reddish colour; those parts, which had a depending situation, as in the bottom of the pelvis, and upon the loins, had this in a greater degree than the others; this evidently arose from the fluid state of the blood. The stomach was rather relaxed, but the internal surface was entirely free from any appearance of disease; the orifice at the pylorus was uncommonly open. The gall-bladder contained five or six small stones, of a light yellow colour. The liver and the other viscera exhibited nothing unusual in their appearance.

The cartilages of the ribs had in many places become bone, requiring a saw to divide them. There was no water in the cavity, or the chest, and the lungs of the right side were uncommonly healthy; but those of the left had very strong adhesions to the pleura, extending over a considerable surface, more especially towards the sternum.

The pericardium was very unusually thickened, which did not allow it to collapse upon being opened; the quantity of water contained in it was scarcely more than is frequently met with, although it might probably exceed that which occurs in the most healthy state of these parts.

The heart itself was very small, appearing too little for the cavity in which it lay, and did not give the idea of its being the effect of an unusual degree of contraction, but more of its having shrunk in its size. Upon the under surface of the left auricle and ventricle, there were two spaces nearly an inch and a half square, which were of a white colour, with an opaque appearance, and entirely distinct from the general surface of the heart: these two spaces were covered by an exudation of coagulating lymph, which at some former period had been the result of inflammation there. The muscular structure of the heart was paler and looser in its texture than the other muscles in the body. There were no coagula in any of its cavities. The coronary arteries had their branches which ramify through the substances of the heart in the state of bony tubes, which were with difficulty divided by the knife, and their transverse sections did not collapse, but remained open. The valvulæ mitrales, where they come off from the lower edge of the auricle, were in many places ossified, forming an imperfectly bony margin of different thicknesses, and in one spot so thick as to form a knob; but these ossifications were not continued down upon the valve towards the chordæ tendineæ.

The semilunar valves of the aorta had lost their natural pliancy, the previous stage to becoming bone and in several spots there were evident ossifications.

The aorta immediately beyond the semilunar valves had its cavity larger than usual, putting on the appearance of an incipient aneurism; this unusual dilatation extended for some way along the ascending aorta, but did not reach so far as the common trunk of the axillary and carotid artery. The increase of capacity of the artery might be about one-third of its natural area; and the internal membrane of this part had lost entirely the natural polish, and was studded over with opaque white spots, raised higher than the general surface.

CORONARY OCCLUSION

Adam Hammer

The first case of coronary occlusion correctly diagnosed during life was reported by Dr. Adam Hammer of St. Louis. Adam Hammer was born in the little town of Mingalsheim, Baden, in 1818. He received his preliminary education at the gymnasium of Bruchsal and in 1837 entered the University of Heidelberg where he had a brilliant career as a student. In 1842 he received his M.D. at Heidelberg, spent three years in the army and then began practice at Mannheim. In 1848 he took part in the Revolution in Germany and on account of its failure was forced to seek an asylum abroad. He emigrated to America and reached St. Louis in October of the same year.

Hammer began practice in St. Louis and was immediately impressed with the need for reform in medical education. In 1850 the Legislature of Missouri chartered an institution which was organized to carry out Hammer's ideas. This institution was the first in the United States to have high preliminary requirements, a graded curriculum, and four courses of lectures. In the curriculum were courses in Microscopic Anatomy, Experimental Physiology, and Embryology. This college survived only one year. In 1859 Dr. Hammer opened the "Humboldt Institut" an institution unique in the history of American medicine since the instruction was entirely in the German language. This institution also had high preliminary requirements, a graded curriculum, and four courses of lectures and carried on until 1869. In 1877 Dr. Hammer left for Europe; in 1878 he was in Vienna and the same year he died.

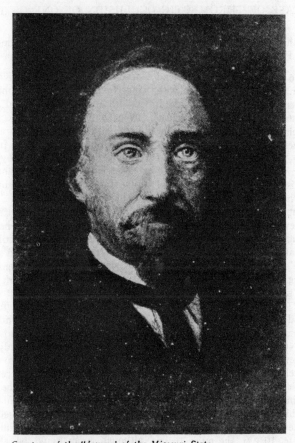

Courtesy of the "Journal of the Missouri State Medical Association"

ADAM HAMMER (1818-1878)
From a painting by Dr. Adolf Neubert

Hammer was a man of high ideals, an able surgeon, and a pioneer in American medical education. He and his colleagues in St. Louis were men of culture, graduates of famous German universities, men who had fled for political reasons, and carried their zeal for learning into America. They wished to establish at St. Louis a medical school the equal of those they knew in Heidelberg, Vienna, and Prague. They wished to do in the fifties in St. Louis what Gilman was not able to do in Baltimore until the nineties.

Hammer was not only an able surgeon but also a good pathologist and internist, as the following selection proves. Although he must have been disappointed at the failure of his educational projects he was rewarded by the great esteem and confidence in which he was held. The *Journal of the Missouri State Medical Association* for September, 1909, contains an article on Dr. Hammer by Dr. James M. Ball in which the essential details and achievements of his life are presented.

A CASE OF THROMBOTIC OCCLUSION OF ONE OF THE CORONARY ARTERIES OF THE HEART*

At the bedside diagnosed and communicated by Dr. A. Hammer, Professor of Surgery from St. Louis, at present in Vienna

On May 4, 1876 at 9 A.M. my young friend and colleague, Dr. Wichmann, took me with him to see a patient, whom, as he remarked, he did not understand. Concerning the cause of his illness he related the following: Patient Jacob Schrier, merchant, married, 34 years old, strongly built, a heavy beer drinker, had suffered for a year from frequent attacks of articular rheumatism. He had never detected changes in the heart valves. Four weeks before the patient had a very acute attack which involved several joints. Improvement set in gradually and recently complete convalescence had taken place; pulse rate 80 to the minute. Yesterday (May 3) he insisted upon getting out of bed, got up shortly before noon and sat down in an arm chair. At one o'clock (1¼ hours later) the patient suddenly collapsed in his chair. A half hour later Dr. Wichmann came and found the pulse weak, only 40 beats to the minute, the lips pale and somewhat cyanotic, slight dyspnoea, but absolutely no pain. He thought at first that the collapse was due to a sudden massive effusion into the pericardial sac, but later abandoned this idea. At 6 P.M. the same condition, save the pulse was slower, only 23 beats to the minute. 10 P.M. the pulse 16 to the minute, otherwise everything unchanged.

Status prasens: I found the patient in the following condition: body stretched out in bed, slightly elevated, his hands resting on the covers. Pulse, 8 beats to the minute (half as frequent as on the preceding evening at 10 o'clock) at regular intervals, that is, one contraction of the heart every 8 seconds. Face and skin of the entire body pale, cool and covered with sticky sweat. The eyes clear, pupils of moderate size, reacting easily,

around the lips a light tinge of cyanotic coloring, tongue and mucous membranes of the mouth and throat pale and anemic, no dyspnoea, no cough, no expectoration and no pain in any place. Respirations 24 to the minute. Sensorium quite free. The patient produces the impression, by his bearing, the expression of his countenance and conversation, that he has no idea of the seriousness of his malady.

Physical Examination: The percussion of the cardiac area showed no abnormal dullness, the heart could be outlined on the chest without great difficulty and as far as position and size were concerned must be considered as normal. Percussion of the lungs also showed no dullness, so that one was justified in excluding a pleuritic effusion as well as pneumonia or any other infiltration. Auscultation of the lungs showed everywhere normal respiratory sounds, only here and there were a few fine râles, such as commonly occur in a very marked hyperemia of the lungs.

The auscultation of the heart however showed some remarkable findings. The heart beat weak, one every 8 seconds. Upon the sound of each systole and diastole which although weak could be clearly made out and were without any murmur, there followed immediately a clonic spasm of the heart, which beat forcibly upon the applied ear with a sort of rustling, lasted exactly 5 seconds with the same intensity and then ceased as if cut off. I can compare these rapid successive twitchings of the heart muscle with nothing better than with the marked tremor of the hand of a man who is suffering from delirium tremens.

* * *

What impressed me particularly about this

Wien. med. Wchnschr., 1878, XXVIII, 102.

case and attracted my attention in the highest degree, was the sudden appearance and the steadily progressive course of the collapse. I thought that only a sudden, progressively increasing disturbance in the nutrition of the heart itself such as a cutting off of the supply of nourishment could produce such changes as this case showed, and that such an obstruction could be produced only by a thrombotic occlusion of at least one of the coronary arteries. From lack of ground for any other satisfactory explanation, I was carried away by this thought.

* * *

I mentioned my conviction to my colleague at the bed side. He however had a non-plussed expression and burst out "I have never heard of such a diagnosis in my whole life." and I answered "Nor I also."

* * *

As the patient had only a few hours to live, we could be certain by an autopsy; he therefore took great pains to obtain permission from the relatives for an autopsy. (This last remark may be explained by the fact that at the present time the obtaining of an autopsy in America is attended by great difficulties. How often have I purchased this permission by giving up my fee for professional services! Indeed in certain cases I have had to pay money out of my pocket in order to succeed. Before this universal medium even the most subtle misgivings, even the religious ones, soften.)

Remarkable to relate, the patient lived 19 hours longer, he died early on May 5. Dr. Wichmann obtained permission to examine the body but only to a limited extent. We were permitted only to remove the heart, but not to disturb any other organ. For our purpose that was sufficient and we were satisfied to have obtained so much. On May 6 (29 hours after death) at 11 A.M. we carried out a partial autopsy, while the body was already in its coffin.

Autopsy findings . . . The outer surface of the pericardium showed nothing abnormal. In the sac there was ½ ounce of clear, yellow serum, its walls were smooth and shiny. The heart in its proper position, of normal size and shape, markedly distended. Its surface smooth and shiny, and except for an abundant layer of fat in the sulcus, no trace of spots or of any other exudate.

After the heart was removed its interior was investigated. The right auricle and ventricle was filled with thick coagulated black blood, containing massive clots of fibrin and globular vegetations (post mortem or agonal). The cavities of the auricle and ventricle of normal size, the tricuspid and pulmonary valves intact: the color of the muscle on cut section pale, with a slight tendency to a brownish yellow; the wall of the ventricle of normal thickness, the endocardium unchanged.

All that was said of the right auricle and ventricle and their valves, holds also for the left auricle, ventricle and valves with the single exception of the aortic valves. Upon these there were remarkable changes which could be detected as soon as one looked through the trunk of the aorta. In order to examine these more closely, I split the aorta and extended the incision through the commissure of the *right* and *left* valves, which later proved to be very useful. Had I carried out the incision in the usual manner through the commissure of the *posterior* and *right* valve an important part of the findings would have been destroyed and an exact view of the beginning and further development of the pathological process would have been obscured. What first and principally struck one's view was the marked tension and stretching of the right valve by a mass which not only filled the right sinus of Valsalva but also bulged out like a half sphere. On removing this mass carefully and examining it carefully, it was found that the upper layers from above to the origin of the coronary arteries inside the sinus were composed of fresh, coagulated, jelly-like, whitish-yellow material mixed with blood. . . . On the right and left valves there were fresh white, soft endocarditic excrescences.

* * *

The autopsy finding confirmed the diagnosis in the most convincing manner; and also explains most satisfactorily the peculiar progressive course of the disease picture. There can be no doubt that during the formation of the thrombus in the right sinus of Valsalva and so long as it did not reach the level of the exit of the coronary artery, the patient felt relatively well, but that with the beginning occlusion of the lumen of the artery collapse appeared, and that the constant diminution of the pulse rate was directly caused by the constant growth of the thrombus until complete closure appeared.

* * *

This case will interest particularly the clear-sighted and clever Cohnhein, as he wrote in his *Lectures on General Pathology,* which appeared in print at the end of the year 1877 on page 24 "In fact Bezold by closing the coronary arteries with a clamp and Panum by producing an embolus in the same with a thin wax emulsion were able to stop the heart; but whether a similar event in human pathology will ever be observed, is to me improbable enough." He did not know, and indeed also could not know, that this occurrence had indeed been observed 18 months before.

The specimen is in the possession of my friend Dr. Wichmann.

Vienna the 22nd of January 1878.

George Dock

George Dock has been for many years an outstanding internist, teacher and investigator. He was born in Hopewell, Pennsylvania, in 1860 and received the degree of M.D. from the University of Pennsylvania in 1884. From 1887 to 1888 he was assistant in medicine at his Alma Mater, under William Osler. Osler, writing years later of his experiences at Pennsylvania, said "there was no clinical laboratory, only an improvised room under the amphitheatre, which was very active the year George Dock was in charge."

From 1889 to 1891 he was professor of pathology and of clinical medicine at Galveston. In 1891 he was called to the chair of medicine at the University of Michigan where he remained until 1908. While at the University of Michigan he published in 1896 the first account of a case of coronary thrombosis in America diagnosed during life and confirmed by autopsy findings. From 1908 until 1910 he was professor of medicine at Tulane and in 1910 became professor of medicine at Washington University. He resigned from this position in 1922 and moved to Pasadena, California, where he has since engaged in private practice.

Dock is a gifted and inspiring teacher and has left his impress upon all his students and upon the medical schools with which he has been associated. His medical articles cover a wide range of subjects and are characterized by clarity of expression and charm in diction. In addition to his purely medical writings he has contributed to medical history many interesting and important studies. The late Victor C. Vaughan in his delightful *A Doctor's Memories* wrote "From 1891 to 1908 George Dock served as professor of the theory and practise of medicine, and I am sure that in this capacity he had but few equals and no superiors. He lived in the laboratory and in the wards of the hospital. His original contributions to scientific medicine won recognition throughout the world. As a teacher he initiated his students in scientific investigations and demonstrated the value of research work in the treatment of disease."

NOTES ON THE CORONARY ARTERIES*

One nundred years ago all of cardiac path-

* Dock, George, *Notes on the Coronary Arteries,* Ann Arbor, Michigan, The Inland Press, 1896.

ology was chaos. Corvisart had not revived the discovery of Auenbrugger, and enriched percussion with the results of his own indefatigable observations at the bedside and on the post-mortem table. Laennec had not, accidentally and from his keen sense of decorum, made the immortal discovery that soon revolutionized medical diagnosis. As Corvisart says, many so-called physicians of that day "looked on attempts at an exact diagnosis in heart-disease as useless, because those diseases are incurable." With neat sarcasm he says, in reference to such men, that

attacks, he led an unquiet and anxious life. By-and-by he became cachectic and dropsical, and, finally, grievously distressed, he died in one of his paroxysms. In the body we found the wall of the left ventricle ruptured, having a rent in it of a size sufficient to admit any one of my fingers, although the wall itself appeared sufficiently thick and strong." The explanation Harvey gave, that "the laceration

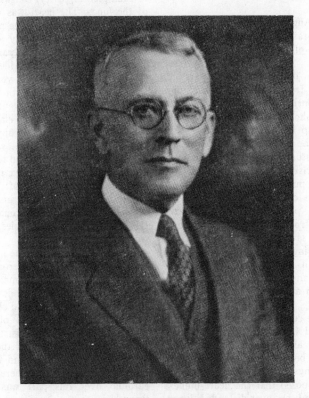

GEORGE DOCK (1860-)

"art is short, experience silent, and judgment weak."

Yet post-mortem observations on diseases of the coronary, and of the heart-muscle in consequence, are among the oldest in medical literature. Harvey himself (Second Disquisition addressed to Riolan, Jr.,) has recorded a case that must have been one of atheroma of a coronary artery. "Sir Robert Darcy, when he reached about the middle period of life, made frequent complaints of a certain distressing pain in the chest, especially in the night season; so that dreading at one time syncope, at another suffocation in his

had apparently been caused by an impediment to the passage of the blood from the left ventricle into the arteries," is evidently insufficient, but points strongly to aortic disease, in which the coronaries are often affected.

At the end of the last century a few, at least, of the choicer spirits of medicine had a knowledge of myocardial disease by no means inconsiderable, and far in advance of their knowledge of valvular disease. The most illustrious example of this is furnished by the oft-cited case of John Hunter. The acute Jenner correctly diagnosed the calcification of the coronary arteries and referred to them the anginal attacks of his friend and teacher. Parry, too, in several cases was able to make similar predictions, verified post-mortem. On the whole, such cases were not common enough to soon make an impression on the profession as a whole, and it is not surprising that later writers allowed the subject to escape them.

* * *

CASE IV.—Angina pectoris; dyspnea; double hydrothorax; sudden death. Atheroma and obstruction of coronaries; infarction of the heart.

Mr. B., lumber dealer, sixty-four years old, a man of large frame, was never sick until about three months before death. He then began to notice shortness of breath, especially when walking up hill. A week before death severe pain in the heart region began. There was no clear history of radiating pain. Soon after this, in rising suddenly, the patient fainted, became pulseless and very dyspneic. Dr. Breakey was called in and made a diagnosis of angina pectoris, prescribing nitroglycerine and strophanthus. The symptoms continued and I saw the patient a week later. He was then lying propped up in bed, but anxious to get out. There was slight cyanosis; breathing rapid and superficial; pulse eighty, small, quick; no atheroma of the peripheral arteries.

The apex-beat could not be felt. The heart dulness extended from the fourth rib to the fifth interspace, and from the left edge of the sternum to beyond the left parasternal line. As the lungs gave a very tympanitic note, it was supposed that the heart dulness might be masked by over-distended lungs. The sounds over the heart were faint but clear. Over the apex-region a loud double friction-sound was audible. There was a small area of moveable dulness in each side, which had been present for two or three days. Loud moist râles obscured the respiratory murmur. The abdomen was considerably distended, the tongue coated; constipation had existed for some time. Repeated examinations of the urine were negative.

The diagnosis was myomalacia following coronary sclerosis, with secondary pericarditis. This was based on the history of increasing dyspnea and heart pain, without evidence of disease in lungs or kidneys, or other (valvular) disease of the heart, the history

of the acute attack indicating infarction, and the acute onset of pericarditis without other cause.

The same day, against explicit orders and explanations of the danger from exertion of any kind, the patient insisted on being helped out of bed to defecate. While straining at stool he suddenly expired.

Autopsy showed about a pint of clear fluid in each pleural cavity, congestion and edema of the lungs. The heart was enlarged, reaching the left nipple line. The pericardium was adherent over the apex by a thin, greenish fibrinous exudate, easily separated. The pericardium was uniformly reddened and rough.

The surface of the left ventricle, beneath the thin exudate, was mottled red and green in irregular spots. Both ventricles were dilated, the left being 10.3 cm. long, its wall fifteen mm. thick at the upper part, seven mm. thick at the apex. The walls of the right ventricle were five mm. and three mm. thick, at the upper part and apex respectively. All the chambers contained soft, dark-red clots.

The aorta, seven cm. in circumference, showed a few atheromatous areas around the orifices of the coronaries, but the latter were not obstructed.

Just below the orifice the left coronary artery became extremely atheromatous, nodules of two to three mm. in diameter, in the walls, obstructing the lumen. The descending branch was narrowed, calcified, and about the middle of the anterior wall was obstructed by a red thrombus. Below this the artery was smooth. From the level of the thrombus the muscle was dry, yellow and red in irregular areas, and tore easily. Adherent to the endocardium over this part was a thin mixed thrombus.

The circumflex branch was nodular, but its lumen was free as far as the first branch, 2.5 cm. from its origin. Here it was completely obstructed by nodular arteritis for a distance of three mm. Beyond this, the lumen of the circumflex proper was free, but the next large descending branch was also totally obstructed. The wall of the left ventricle from this point, i.e., from the anterior papillary muscle, to the septum, the posterior part of which was involved, and from near the ring to the apex, was the seat of a recent infarction. Only a thin layer, under the epicardium, from one to two mm. in thickness, was not necrosed, and it was red, swollen, the fibres cloudy and granular. The noninfarcted parts of the heart showed brown atrophy, fibroid degeneration and fatty change.

In this case the relation of the coronary sclerosis to the gradually developing dyspnea, and of the infarction to the acute attack a week before death is clear. The case illustrates also the fact that a heart extensively necrosed may continue to act for some time fairly well, if exposed to no sudden strain, thus explaining the early stages of those cases in which large fibrous areas are found *postmortem* in the heart. It is also a fine example of atheroma limited almost entirely to the coronary vessels. Usually there are other evidences, but in rare cases only one set of vessels is involved, a point brought out prominently in the diagnosis of this case.

I have not intended to speak in detail of the symptoms of coronary artery disease, nor even to touch on the important points of prognosis and treatment. If I have been able to interest you in the subject in such a way that new light will be thrown upon it, I shall have additional cause for congratulating myself on being with you to-day.

William Osler

THE LUMLEIAN LECTURES ON ANGINA PECTORIS
Delivered before the Royal College of Physicians of London by
WILLIAM OSLER, M.D., F.R.S., Regius Professor of
Medicine in the University of Oxford

LECTURE II*

Delivered on March 15
PATHOLOGY

Mr. President and Fellows,

Had Heberden listened to my first lecture he could have remarked very justly: "Well! they have not got much ahead since my day." In descriptive symptomatology we have not, and among 100 cases of angina pectoris there is no reason why Heberden should not have met all the important anomalies and complications. He had the good sense not to say much about the cause of the disease, and the good fortune to get very close to the truth in what he did say. I do not propose to weary you in a vain repetition of the scores of explanations which have been offered since his day. The older ones are to be found in the monographs of Parry and Jurine, the more recent in the *Traité* of Huchard, in the writings of our President, and in those of Allbutt, Bramwell, Gibson, Morrison, Mackenzie, and others. At the outset let us frankly face certain obscurities which have not yet been cleared up. Why is it more common in the upper classes? Why do we not see it more often in hospital practice? Worry and work are the lot and portion of the poor, among whom vascular degeneration is more widespread. It is as though only a special strain of tissue reacted *anginally*, so to speak, a

* The Lancet, 1910, p. 839.

type evolved amid special surroundings which existed in certain families. Or there may be a perverted secretion which favours spasm of the arteries, as Harvey at Cambridge has shown to be the case with pituitary extract and the coronary vessels. And a case of aortic valve disease is reported in which the use of this extract caused anginal attacks. This suggestion is supported by the fact that in myxoedema anginal attacks may be caused by thyroid extract. I saw last year a patient of Dr. Lafleur's of Montreal with this most distressing peculiarity, which was mentioned to me also by Dr. Allan Starr of New York. The disease may occur in three generations, as in the Arnolds, and a father and four children have been affected. In three instances of my series father and son were attacked; in two, brothers, and in one, a brother and sister. It is not the delicate neurotic person who is prone to angina, but the robust, the vigorous in mind and body, the keen and ambitious man, the indicator of whose engines is always at "full speed ahead." There is, indeed, a frame and facies at once suggestive of angina —the well "set" man of from 45 to 55 years of age, with military bearing, iron grey hair, and florid complexion. More than once as such a man entered my consulting room the suggested diagnosis of angina has flashed through my mind. Still more extraordinary and inexplicable is an imitative feature, if one may so speak of it, by which the repeated witnessing of attacks may induce one in the observer. The case of Senator Sumner attracted widespread interest on account of his distinguished public position. Two weeks after his death Dr. Hitchcock, his physician, died in an attack with coronary artery disease and acute infarct of the myocardium. Tabor Johnson, his other physician, at that time a young man, had two attacks, diagnosed by Brown-Séquard as angina, and he had seen some twenty cases of what may be called the manufactured variety. Straus died not long after his friend Charcot. A young man, aged 28, whose father, a very vigorous planter, had through the spring and summer of 1900 severe attacks and died in one September 28th, consulted me the following January for angina. I had seen the father, and had been a witness to the devotion of the son during the terrible paroxysms. Within a month of the death of the father he began to have severe pain in the chest, with pallor, sweating, the pains down the left arm, which became numb and tingled. The sister said the paroxysms were identical with those of the father, and naturally the family were greatly distressed. The patient was a healthy robust fellow, very neurotic and almost frightened to death. A reassuring prognosis was all the treatment he required. He has had no further attacks. A woman, aged 38, after her father's death from angina, had severe pains about the heart, and attacks which she insisted were of the same character, but she too, got well. A still more remarkable illustration of the imitative, emotional influence was seen in the outbreak of angina-like attacks among the sailors of the French corvette *L'Embuscade* reported by Gelineau.

There are two primary features of the disease, pain and sudden death—pain, paroxysmal, intense, peculiar, usually pectoral, and with the well-known lines of radiation—death in a higher percentage than any known disorder, and usually sudden. Often, indeed, it is as the poet says, "Life struck sharp on death." The problems for solution are: What is the cause of the pain? Why the sudden death? The secondary features of the attack, the vaso-motor phenomena, the radiation of the pain, the cardiac, respiratory, and gastric symptoms are of subsidiary interest.

Morbid Anatomy

Naturally in the presence of a disease with such startling characters, men have sought an explanation in the bodies of its victims.

And angina pectoris has a very definite morbid anatomy, few affections more so, since in practically all cases vascular disease exists. With Morgagni, Jenner, Fothergill, and Parry, a majority of authors have correlated the fatal symptoms with the arterial disease; others have reached the less satisfactory, if more philosophical, position of Rougnon who, taking all the circumstances into consideration, concluded, "Monsieur Charles est mort parce qu'il est mort." Not a hospital disease, one naturally does not see many necropsies. I have notes of 17 post-mortem examinations, all in men, 8 of them in men under 40 and 4 of them with a history of syphilis, and dying at the ages of 34, 38, 37, 39. They fall in three groups—aortitis, coronary artery disease and a negative case.

A. *Aortitis.*—From the publication of Morgagni's famous case writers have recognized the importance of aortic changes at its root. The special importance of this has been dwelt upon by my brother regius of Cambridge, whose many publications upon the subject, dating from his remarkable study of syphilitic arteritis in 1868, have edified his colleague and students. For our purposes here there is but one aortitis—the syphilitic. Occasionally a fairly acute process occurs at the root of the aorta in the specific fevers, but this is very uncommon, except in connection with endocarditis. Chronic atheromatous changes in the aorta of the aged are very rarely associated with angina unless the coronary arteries are involved. Syphilitic aortitis is a most distinctive lesion. I pass round the beautiful plate of Corrigan's paper, in which he brings out for the first time I think, and with great clearness, the connexion of the disease with this lesion. The frontispiece of Balfour's book on *The Senile Heart*, gives an equally good representation. Upon its anatomical features I need not dwell further than to refer to its predilection for the supra-sigmoidal region, the sectional limitation, and the great frequency of its association with aneurysm.

Of the post-mortem examinations of my series only one offered a good illustration of the supra-sigmoidal type; a negro, aged 38, who had had syphilis about a year before. The attacks of angina began in December, 1904, they lasted for from 15 minutes to half an hour, with very characteristic distribution of the pain; in severer paroxysms he had fallen unconscious. The attacks recurred even when he was in bed and quiet. There was diffuse cardiac impulse, the area of flatness was increased, but there were no murmurs; the blood pressure was 188 mm. Hg. On the evening of admission he had a very sharp attack, and another at 1:30 A.M., in which the pain was chiefly epigastric; he sweated profusely and became very weak, and at 2:30 was found unconscious, and died at 4 A.M. The heart weighed 490 grammes, the free edges of the valves were a little thickened; the only important lesion was an extensive fresh-looking aortitis, involving the root of the vessel and narrowing the orifice of the left coronary. The right coronary orifice was normal; the coronary arteries themselves were not affected.

Another syphilitic patient, W.A.M., aged 38, admitted February 20th, 1895, had very severe paroxysms of angina, with aortic insufficiency. The aortic segments were thickened and curled; the coronary arteries were small but healthy; there was the characteristic sclerotic aortitis not confined to the root. The smaller arteries of the body, particularly the splanchnic, were tortuous and thickened.

In a third syphilitic case, J. W., a negro, aged 34, admitted May 25th, 1897, the paroxysms were most characteristic, and had recurred since March: in several attacks he had become unconscious, and following them he had transient weakness of the left arm. During the fortnight he was in hospital he had several severe attacks; the left arm was distinctly weaker than the right, particularly the grasp of the hand; the heart appeared to be normal. On June 8th he complained of a great deal of coldness of the hands and feet; at 6:10 in the evening he threw up his hands suddenly and died within a few minutes. Widespread aortitis of the sclerotic type, with here and there plaques of atheroma, were the only lesions. The coronary arteries were not involved; they looked small, the walls thin, but there was no occlusion.

B. *Coronary arteries.*—We are all united in the acceptance of the Jennerian view of the close connexion of lesions of the coronary arteries with the disease. As shown in the extensive analysis by Huchard, a very large proportion of all of the cases show changes in these vessels. Of the 17 necropsies of my list, 13 illustrated all the varieties of the lesions.

(a) Narrowing of the orifices is a very common occurrence, particularly in the syphilitic aortitis, but not often met with without some involvement of the branches. In the case of a man who died suddenly in my wards after recurring attacks the sclerosis of the ascending part of the arch was marked and the orifices of the coronary arteries were extensively contracted; as the post-mortem report states, "they admitted only a bristle." The arteries beyond were nearly normal, showing only slight sclerotic change.

(b) Blocking of a branch with a fresh thrombus is very common in cases of sudden death in angina. In my post-mortem experience this has been more frequent in the medico-legal cases of sudden death without symptoms of agina. One of the main stems or a small branch may be plugged with the formation of fresh infarct. In patients who live some time the infarct may soften and pericarditis may be excited. A specimen in McGill College, from a man who died suddenly the day after an attack, shows the left coronary artery blocked by the thrombus and perforation of the softened anterior wall of the ventricle.

(c) Obliterative endarteritis, if we may judge from the reports of fatal cases collected by Huchard and others, is the lesion of the disease; it was present in nine case of my series. The most remarkable peculiarity is the variation in the extent of involvement. The angina may be associated with obliteration of a comparatively small branch, or with a most widespread involvement of all the vessels. In the younger subjects the process is a gradual endarteritis with narrowing, and even complete occlusion of the vessel. In older subjects, the arteries may be converted, as in John Hunter and in William Pepper, into "open bony tubes." In one instance of my series the vessels were calcified to their smallest branches. Four cases showed disease of the coronary arteries alone; five in connexion with aortitis. In looking over these notes one is astonished at the comparatively small extent of coronary tubing which is sufficient to carry on the myocardial circulation. Mr. G., aged 39 years, had read an important paper at a college society and died the following night in an attack. Not more than a third of his coronary vessels were in use. It has long been known that advanced coronary artery disease may be present without much disturbance of the function of the heart. There is not a clinician among us who could not furnish from his notes a dozen cases of this kind. A man may get on very comfortably with only the main branch of one coronary, practically a fourth of the whole system. A heart once in my possession showed almost complete obliteration of the left coronary, only a pin-point channel could be traced for a short distance. Of the right branch, the main division passing between the auricle and the ventricle was completely obliterated, so that the only one of full size passed in the posterior interventricular groove. The heart came from a large, very muscular imbecile, aged 36, an inmate of the Institution for the Feeble-Minded, at Elwin. I knew him well; a good-natured, helpful fellow, constantly employed in carrying about, and attending to, the more helpless children. He died suddenly one day in a fit. The coronaries are not endarteries in the sense of Cohnheim, and disease of their branches is not necessarily associated with angina.

(d) And in a few fatal cases no lesions whatever are found; we must accept the fact that angina pectoris may kill without signs of obvious disease in heart or blood-vessels. Such an instance has been reported by Dr. Bullard and myself. The case was regarded by all who saw it as one of so-called functional angina. The patient, aged 26, was very strong and robust, devoted to athletics, and a heavy smoker. He had served in the United States Army, but was discharged in the spring of 1896 for attacks of angina. The chief feature was pain in the heart, and "awful cramps," as he described them, in his arms. The attacks were so severe that at times he became unconscious, and after one he was thought to be dead, and was about to be removed to the dead-house. The attacks were brought on by cold and exertion. The pain was evidently very severe, and in the major paroxysms respiration would cease, and his pulse would become so feeble that he seemed to be dead. Only chloroform and morphia were of any avail in the attacks. He had an extraordinary number of attacks in 1896-7; Dr. Bullard had notes of 105. In 1989 he was better and had not nearly so many attacks, and was able to be at work. On November 27th at 11:30 he had an attack of great severity; at 12:55 the doctor gave him choloroform; the attack was very prolonged, and the muscles of the chest became fixed, and remained so; he had a series of paroxysms and died at 6:40 in the morning. Except a few pleural adhesions, there was nothing special to be noted. The heart weighed 14 ounces; the muscle and the valves were normal. Just above the ring the aorta measured not quite 6 centimeters, a small vessel for a man of 5 feet 10 inches, weighing just over 13 stones. There was no disease except a flake here and there of atheroma. There was no thickening about the pericardium, and the sections showed no changes in the cardiac nerves.

James B. Herrick

James Bryan Herrick, one of the best known clinicians in the United States, was born at Oak Park, Illinois, in 1861. He received the degree of A.B. from the University of Michigan in 1882 and the degree of M.D. from Rush Medical College in 1888. The following year and a half he served as interne in the Cook County Hospital and in 1890 became instructor in medicine in his alma mater. In 1894 he was promoted to the rank of adjunct professor and in 1900 was appointed professor of medicine.

Dr. Herrick's numerous important contributions to medical literature are characterized by painstaking study of clinical symptoms and by accurate and logical deductions. His outstanding contributions are his original description of sickle cell anemia and his classic work on coronary occlusion. While this latter condition had been noted before the appearance of Herrick's paper, his masterful studies have cleared up the confusion surrounding this disease and have sharply delineated this most important syndrome.

Dr. Herrick was President of the Association of American Physicians in 1923 and in 1930 received the Kober medal. On the occasion of the presentation of this medal Dr. Kober expressed "the hope that your days of usefulness and happiness may still be many, and that the coming years may be as fruitful in achievements as they have been in the past"—a hope that is echoed by his numerous friends and admirers, both within and without the medical profession.

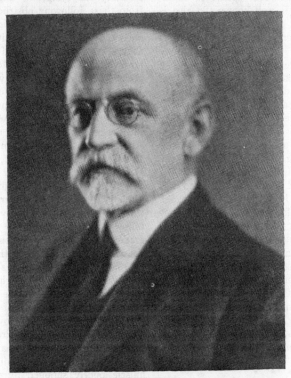

JAMES B. HERRICK (1861-   )
Photograph by Wallinger, Chicago

CLINICAL FEATURES OF SUDDEN OBSTRUCTION OF THE CORONARY ARTERIES*

James B. Herrick, M.D., Chicago

Obstruction of a coronary artery or any of its large branches has long been regarded as a serous accident. Several events contributed toward the prevalence of the view that this condition was almost always suddenly fatal. Parry's writings on angina pectoris and its relation to coronary disease, Jenner's observations on the same condition centering about John Hunter's case, Thorvaldsen's tragic death in the theater in Copenhagen, with the finding of a plugged coronary, sharply attracted attention to the relation be-

tween the coronary and sudden death. In Germany Cohnheim supported the views of Hyrtl and Henle as to lack of considerable anastomosis, and as late as 1881 lent the influence of his name to the doctrine that the coronary arteries were endarteries; his Leipsic necropsy experience, as well as experiments on dogs, forced him to conclude that the sudden occlusion of one of these vessels or of one of the larger branches, such as the ramus descendens of the left coronary, meant death within a few minutes. Others emphasized the same view.

No one at all familiar with the clinical,

* *J.A.M.A.*, 1912, LIX, 2015.

pathological or experimental features of cardiac disease can question the importance of the coronaries. The influence of sclerosis and fibrosis of the myocardium, with such possible results as aneurysm, rupture or dilatation of the heart, is well known. So also is the relation of the coronaries to many cases of angina pectoris, and to cardiac disturbances rather indefinitely classed as chronic myocarditis, cardiac irregularities, etc. It must be admitted, also, that the reputation of the descending branch of the left coronary as the artery of sudden death is not undeserved.

But there are reasons for believing that even large branches of the coronary arteries may be occluded—at times acutely occluded —without resulting death, at least without death in the immediate future. Even the main trunk may at times be obstructed and the patient live. It is the object of this paper to present a few facts along this line, and particularly to describe some of the clinical manifestations of sudden yet not immediately fatal cases of coronary obstruction.

Before presenting the clinical features of coronary obstruction, it may be well to consider certain facts that go to prove that sudden obstruction is not necessarily fatal. Such proof is afforded by a study of the anatomy of the normal as well as the diseased heart, by animal experiment and by bedside experience.

* * *

The clinical manifestations of coronary obstruction will evidently vary greatly, depending on the size, location and number of vessels occluded. The symptoms and end-results must also be influenced by blood-pressure, by the condition of the myocardium not immediately affected by the obstruction, and by the ability of the remaining vessels properly to carry on their work, as determined by their health or disease. No simple picture of the condition can, therefore, be drawn. All attempts at dividing these clinical manifestations into groups must be artificial and more or less imperfect. Yet such an attempt is not without value, as it enables one the better to understand the gravity of an obstructive accident, to differentiate it from other conditions presenting somewhat similar symptoms, and to employ a more rational therapy that may, to a slight extent at least, be more efficient.

The variations in the results are to be accounted for in part by variations in the freedom with which anastomosing branches occur. Presumably, too, symptoms will vary with the vessel or branches occluded. It is conceivable that with occlusion of the right coronary the symptoms might be different from those following obstruction of the left artery; systemic edema might be a consequence of the former condition and pulmonary edema of the latter. These points, are however, by no means settled either by experimental or clinical observation. The condition of the remaining vessels as to patency and presence of sclerosis must play an important part in deciding how much they are capable of doing in the way of compensatory nutrition to the anemic myocardium; the strength of the heart itself, as determined, perhaps, by old valvular or myocardial disease, would also have it influence. And presumably a sudden overwhelming obstruction, with comparatively normal vessels, would be followed by a profounder shock than the gradual narrowing of a lumen through sclerosis which has accustomed the heart to this pathologic condition and has perhaps caused collateral circulation through neighboring or anastomosing vessels to be compensatorily increased. The influence of the vessels of Thebesius is also not to be overlooked in this connection; compensatory circulation through these accessory channels may be of considerable importance in nourishing areas of heart muscle poorly supplied by sclerotic or obstructed arteries.

Attempts to group these cases of coronary obstruction according to clinical manifestations must be more or less unsatisfactory, yet, imperfect as these groups are, the cases may be roughly classified.

One group will include cases in which death is sudden, seemingly instantaneous and perhaps painless. Krehl has emphasized the peculiarities of the sudden death of this type, the lack of terminal respiratory agony, of distortion of the features, of muscular contractions.

A second group includes those cases in which the attack is anginal, the pain severe, the shock profound and death follows in a few minutes or several minutes at the most.

In a third group may be placed non-fatal cases with mild symptoms. Slight anginal attacks without the ordinary causes (such as walking), perhaps some of the stitch pains in the precordia, may well be due to obstruction of small coronary twigs. Such an interpretation of these phenomena is, however, only a surmise based on the fact that other causes for the pains are lacking and that the patchy fibrosis of the myocardium that is later found at autopsy may have originated in obstruction of the sclerotic vessels; and such obstruction in small vessels may well have produced symptoms differing chiefly in degree from those caused by obstruction of larger arteries of the heart.

In a fourth group are the cases in which the symptoms are severe, are distinctive enough to enable them to be recognized as cardiac, and on which the accident is usually fatal, but not immediately, and perhaps not necessarily so. It is to the clinical features of this group that attention is directed in what follows.

By way of introduction, I give in outline the history of a case, experience with which acutely attracted my attention to this subject.

Case 1. *History.*—A man, aged 55, supposedly in good health, was seized an hour after a moderately full meal with severe pain in the lower precordial region. He was nauseated and believing that something he had just eaten had disagreed with he, he induced vomiting by thickling his throat. The pain continued however, and his physician was called, who found him cold, nauseated, with small rapid pulse, and suffering extreme pain. The stomach was washed out and morphine given hypodermically. The pain did not cease until three hours had passed. From this time the patient remained in bed, free from pain, but the pulse continued rapid and small, and numerous râles appeared in the chest. When I saw him twelve hours from the painful attack his mind was clear and calm; a moderate cyanosis and a mild dyspnea were present. The chest was full of fine and coarse-moist râles; there was a running feeble pulse of 140. The heart tones were very faint and there was a most startling and confusing hyperresonance over the chest, the area of the heart dulness being entirely obscured. The abdomen was tympanitic. The urine was scanty, of high specific gravity, and contained a small amount of albumin and a few casts. The temperature was subnormal, later going to 99 F. Occasionally there was nausea and twice a sudden projectile vomiting of considerable fluid material. The condition remained with slight variations up to the time of death, fifty-two hours after the onset of the pain, though at one time the râles seemed nearly to have disappeared. A few hours before death the patient described a slight pain in the heart region, but said it did not amount to much. A remarkable circumstance, and one that occasioned surprise in those who saw the patient and who realized from the almost imperceptible pulse and the feeble heart tones how weak the heart must be, was the fact that he frequently indulged in active muscular effort without evident harm. He rolled vigorously from side to side in the bed, sat suddenly bold upright, or reached out to take things from the table near by; and once, feeling a sudden nausea, he jumped out of bed, dodged the nurse and ran into the bathroom, where he vomited; and yet he seemed none the worse for these exertions.

Necropsy (Dr. Hektoen).—The heart was of normal size, but both coronary arteries were markedly sclerotic, with calcareous districts and narrowing of the lumen. A short distance from its origin the left coronary artery was completely obliterated by a red thrombus that had formed at a point of great narrowing. The wall of the left ventricle showed well-marked areas of yellowish and reddish softening, especially extensive in the interventricular septum. At the very apex the muscle was decidedly softer than elsewhere. The beginning of the aorta showed a few yellowish spots, these areas becoming less marked as the descending part was reached. An acute fibrinous pericardial deposit, which showed no bacteria in smears; was found over the left ventricle. (The pericarditis probably explains the slighter pain complained of a few hours before death.) There was marked edema of the lungs. In other respects the anatomic findings were those of health.

DIGITALIS

William Withering

Digitalis is without question the most valuable cardiac drug ever discovered and one of the most valuable drugs in the entire pharmacopoeia. The introduction of digitalis was one of the landmarks in the history of cardiac disease.

William Withering, who introduced digitalis into the practice of medicine,

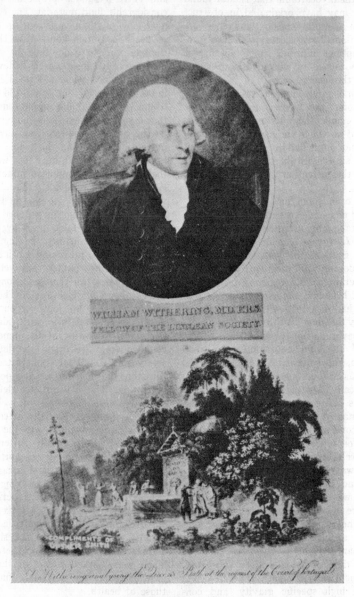

WILLIAM WITHERING (1741-1799)
Kindness of Upshur Smith

was born in Wellington, Shropshire, England, in 1741. His father was an apothecary-surgeon, who enjoyed a good practice in Shropshire. William Withering received his first education at the school of his native town and later went to Edinburgh where he took the degree of M.D. in 1766. The following year he commenced practice in Stafford, but does not seem to have been unusually successful since he wrote that his "professional engagements scarcely produced on the average of six years one hundred pounds per annum." Presently he left Stafford and moved to Birmingham, taking over the practice of Dr. Small. In 1776 we learn that his practice had become considerable and his receipts increased to more than one thousand pounds a year. He gave free advice to the poor at his home on certain days and aided the poor and unfortunate in many ways. His extensive practice caused him to travel both day and night, and during these trips he read and wrote. His carriage was equipped with a light so he could study while travelling along the countryside at night. His first published work was *A Botanical Arrangement of All the Vegetables Growing in Great Britain According to the System of the Celebrated Linnaeus; with an easy introduction to the study of Botany*. He remained all his life an ardent student of botany, and later became much interested in chemistry and mineralogy. In Birmingham he became a member of the Lunar Society, a scientific body so named because it met once a month, and which numbered among its members such celebrities as Priestley and Watt.

Withering's *Account of the Foxglove and Some of Its Medical Uses* was published in 1785, and immediately attracted great attention. This work was the fruit of many years of observation, and on its title page appears the appropriate quotation from Horace, *Nonumque prematur in annum* (let it be suppressed for nine years). The year of its publication he was made a fellow of the Royal Society and received a diploma from the Medical Society of London. This book of Withering is one of the classics of medical literature and greatly prized by collectors. It sold when published for five shillings with the colored plate of the foxglove. A copy sold in 1943 for $275.00.

The use of digitalis in practice was condemned by Dr. John Coakley Lettsom, who enjoyed the largest and most remunerative practice in London. Lettsom was a man of marked literary ability, a skillful physician, and a great philanthropist. Lettsom, on the recommendation of Withering, had prescribed digitalis and in eight instances the illness had terminated fatally. Among these patients was Charles James Fox, the English statesman, who was suffering from cirrhosis of the liver with ascites, and in whom it had apparently produced a fatal effect. Withering, in a letter answering Lettsom's strictures, complains that "No one could compare Lettsom's choice of patients with my declaration of the fit and unfit, or the doses he prescribed, and the perseverance he enjoined, with my doses, rules, and cautions."

Withering suffered for twenty years from bronchiectasis or possibly tuberculosis and died in 1799, age 58. He is buried in the Parish Church at Edgbaston, his tomb being adorned with the staff of Aesculapius, around which are entwined the serpent and the foxglove. Withering lived to see digitalis admitted into the *Edinburgh Pharmacopoeia* and its merits generally recognized.

Dr. Erasmus Darwin, the grandfather of Charles Darwin, employed digitalis to good effect and sought to immortalize it in the following verses:

> Bolster'd with down, amid a thousand wants,
> Pale Dropsy rears his bloated form, and pants;
> "Quench me ye cool pellucid rills," he cries,

Wets his parched tongue and rolls his hollow eyes.
So bends tormented Tantalus to drink
While from his lips the refluent waters shrink;
Again the rising stream his bosom laves
And thirst consumes him mid circumfluent waves.
Divine Hygeia from the bending sky
Descending, listens to his piercing cry;
Assumes bright Digitalis dress and air;
Her ruby cheek, white neck and raven hair;
Four youths protect her from the circling throng,
And like the Nymph the Goddess steps along.
O'er him she waves her serpent wreathed wand,
Cheers with her voice and raises with her hand
Warms with rekindling bloom his visage wan,
And charms the shapeless monster into man.

BOTANIC GARDEN. Part 2. Canto. 2.

AN ACCOUNT OF THE INTRODUCTION OF FOXGLOVE INTO MODERN PRACTICE*

As the more obvious and sensible properties of plants, such as colour, taste, and smell, have but little connexion with the diseases they are adapted to cure; so their peculiar qualities have no certain dependence upon their external configuration. Their chemical examination by fire, after an immense waste of time and labour, having been found useless, is now abandoned by general consent. Possibly other modes of analysis will be found out, which may turn to better account; but we have hitherto made only a very small progress in the chemistry of animal and vegetable substances. Their virtues must therefore be learnt, either from observing their effects upon insects and quadrupeds; from analogy, deduced from the already known powers of some of their congenera, or from the empirical usages and experience of the populace.

The first method has not yet been much attended to; and the second can only be perfected in proportion as we approach towards the discovery of a truly natural system; but the last, as far as it extends, lies within the reach of every one who is open to information, regardless of the source from whence it springs.

It was a circumstance of this kind which first fixed my attention on the Foxglove.

In the year 1775, my opinion was asked concerning a family receipt for the cure of

the dropsy. I was told that it had long been kept a secret by an old woman in Shropshire, who had sometimes made cures after the more regular practitioners had failed. I was informed also, that the effects produced were violent vomiting and purging; for the diuretic effects seemed to have been overlooked. This medicine was composed of twenty or more different herbs; but it was not very difficult for one conversant in these subjects, to perceive, that the active herb could be no other than the Foxglove.

My worthy predecessor in this place, the very humane and ingenious Dr. Small, has made it a practice to give his advice to the poor during one hour in a day. This practice, which I continued until we had an Hospital opened for the reception of the sick poor, gave me an opportunity of putting my ideas into execution in a variety of cases; for the number of poor who thus applied for advice, amounted to between two and three thousand annually. I soon found the Foxglove to be a very powerful diuretic; but then, and for a considerable time afterwards, I gave it in doses very much too large, and urged its continuance too long; for misled by reasoning from the effects of the squill, which generally acts best upon the kidneys when it excites nausea, I wished to produce the same effect by the Foxglove. In this mode of prescribing, when I had so many patients to attend to in the space of one, or at most of two hours, it will not be expected that I

* Withering, William, *An Account of the Foxglove and Some of its Medical Uses,* Birmingham, Swinney, 1785, p. 1, p. 11.

could be very particular, much less could I take notes of all the cases which occurred. Two or three of them only, in which the medicine succeeded, I find mentioned amongst my papers. It was from this kind of experience that I ventured to assert, in the Botanical Arrangement published in the course of the following spring, that the Digitalis purpurea "merited more attention than modern practice bestowed upon it."

I had not, however, yet introduced it into the more regular mode of prescription; but a circumstance happened which accelerated that event. My truly valuable and respectable friend, Dr. Ash, informed me that Dr. Crawley, then principal of Brazen Nose College, Oxford, has been cured of a Hydrops Pectoris, by an empirical exhibition of the root of the Foxglove, after some of the first physicians of the age had declared they could do no more for him. I was now determined to pursue my former ideas more vigorously than before, but was too well aware of the uncertainty which must attend on the exhibition of the *root* of a *biennial* plant, and therefore continued to use the *leaves*. These I had found to vary much as to dose, at different seasons of the year; but I expected, if gathered always in one condition of the plant, viz., when it was in its flowering state, and carefully dried, that the dose might be ascertained as exactly as that of any other medicine; nor have I been disappointed in this expectation. The more I saw of the great powers of this plant, the more it seemed necessary to bring the doses of it to the greatest possible accuracy. I suspected that this degree of accuracy was not reconcilable with the use of a decoction, as it depended not only upon the care of those who had the preparation of it, but it was easy to conceive from the analogy of another plant of the same natural order, the tobacco, that its active properties might be impaired by long boiling. The decoction was therefore discarded, and the *infusion* substituted in its place. After this I began to use the leaves in *powder*, but I still very often prescribe the infusion.

Further experience convinced me, that the *dieuretic* effects of this medicine do not at all depend upon its exciting a nausea or vomiting; but on the contrary, that though the increased secretion of urine will frequently succeed to, or exist along with these circumstances, yet they are so far from being friendly or necessary, that I have often known the discharge of urine checked, when the doses have been imprudently urged so as to occasion sickness.

If the medicine purges, it is almost certain to fail in its desired effect; but this having been the case, I have seen it afterwards succeed when joined with small doses of opium, so as to restrain its action on the bowels.

In the summer of the year 1776, I ordered a quantity of the leaves to be dried, and as it then became possible to ascertain its doses, it was gradually adopted by the medical practitioners in the circle of my acquaintance.

* * *

Cases,

CASES, IN WHICH THE DIGITALIS WAS GIVEN BY THE DIRECTION OF THE AUTHOR

1775.

It was in the course of this year that I began to use the Digitalis in dropsical cases. The patients were such as applied at my house for advice gratis. I cannot pretend to charge my memory with particular cases, or particular effects, and I had not leisure to make notes. Upon the whole, however, it may be concluded, that the medicine was found useful, or I should not have continued to employ it.

CASE I.

December 8th. A man about fifty years of age, who had formerly been a builder, but was now much reduced in his circumstances, complained to me of an asthma which first attacked him about the latter end of autumn. His breath was very short, his countenance was sunken, his belly large; and, upon examination, a fluctuation in it was very perceptible. His urine for some time past had been small in quantity. I directed a docoction of Fol. Digital. recent. which made him very sick, the sickness recurring at intervals for several days, during which time he made a large quantity of water. His breath gradually drew easier, his belly subsided, and in about ten days he begun to eat with a keen appetite. He afterwards took steel and bitters.

1776.
CASE II.

January 14th. A poor man labouring under an ascites and anasarca, was directed to take a decoction of Digitalis every four hours. It purged him smartly, but did not relieve him.

An opiate was now ordered with each dose of the medicine, which then acted upon the kidneys very freely, and he soon lost all his complaints.

CASE III.

March 15th. A poor boy, about nine years of age, was brought for my advice. His countenance was pale, his pulse quick and feeble, his body greatly emaciated, except his belly, which was very large, and, upon examination, contained a fluid. The case had been considered as arising from worms. He was directed to take the decoction of Digitalis night and morning. It operated as a diuretic, never made him sick, and he got well without any other medicine.

CASE IV.

July 25th. Mrs. H...., of A...., near N...., between forty and fifty years of age, a few weeks ago, after some previous indisposition, was attacked by a severe cold shivering fit, succeeded by fever; great pain in her left side, shortness of breath, perpetual cough, and, after some days, copious expectoration. On the 4th of *June,* Dr. Darwin,* was called to her. I have not heard what was then done for her, but, between the 15th of *June* and 25th of *July,* the Doctor, at his different visits, gave her various medicines of the deobstruent, tonic, anti-spasmodic, diuretic, and evacuant kinds.

On the 25th of *July* I was desired to meet Dr. Darwin at the lady's house. I found her nearly in a state of suffocation; her pulse extremely weak and irregular, her breath very short and laborious, her countenance sunk, her arms of a leaden colour, clammy and cold. She could not lye down in bed, and had neither strength nor appetite, but was extremely thirsty. Her stomach, legs, and thighs were greatly swollen; her urine very small in quantity, not more than a spoonful at a time, and that very seldom. It had been proposed to scarify her legs, but the proposition was not acceded to.

She had experienced no relief from any means that had been used, except from ipecacoanha vomits; the dose of which had been gradually increased from 15 to 40 grains, but such was the insensible state of her stomach for the last few days, that even those very large doses failed to make her sick,

* Then resident at Lichfield, now at Derby.

and consequently purged her. In this situation of things I knew of nothing likely to avail us, except the Digitalis: but this I hesitated to propose, from an apprehension that little could be expected from any thing; that an unfavourable termination would tend to discredit a medicine which promised to be of great benefit to mankind, and I might be censured for a prescription which could not be countenanced by the experience of any other regular practitioner. But these considerations soon gave way to the desire of preserving the life of this valuable woman, and accordingly I proposed the Digitalis to be tried; adding, that I sometimes had found it to succeed when other, even the most judicious methods, had failed. Dr. Darwin very politely, acceded immediately to my proposition, and, as he had never seen it given, left the preparation and the dose to my direction. We therefore prescribed as follows:

R. Fol. Digital. purp. recent. oz iv. coque ex

Aq. fontan. purae lb iss ad lb i. et cola.
R. Decot. Digital. oz iss.

Aq. Nuc. Moschat. oz ii. M. fiat. haust. 2 dis horis sumend.

The patient took five of these draughts, which made her very sick, and acted very powerful upon the kidneys, for within the first twenty-four hours she made upwards of eight quarts of water. The sense of fulness and oppression across her stomach was greatly diminished, her breath was eased, her pulse became more full and more regular, and the swellings of her legs subsided.

26th. Our patient being thus snatched from impending destruction, Dr. Darwin proposed to give her a decoction of pareira brava and guiacum shavings, with pills of myrrh and white vitriol; and, if costive, a pill with calomel and aloes. To these propositions I gave a ready assent.

30th. This day Dr. Darwin saw her, and directed a continuation of the medicines last prescribed.

August 1st. I found the patient perfectly free from every appearance of dropsy, her breath quite easy, her appetite much improved, but still very weak. Having some suspicion of a diseased liver, I directed pills of soap, rhubarb, tartar of vitriol, and calomel to be taken twice a day, with a neutral saline draught.

9th. We visited our patient together, and

repeated the draughts directed on the 26th of *June,* with the addition of tincture of bark, and also ordered pills of aloes, guiacum, and sal martis to be taken if costive.

September 10th. From this time the management of the case fell entirely under my direction, and perceiving symptoms of effusion going forwards, I desired that a solution of merc. subl. corr, might be given twice a day.

19th. The increase of the dropsical symptoms now made it necessary to repeat the Digitalis. The dried leaves were used in infusion, and the water was presently evacuated, as before.

It is now almost nine years since the Digitalis was first prescribed for this lady, and

notwithstanding I have tried every preventive method I could devise, the dropsy still continues to recur at times; but is never allowed to increase so as to cause much distress, for she occasionally takes the infusion and relieves herself whenever she chooses. Since the first exhibition of that medicine, very small doses have been always found sufficient to promote the flow of urine.

I have been more particular in the narrative of this case, partly because Dr. Darwin has related it rather imperfectly in the notes of his son's posthumous publication, trusting, I imagine, to memory, and partly because it was a case which gave rise to a very general use of the medicine in that part of Shropshire.

ANEURYSM

Jean Fernel

An aneurism is the dilatation of an artery full of spiritous blood. It sometimes occurs externally, as in the hands and feet, or about the throat and chest; differing in this respect from a varix, that it is large, swollen, and has often an annoying pulsation. On the tumour being pressed upon, the matter contained within it disappears. It also sometimes occurs in the internal arteries, especially in the chest, or about the spleen and mesentery, where a violent throbbing is frequently observable.

It is scarcely credible that some imagine that in these affections the vein or artery is ruptured or opened; for if the blood had escaped from the vein or artery, it would soon putrefy, and give rise to a tumor of a different kind.*

*Jo. Fernelius Ambiana, *Universa Medicina,* Frankfurt, Andreas Wechel, 1581, p. 652. Translated by John E. Erichsen, *Observations on Aneurysm,* London, Sydenham Society, 1844, p. 36

Ambroise Paré

Ambroise Paré, one of the most interesting and attractive personages in the history of surgery, was born at Bourg Hersent, a little village in the old French province of Maine, in 1510. His father was a valet and barber, and several of his near relatives were in medical occupations. His brother-in-law was a master barber surgeon of Paris and his brother Jean was a master barber surgeon at Vitré.

Paré studied first with his brother Jean and in 1532 was apprenticed to a barber-surgeon in Paris. After his apprenticeship was ended he became an interne at the Hôtel-Dieu, then the only public hospital in Paris, where he served four years. His first opportunities in the practice of military surgery came during the campaign of Francis I in Piedmont. During this campaign, he treated the wounded with boiling oil, but as the supply of oil gave out, he was forced to treat many with a mixture of egg-yolk, oil of roses, and turpentine. Finding that the wounded treated with the bland mixtures did very much better he "determined never again to burn thus so cruelly the poor wounded by arquebuses."

After the campaign was over Paré returned to Paris and studied hard, especially anatomy. In 1541 he passed his examinations and became a master barber-surgeon. From 1543 to 1545 Paré served with the army and in 1545 published his first work on the treatment of wounds. After his return to Paris,

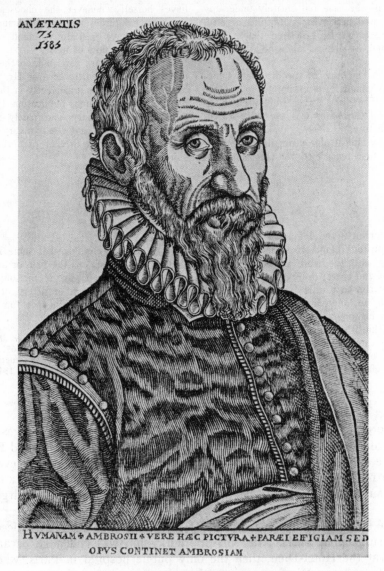

AN'ÆTATIS
73
1585

HVMANAM ✦ AMBROSII ✦ VERE HÆC PICTVRA ✦ PARÆI EFIGIAM SED
OPVS CONTINET AMBROSIAM

AMBROISE PARÉ (1510-1590)

A portrait of Paré at the age of seventy-five. From
Les œuvres d'Ambroise Paré (Lyon, 1633)

he worked hard at anatomy and in 1552 again saw military service, this time in Germany. His reputation gradually grew and he became surgeon successively to Henry II, Francis II, and Charles IX. He was present at the Massacre of Saint Bartholomew and dressed Admiral Coligny's wounds when the Protestant chief was wounded a few hours before the general massacre began. Paré was strongly suspected of being a Huguenot, and Brantôme and Sully stated that he was the only Protestant spared by royal mandate. Paré's religion has been the occasion of much dispute and while he conformed externally to the Catholic faith, there are strong reasons for believing that he was at heart a Huguenot.

On the death of Charles IX, Paré became surgeon to Henry III and was also appointed "valet de chambre du roi." In 1575 Paré published the first collected edition of his works, written in French and dedicated to the King. Paré died in 1590 at the age of eighty.

Paré's contributions to surgery were of capital importance. He devised many new surgical instruments, re-introduced the ligature, introduced massage, artificial limbs, and artificial eyes. One of his frequent and oft quoted remarks "Je le pansay, Dieu le guarist" (I dress him, God cures him) expressed his belief in the boundless healing powers of nature.

The following brief treatise on aneurysms is from the well-known English translation of Paré's works by Thomas Johnson, first published at London in 1634.

CHAP. XXXII*

OF AN ANEURISMA, THAT IS, THE DILATATION, OR SPRINGING
OF AN ARTERY, VEINE, OR SINEW

An *Aneurisma* is a soft tumor yielding to the touch, made by the blood and What it is spirit powred forth under the flesh and Muscles, by the dilatation or relaxation of an Artery. Yet the Author of the definitions seems to call any dilatation of any venous vessell by the name of an *Aneurisma*. *Gallen* calls an *Aneurisma* an opening made of the *Anastomasis*, of an Artery. Also an *Aneurisma* is made when an Artery that is wounded closeth too slowly, the In what parts they substance which is above it being chiefly in the mean time agglutinated, happen filled with flesh and cicatrized, which doth not seldome happen in opening of Arteries unskillfully performed and negligently cured; therefore *Aneurismaes* are absolutely made by the *Anastomasis*, springing, breaking, *Erosion*, and wounding of the Arteries. These happen in all parts of the body, but more frequently in the throat, especially in women after a painfull travail. For when as they more strongly strive to hold their breath, for the more powerful expulsion of the birth, it happens that the Artery is dilated and broken, whence follows an effusion of blood and spirits under the skin. The signs are, a swelling one while great, another small, with a pulsation and a colour not varying from the native constitution of the skin. It is a soft tumor, and so yeelding to the impression of the fingers that if it peradventure be small, it wholly vanisheth, the Arterious blood and spirits flying back into the body of the Artery, but presently as soon as you take your fingers away, they return again with like celerity. Some *Aneurismaes* do not only when they are pressed, but also of themselves make a sensible hissing, if you lay your ear near to them, by reason of the motion of the vitall spirits rushing with great violence through the straitness of the passage. Prognostick Wherefore in *Aneurismaes* in which there is a great rupture of the Artery, such a noise is not heard, because the spirit is carryed through a larger passage. Great *Aneurismaes* under the Arm pits, in the Groins and other partt wherein there are large vessels, admit no cure, because so great an eruption of blood and spirit often follows upon such an incision, that death prevents both Art and Cure. Which A History I observed a few years ago in a certain Priest of Saint *Andrews* of the Arches, Mr. *John Maillet,* dwelling with

* Paré, Ambroise. *The Workes of that famous Chirurgion Ambrose Parey.* Translated out of the Latine and compared with the French by Th. Johnson, London, Cotes, 1649, p. 224.

a Chief President *Christopher de Thou.* Who having an *Aneurisma* at the setting on of the shoulder about the bigness of a Wall-nut, I

Aneurismaes must not rashly be opened

charged him, he should not let it be opened, for if he did it would bring him into manifest danger of his life, and that it would be more safe for him to break the violence thereof with double clothes steeped in the juyce of Night-Shade & Housleek, with new and wheyey cheese mixt therewith: Or with *Vnguentum de Bolo* or *Emplastrum contra rupturam* and such other refrigerating and astringent medicines, if he would lay upon it a thin plate of Lead, and would use shorter breeches that his doublet might serve to hold it too, to which he might fasten his breeches in stead of a swath, & in the mean time he should eschew all things which attenuate and inflame the blood, but especially he should keep himself from all great straining of his voice. Although he had used his diet for a yeer, yet he could not so handle the matter but that the tumor increased, which he observing goes to a Barber, who supposing the tumor to be of the kind of vulgar impostumes, applies to it in the Evening a Caustick causing an eschar so to open it. In the Morning such an abundance of blood flowed forth from the tumor being opened, that he therewith astonished, implores all possible ayd, and bids that I should be called to stay this his great bleeding, and he repented that he had not followed my directions. Wherefore I am called, but when I was scarce over the threshold, he gave up his ghost with his blood. Wherefore I diligently admonish the young Chirurgeon that he do not rashly open *Aneurismaes* unless they be smal in an ignoble part, aand not indued with large vessels, but rather let him perform the cure after this manner. Cut the skin which

How they must be cured

lyes over it until the Artery appear, and then separate it with your knife from the particles about it, then thrust a blunt and crooked needle with a thred in it under it, bind it, then cut it off and so expect the falling off of the thred of its self while nature covers the orifices of the cut Artery with new flesh, then the residue of the cure may be performed after the manner of simple

These of the inward parts incurable

wounds. The *Aneurismaes* which happen in the internall parts are incurable. Such as frequently happen to those who have often had

the unction and sweat for the cure of French disease, because the blood being so attenuated and heated therewith that it cannot be contained in the receptacles of the Artery, it distends it to that largeness as to hold a mans Fist; Which I have observed in the dead body of a certain Taylor, who had an

A History

Aneurisma of the Arterious vein suddenly whilst he was playing at Tennis fell dead, the vessel being broken: his body opened I found a great quantity of blood powred forth into the capacity of the Chest, but the body of the Artery was dilated to that largness I formerly mentioned, and the inner coat thereof was bony. For which cause within a while after I shewed it to the great admiration of the beholders in the Physitians School whilest I publiquely dissected a body there; the whilst he lived said he felt a beating and a great heat over all his body by the force of the pulsation of all the Arteries, by occasion whereof he often swounded. Doctor *Syluius* the Kingsprofessor of Physick at that time forbad him the use of Wine, and wished him to use boyled water for his drink, and Curds and new Cheeses for his meat, and to apply them in form of Cataplasms upon the grieved and swoln part. At night he used a ptisan of Barly meal and Poppy-seeds, and was purged now and then with a Clyster of refrigerating and emollient things, or with Cassia alone, by which medicines he said he found himself much better. The cause of such a bony constitution of the Arteries by *Aneurismaes* is, for that the hot and fervid blood first dilates the Coats of an Artery, then breaks them; which when it happens, it then borrows from the neighbouring bodies a fit matter to restore the loosed continuity thereof.

This matter whilst little and little it is dryed and hardened, it degenerates into a gristly or else a bony substance, just by the force of the same materiall and efficient causes, by which stones are generated in the reins and bladder. For the more terrestriall portion of the blood is dryed and condensed by the power of the unnaturall heat contained in the part affected with an *Aneuisma;* whereby it comes to pass that the substance added to the dilated and broken Artery is turned into a body of a bony consistence. In which the singular providence of nature, the handmaid of God is shewed, as that which, as it were by making and opposing a new wall or bank, would hinder and break the violence of the raging blood swelling with the abundance of the vitall spirits; unless any had rather to refer the cause of that hardness to the continuall application of refrigerating and astringent medicines. Which have power to condensate and harden, as may not obscurely be gathered by the writings of *Galen*. But beware you be not deceived by the fore-mentioned signs; for sometimes in large *Aneurismaes* you can perceive no pulsation, neither can you force the blood into the Artery by

Lib 4. Cap. ult de praes ex pulsa

the pressure of your fingers, either because the quantity of such blood is greater than which can be contained in the ancient receptacles of the Artery, or because it is condensate and concrete into clods, whereupon wanting the benefit of ventilation from the heart, it presently putrefies; Thence ensue great pain, a Gangren, and mortification of the part, and lastly the death of the Creature.

A Caution in the knowing of Aneurismaes

Richard Wiseman

CHAPTER XVI*
OF AN ANEURISMA

An *Aneurisma,* according to my Description, is an *Ecchymosis*, and indeed the highest Species of it. But since Authors have given another account of that Tumour, and have allowed it a peculiar Chapter I have done so too; the rather, because the nature of the Vessel through which the Effusion is made doth require a different method of Cure.

It is a Tumour soft, white, and yielding to the touch, but riseth again on removal of your finger; and is for the most part, accompanied with pulsation of the Artery.

It is raised, according to the Opinion of Authors, by dilatation or relaxation of the Artery; they supposing the Bloud to have burst its passage through the first Coat, and dilated the second, thereby raising the Tumour. And this some of them have delivered to us so positively, as if they had in opening found the exteriour Coat so dilated. This I my self was taught, and some while believed: but not having been able by my practice to discover one *Aneurisma* made by dilatation or relaxation of the outward Coat, I am apt to believe that there is no such thing, but that it takes its rise from Bloud bursting quite through the Artery into the interstices of the Muscles, where it raiseth a Tumour suitable to the Cavity it findeth, growing bigger or less, of this or that shape, as the Muscles give way. But this Tumour consists of Bloud extravasated, the Artery lying undilated the while. I

Description

Opinion of the ancients

do therefore, suspect the possibility of an *Aneurisma* by the dilatation of the outward or softer Coat of the Artery, because it seems improbable that a force big enough to burst the inward Coat, which is so tough and firm, should leave the exteriour being softer and weaker, whole, and go out so leisurely into it as to give it time for dilatation. Those which I have met with did all come from downright eruption through both the Coats: and those that come from external Punctures must of necessity begin with a breach of external Coat first, it being next the Lancet, or other Weapon that made the division. *Sennertus* would have it to heal again, though contrary to my experience, who have always found it open as well as the internal: and indeed reason must tell us, that the constant eruptions of the bloud out of the Artery in every Pulse must needs keep it open; nay, the Bloud keeps not within the bounds of any one Membrane, but I have seen it extravasated through all the intersitices of the Muscles of the whole Arm.

The Causes of Aneurisma's are divers, internal, or external. 1. The internal Cause is, the impetuousity of the Bloud, which moving with greater violence in its Chanels than the Artery can sustain, doth force its way through the side of the Vessel, and bursting a hole in it, doth issue into the space that lieth between it and the neighbouring Muscles, there incrassating the Membranes of the Muscles and framing it self a nest.

Causes

This *Impetus* may rise first from the quantity of the Bloud. Either when it is more than the Vessel can contain, a case that sel-

* Richard Wiseman, *Eight Chirurgical Treatises*, III Ed., London, Tooke and Meredith, 1696, p. 70.

dom happens to produce an *Aneurisma* in any conspicuous Vessel; but if any such thing be, it opens at the Nose or Lungs, or in the Brain, (there causing an Apoplexy;) or in the Stomach, Guts, *Anus, &c.* Or else when this Bloud is not really more than the whole Body naturally should contain, but by violent Passion or Motion in stirring, is too forcibly driven forwards from the Heart towards some peculiar Artery; when the farther progress being (it may be) intercepted by some violent contraction of the Muscles through which it must pass, it of necessity breaks the Vessel: and thus in violent Vomiting and other Straining *Aneurisma's* are often made in the Neck, Arms, Legs, &c.

Secondly, from the quality of the Bloud, which being too sharp or thin, erodes the Vessel; or, being highly fermented by other causes, bursts through all.

This Bloud, though extravasated, doth usually pulse: partly, because the body of the Artery from which it breaks doth pass through it, and by its Pulse doth agitate that; and partly, because in every such Pulse some addition of Bloud is made to the Tumour. Yet this Pulse is chiefly in small *Aneurisma's* or superficial ones; for in the greater the motion of the Artery is not always felt.

2. The external Causes are puncture by Lancet or Weapon, cutting, bruising, erosion, or whatever else may divide the Coats of the Arteries.

The *Differences* of an *Aneurisma* are either from its magnitude, situation, or shape. From the Magnitude it is denominated great or small, possessing the whole member or part. From its Situation, it is superficial near the Skin, or deep in the Muscles. From its Shape: either it keeps the shape of the Part; which usually happens when the Orfice in the Artery is small, so that the Bloud comes out leisurely, and finds the neighbour Membranes so well united as to keep it within a certain channel, which Membranes are also fortified by an addition of a *Serum* coagulated from the extravasated Bloud: or else it alters its form, when it groweth suddenly or irregularly the Eruption being so great that it cannot be kept within bounds; or when it is by an ignorant Chirurgeon treated with Lenients and Discutients, being mistaken for some other Disease; for in this case the Membranes are relaxed, and give way to the Tumour.

From these Differences the *Signs* of an *Aneurisma* may be taken. If the Tumour be small and superficial, a Pulsation may easily be felt in every part of it. If it be great and rise suddenly, and was white and soft from its first appearance, though there be no Pulsation to be felt, yet you may conclude it an *Aneurisma*, there being not any Humour save that of the Bloud which can so suddenly raise such a Tumour. The often increase and diminution of the Tumour is also a Sign of an *Aneurisma;* the diminution of it being the return of the Bloud into the Artery, whence it as often cometh out again.

Signs

If it happened from a Puncture of a Lancet, the manner of the spurting out of the Bloud, will shew it; and if it do not bleed, yet a sudden Tumour thrusts up under your Finger, with Pulsation, the bloud breaking out into the interstices of the Muscles, though not quite into the Skin.

The Tumour is more compact or scattered according as there was care taken at first to restrain it within compass. In some of these there is a redness and Inflammation, by reason of the expansion of the Parts beyond their capacity, or from the putrefaction of the Bloud: in which latter case Fever and Fainting for the most part accompany it.

All *Aneurisma's* are difficult of Cure. Those which are large, and arise from Arteries deep in the Muscles, to which you cannot make your Applications, are incurable: and if they be unadvisedly opened, the Patient is in great danger of his life. But if the *Aneurisma* be in such a Part is capable of Bandage and application of Medicaments, the Cure is feasible; or the Disease may be palliated to the ease of the Patient.

Prognostick

Giovanni Maria Lancisi

Giovanni Maria Lancisi was born in Rome in 1654, the son of parents of the middle class. He studied theology first, but later became interested in medicine and studied anatomy, chemistry, geometry, and botany at the Collegio de Sapienza. He received his doctor's degree when eighteen years of age and four years later was appointed assistant physician to the San Spirito Hospital. In 1684 he became Professor of Anatomy at the Collegio de Sapienza, holding this position until 1697 when he was appointed Professor of the Theory and Practice of Medicine. The latter position he held until his death in 1720, at the age of sixty-six.

Lancisi was appointed a papal physician in 1688 by Innocent and in 1700

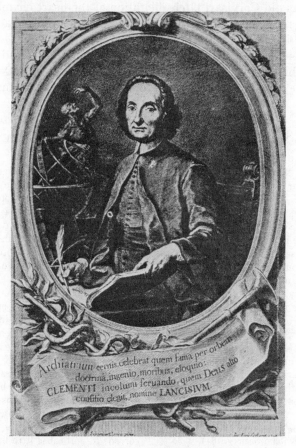

GIOVANNI MARIA LANCISI (1654-1720)
Etching by Sebastian Conra

became first physician. In 1714 at the request of Pope Clement he published the superb anatomical plates of Eustachius, which had remained unprinted in the Papal Library for one hundred and sixty-two years. These were the first anatomic plates on copper.

Lancisi was the greatest Italian clinician of his time, as well as a great epidemiologist. He described the epidemics of influenza and cattle plague, and in his work on malarial fevers mentions the possibility of their transmission by mosquitoes.

The best known works of Lancisi are his *De subitaneis mortis* (on sudden death) published at Rome in 1707 and his *De motu cordis et aneurysmatibus* (on motion of the heart and aneurysms) published at Naples in 1738, eighteen years after his death. The first work was written at the request of Pope Clement XI, on account of the terror of the Roman public, caused by the large number of sudden deaths in 1705. In this work, he notes heart diseases as a common cause of sudden death, describes vegetations on heart valves, and gives a classification of heart disease. In his work on aneurysms, he notes syphilis as a cause of aortic aneurysm. Under the term aneurysm of the heart, he described, as did Corvisart later, dilatation of the heart chambers. He noted the value of percussion of the sternum in the diagnosis of cardiac dilatation, an observation which makes him a forerunner of Auenbrugger.

Lancisi was very eloquent and impressive in public life, and in private life was very sociable and charming. He collected a library of 20,000 volumes which he gave to the San Spirito Hospital for the use of physicians and medical students.

PROPOSITION XXXII.—ON THE MODE OF FORMATION, THE CAUSES AND SYMPTOMS OF A SYPHILITIC ANEURISM*

As an acrid fluid, distilling from the aneurismal cyst or sac, may penetrate as far as the bones of ligaments, which it may gradually corrode, and wear away; so, on the contrary, it may sometimes happen that the lymph, abounding in syphilitic humours, may, first of all, give rise to congestion in the bones and ligaments; but by and by, having become more acrid, and settling in the external coat of the artery, it may begin to corrode, and thus to dilate it into an aneurism; which being produced both by compression and erosion, is much worse than the others, more particularly as physicians, being formerly but imperfectly acquainted with its nature, were most generally accustomed to treat it by bloodletting and the administration of whey, when, on the contrary, the proper method

of cure consists entirely in acting upon it with particular and appropriate remedies, so as to promote the transpiration and the diuresis of the venereal lymph, as will clearly be shown by the subjoined cases. Marcus Aurelius Severinus has also stated, in his treatise 'De Novissima Observatione Abscessus,' that aneurisms arise from syphilitic cachexy.

A venereal aneurism may be known not only by the suspicious connexion and the appearance of syphilitic infection in other parts of the body, by which it has been preceded, but more especially by the manner in which any particular vessel becomes affected with aneurism; for the pulsation of the artery is not suddenly perceived, but it is preceded, especially at night, by pains in the joints and bones, which gradually projecting in the form of a tumour, press upon the subjacent artery, corrode it, and cause it to begin to pulsate.

* *Observations on Aneurysm,* John E. Erichson, London, Syndenham Society, 1844, p. 36.

Giovanni Battista Morgagni

BOOK II. OF THE DISEASES OF THE THORAX
LETTER XXVI*

5. A young man, of about twenty-seven years of age, had been afflicted, already, for

* Morgagni. J. B., *The Seats and Causes of Diseases,* translated by Benjamin Alexander, M.D., London, Millar and Cadell, 1769, I, p. 795, 799, 800, 806-809.

a long time with a pulsating kind of tumour in the right part of the thorax, betwixt the third and fourth rib; in which tumour, while he turn'd himself from one side to the other, he felt a fluctuating matter that was acted upon by that motion; in the mean while, he had been often seiz'd with a shortness of breath; which, however, in a short time after a vein was open'd, remitted. One day, as he was at his devotions, he fell down suddenly; his face was pale, he could scarcely speak; he soon died.

In the thorax was seen a large aneurism. For where the carotid arteries came off from

out, and then render'd rough and unequal. Finally, it came within the pericardium, where, being ruptur'd, it had fill'd all the cavity of it with blood. There was no polypous concretion in the heart.

* * *

13. A strumpet of eight-and-twenty years

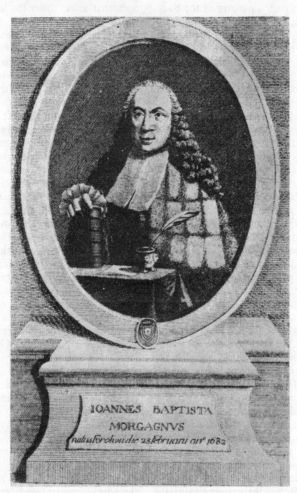

GIOVANNI BATTISTA MORGAGNI (1682-1771)
From the frontispiece to *De sedibus et causis morborum*, 1761

the aorta, it began; and extending itself to the sternum, to which it then strongly adher'd, so that it could not be separated without laceration. It was also produc'd under the right clavical to the third and fourth rib, the internal surface of which had hollow'd

of age, of a lean habit, having complain'd for some months, and particularly for the last fifteen days, of a certain lassitude, and a loathing of food, and almost of everything, for this reason made less use of other aliments and more of unmix'd wine; to the use of which she had always been too much addicted. A certain debauchee having gone into the house to her, and after a little time having come out, with a confus'd and disturb'd countenance and she not having appear'd for two or three hours after, the neighbours, who had observed these things, entering in, found her not only dead but cold; lying in bed with such a posture of the body, that it could not be doubted what business she had been about when she died, especially as the semen verile was seen to have flow'd down from the organs of generation. I was, therefore ask'd, whether I desired to have the genitals or not? and whether I would have the other viscera also? In answer'd, that I should be glad of both; not that I expected to see any thing particular in the organs of generation, now that the semen had flow'd out, but that I wish'd to take fresh notice of some things which I had often observ'd; for I conjectur'd, as I then said, that the cause of this sudden death would certainly be found to consist in the rupture of some large vessel. It was at this time extremely hot, it being June of the year 1725, nor were we allow'd to dissect the body till about the later end of the following day. For which reason, changing my design I sent my friend Mediavia to examine all the parts; and to take care to bring home the principal of them only to me.

The neck was livid under the chin, yet without any marks of force having been externally applied. The back was also somewhat livid. The abdomen was tense and did not shew any mark of the woman's having ever been pregnant. The uterus being taken away, the small intestines appear'd very red. The large intestines, and especially the lower ones, were full of excrements: the stomach was very large although almost empty. There was serum extravasated in the belly, to about the quantity of a pint, not unlike turbid water in which fresh meat had been wash'd, and so acrid, that it effected the extremities of the fingers with the sense of a kind of heat. In the thorax, the lungs were so far off their natural colour, that they were not black even on the posterior part. But the pericardium was so distended, that no sooner was a little wound made into it, but a serum burst forth, of the same nature with that which had been seen in the belly. Yet still a great quantity remain'd, and under it a black and firmly-concreted blood cover'd the surface of the heart. Which being brought to me on the

following day, in the morning, together with the large vessels and the genitals, I observ'd, before I cut into them, that neither the heart itself, nor the trunk of the great artery, was dilated; and even that both of them, by their smallness, corresponded very well with the stature of the woman, which they said had been rather small. Being then about to lay open that artery from the inferior extremity, which was at the septum transversum, and having seen that one side of it, not much higher, was black to the extent of five or six fingers breath; I found that this was owing merely to the effusion of blood into the cells of the external coat; for the other parts were quite in their natural state. But an internal disease began from the left extremity of the curvature of the aorta, and going from thence quite to the heart, became so much the larger in proportion as the artery came nearer to the heart. That is to say, in some places whitish marks of a future ossification occur'd; in others, some small foramina, as it were, had begun to be form'd, and in still other places were parallel furrows, drawn longitudinally: and in this manner was the surface of the artery unequal here and there. But when I came near to the semilunar valves, which seem'd to be lank and contracted, at the distance of half an inch above that which lies on the back-part, was an orifice that would have admitted the end of a man's thumb by means of which the aorta communicated with a roundish aneurism, that hung to it in the form of a sacculus. This sacculus exceeded the size of a walnut before it is stripp'd of its green coat; and was so plac'd in the back of the aorta, that, as it inclin'd a little to the left side, it seem'd that it could not happen otherwise, but it must have obstructed the offices of the left auricle, or the adjoining sinus. And it had been ruptur'd in the upper part by the blood flowing from thence into the pericardium through a small foramen, the edges of which were lacerated and black. The internal surface of the sacculus was invested with red and polypous pellicles, which, like the texture of an onion, you might divide into as many strata or lamina as you pleas'd. But in the auricles and the ventricles of the heart, neither was there any polypous concretion, nor did the least quantity of blood remain.

* * *

21. A Venetian woman, of the same age as the last I have describ'd; of a stature, colour,

and habit of body that were laudable, but rather fattish; being the mother of many children; and having been, ten years before, seiz'd with a palsy of the lower limbs, was said to be made sound by the use of rosemary; or at least, she had been subject to no inconvenience from that time, which was worthy of remark, but, for some months past, had labour'd under a difficulty in breathing, which, however, was not continual; and besides this, with a pulsating tumour that ran upon the neck, longitudinally, in the region of the right carotid artery, yet never, (which you will remark, on account of those things which we found in the dead body), did she complain of any pain, numbness, or tumour of the right arm. But four or five days before her death, she complain'd of a troublesome kind of sensation, just as if her ribs, as she said, had fall'n towards the abdomen, when, on a sudden, about the middle of December, in the year 1708, being seiz'd with a kind of fainting, and affirming that she should die, she was with great difficulty supported by the women, who ran to her, and plac'd her in bed; where, her face, and particularly her lips, being livid; she, being cold and senseless, with a very small pulse, a difficult and slow respiration, departed from this life, in less than a quarter of an hour from the time of her being attacked.

Upon inspecting the body, it exhibited no oedematous tumor in any part, or any thing else that was worthy of remark, but when the belly was opened, some parts of the intestines appear'd to be, as it were, inflamed, if you attended to the colour; which colour was soon after obvious in the pancreas also. But upon examining the small intestines more attentively in one part of them, to the length of a man's hand, appear'd some very small and innumerable tubercles of an obscure kind, which were nothing else but tokens of the cells, that being distended with air, betwixt the fleshy coat and that which lay beneath it, lifted it up outwards; the air, therefore, having escap'd, by means of wounds in the nearest sanguiferious vessels, these cells collaps'd.

In the gall-bladder were four or five little stones, of an unequal magnitude among themselves, which being applied to the flame took fire. From the vena cava, when cut into, a considerable quantity of blood flow'd down; but from the great artery only a small quantity. The viscera of the belly being now suf-

ficiently inspected, and for that reason remov'd, it was evident that the diaphragm did not ascend, on both sides, in the form of a vaulted roof; but that it rather fell downwards.

When the thorax was open'd, we saw that a very bloody serum had been extravasated in both the cavities of it, to the quantity of a few ounces: but that the lungs were sound, although somewhat turgid; for the bronchia, and especially the left, as I afterwards saw, were fill'd with a serum like that I just now spoke of. In the mean while, the pericardium, by its tumid and livid appearance, had given marks of having blood extravasated in it: with which, however, it was not full; but contain'd somewhat less than a pound: about two ounces of which were a bloody serum; the remaining part of the blood having form'd itself into a thick and pretty firm lamina: whereas all the blood that I saw in this body was black, indeed, like this, but quite fluid. The blood being taken from the pericardium, as we saw that the aorta, as soon as ever it came out from the heart, was manifestly dilated, by pursuing the trunk and the principal branches thereof, I found that the former of them was dilated almost quite to the emulgent arteries, and that the branch of the aorta, which is of itself a common trunk of the right cartoid and subclavian, and, in like manner, that both of these branches were so dilated, as to make the breadth of the carotid, from the beginning of it quite to the division, more than twice as large as it ought naturally to be; and the subclavian artery, to the extent of three inches, was not expanded equally on all sides indeed, but had its posterior and superior paries only curv'd out into a prominent aneurism; by means of which, nothing at all being interpos'd, two or three nerves, of those that go from the neck into the upper limb, were compress'd. From this aneurism, which would have admitted my thumb, two arteries proceeded: these having a broader beginning than they naturally have, put on the form of a cone, and the farther they proceeded the more they were contracted; till having measured out the space of an inch and a half, they were reduced to their natural dimensions. One of these went to the thyroid gland, which was in this woman large, and some places hard.

After having examin'd all these parts externally, I began to lay open all these vessels, and even that part of the aorta which had been in the belly, in a longitudinal direction, beginning with the iliacs. And from these arteries quite to the emulgents, I found no appearance of disease, except whitish spots in some places, and very small furrows here and there. But as the dilatation of the trunk began above the emulgents, so from thence. quite to the heart, the parietes of the artery were much thicker then they usually are; yet not equally in every place, and were, in like manner, more hard and rigid than usual; although I found no where any appearance of ossification; but in some places whitish spots, in other very considerable parellel sulci, drawn in a longitudinal direction, and so much the more remarkable, as they were interrupted, after having run over a short space, by other transverse sulci, the direction of which was not near so strait; after that others follow'd, similar to the former, which were presently interrupted by transverse furrows; and after these still others in the same manner, so that in this morbid constitution a kind of elegant order was preserv'd, quite to the whole arch of the aorta; and, indeed, it was continu'd from this curvature into the left subclavian to the extent of an inch; into the neighboring carotid to the extent of two inches; but into the other through the whole of it, together with the spots, the thickness and hardness of the coats. But that aneurism of the subclavian resembl'd the structure of an auricle, as it were, of the heart, form'd of an unequal, hard, and thick coat, not internally lin'd with polypous laminae, or strata. but only having a very small, whitish, and oblong jagged concretion adhering to it; besides which I found no other polypous concretion in the whole body.

Finally, the trunk of the aorta itself, from that place where it sends off its first branch to the upper parts quite to the heart, was both distinguish'd with spots, and marked out into furrows; but these were so confus'd and irregular that nothing but a perpetual and very great inequality of the surface appear'd. Yet, besides this, a kind of ulceration, as it were, was found about two inches above the semilunar valves, where the artery looks toward the right and posterior parts; and in that ulceration were three or four very deep foramina, very near to each other, each of them of the bigness of a lentil, but of an angular form rather than round. From these foramina, winding sinusses were carried

obliquely outwards, and reach'd to the external lamina of the aorta; which was in that place, therefore, of a brownish colour mix'd with red, as if in consequence of inflammation, and because much thicken'd by a great flow of moisture, and in the middle of that redness, the lamina being at length lacerated, the blood had made a way for itself into the pericardium, by a foramen similar to the internal foramina, and almost of the same magnitude.

The left ventricle of the heart was greatly dilated; but the auricle that lay close to it. was very much contracted and thin. In that ventricle, and in the right, blood was not wanting; and in the pulmonary artery there was a great quantity; nor were the carotids, nor the jugular veins, devoid of it.

Finally, I found the cerebrum and cerebellum to be very lax, notwithstanding there was no water in the ventricles, a very little of which was found in some places only under the pia mater. The vessels of this membrane were somewhat turgid with blood. The vertebral arteries, where they enter'd the cranium, seem'd to be a little wider than usual. The other circumstances that were remark'd in this body by me, and by my friends, that assisted me in the dissection of it, relate to other subjects.

22. There were found in this woman four aneurisms at least; one of the left ventricle of the heart, one of the greater part of the aorta, and one of the right subclavian, and one of the carotid on the same side; so that there not only appears to have been sufficient causes for the symptoms with which the woman was troubl'd, but it is even surprising, that she had not been afflicted with more. As to the aneurism of the carotid, which discover'd itself by its prominence and pulsation, although I readily confess that these arteries are sometimes dilated, from peculiar causes that affect them in particular; yet that their dilation is join'd more frequently with the dilation of the aorta, and is even a propagation and effect of it; nobody since the time that the causes of diseases were begun to be enquir'd into, by frequent dissections, will deny. The ancient physicians, indeed, being in want of this assistance to their enquiries, seemed to suspect nothing of that kind; and thought that they had nothing else to do in an aneurism of the carotids, than to make a revulsion of the blood; to diminish and correct the acrid particles in it; and,

finally, to apply such things as had a property of contracting and constringing the coats of the arteries; as you will very clearly perceive from reading that chapter of Arantius[q], in which he particularly treats of this aneurism. But if any one attempt to constringe the artery, when it is a production or

effect of an aneurism of the great artery, he will increase the latter, and not remove the former; but he even will not be able to effect this, when it is only from an eroding cause, as Lancisi[r] shows, by producing an example of a noble matron.

[q] De Tumor. Praet. nat. c. 38.

[r] De Aneur. Propos. 31.

Jean Nicholas Corvisart

IV. SIGNS OF ANEURYSM OF THE AORTA*

The exposition of the signs of the aneurysm of the aorta is in close accord with the symptoms described in the observations reported above, and how to summarize the findings, which I have discussed in the preceding article, the state in which the aneurysmal tumors of the aorta are found, modifies markedly the degree of the certainty in the signs of these affections. The diagnosis presents always some obscurity when the dilation does not show itself without, while it becomes evident when the tumor presents itself to the eye and to the touch of a physician. In the first case, where the dilatation produces no tumor without most of the signs of the aneurysm of the aorta, can be confused with those of certain other affections of the chest. Since I have, so to say, enumerated these signs in reporting observations of this disease, I shall content myself with indicating those which can, although the aneurysm is not visible, indicate or indeed prove its existence and distinguish it from other similar affections. Along with these signs, so to say, pathognomonic, I place a sort of peculiar whistling, of which I have spoken in the article on effects. The whistling does not exist except when the tumor produces compression of the trachea, that is to say, when the aneurysm is located on the arch of the aorta. I ought not, moreover, fail to say that aneurysm of the arch of the aorta is not the only tumor which produces this particular whistling; here is a case, which causes the wise reservation on this subject:

Observation 51—A woman, still young, wishing to grasp a kitchen utensil above her head, threw her head forward violently, from fear of falling, the same instant of this movement she felt inside the lower part of the

neck a sort of tearing, which caused her very acute pain. This pain, for several days, remained located in the place where she first noticed it. Her voice commenced soon afterwards to become hoarse and soon there followed a complete aphonia. In addition to these symptoms of an extraordinary difficulty in breathing; and a marked loss of weight, there was added the distinct sensation to the patient of a hard body placed behind the sternum, to which she attributed her dyspnoea. During respiration we heard this type of whistling of which I have spoken, but in this patient it was very much more marked than in other cases; the pulse was also feeble, but regular. The chest was resonant throughout. The attentive consideration of all signs, and the absence of all other signs of aneurysm, made me suspect that a substance of some peculiar nature, pressed upon the trachea near its termination. After a long time, the patient, as it could be easily predicted, succumbed to this affection, and I saw on opening the body that I was not mistaken in my diagnosis, and that a tumor like a hard bronchial gland, of the form and size of an almond, had not only compressed the trachea, but had destroyed several of the cartilaginous rings of this structure.

I return to the signs of the affection of which I am discussing. A peculiar thrill, which is sometimes felt above the place where the heart is normally situated, this organ beating in its normal place; the dullness of tone, which the upper and middle part of the chest gives when one percusses, the smallness of the pulse and its irregularity in certain cases; in other cases its inequality on the two arms are a phenomena, which one can count among the number of signs, which are to a certain extent, pathognomonic of eneurysms of the aorta; because the majority of them belong exclusively or are common only to

* Corvisart, J. N., *Essai sur les maladies et les lésions organiques du cœur*, Paris, Migneret, 1806, p. 343.

analogous affections of the central organ of circulation.

I am now going to report an observation in which we find together the greatest number of signs of aneurysm of this artery.

Observation 52—A man aged forty-nine years, with healthy complexion, entered the hospital on the 22nd of October, 1798. Ten years before this time he began to notice palpitation of the heart, which returned about every fifteen days and lasted some times for several days. For three years he had none of these palpitations; his respiration nevertheless, remained markedly impaired and the patient had attacks of suffocation; although he took little exercise. Furthermore, the other functions were normal enough.

Four months after this man entered the hospital, his embarrassment of respiration was increased to such a point that he could not lie down flat without being menaced with suffocation. He had very often been obliged to pass the night seated in an arm chair, without undressing himself, which had helped not a little to cause the swelling of his lower extremities. When he presented himself at the hospital his face was a little reddish and bloated. His chest was resonant in the posterior portions, but gave a dull note on its anterior and superior position. Respiration was halting, high, difficult and whistling; his cough produced with difficulty, the expectoration of a viscid sputum; application of the hand over the region of the heart and above, allowed one to feel clearly a strong, frequent and vigorous beating, although the pulsations of the radial and cubital arteries were feeble, small and suppressed; irregular and frequent. The pulse showed the same phenomena on both sides. The urine was of sufficient quantity, dark reddish in color.

I carried out a bleeding of two palettes.*

*A palette was a bleeding cup holding three ounces.

I prescribed wine of scilla and nitrated hydromel. The bleeding produced a very marked relief. The respiration became much less whistling; the patient was able to take a little rest, the beating in the region of the heart was felt over a smaller area, but it continued nevertheless to spread out over the upper part of the chest; the pulse became less feeble; infiltration of the lower extremities disappeared; he seemed better than for several days. The patient was able to work and sleep well enough, when the 3rd of November, towards eight o'clock in the evening, he was seized with a violent coughing, accompanied by expectoration of blood, which suffocated him promptly. The blood which came by expectoration could be evaluated by three palettes, it was of a reddish vermillion color and contained a great deal of air.

At the opening of the body, the mouth was full of foaming saliva, which was not bloody. The larynx and trachea did not contain any blood clots, but a reddish serous fluid ran from them; the lungs were perfectly healthy and showed no adhesions to the pleura; there was a small amount of yellowish serous fluid effused into the left cavity of the chest. The substernal tissue was emphysematous; the heart was normal, but the arch of the aorta formed a tumor a little less than twice as large as the heart itself, in the middle of which emerged the sub-clavicular and carotid arteries. The pulmonary artery was adherent through a rough cellular tissue to the right side of this tumor. The descending aorta showed nothing remarkable.

I could not discover on the walls of the aneurysm any lesions through which we thought the blood had escaped. The trachea in that part, which increased by the dilatation of the aorta, had been compressed and pushed from left to right in such a manner it had taken the form of a Roman S.

William Silver Oliver

The following obituary notice is from the *British Medical Journal*, May, 1908.

(It is noteworthy that while Oliver's military career was given in some detail there is nothing about his discovery of the tracheal tug.)

Surgeon-General William Silver Oliver, M.D., late of the Army Medical Department, died on April 27th, at Farnborough Park, at the age of 72. He was an M.D. of Halifax, Nova Scotia, and entered the service as an Assistant Surgeon, September 15, 1857, becoming Surgeon, February 3, 1872; Surgeon-Major, March 1, 1873; Brigade Surgeon, August 23, 1882; and Honorary Deputy Surgeon-General on retirement, May 1, 1883. His war record was as follows: Indian Mutiny, 1858—Campaign in Rohilcund: actions of Bugawalla and Nugena; relief of Moradobod; action on the Dojura; assault and capture of Bareilly; attack, bombardment, and relief of Shahjehanpore; capture of Fort Bunnai; pursuit of the enemy to the left bank of the Goomtee; destruction of the fort of Mahomdee; attack on and destruction of Shahabad; action of Bungkagong. Campaign in Oude—Actions of Pusagon and Rissoolpore; attack and capture of fort Mittowlie; and actions at Mehundee and Biswah (mentioned in dispatches; medal).

PHYSICAL DIAGNOSIS OF THORACIC ANEURISM*

To the Editor of the Lancet

Sir,—as the diagnosis of thoracic aneurism of the aorta is often difficult and obscure, notwithstanding the various physical means we have now at our disposal for detecting it, I am desirous of mentioning a method of examination which has afforded me material assistance in diagnosing this disease (or even simple dilatation of the vessel), when it occurs, as is most generally the case, either in the ascending or the first part of the transverse portion of the arch.

Lancet, 1878, II, p. 406.

The process is as follows:—Place the patient in the erect position, and direct him to close his mouth, and elevate his chin to the fullest extent, then grasp the cricoid cartilage between the finger and thumb, and use gentle upward pressure on it, when if dilatation or aneurism exist, the pulsation of the aorta will be distinctly felt transmitted through the trachea to the hand. The act of examination will increase laryngeal distress should this accompany the disease.

Yours, &c,

W. S. Oliver, M.D., Surgeon-Major.
Sept. 13th, 1878.

ENDOCARDITIS

According to Laënnec, the first description of endocarditis in medical literature is found in the medical works of Lazarus Riverius. His description of a patient who showed at autopsy, carbuncles like hazlenuts which projected into the aorta, most probably had vegetations on the aortic valves. Morgagni's patient with excrescences on the valves of the heart was unquestionably an example of vegetative endocarditis, probably of gonorrheal origin. The spleen of this patient also showed an old healed infarct. Bouillaud gave a clear description of vegetative endocarditis. Bouillaud was, as Herrick notes, "the first accurately to describe the endocardium (the name is his); the first to conceive of this membrane as the seat of an inflammation, which he called endocarditis, and the first clearly to describe the stages of this inflammation."

Virchow, in the first volume of his *Archiv*, described several cases of endocarditis associated with embolism. In his classic work on "Embolism and Thrombosis," published in his *Gesammelte Abhandlungen* in 1856, he emphasized anew the role of valvular vegetations in the production of emboli and pointed out that the vegetations on the heart valves were not solely deposits of fibrin from the blood but also new growths on the surfaces of the valves.

Kirkes published one of the earliest and clearest accounts of infectious endocarditis associated with embolism. His paper and the later paper of Wilks brought this disease to the attention of English speaking physicians. Winge's account leaves little doubt that he saw streptococci in the valves of a patient dying from endocarditis, the first demonstration of the bacterial origin of this disease.

Lazarus Riverius

CENTURY IV OBSERVATION XXI

Palpitation of the heart and unequal pulse*

Master de Becheran, Councillor in the Chamber of Assessors and Reserves and of the Royal Treasury, came to me in the early part of November in the year 1646 complaining of palpitation of the heart which had troubled him for several days. I found the pulse small, irregular with every variety of irregularity, so that I immediately called to mind that history of the physician Antipater in Galen, who was judged to have obstructions or a soft tubercle in the smaller arteries. At that time there was no difficulty in respiration, & the patient attended to his customary duties, daily going to the Chamber, he neither wished any remedy nor desired to take advantage of holidays. I prescribed immediately repeated venesections and then purgations, after which he was somewhat better.

After ten or twelve days he complained again of the same trouble, various attenuating remedies & cupping were prescribed, avoiding the application of heat which is not customary. Various measures were employed. Then at the beginning of the month of December he took to his bed, he began to suffer with difficulty in breathing & his legs appeared swollen. Then, for a time, he employed the aforesaid remedies with repeated Phlebotomy, which though continued for twelve days produced no results. The disease continually grew worse and a consultation with other physicians was called, the opinion of whom was that it was the same disease described by Galen (4. de loc. affect. cap 8. concerning the physician Antipater) & thus to be combated with cuppings and attenuating remedies. Various formulae of medicines were prescribed for this purpose, to enumerate which would be superfluous. These aided not at all and the patient grew steadily worse,

suffered from the greatest difficulty in breathing, & no pulse appeared at the Wrist, and when the hand was applied over the region of the heart, a most rapid, weak and irregular palpitation was felt. Presently the swelling of the legs increased so that now the thighs were involved. Remedies similar to the former ones were prescribed to which were added internal and external cardiac remedies. After two days the patient seemed in extremis, great suffocation seized him & there was no pulse in the arm and it could be perceived only with difficulty in the heart. The same day he was thought dying. I ordered a cupping glass applied to the region of the heart with scarification, the value of which in relieving dangerous palpitations of the heart is praised by Zacutus Lusitanus. He was slightly better, & the following night began to expel a black thick bloody sputum in balls with a troublesome cough, then he began to breathe easier. . . . Later the difficulty in respiration increased by day, the bloody sputum increased, the eighth day he died in the hours of evening.

On opening the body the ventricle of the heart was found to be filled with a bloody mass and the whole lung was filled with much blood from which the suffocation of the natural beat spread to each part. A few days before death the predisposing cause of this morbid state became apparent, which the patient never related; certainly the great terror, into which he was seized while travelling to Arles and was thrown in danger of shipwreck near Rhodes. After this terror, the retracted blood was forced in large amounts towards the heart so that it could not be controlled but curdled in the ventricles; and so the heart attempting to cast out the heavy load, put forth palpitating, tremulous and irregular movements. For the blood ascending continually by the vena cava not coming

* Riverius, Lazarus, *Opera omnia*, Venice, Viezzeri, 1723, p. 526.

freely to the heart overflowed in the lung and filled it up.

Moreover in the left ventricle of the heart round carbuncles were found like the substance of the lungs, the larger of which resembled a cluster of hazlenuts & filled up the opening of the aorta, which I judged caused the failure of pulsations in the arteries. Now these carbuncles I thought were caused by the excessive blood which the marked heat of the ventricle hardened & in this manner changed its substance. A similar and much greater carbuncle was found eight days ago in the right ventricle of the heart of a soldier who was dissected in the Anatomical Theatre after he had been killed by another soldier.

LETTER THE TWENTY-FOURTH
Treats of Preternatural Pulses*

* * *

A man about six-and-thirty years of age, of a large stature, and who was servant to a miller, fell into a disease which seemed to be a dropsy of the thorax. For which reason, his legs being swell'd, his pulse being very low, and a virulent gonorrhea, moreover, afflicting him, he died.

There was not only water in the thorax, but in the belly also, as they who had remov'd the viscera related; and besides this, that the larger intestines were in some places inflam'd, and had a very strong smell, for which reason they had not been sent together with the other viscera. And that these circumstances were true, was confirm'd by the disagreeable odour of those which had been brought, particularly by the viscera of the belly, and not a little, indeed, by the viscera of the thorax. Wherefore, passing over the lungs, which were extremely heavy, I very accurately enquir'd into the state of the heart and the vessels, into which I happen'd at that time to be desirous of making some particular enquiries. Some whitish polypous concretions, some of which kind were also in the vena portarum and the inferior cava, being taken away from the right auricle, and no concretion of this kind being found in the other cavities of the heart, and no disorder appearing in any part of the viscus, or its vessels, except in the valves of the great artery, and that being very considerable, upon looking upon and examining it very attentively, I found it thus: All these valves, on the upper part of their border, and on the neighbouring part of that surface with which they look upon each other, swell'd out

into short and unequal excrescences; by the load of which being weigh'd down, they were all brought so near together by this means, as to leave but a very narrow passage betwixt each other through which the blood might pass out. But when I examin'd each valve in particular, I saw that the right had its border much shorter than usual, or was become less transversely; and that the left was ruptur'd through the middle, from the border quite to the lower part; and that from the very lips of this rupture other excrescences were protuberant. The substance of all these valves was in part lax and flaccid, so that it might be very easily pull'd away by the fingers and by the nails; and yet it was partly harder than usual, also; so that when you rubb'd it betwixt your fingers, you would perceive some particles to be mix'd with it, which approach'd, in some measure, to the nature of a cartilage. These excrescences being taken away, the substance of the valves remain'd, but was contracted and deficient, and confirm'd what had appear'd at first sight; I mean, that this disorder had taken its rise from a kind of erosion, especially as the internal surface of the ventricles, where it border'd upon the valves, shew'd itself also some marks of erosion. Having seen these things, and other preternatural appearances being look'd for in vain in the aorta and the other vessels, and in the whole heart itself; and the borders of the mitral valves being only somewhat thicker here and there than they generally are, and being at the same time observ'd to be harder than usual; I went on to examine into the remaining parts.

Some of the viscera of the belly had only these few things which were worthy of remark. The liver was large, and yet not to an immoderate degree, of a palish complexion; and in its whole external surface there

---

* Morgagni, John Baptist, *The Seat and Causes of Diseases*, Translated by Benjamin Alexander, London, Millar and Cadell, 1769, Vol. I, Book II, Letter XXIV, Article 18, p. 730.

appear'd a kind of brownish network, and which some very small and white spots were mix'd. The spleen, being internally soft, had on the external surface some thick adipose ramifications, as it were, if our eyes were to be believ'd; but the substance of them was of a tendinous firmness, and even of a middle nature betwixt a cartilage and a ligament. The glands in the centre of the mesentery, and at the trunk of the vena portarum, were enlarg'd.

J. Bouillaud

CHAPTER III

Concerning Endocarditis (Inflammation of the Inner Membrane and of the Valves of the Heart) and of their Results*

1. The disease, the history of which we propose to sketch here, is one of the most common: it is at least as frequent as pericarditis or pleurisy, but before our work it was so little known that it had not even received a particular name. The name *endocarditis*, which I have given to inflammation of the inner membrane of the heart in general, appears to me, according to all reports, to conform to the principles of nomenclature universally adopted today. I will propose that of *cardiovalvulitis* to designate especially inflammation of the valves of the heart, which are, as everyone knows, essentially formed of a fibrous tissue upon which is folded back the *endocardium* or internal membrane of the heart. One can thus give to this local disease the name *valvular endocarditis*.

In 1824 and in 1826, I possessed already a sufficiently large number of facts to get a glimpse of the importance of inflammation of the internal membrane of the heart and of the large vessels. But they did not relate to the most important type of endocarditis, to the *rheumatic* endocarditis, which we had the honor of discovering later, and which occupies today such a large place in the classification of diseases. Also, these early facts, moreover incomplete, did not allow me to treat with all the proper detail this rich and fruitful material.

However that may be, the first ideas which I suggested were considered by many physicians of great authority as purely systematic. But the objections of these physicians convinced us not at all of our supposed systematic error, but that most of these objections were false. . . .

Since our first investigations we have lost no opportunity to collect new facts on the subject which we are considering. In 1828 and 1829, we examined the internal membrane of the heart and of the vessels in more than a hundred patients who died on the different services of medicine and surgery in the Charity Hospital, and we have preserved accurate notes of these examinations. This work allows us to determine with more precision in which cases the redness of this membrane could be attributed to an inflammatory state, and in which of those, on the contrary, the redness was the simple result of cadaveric imbibition.

Finally, during the past eight years while we have been in charge of clinical instruction, we have collected on the inflammation of the vascular system in general, and especially on acute endocarditis, numerous observations by means of which we hope to be able to fill one of the large gaps which still remain in pathology. We recommend this chapter of our work to the impartial attention of our readers, and we beg of them to be well assured that in all we say of inflammation of the endocardium, we have not been guided by any preconceived theory, but, on the contrary, the theory followed only in the train of numerous facts, I repeat, and so patiently observed that we cannot but accord them the term exact.

* * *

More fortunate or at least richer in material, than at the time of the first edition of this Treatise, I can place in the first category, many new observations of endocarditis with anatomical lesions quite as clear-cut as those of pericarditis, the observations on which have been placed by us in the same category. We will begin with these.

---

* J. Bouillaud, *Traité Clinique des Maladies du Coeur*, II Edition, Paris, J-B. Ballière, 1841, Vol. II, p. 1.

But before reporting these new observations, some of which have been already inserted in my *Traité clinique du rhumatisme articulaire*, permit me to recall here the one which I have already related in the first volume of the present Treatise, under number 14. In this case collected by me, during the year 1832, *the mitral valve, thinned out and adherent to the internal surface of the heart,* *warts, composed of a fibrous, friable material, crumbling easily under the blade was sprinkled and covered with numerous, confluent vegetations similar to venereal of the scalpel, etc.—A bellows murmur of the heart had accompanied the valvular lesion.* Before 1832, no observation of endocarditis, so complete, had yet been published.

Rudolf Virchow

CONCERNING THE ACUTE INFLAMMATION OF ARTERIES*

* * *

Case VII. Thickening and narrowing of the mitral valve, fibrous softening coagulum on the valve. Emboli in the cerebral carotid artery, the left femoral artery and the left iliac. Hemorrhagic infarctions of the spleen.

Franz Kruse, merchant, 27 years old, was admitted on October 29, 1845, to the University Clinic in the Charite (Geh. Rath. Schönlein). After he had been feverish for five weeks, a condition diagnosed by his physician as rheumatic, he was suddenly seized, on the day before his admission, with incoherence of speech. On admission he was quite unable to give any information concerning himself; very confused, hot, the pupils markedly contracted, entirely immovable; body collapsed, soft, somewhat painful; bowels moved the day before. Retention of urine, on catherization a clear urine. Pulse 100.

Oct. 31. Slept well. In the morning head clearer, pupils unchanged. Tongue dry, body collapsed, quite without pain. Urine scanty. Pulse 80, evening 84.

(Here follows a daily account of the patient's condition. Only a few entries are reproduced here.)

Nov. 1. Head clearer, convergent strabismus. Skin moderately hot, urine dark, tip of tongue dry, a mushy stool. Pulse 100. Evening very confused, pupils contracted, pulse 102.

Nov. 3. Slept well, some perspiring. Dizziness, confusion. Tongue moist with a red, dry triangle; body drawn together and tense, not painful, borborygmi. Skin moderately hot and dry. Pulse 104. Evening, skin burn-

Arch. f. path. Anat. u. Physiol. und f. klin. Med., Berlin, 1847, I, 272.

ing hot but soft; pulse 116. Slight cough, respiratory sounds normal. *One hears a bellows murmur with the first heart tone,* which the second tone closely follows.

Nov. 10. Since yesterday evening severe pains on the inner side of the left foot, so that he cannot stand on it; on pressure great sensitiveness. Sleeps fairly well, night sweats. Towards morning pain in the right temple. Body distended, two thin sediment-like stools. Pulse 100, tense, full. Evening, headache moderate, dizziness, buzzing in his ears and sparks before his eyes. Pains in foot on the plantar surface and inner side continue. Poor appetite. Great thirst. Pulse 120.

Nov. 18. On the left leg, especially on the outer surface, a kind of exanthema appears, which began with *dark red, bluish spots around the roots of the hairs,* soon appeared more like an eczema, great hyperesthesia of the skin.

Nov. 19. The spots grow larger like extravasations. Towards evening great uneasiness, hasty aund uncontrolled movements. Pulse 132.

Nov. 30. Urine scanty, sediment present. Very loud bellones murmur. *Gangrenous separation of the skin of the left leg; toes cold and bloodless.* Pulse 132. In the evening at six, he became suddenly stuporous, could not be aroused, even by pressure on the painful leg. However he swallowed a drink when offered, respiration was even although somewhat rapid; the body, especially the head, was covered with warm watery sweat. The urine showed uric acid sediment. The pulse increased to 156, the respiration rattling, the pupils fixed and immovable, gradually foam appeared on his mouth, his sweat became colder. Thus he continued until December 2 when he died at 5 A.M. without a clear moment.

Autopsy after 31 hours: skull normal, on the left atrophied by a large Pacchionian granulation. Sinus with a fresh, firm coagulum. Membranes normal. On cutting the right cerebral carotid, there was pulled out a long, rather firm reddish white, spotted thrombus, ¾" long, which was fairly firmly adherent to the under wall. The carotid in the Sulcus sphenoid was quite free, also the arteries of the Sylvian fossa and the corpus callosum, however the part from the opening of the ophthalmic artery to the point of division showed thickened cloudy opaque walls, without, however, narrowing. The remaining vessels were free. The brain substance which was supplied by the branch arteries, the operculum, insula Reilii, etc. softened, easily depressed with the finger, somewhat whiter than the rest of the brain substance; the softened area about the size of a large apple. The rest of the brain, ventricles, etc. normal.

Pericardial sac normal. The heart somewhat enlarged, the wall of the left ventricle very thick. Small amount of dark blood, not very fibrinous. The mitral somewhat narrowed, much thickened especially the posterior flap, and on this a ragged, fringed, hanging, fibrous coagulum, 4" long, which was partly firmly attached to the swollen margin of the valve, and in some places degenerated into a reddish, pus-like pulp. The other valves were not essentially changed, only the aortic valves somewhat thickened.

* * *

The spleen was so firmly attached to the diaphragm and colon that it could not be separated without tearing; in the lower part there was a large, hard, dry, not friable yellowish white infarct (fibrous tissue wedge) the size of a goose egg; in the upper part there was a coarse meshed loose tissue, partly filled with serous fluid and edematous, partly with a decolorized, brownish red pulpy mass. The remainder of the spleen was not enlarged, soft, coarsely granular and dirty reddish brown.

The veins of the body were normal, only on the legs somewhat varicose. The arteries of the left leg, namely the posterior tibial and peroneal, unchanged but at the point of division of the popliteal, there was a coarse. elastic, colorless translucent almost cartilagenous embolus, firmly adherent to the vessel wall, besides which the circulation had been re-established and which showed an advanced state of thrombus metamorphosis. At the division of the femoral artery where the deep femoral originates, there was a thrombus more than 1½" long, which in the center was liquified into pus and which from beginning to end was sharply limited, and could be followed into an inner layer adherent to the vessel wall; in the middle there was a white, firm pus-like mass, the inner lining was necrotic, partly destroyed, so that the middle layer was visible. From here to the embolus in the popliteal the vessel was empty, shrunken, diminished in size: the wall the entire length of the femoral was not injected but thickened and so grown to the surrounding tissues that the artery was dissected only with the greatest difficulty. In the right common iliac at the point of division a similar embolus, also purulent, but still clearly marked by layers of coagulum and the cortical layer could be separated from the vessel. The walls of the vessel were not essentially altered.

William Senhouse Kirkes, M.D., F.R.C.P.

"We deeply regret to announce the premature demise of Dr. William Senhouse Kirkes, Physician to St. Bartholomew's Hospital and Lecturer on Medicine in the Medical School. Dr. Kirkes was one of the most amiable, upright, and respected of metropolitan physicians. He was educated at the hospital and distinguished himself in his physiological studies. His *Handbook of Physiology* was one of the clearest, ablest, and most accurate of books, had great popularity, and was deservedly held as an authority. Among the most important of his contributions to the science of medicine were his papers on

The Detachment of Fibrinous Deposits from the Interior of the Heart, and their Mixture with the Circulating Blood. Together with the eminent Virchow, the name of Kirkes stands firmly connected with the subject of Embolism, one of the most fruitful inquiries in modern pathology. Dr. Kirkes was one of the

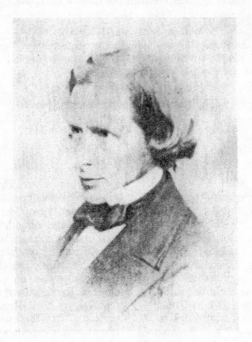

WILLIAM SENHOUSE KIRKES (1823-1864)
Courtesy of Dr. George Blumer

Commission whom we recently announced as nominated by the Admiralty and Horse Guards to inquire into the nature, treatment and prevention of veneral disease. He had attended the last meeting of the committee in the commencement of the week, and came home complaining of a feeling of cold and depression. He became rapidly worse; pleurisy developed itself; with this, we believe, pericarditis and haematuria. Dr. Kirkes had the benefit of the skill of his distinguished friend and colleague, Dr. Burrows; but he never rallied. He has been cut off this suddenly in the early prime of a career full of promise and of the first fruits of labour, and his loss under such a painfully sudden visitation will be felt keenly. Consequent on his death will probably be the promotion of Dr. Martin to the office of Physician, leaving a vacancy among the assistant physicians."*

* Obituary Notice in the *Lancet,* December 19, 1864.

* * *

On some of the
Principal Effects Resulting from the
DETACHMENT OF FIBRINOUS DEPOSITS
from
THE INTERIOR OF THE HEART
and Their Mixture with the Circulating Blood.†
by
William Senhouse Kirks, M.D.
Licentiate of the Royal College of Physicians, Registrar and Demonstrator of
Morbid Anatomy at St. Bartholomew's Hospital
Communicated by
George Burrows, M.D., F.R.S.
Physician to St. Bartholomew's Hospital

Received April 12th—Read May 25th, 1852

* * *

Case I.—Margaret Shaw, aet, 34, a pale, weakly-looking woman; admitted into St. Bartholomew's Hospital, under Dr. Roupell, about the middle of July, 1850, on account of pains in her lower limbs, and general debility. A loud systolic murmur was heard all over the cardiac region. No material change ensued in her condition until August 7th, when, while sitting up in bed eating her dinner, she suddenly fell back as if fainting, vomited a little, and when attended to was found speechless, though not unconscious, and partially hemiplegic on the left side. The hemiplegia increased, involving the left side of the face as well as the limbs, and gradually became complete in regard to motion, while sensation seemed to remain unimpaired. She continued speechless and hemiplegic, but without loss of consciousness for five days, when she quietly died.

On examining the body, six hours after death, the skull and dura mater were found natural; but the small vessels of the pia mater were much congested, the congestion amounting in some places, almost to ecchymoses. The right corpus stiatum was softened to an extreme degree, being reduced to a complete pulp of a dirty greyish-white tint, and without any remains of its characteristic striated structure. The corresponding optic thalamus was healthy; but a condition of pale softening, similar to that affecting the corpus striatum, existed also to a considerable extent in the posterior lobe of the right

cerebral hemisphere. The rest of the cerebral substance of this hemisphere was softer than natural, and appeared to contain less blood than ordinary. All other parts of the brain were healthy. The right middle cerebral artery just at its commencement was plugged up by a small nodule of firm, whitish, fibrinous-looking substance, which, although not adherent to the walls of the vessel, must have rendered its canal almost, if not quite, impervious. With the exception of a speck or two of yellow deposit in their coats, the rest of the vessels at the base of the brain were healthy and filled with dark blood.

The heart was enlarged; on its exterior were several broad white patches of old false membrane. The right cavities and left auricle contained recent separated coagula; the fibrine firm and whitish. The right valves were healthy; so also were the aortic, with the exception of slight increase of thickness. The mitral valve was much diseased, the auricular surface of its large cusp being beset with large warty excrescences of adherent blood-stained fibrine. There were a few scattered deposits in the coats of the aorta. The right common iliac artery, about an inch above the origin of its internal branch, was blocked up by a firm, pale, laminated coagulum, which extended into the internal iliac, and for about a quarter of an inch down the external iliac, where it terminated rather abruptly. The lower portion of the coagulum was colourless, and softer and more crumbling that the upper, which was also more blood-stained and laminated. There was no adhe-

† Med.-Chir. Tr., London, 1852, xxxv, 281.

sion of the coagulum to the walls of the vessels. No similar clot existed in the iliac vessels on the opposite side. The pleurae were adherent in places; the lungs oedematous, and in places solidified by compact greyish-white masses, such as might result from uncured pneumonia. The pulmonary vessels were free from old coagula.

The liver and intestinal canal were healthy. The spleen was large, pale, and soft. One large portion, about a fourth of the organ, was converted into a mass of firm, yellowish white, cheesy substance. The kidneys were pale, rough, and granular. Within the cortex of the right were several large masses of yellow deposit, surrounded by patches of redness. The portions of medullary structure passing to these deposits were compact, dryish, and yellow.

* * *

Case II.--Louisa Richards, aged 24 a thin, pale young woman, was admitted into St. Bartholomew's Hospital, under Dr. Burrows, in November, 1851, on account of hemiplegia on the right side, which had ensued suddenly, while at dinner, five days previously. The loss of motion was complete, that of sensation partial. Her intelligence was tolerably clear, though her articulation and memory of words were impaired. She appeared to have been in tolerable health at the time of the seizure, but had latterly been exposed to great privations. On auscultation a loud systolic murmur was heard at the apex of the heart; the sounds clear at the base. At first the symptoms amended; but in a fortnight headache, vertigo, and increased difficulty of speech returned, and there was no steady improvement afterwards, but increasing emaciation, debility, and unconsciousness until her death, in a state of coma, three months after admission. A few petechial spots appeared on the body a few days before death, together with swelling of the right hand and foot. Throughout its progress, the case was regarded by Dr. Burrows as one of gradually-advancing softening of the left side of the brain; and the evident co-existence of extreme mitral disease invested the autopsy with unusual interest.

Examined 32 hours after death, the body was found extremely emaciated. Numerous minute petechial spots existed on the neck, chest, and extremities, and several dusky-red blotches on the ankles. The skull was thin,

light, and deficient in blood. The tissue of the pia mater, over almost every part of the brain, was spotted and mottled by dark-red and pinkish blotches of extreme congestion, amounting in places almost to ecchymoses. In the midst of a few of these engorged patches were streaks of yellowish material, as if the neighbouring tissue was infiltrated with pus; but on microscopic examination, the yellowish material was found to consist of multitudes of minute glistening granules like particles of fat: nothing like pus-corpuscles could be found, and it is probable, therefore, that the yellow material was composed merely of degenerated blood or fibrine. The surfaces of the arachnoid were smeared over by a layer of soft pinkish material, like thin mucilage. There was considerable excess of watery fluid in the cavity of the arachnoid and in the tissue of the pia mater. The general substance of the brain was soft and watery, and of about ordinary vascularity. The left corpus striatum, and the portion of cerebral hemisphere immediately around it, were reduced to a soft, shreddy, almost diffluent pulp, of a pale greyish or dull white colour. The left optic thalamus appeared of ordinary consistence, as did also the corpus striatum and optic thalamus on the opposite side. The septum lucidum was entire; the fluid in the lateral ventricles pale, rather turbid. No trace of either old or recent hemorrhagic cyst could be found. The left middle cerebral artery, immediately after its origin, was completely plugged up by a firm, whitish, oval mass, about the size and form of a grain of wheat: this mass was tightly impacted within the vessel, the canal of which it completely obliterated, while it loosely adhered to its interior. The branches immediately beyond the obstruction were reduced to firm, narrow, yellowish or rust-coloured cords. These obliterated vessels were imbedded in the pulpy, diffluent, cerebral substance immediately below and in front of the softened corpus striatum already described. A similar though smaller fibrinous plug existed in the right middle cerebral artery, but did not quite block up the canal of the vessel. There was no trace of atheromatous disease of the arteries of the brain, nor of any other part of the arterial system examined. There were no old coagula in any of the cerebral sinuses, which contained recent clotted and fluid blood.

The pericardium contained a few drachms

of clear fluid; there were several white patches of old lymph on the surface of the heart, and a few petechial spots. The heart was much enlarged, especially when contrasted with the general wasting of the rest of the body. The right cavities and valves were healthy; the left ventricle much hyper-trophied. The mitral valve was the seat of numerous large fungous or condylomatous growths, consisting of pale, tolerably firm masses of fibrine, heaped up in warty ex-crescences heaped up along the auricular bor-der of the valve, and extending for some distance along the posterior part of the in-terior of the auricle. The individual masses of fibrine were of various shapes and lengths, some nearly half an inch long; they were pretty firmly attached to the thick and roughened surface of the valve, yet portions could be readily detached, and, when sub-mitted to pressure, crumbled down beneath the finger. Several of the masses extended among the tendinous cords, which were thick-ened and united together in bundles; one of the thickened cords was distinctly ulcerated across, while portions of fibrine adhered rather firmly to each of the separated ends.

* * *

Case III.—William Purdy, aet. 24, a gas-fitter, of intemperate habits, was admitted into St. Bartholomew's Hospital, under Dr. Roupell, January 22nd, 1852, in a state of extreme emaciation and debility, with sloughs on his back, and hemiplegia of the left side. Both feet and legs were much swol-len, while the femoral vein in each groin was found hard, cord-like, and painful on pres-sure. Several dusky blotches, composed of distended capillaries, were also observed on the right thigh. On ausculation a prolonged, harsh, systolic murmur was heard at the apex of the heart, fading towards the base, where the second sound was clear. It was learnt that three months previously, after exposure to cold, he was attacked with diarrhoea, to which he was subject, and severe pain across the back. He continued ill and under treat-ment for about two months, suffering with diarrhoea and obscure pains in his joints, which his medical attendant considered to be rheumatic. At the end of this time he was suddenly attacked with severe pain in the re-gion of the heart, accompanied by palpitation, both of which symptoms were relieved by the application of leeches and blisters, and

in a week had almost disappeared; but he still continued too ill to leave his bed. One night, about a fortnight after the commence-ment of the cardiac symptoms, he suddenly got out of bed, quite contrary to his usual custom, and left the room, apparently for the purpose of relieving his bowels. His wife immediately followed, and found him in a confused, bewildered state, with his left hand and arm paralysed, his face drawn to one side, and his speech impaired. Shortly after being placed in bed the left leg became pow-erless like the arm, and both continued so un-til his admission to the hospital a fortnight afterwards, at which time the loss of motion was complete, though sensation was not much impaired. He had complained of headache a few days before the seizure, but at the time of the attack did not lose his consciousness, and he had no fit either previous or subse-quent to the paralysis.

The swelling of the ankles had existed about three days previous to admission, hav-ing been preceded by pain in each thigh.

For a few days after admission he seemed to rally under the influence of tonics, nutri-tious diet, and wine, while the pain in the thighs was relieved by the application of leeches over the femoral veins. The amend-ment, however, was but temporary, and he died in ten days after admission.

An examination of the body was made twenty-eight hours after death. The emacia-tion was considerable. The lower limbs re-mained oedematous, especially the left, the foot of which was of a dark, livid colour. The tissues generally were very pale, especially about the scalp. The skull was pale and light. The membranes of the brain were healthy, but pale, while there was a considerable ex-cess of clear fluid in the cavity of the arach-noid and the tissue of the pia mater. The vessels of the pia mater were unusually de-ficient in blood, almost empty. The sub-stance of the brain was remarkably pale, soft, and watery in every part; there was no trace of a clot, or any manifest product of inflammation. Impacted within the right mid-dle cerebral artery, just at its origin, was a firm plug of pale fibrinous substance, about the size of a hemp-seed, completely blocking up the canal of the vessel, while the branches immediately beyond the obstruction were narrow, but filled with dark stagnant-looking blood, which had quite a different character to that in the other cerebral vessels. There was no trace of any disease in the coats of the cerebral arteries, and no obstruction in the left middle cerebral. Within the left lateral sinus was a large mass of old dryish colourless fibrine, somewhat adherent to the lining membrane, which was spotted red. A piece of similar fibrine existed also in the left internal jugular, but not connected with the mass in the lateral sinus. The other cerebral sinuses and right internal jugular were free from old coagula. The pericardium was healthy within, but externally it adhered to the left pleura. The heart was about natural size, but much diseased in its interior, the tricuspid, mitral, and aortic valves being encrusted over with large, firm, warty vegetations. On the tricuspid valve these growths were attached along the auricular surface, just above its free border. They varied considerably in size and number at different parts of the valve; many of the masses consisted of small compact roundish or oval bodies about the size of hemp-seeds, or bigger, attached singly or in clusters to the edge of the valve and to the tendinous cords to which they more or less tightly adhered. In structure they were firm and solid throughout, of a yellowish-white colour, and evidently composed of a dense fibrinous substance. The free border of the mitral valve was thickly studded with a continuous ridge of rough cauliflower-like masses of firm white fibrine, which formed warty excrescences of various sizes and shapes. One mass was nearly as big as a hazel nut, firm, elastic, and solid throughout, and of a mottled yellow and red colour on section.

The aortic valves were studded by a similar crop of smaller warty vegetations. Lying loose in the cavity of the ventricle were several small brownish nodules of old blood-stained fibrine. The muscular tissue of the heart was generally healthy; but just beneath the lining membrane of the left ventricle, and occasionally deep within its substance, were numerous pale yellow or bluff-coloured blotches and streaks surrounded by red borders, and having the general appearance of the changes described under the term of capillary phlebitis. The coronary arteries were healthy; so also was the general arterial system, though the aorta and its main branches were very narrow. The principal venous trunks contained recent coagula, but the two external and internal iliac veins, and both femoral veins, were blocked up by old variously-discoloured masses of firm, friable fibrine. These old coagula were very large, and produced great distension of the veins in which they occurred. There appeared to be no disease of the coats of the veins, and the coagula were nowhere adherent to them; and the arteries leading to the lower extremities were free from old coagula.

Sir Samuel Wilks

Sir Samuel Wilks, whose long life was a link between the days of Addison, Bright, Hodgkin and the present, was born at Camberwell in 1824. He received his preliminary education at the Sedenham Grammar School and then entered London University. In 1841 he entered Guy's Hospital as a medical student. He received his M.B. from London University in 1848 and his M.D. degree in 1850. Wilks was elected a fellow of the Royal Society in 1870 and was created a baronet in 1897. He died in 1911 at the advanced age of eighty-eight.

Wilks' reputation was established by his book *Pathological Anatomy*, which first appeared in 1859. This work laid the foundation of scientific pathology in England and had a profound influence on medical thought among English speaking students. Sir William Osler wrote in later years that in 1871, "It was my habit to pester Dr. Palmer Howard for information and literature, and one day he handed to me Wilks' *Lectures on Morbid Anatomy,* and from that time everything was plain sailing, as all the ordinary appearances met with were fully described."

Wilks was connected with Guy's Hospital for nearly sixty years. He often said that Guy's was his life and no one was ever devoted to it or added more to its reputation. Wilks became full physician to Guy's Hospital in 1867, succeeding Sir William Gull and, until his retirement from this position in 1885, was one of the most brilliant and the most popular teacher in London. His love and veneration of Guy's Hospital breathes forth from every page of his

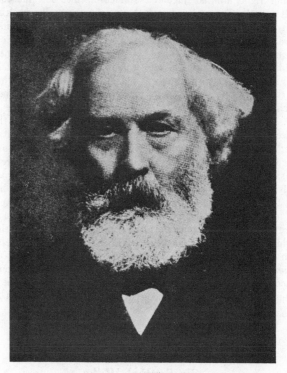

SIR SAMUEL WILKS (1824-1911)
Courtesy of Surgeon General's Library, Washington

charming *History of Guy's Hospital,* published in collaboration with G. T. Bettany, in 1892. This work emphasizes the great discoveries of Bright, Addison, and Hodgkin and, with his other writings, is largely responsible for the fact that the diseases called after these men have taken their place as clinical entities.

Wilks was idolized by his colleagues and students. He was a man of charming personality, of great frankness, integrity and honesty. Osler wrote, "he had a remarkably attractive personality, which age so adorned, that at three score and ten there was no handsomer man in London." Innumerable artists and sculptors, fascinated by his appearance, tried to reproduce his features, but with indifferent success.

Sir Samuel Wilks published a great many papers on medical and pathological subjects, one of which contains an early account of subacute bacterial endocarditis.

* * *

ABSTRACT OF A CLINICAL LECTURE
on
PYAEMIA AS A RESULT OF ENDOCARDITIS*

By SAMUEL WILKS, M.D.
Physician to Guy's Hospital.

The following is an abstract of a very full report of the case taken by Mr. J. R. Stocker.

Alfred F., aged 25, was admitted on Jan. 1st, 1868, for heart-disease. He stated that he had rheumatic fever in 1851; and that the doctor then informed him that his heart was affected, but he had no symptoms referable to it until four months ago. He then became very ill, with shortness of breath, palpitation, etc., followed by some swelling and pains of the joints. On admission, he was seen to be very ill, having sallow countenance, and suffering great distress from shortness of breath and palpitation. The heart was most irregular and rapid in its action, with a loud systolic murmur, heard loudest over the apex. The urine had a good specific gravity, and was slightly albuminous. The legs were somewhat oedematous. He was ordered a saline mixture, with a pill of digitalis, squills and mercury.

In four days he was much better; the breathing being less oppressed, and heart's action checked. He was then ordered to take ferrum tartaratum.

On January 14th, he suddenly felt giddy, and afterwards had intense headache.

On the 24th, there was an aggravation of the original symptoms, and great irregularity of the heart's action, with dyspnoea.

On the 31st, he found his right arm and leg very weak and numb. After four days, this weakness had increased; and at the same time there was some hesitation in his speech and forgetfulness of words. He had also pain and swelling of the joints.

On February 14th, he lay in a most precarious state. There was great irregularity of the heart's action. He had complete right hemiplegia, with partial aphasia; that is, a forgetfulness of many words. Thus, being told the name of a key, he would use the word "key" for every object presented to him;

and being shewn his grapes, and various names for them suggested to him, and amongst them the correct appellation, he would not assent to any of them. He could read certain words on his bed-card, but not others. He thus continued in a barely living condition until March 1st, when he died.

POST MORTEM EXAMINATION.—The left middle cerebral artery was plugged, and a large part of the left hemisphere disorganised by an abscess; the pus being green and thick. The lungs were in a state of splenisation. The heart showed the mitral valve much diseased, the columns and cords covered with vegetation and shreds of fibrine. The liver contained throughout minute points of pus. The spleen had several fibrinous masses which were softening, and some were purulent—indeed, were distinct abscesses. The kidneys contained fibrinous masses not softening.

I bring this case before your notice, because it is the most marked which I have ever seen of the pyaemic process in connection with endocarditis. This disease is one of great interest pathologically, but has scarcely received a full recognition at the bedside of the patient. Although isolated cases of the disease may be found scattered through the journals, it has never been systematically treated of in the textbooks of medicine. You know that, by the term pyaemia, we generally understand that form of disease in which the blood is infected by some purulent or kindred fluids; and that certain marked symptoms result, with a tendency to abscess in various parts of the body. The source of infection is to be found on the surface of the body, and the deleterious matter is taken up into the veins. But now I have to tell you (in a clinical lecture, as I have been doing for many years past in the pathological lectures), that the arterial blood may be in a like manner primarily infected at the very centre of the circulation. Just as, in ordinary pyaemia, the poisoned blood travels from

* Brit. M. J., 1868, I, 297.

the circumference to the centre so here the converse process is in operation, the seat of the infection being the heart itself.

I should tell you that it has long been known that fibrinous masses have been found in the kidneys and spleen of those who have died of cardiac disease, and various theories have been mooted in explanation of their origin; the term capillary phlebitis having been much used of late years, after Rokitansky. We are indebted, however, more especially to the late much to be lamented Dr. Kirkes for unravelling this subect in a most masterly manner. If you refer to his paper, you will find that he had discovered the fact that, if particles of fibrine or vegetations were washed off the valves of the heart, they would be carried into the blood and plug up the vessels; they thus might lead to the destruction of any part, as of the brain or a limb, by the occlusion of the artery proceeding thereto. A case of this kind is now known by the term embolism. It was also stated by Dr. Kirkes, that the fibrinous masses just spoken of as occurring in the kidneys and spleen were also owing to small particles of fibrine blocking up the smaller arterial twigs; and he also showed that, with these formations the blood was necessarily deleteriously affected, and that the patient suffered from symptoms of pyaemia. Now, it has so happened that the first named facts contained in the doctrine inculcated by Dr. Kirkes have received the attention of the profession; but the latter have been too much disregarded, although equally important. The case of plugging of a large vessel and its effects are so manifest, that the case of blood-poisoning by smaller particles of disintegrating fibrine have been overlooked except by a few pathologists, who have now and then published isolated cases of the affection. Thus cases by myself and others may be found in the *Transactions of the Pathological Society* and in the *Guy's Hospital Reports*. I might say that Dr. Kirkes and myself had, some years ago, some interesting correspondence on the subject.

In an ordinary case of pyaemia, death is most frequently due to a poisoned state of the blood, without any sufficient disease of a vital organ to account for the event; but we have no difficulty in pronouncing upon the character of the disease, from the peculiarity of the symptoms and the existence of a wound on the surface of the body. In the case, how-

ever, of pyaemia of the arterial system, arising from infection at the centre of the circulation, no such manifest cause may exist; and, after death, when the fibrinous masses or infarctions are found in the viscera, they are believed to be inert, and the valvular disease is considered sufficient to account for all the symptoms and the ultimate issue of the case. Sometimes, however, the cardiac distress is but slight, whilst the symptoms of blood-infection are most marked, and then we begin to gain an insight into the importance of this variety of embolism. Thus, in a case which I published in the *Transaction of the Pathological Society* four or five years ago, the man had gangrene of the leg from the impaction of a plug of fibrine in his femoral artery; but, previous to this, he had several attacks of severe illness, accompanied by pains and swelling of the joints called rheumatic, but which were in reality of a pyaemic origin.

In the case of ordinary pyaemia, an abscess may form in the brain, lung, or other organ, and so lead to death; but far commoner is it for these organs to show a lesser disease indicative of the morbid process in operation, whilst death is due directly to the altered state of the blood. So, in embolism, there are the striking instances of the embedding of a plug in a vessel, leading to the destruction of the organ which it supplies; but there are also the other cases where the changes in the organ merely point to the blood-infection which is the real cause of the fatal issue. Why in one case the symptoms are more severe than in another, may be due to the state of softening or disintegration of the fibrin. In one case the deposits are hard; in another they may have softened into a creamy fluid. I had until lately held the opinion that the material into which fibrinous matter softened was not true pus, but only pus-like; for if examined by the microscope, no cells are seen; and that, if true pus were found either at the source of infection in the heart or in the viscera, endocardial ulceration must have taken place, and the tissues beneath must have been involved. In the present case, however, there was no proof of this deep-seated implication of the tissues; but yet the spleen and brain contained actual and well formed abscesses. I have never before seen so true an example of pyaemia from such a case.

I wish you principally to remember the

fact that the blood may be infected from disintegrating fibrine in the heart; and that all the symptoms of pyaemia may result, as violent rigors, followed by sweating, great prostration, sallow skin, pains and swelling of the joints, etc. (See the case of Dr. Ray, in the Journal for March 7th, 1868.) I do not know that suppuration is necessary to the production of rigors, although it generally implies the introduction of a deleterious substance into the blood. Some of the most striking instances of this were those related in the *London Hospital Reports*, in which transfusion of fluid into the veins was performed. I have very little doubt that many of the symptoms which we witness in heart-disease are really due to the state of the blood, although overlooked from the greater attention given to the condition of the mechanism of the heart. Thus, in this very case, the patient is said to have had rheumatic pains and swelling of the joints, but these were probably pyaemic; and, carrying my memory back to other cases where death occurred after rheumatic endocarditis, I believe now that death was due to blood-poisoning, although at the time we thought the derangement of the affected valve sufficient cause for the event. In other diseases, too, it may give us a clue to the occurrence of certain symptoms; as for instance, in scarlatina. Here there is the well-known rheumatic affection constantly occurring as a sequel to the disease, and at the same time endocarditis. Also, on post-mortem examination, as I have elsewhere shown, these fibrinous masses already mentioned may be found.

The purport of these remarks is that, in endocarditis or valvular disease of the heart attended by the presence of vegetations or fibrinous coagula, a blood poisoning may occur, giving rise to all the symptoms of pyaemia; and also that these may exist to a lesser degree in the form merely of pyrexia, prostration, pain in the joints. The facts are pathologically known but are not sufficiently recognized from a clinical point of view, owing to the attention being too exclusively confined to the mere deranged mechanism of the heart.

I would also say that these symptoms by no means imply a fatal result. They come and go; the proof of this being found eventually in the cicatrices and remnants of deposits met with in the organs of the bodies of those who have died with heart-disease.

MYCOSIS ENDOCARDII

Emanuel Fredrik Hagbarth Winge

E. F. H. Winge was born in Fredriksvaern, Norway, in 1827. In 1851 he was certified as a practicing physician and later became a ship's surgeon. He spent the years 1857 and 1858 in Berlin, Prague, Vienna and Paris. In Berlin he was a student of Virchow, Traube and Hoppe-Seyler and, on his return to Christiania, he became assistant in the medical clinic. In 1859, he was appointed prosector in the newly established pathological laboratory of the Reichshospital in Christiania. In 1866, he became professor of pathology and, in 1869, professor of internal medicine. In 1877, he received the title of M.D. from the University of Upsala. He died in 1894.

Winge made many important observations in the field of pathological anatomy and internal medicine. In 1869, he described a case of endocarditis with thrombosis which showed microorganisms in the endocardial lesions and also in the thrombi. This was the first proof of the bacterial origin of ulcerative endocarditis.

MYCOSIS ENDOCARDII*

A. A., laborer, 42 years old, previously well, had a corn at the base of his right little toe which he tore off because it pained him; under it he found a small abscess. 5 days later he had a severe chill, which lasted two hours; this was repeated every day during the following three weeks, appeared at the same time; after the chill, cough, sweating, headache, and usually at the same time lassitude, dyspnea, later mild diarrhea, and the

sized ulcer at the base of the little toe, with a sound one could probe ½ to 1″ in several directions under the skin, small amount thin, blood-colored pus. Urine contained a trace of albumin. During his stay in the hospital, where he lay 5 days, his strength declined steadily, the fever continued unchanged (temperature 39° to 40°), no chills, some delirium, last day petechia over the greater part of the body. When the abscess

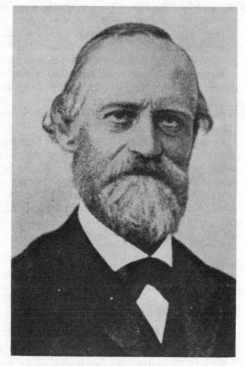

E. F. H. WINGE (1827-1894)
Courtesy of Dr. George Blumer

last days cough with clear sputum, pains in both knees and shoulders. On admission, 20 days after the first chill, he was weak, stuporous, had severe dyspnea, R. 40, P. 108, T. 39.59. No pain in chest, cough occasionally, sputum clear with some light blood streaks, 1st heart sound prolonged, nothing else abnormal found in the chest. Light effusion in the left knee, also local heat and redness on the inferior patellar ligament, also on the right local heat and redness without effusion. Slight edema on the dorsum of the right foot and about the ankle, a pea-

opened, the pain diminished, and the red spots on the legs disappeared.

At autopsy an abscess was found lying under the skin, whose walls were light gray in color, the blood was fluid in the veins on the back of the foot as well as over the entire extremity. In both knee joints the synovial membrane showed ecchymoses like flea-bites with a greyish yellow center. The synovial fluid was quite clear and slightly increased in amount. Nothing in the shoulder joints. The lungs edematous and congested, and a pair of fresh hemorrhagic infarcts and fresh pleurisy on the left side; in the arterial branches, which led to the infarcts there were half softened thrombi. The heart on

* Hygiea. Medicinsk och farmaceutisk manadsskrift, 1870, XXXII, 172. Translated by Dr. Hjalmar E. Carlson.

the whole somewhat enlarged, liquid blood in the venous trunks and in the right heart, soft clots in the left. On the aortic valves there were present nodules varying from the size of a pea to a bean, 1 to 2" thick, gray, irregular and somewhat thickened, thrombotic masses, which can be easily scraped off. endocardium under same was uncovered did not show the substance clearly. On the border and underside of the tricuspid valves large, clear, flat masses, from which hung down one 5" long triangular piece between the anterior and medial valve leaf. On the endocardium superficial ulcerations were seen of varying size, covered with small greenish crusts. At insertion of valve near the trabecula on the anterior wall of the right ventricle a small plaque of the same material. In the heart muscle under the endocardium especially on the conus arteriosis there was a mass of round or oval gray-white spots not quite as large as the head of a pin, some of which are surrounded by red halo. In the left kidney two wedge-shaped gray infarcts with a red halo and in the corresponding artery a softened thrombus mass. Spleen and liver swollen, in the spleen a pair of hemorrhagic wedges.

After what has been discribed up to this time, the observation cannot be criticized that the endocarditis was most developed on the right side. That ulcerative endocarditis can be found with pyemia is a known fact, if it occurs with an infection such as the present infection cne could regard it as a secondary phenomenon and put it in the class of metastatic processes, or as the origin of the infection. In three cases of ulcerative endocarditis, which I previously have had occasion to see (two of which are referred to in the autopsy protocoll in Magazinet Volume XIX, page 344, the third was admitted to the medical devision a little over a year ago), this endocarditis was primary, in these cases no other infectious process was found, all died with the picture of typhoid and at autopsy fresh endocarditis was found with a large number of miliary abscesses and hemorrhages in the serous membranes, skin, wall of the heart, kidneys, etc. In the present case it is possible to show an infectious process, the illness progressing with the picture of a pyemic fever with striking intermittent chills. The endocarditis could, with some reason, also be considered as a pyemic secondary process, and certainly can be considered the point of origin for later pathological processes (in the lungs from the right heart, in the kidneys, heart muscle, synovial membranes and skin from the left heart). The further study of the lesions on the heart valves gave an unexpected result, which will not give any positive explanation of the development of the endocarditis from the infection present, however the occurrence merits our attention. It was demonstrated that the thrombi produced by the lesions of the endocarditis for the most part were not composed of fibrin of the components of the blood, but of a parasitic vegetation. They appeared under the microscope, at first glance as a mesh of fine threads of fibrin with a finely granular mass of detritus, but on close inspection the threads were found to be fine cross striations, and on greater magnification (oil immersion) they were seen to be composed of short, rod-shaped or round bodies, they were partly branched, also the grains of the short rods had the appearance of small bacteria, while the threads appeared like the mycelium of leptothrix. The same structure was found in the emboli in the arteries of the kidney as well as in the small foci in the heart, with the exception of blood and detritus there were the same threads and grains, with the exception that these could be shown to lie in the great vessels. On further study of the abscess of the little toe no such structures were found, the lungs were unfortunately not examined further. It should also be noted that none could be found in the small foci of the synovial membranes of skin.

It is claimed now that plant parasites play a large role in the etiology of infectious diseases, with what right the future will show. As far as I know, no one has definitely shown any parasite in pyemia especially with that form associated with endocarditis, and it is therefore certainly of interest that in the present case there appear to be a parasitic process. Threads and grains varying both in size (no measurements were made) and appearance from those elements previously found by Klebs in cholera. The fine grained appearance of the embolic plugs in the small arteries of the kidney, which I had previously found in ulcerative endocarditis, was found in the small foci in the heart muscle; but since I did not make preparations of the older cases, I cannot say positively that there were similar parasites in the other cases, it is something future observers may demonstrate. Rindfleisch states in his Pathological Histology, that the small metastatic abscesses, which he has encountered in the heart, may consist of vibrions, but never himself, refers to the complication in such cases of endocarditis.

In the present case there can be no basis for confusion, I must say for certain (in addition to the microscopic structure chemical reaction speaks for the correctness of my view, neither acid nor alkali dissolve the threads) that this is not a postmorten artifact.

APOPLEXY

Johann Jakob Wepfer

Johann Jakob Wepfer was born in 1620 at Schaffhausen, Switzerland, the son of Johann Jakob Wepfer, Councillor of the Canton. He studied at Basle and Strassburg, then spent two years in Italy and returned to Basle, where he took his doctor's degree in 1647. He was an ardent champion of Harvey's doctrine on the circulation of the blood, and his doctor's thesis of 1647, *de palpitatione cordis,* defends the Harveian conception. He settled at Schaffhausen, became the town physician, and acquired such a reputation that he became known as the "Hippocrates of Helvetia." Wepfer was physician to the Duke of Wurtemberg and was called to be physician to Louis XIV but declined. He was a most industrious worker and reader. He rarely retired before eleven and usually rose about four in the morning. Sunrise found him in his study, where he spent the first part of the day in prayer and in reading the Scriptures. He was never idle, even during his meals poring over some book or busy with his correspondence. He took very sparingly of both food and drink, taking wine only with his meals, and then highly diluted.

Wepfer's name is known to posterity not because he was the physician of kings and dukes, nor because he had a very extensive practice, but because he demonstrated the fact that apoplexy is due to cerebral hemorrhage. His *Historiae apoplecticorum* first appeared in 1658, his first case having been studied and autopsied in 1655. This book begins with a description of four cases, which are then discussed in great detail. Wepfer died in 1695. His son, Johann Conrad Wepfer, and grandson, Georg Michael Wepfer, were also physicians. Johann Jakob Wepfer's library and correspondence were purchased by the University of Leyden in 1774 for 400 gold florins.

The first selection is a description of the first case recorded in his *historiae.* The second selection is of particular interest since it is a description of the last illness and death of the celebrated Marcello Malpighi with a brief protocol of the autopsy findings. These observations were made by Baglivi but are included by Wepfer in his work. The English translation is taken from an English edition of Bagvili's *Practice of Physick* published in London in 1704.

HISTORIAE APOPLECTICORUM

I

Johann Jacobus Reiter Kenzinga-Brisgojus, age about 45 years, with a slender build, endowed with yellow and curly hair, naturally strong; of honest parents, indeed descended from the Consul; from boyhood he gave attention to letters, and would have been able to have lived splendidly, except that pitiable and devastating misfortune struck all Germany; and which overwhelmed the country in a general calamity, enduring these vicissi-

school master for several years; at length he came to the Most Reverend and Most Distinguished Lord D. Bernhard a Freiburg, the most deserving Head of that most celebrated Monastery; My Lord having the very highest renown, he was admitted into the

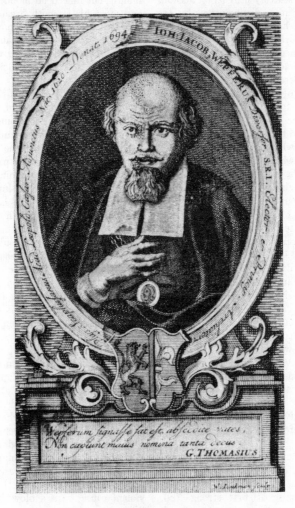

JOHANN JAKOB WEPFER (1620-1693)
From *Historiae apoplecticorum* (Amsterdam, Jassonio-Waesbergios, 1724)

tudes, the chief of which was the grim sway of famine experienced most gravely in the year 1634, which led him ill-advisedly, to stuff himself with food, which nature, at other times is accustomed to abhor. Then after many hazards and various mishaps he reached Rheinovium where he acted as a

Monastery, where he performed faithfully the post of chamber servant for many years.

Always moderate, he ate more during this new state of affairs, he indulged to be sure more in the cup, but however he did by no means worship Bacchus particularly. Little inclined to anger, yet not loving brawls, nor making quarrels from disputes. At different times, living in this Monastery, he was tormented by gout, which during the first years vented its rage in the joints of the feet, subsequently he suffered also further in the remaining joints; when he struggled with this disease, he could scarcely bear it, on account of which indeed, it is distinguished by the name of podagra, he bore nothing. From the actual year in which it appeared, until death he never felt its accustomed cruelty whether because of the practice of taking medicines secretely or if because of the weakness of nature, the virus of the disease was not able to extend further to the joints, as if to push further to ignoble places. Then about this time he was vexed by day by a most troublesome cough, for which reason they believed he had phthisis, which they attributed to a suppression of the gout. But however, the proper remedies being given by me, the cough ceased & in the course of about a whole year he duly regained his strength sufficiently, if we except an intestinal hernia, which the violent coughing caused.

In the year 1655, the seventh day of November, the fifth day after the full moon, in the morning sane and sound, he did much of everything—he assisted the Most Reverend Lord Abbot in the carrying out of sacraments, accomplishing which, he gathered up things in the dining-room, according to his custom; the Abbot by chance wished to decide with him the fate of the servants, found him prostrate upon the ground, insensible to shouts, to shaking & pinching of the body, the same in the trunk, senseless; there was hurry, anti-apoplectic water given and other things which were at hand, were tried but all in vain, & I was summoned:

I arrived in about half an hour, I saw him livid from pallor, deprived of all sensation & animate motion, with his nostrils cold to the touch. His pulse at first strong, full, quick, soon afterwards weaker, smaller & more frequent, his breathing also more laborious, soon it became irregular, and many times it appeared about to cease from within.

No kind of suitable remedies were omitted, however in his weak condition and about to soon expire, I did not dare cut his vein. At the tenth hour, before midday his body was shaken albeit by a movement and much sputum white, viscid, tenacious passed from his mouth, but indeed no blood: after this more and more his strength began to weaken and his extremities to become more cold: The first hour after midday of the same day he ceased to live. And immediately he was carried away by disease. He excreted much black sediment by his bowels, which was ascribed to the chabybeate (iron) wine, which, for some time, from the ignorant counsel of this Empiric and until his end he was accustomed to drink alone a ladle-full each morning and evening.

By the indulgence of the Most Reverend Lord Abbot for a long time past the renowned exalted patron of all learning and fine arts, I opened the head: the skull removed and the dura mater being cut into pieces much blood flowed from the space, which is very roomy between this and the thin meninges, copiously, that is, from all sides & everywhere it poured forth; Nor truly had the blood collected solely about the base of the brain, but covered it all over to the top both anteriorially and posteriorially, indeed it had forced itself into nearly all the windings of the brain, as many as there are. The ventricles laid open I found them all filled up with blood; but a portion of them excepted, the lateral ones for the floor was badly torn as it were, as if the fissures were stretched apart by too great a quantity of blood. I was able without difficulty to estimate the weight of the quantity of extravasated blood to have totalled two pounds. The whole brain, ventricles & surface were contaminated by blood in large amounts & crumbly; there was nothing further to observe, I was able to find no ruptured vein or artery. This however is certain, no external violent cause, be it a blow, be it a fall, was the cause of such ruptures of the blood-vessels; to settle this point, with his hair cut and skin washed off he showed not the slightest trace of any contusion whatever.

* * *

THE HISTORY OF THE SICKNESS OF MARCELLUS MALPIGHI, THE POPE'S PHYSICIAN; WITH AN ACCOUNT OF THE DISSECTION OF HIS CORPS*

Having been intimately acquainted with

Dr. *Malpighi* at *Bologna*, and waited upon him in his last Illness at *Rome*, I shall here oblige the learned World with a History of the

* Baglivi, George, *The Practice of Physick*, London, Bell, 1704, p. 461.

Disease, and an Account of the Dissection of the Corps of that excellent Anatomist.

Marcellus Malpighi was of a Constitution that tended to a Dryness, an indifferent Habit of Body, and a middling Stature: He had been subject for many Years to Vomiting, bilious Stools, Palpitations of the Heart, Stones in the Kidneys and Bladder, a pissing of Blood, and some light Touches of the Gout. Upon his coming to *Rome*, all these Disorders were inflam'd; especially the Palpitation of the Heart, the Stone in the Kidneys, and very sharp biting Night Sweats. Such was the Condition of *Malpighi*, July 25th, 1694; at which Time he was seiz'd, in the 66th Year of his Age, about 1 a Clock in the Afternoon, with an Apoplexy, usher'd in With Care, Passions of the Mind, *etc.* The Apoplexy was attended with a Palsie of the whole right Side, and a Distortion of the Mouth and right Eye. Presently we try'd several Remedies, particularly Bleeding in the left Arm: If it had not been for the contrary Sentiments of the Physicians that consulted with me, I would have order'd the Blood to be drawn from the paralytick Arm; upon the Consideration, That the defective Circulation of the Fluids of the Part affected, is not retriev'd by any speedier Method than that of opening a Vein in the same; as it appears plainly from the mechanical Principles of Resistance and Motion. We prescrib'd at the same time scarrify'd Cupping-Glasies, to be applied to the Shoulder-Blades; the Powder of *Cornachini, Sinapismus's* to be apply'd to the Soles of the Feet; and several other spirituous, cephalick, and specifick Remedies; by the Use of which, after struggling 40 Days with a long Train of grievous Symptoms, particularly a Light-Headedness, a *Capiplenium*, and other Accidents, he got clear of the Apoplexy, and Palsie, and the above-mention'd Symptoms. But as Evils use to spread and gain Ground, so this famous Man suffer'd much by the fore-going Disease in his Memory and Reason, and melted into Tears upon the slightest Occasion. He was troubled by Intervals with Inappetency, a Want of Digestion in the Ventricle, a subsultory Motion of the Muscles, and slight Fits of a Giddiness. In fine, being worn out with these and other Symptoms, he was seiz'd, *Nov.* 29, with a fresh fit of an Apoplexy, after the Injection of a customary Glyster in the Morning: This new fit was usher'd in by a grievous *Vertigo*, with a fit of the Stone in the Bladder for eight Days, and an Exasperation of the above-mention'd Symptoms. But the Apoplectick Fit was more dismal than all the other Symptoms, for in spite of all Remedies whatsoever, he dy'd four Hours after the Invasion.

THE DISSECTION OF THE CORPS

In Dissecting the Corps, I found the right part of the Lungs somewhat slaggy and livid, especially the hinder part that adheres to the back. The Heart was larger than ordinary, especially the Walls of the left Ventricle, which were as thick as the Breadth of two Fingers. The Gall in the Gall-Bladder was very black: The left Kidney was in a natural State, but the right was half as big again as the left, and the Bason of it was so much dilated, that one might easily thrust 2 Fingers into it. Perhaps this Dilatation of the Pelvis was the Occasion that as soon as the Stones were bred in the Kidneys, they presently slipt into the Bladder, and so sprung out from thence; which our excellent Friend had frequently own'd to me to be a Matter of Fact. In the Bladder we found a little Stone that had descended thither four Days before the Invasion of the last Apoplectick Fit, and by its Descent exasperated his last Vertigoes. The rest of the natural *Viscera* were very well condition'd.

When I open'd his Head, I found, in the Cavity of the right Ventricle of the Brain, an Extravasation of about 2 Pints of black clotted Blood, which was the Cause of his Apoplexy and his Death. In the left Ventricle we found about an Ounce and half of yellowish Water, with a small Quantity of little Grains of Sand mix'd with it. The Blood Vessels of the Brain were dilated and broke on all Hands. The whole Compass of the *dura Mater* adhered tenaciously and praeternaturally to the *Cranium.* And this is the Sum of what I observ'd in Dissecting his Corps, *Dec.* 7, 1694.

RAYNAUD'S DISEASE

Maurice Raynaud

Maurice Raynaud, the son of a distinguished university professor and a nephew of the well-known surgeon Vernois, was born in 1834. He studied medicine in Paris and received his doctor's degree in 1862. He later became professeur agrégé, was made officer of the Legion of Honor in 1871, and was elected to the Academy of Medicine in 1879. His inaugural thesis, *Sur l'asphyxie locale et la gangrène symétrique des extrémités,* which was published in 1862 described

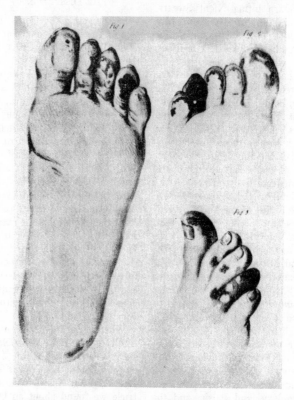

An illustration of gangrene of the extremities from Maurice Raynaud's *De l'asphyxie locale et de la gangrène symétrique des extrémités,* Paris, 1862

the striking local asphyxia and symmetrical gangrene since known as Raynaud's disease.

Raynaud was greatly interested in the history of medicine and his work, *Les Médicins au temps de Molière,* is an interesting and charming account of the practices and customs of the profession that was the target of so many bitter shafts from the great French dramatist, Molière. Raynaud's great ambition was to obtain the chair of medical history at Paris, but this was denied him because, as his friends maintained, of his devotion to the Catholic Church.

He suffered for several years from organic heart disease and in 1881, after dining in apparently good health and playing with his children, was suddenly seized with a heart attack and died three hours later. He was forty-seven years of age at the time of his death.

Raynaud was a man of great integrity, of spotless character, and recognized for unusual intellectual attainments. He was at the same time a physician, a savant, a philosopher, and a man of letters.

CHAPTER II*

OBSERVATIONS

Before giving the observations which form the basis of these memoirs, I ought to say a word about the circumstances which led me to collect them. It was at the beginning of 1860 that one of the cases reported later (Observation IV) attracted strongly my attention. It had to do with the spontaneous gangrene of the four extremities appearing unexpectedly in a young woman of 27 years. During more than one month I saw a series of strange and remarkable phenomena unroll themselves before my eyes—and disconcerted the great experience of many eminent physicians who saw this patient with me. In vain all the organs were minutely explored. In vain all the known or probable causes of gangrene were investigated. It was necessary to admit the presence of some influence up to that time unknown. I started in search of similar cases and once informed of their possibility, there was no delay in observing them. All appear to me to show as a common character, the absence of any appreciable material obstacle to the course of the blood, either arterial or venous. What I had seen, it was impossible that others before me had not seen. In looking up this point of view in the medical literature, I finished by finding a certain number of valuable documents. Thus, I have succeeded in collecting twenty-five observations, of which five are my personal ones.

I am far from attributing the same importance to all of these cases. Some of them are incomplete, some of them are doubtful, which seem to appear at the first glance in contradiction to the conclusion which I wish to draw.

There was a very simple means of avoiding this inconvenience; and that was to unite all the evident cases which presented no difficulty or contention (?) and to suppress all others. There would still remain enough of them to carry a sufficient conviction. But, on one hand it is important to show that a symptomatology more or less analogous to mine has already struck different observers, and on the other hand, I do not wish to be accused of having chosen according to my taste (?) and omitting that which would be unfavorable to my view. I do not tell the truth if I say that I have not certain doubts myself. Always there is a certain interest in collecting in a single bundle facts scattered throughout science. Let the interpretation follow: It can vary without doubt but the facts do not remain any less than what they were.

I have perhaps a prejudicial question to consider, that of the possibility of gangrene without obliteration. I have already had presented that which I think, I refer to the thesis of M. Zombaco which contains on this subject numerous strong proofs; furthermore, there is not, I believe, a single one of these cases which one is going to read that is not an argument in support of this opinion. It will have therefore, a double use.

The order in which I have arranged these observations is not a matter of indifference. I considered the local syncope and asphyxia as the first deliniation of a state which is very much graver, characterized by a coldness carried to the extreme by scaring and the loss of the greater part of the phalanges of the hands and feet. One arrives thus by gradations at the observation which has served to me as typical. It has always seemed to me that this degree in itself need not be the last:

* Maurice Raynaud, *De l'asphyxie locale et de la gangrène symétrique des extrémités,* Paris, Rignoux, 1862, p. 45.

Also I have placed following a certain number of cases in which one has seen, *without known cause,* several segments of the extremities detach themselves by gangrene. I could easily collect more; but as the greater part of them are of ancient date, I should have failed in the rules of healthy criticism if I accepted the recitals already a little circumstantial which are not sufficiently authentic. I have admitted only those which have appeared to me to present striking analogies with my particular cases. So these cases, of which many are known, have not been cited except on account of simple curiosity. They acquire because of their relationship with those which have preceded them, a value which they did not have until now. The cases the most simple, I will say, indeed, the most common, but to those the most surprising by their gravity, are nothing but differences of degree and intensity. It is important to find these intermediaries. First, *syncope and local asphyxia in the simple state.* The most simple degree, which is a condition which all the world is familiar with, although it is not to my knowledge described in any treatise on pathology, corresponds to that which in the ordinary language one designates under the name of *dead finger.* This affection, which constitutes scarcely a slight inconvenience and which often passes unperceived so that it does not require any treatment, is moreover very common. There is scarcely any physician who has not many times had occasion to observe it, and here is an example which has no other object than to summarize accurately what happened in the majority of these cases.

Observation I
The Most Simple Form of Local Syncope

Madame X, 26 years old, had never been ill; but she had shown since her infancy an infirmity which had made her an object of curiosity among those of her acquaintance. Under the influence of cold, indeed very moderate and moreover the strongest in summer, she saw the fingers become exsanguinated, completely insensible and of yellowish white color. This phenomenon appeared often without reason, lasted a very little time and terminated by a period of reaction which was very painful, during which the circulation became established little by little and returned to the normal state. Madame X had no better remedy than to shake her fingers

violently or to dip them in tepid water. The index finger of the left hand showed a greater susceptibility than all the other fingers and was often affected alone. The feet, more tender indeed than the hands, were regularly affected during the hour of dining and for the duration of digestion. Menstruation did not appear to have any influence upon the appearance of the phenomenon, but the thing very curious was, the complete disappearance was always observed by this lady as the first sign of beginning pregnancy.

If one would accept the distinction which I have established above, this state, which I dare scarcely to call a disease, is a local syncope in the most simple form. That which strikes one here is not the passive congestion but rather the momentary absence of local circulation, just as syncope is the suspension of the general circulation.

When this condition is repeated to the point of becoming almost continual, very profound troubles can appear in the nutrition of the arts which are subject to it. The chilblains take hold and the adipose tissue finishes by acquiring an excessive predominance as in all organs which function improperly. That took place in the following case.

Observation II
(Communicated by Dr. Marey)
Local Habitual Syncope with Lesions of Nutrition

Madame X, 25 years old, a young woman of small stature, and a blond; menstruation irregular for many years; after the age of 24 years the menstruation became regular. Slight hysteria, has had several attacks of nerves, with loss of consciousness, sensation of a bolus, tears, involuntary laughter. From 14 to 18 years she suffered a great deal from chilblains which kept her in bed during three months of the winter. She has been very subject for a long time to having *dead fingers.* These became in an instant the seat of coldness, pallor and absolute insensibility. Return of menstruation did not modify this condition. The fingers presented a very peculiar conformation. They were extremely large and soft; the hands themselves appeared edematous and they formed a very striking contrast with the slender wrists and forearms. The nails were not curved. The pulse is perceptible. The feet present the same appearance as the hands. They seem to be entirely skin and adipose tissue.

This young woman died recently of hydatid cyst of the liver.

BUERGER'S DISEASE

Leo Buerger

Leo Buerger was born in Vienna in 1879 and graduated from Columbia University College of Physicians and Surgeons, New York, in 1901. In 1917 he was professor of urologic surgery at the New York Polyclinic and later professor of urology at the College of Medical Evangelists in Los Angeles. Although his professional career was spent in the practice of urology and he devised a well known operating cystoscope, a cystourethoscope and other urologic instruments, he will be best remembered as the discoverer of thromboangiitis obliterans (Buerger's disease). He died October 6, 1943.

THROMBO-ANGIITIS OBLITERANS: A STUDY OF THE VASCULAR LESIONS LEADING TO PRESENILE SPONTANEUS GANGRENE*

By Leo Buerger, M.D., Assistant Adjunct Surgeon and Associate in Surgical Pathology, Mt. Sinai Hospital, New York

There is an interesting group of cases characterized by typical symptoms which the Germans have described under the name of "Spontangangrän." In 1879 von Winiwater published the results of the pathological findings in one case, and reported an obliteration of practically all of the arteries of the leg and by reason of a chronic proliferative process, due, in his opinion, to a new growth of tissue from the intima. He, therefore, proposed a new name for this condition, namely, "endarteritis obliterans." Patients afflicted with this so-called endarteritis obliterans present symptoms which are so characteristic that the diagnosis is not difficult. I have had occasion to observe some thirty cases of this disease, and have made pathological studies on the vessels obtained from eleven amputated limbs.

The disease occurs frequently, although not exclusively, among the Polish and Russian Jews, and it is in the dispensaries and hospitals of New York City that we find a good opportunity for studying it in its two phases, namely, in the period which precedes and that which follows the onset of the gangrene. We usually find it occurring in young adults between the ages of twenty and thirty-five or forty years, and it is because the gangrenous process may begin at an early age that the names presenile and juvenile gangrene have

been employed. In one class of cases there are rather characteristic attacks of ischemia. The patients complain of indefinite pains in the foot, in the calf of the leg, or in the toes, and particularly of a sense of numbness or coldness whenever the weather is unfavorable. Upon examination we see that one or both feet are markedly blanched, almost cadaveric in appearance, cold to the touch, and that neither the dorsalis pedis nor the posterior tibial artery pulsates. When the foot becomes warm some color gradually returns. Some patients complain of rheumatic pains in the leg, others are able to walk but a short distance before the advent of paroxysmal shooting, cramp-like pains in the calf of the leg makes it imperative for them to stop short in their walk. Some of these cases give the typical symptoms of intermittent claudication. After months—or, in some cases—even years have elapsed trophic disturbances make their appearance. It is at this stage that another rather unique symptom makes its appearance: one which gives the foot the appearance typical of erythromelalgia. In the pendent position a bright red blush of the toes in the anterior part of the foot comes on rather rapidly, extending in some cases to the ankle or slightly above. Soon a blister, hemorrhagic bleb, or ulcer develops near the tip of one of the toes, frequently under the nail, and when this condition ensues the local pain becomes intense. Such trophic disturbances

* Amer. J. M. Sc., 1908, cxxxvi, 319.

may at times make little progress and last for months, sometimes, however, the skin in the neighborhood shows cyanotic discoloration, and dry gangrene of the whole toe is an early issue. Even before the gangrene, at the ulcerative stage, amputation may become imperative because of the intensity of the pain. The left leg is usually the first to become affected, although both limbs may show vascular disturbances almost simultaneously, and

process, and before giving out views as to the possible etiology, it may be well to recall some of the more important facts that have been developed by the study of the pathological lesions. These may be summarized as follows: Most of the larger arteries and veins of the amputated limbs were found obliterated over a large extent of their course. The obliterative process can be studied at any stage in its development if enough vessels

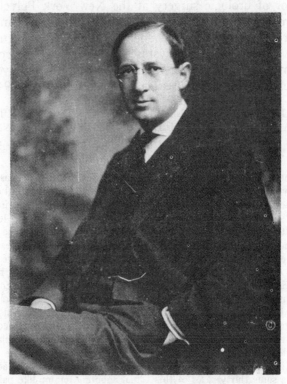

LEO BUERGER (1879-1943)
Photograph by Marceau, New York

when such is the case, the trophic changes, the ischemia or the reddening may give rise to a symptom-complex, often diagnosticated as Raynaud's disease. In short, after longer or shorter periods, characterized by pain, coldness of the feet, ischemia, intermittent claudication, and erythromelalgic symptoms, evidences of trophic disturbances appear which finally pass over into a condition of dry gangrene.

* * *

GENERAL CONSIDERATIONS. Before entering upon a discussion of the genesis of the

are examined. All stages in the occlusive change may occur in the various vessels of an extremity or at times in the same vessel in different parts of its course. The occlusion of the vessels is effected by red obturating thrombi; these become organized, vascularized, and canalized. The recent red thrombosis may involve large portions of arteries or veins and is not secondary to the gangrenous process. It occurs even when no gangrene is present.

Certain changes in the perivascular tissues, in the adventitia, media, and intima, regularly accompany the occluding process.

There is moderate thickening of the intima; this is never sufficient to cause marked narrowing of the lumina of the vessels, and does not seem to play any considerable rôle in the genesis of thrombotic process.

The media and adventitia show cellular infiltration and vascularization whenever thrombosis has occurred. The intensity of the cellular changes seems in general to depend upon the activity of the organization of the clot; however, in some cases it seems to be sufficiently marked to make it appear that the same agent which calls forth the coagulation of the blood is also effective in producing the mesarterial lesion. The occluding masses frequently terminate abruptly in apparently normal vessels. The changes in the media never extend into the walls of the patent portions of the vessels; usually they terminate before the end of the obturating tissue or thrombus is reached; indeed the dependence of the medial changes upon the organization of the thrombi can be demonstrated in many places.

As a result of the dilatation of a central canalizing vessel, and the fibrous change in the occluding tissue, a picture resembling that due to intense proliferation of the intima may be produced. By means of elastic tissue stains and through study of the vessels at many levels it is comparatively easy to show that the obliterative process has its origin in a thrombus and differs in a number of essentials from the occlusive change due to arteriosclerosis.

* * *

Viewing the process from the standpoint of the pathological lesions, and considering certain facts obtained by clinical observation, it would seem more plausible to assume that certain territories of either the arteries or the veins become rather suddenly thrombosed, in a fashion similar to the thrombotic process that occurs in the superficial veins of the lower extremities. Thus, at one time the dorsalis hallucis and dorsalis pedis, or perhaps plantar arteries or veins, could become closed by red clot, and then the process of organization would take place. Perhaps after an interval of weeks or months a similar process would cause extension upward, or affect other arteries and veins, until, after a lapse of many months, or a year or more, practically all the larger vessels would become occluded. It is from a study of the age of the process in the various territories that we are led to this supposition. Here too as in the superficial thrombosis there is more tendency for the larger vessels to be involved than for the very fine ones, and although the process seems to ascend, it probably does not originate in the capilleries or smallest arterioles, but begins in branches of moderate size. The attendent peri-arteritis could be regarded as being either secondary, or possibly, as being produced by the same causes that lead to the thrombosis. Certain it is that the peri-arteritis is intimately linked with the presence of occluding masses.

Taking the true nature of the lesion into consideration, I would suggest that the names *"endarteritis obliterans"* and *"arteriosclerotic gangrene"* be discarded in this connection, and that we adopt the terms *"obliterating thrombo-angiitis"* of the lower extremities when we wish to speak of the disease under discussion.

S. Weir Mitchell

Silas Weir Mitchell was born in Philadelphia in 1830, the son of Dr. John K. Mitchell, a prominent physician of that city, and Professor of Medicine at Jefferson Medical College. He grew up in an atmosphere of culture and, from his earliest youth, was thrown in the company of talented and cultivated people. As a boy he was somewhat bookish, very fond of poetry, and was described as a dreamy child. He graduated in medicine at Jefferson Medical College in 1850, spent a year abroad, chiefly in France, and in 1851, began to practice in Philadelphia. He desired an appointment as interne at the Philadelphia Hospital but was refused the position and began practice as his father's assistant.

Weir Mitchell brought from France an intense desire to experiment and devoted such time as he could spare from his practice to experimental work.

He studied uric acid crystals, investigated the properties of certain alkaloids, and conducted researches upon the venom of the rattlesnake. Research work was then universally held to be incompatible with private practice. One of his revered teachers remarked, "What nonsense to bother yourself about snake poisons," and one of the most eminent physicians in Philadelphia warned him that every experiment would cost him a patient. But Mitchell did not think so and continued his experiments.

During the Civil War he served in the military hospitals of Philadelphia, and in the years following the war built up a large and lucrative practice, but

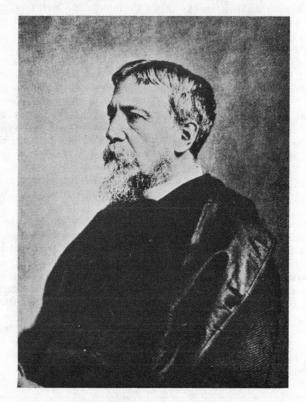

S. WEIR MITCHELL (1830-1914)

kept up his scientific interests and gave an increasing amount of time to literary labors. His first essays, poems, and stories were written anonymously, for he was repeatedly told by his friends that if he used his own name it would be certain to wreck his practice. His literary productions earned for him the respect and friendship of such men as Oliver Wendell Holmes, James Russell Lowell, John G. Whittier, and George Meredith. The height of his literary popularity was attained in 1898 with his novel *Hugh Wynne*, which was for a long time a best seller.

Weir Mitchell is best remembered in medical circles for the Weir Mitchell treatment of functional neuroses and for his original description of erythrome-lalgia—Weir Mitchell's disease.

Weir Mitchell, in summing up his life work, said he had four forms of product: "First, toxicological. Second, I have in my profession made what I may call practical discoveries or inventions. Third, I have written verse, almost all of it since I was fifty. This has yet to be judged seriously by time. Fourth, I have had at last, what always I was sure would come, success as a story-teller."

Weir Mitchell died at the age of eighty-four in 1914, as Sir Launder-Brunton said, "the most accomplished and versatile physician of his time. Of very few men can it be said that as a young man he took first place amongst the physiologists, as a middle-aged man first amongst the physicians and as an elderly man first amongst the novelists of his country."

ARTICLE I

ON A RARE VASO-MOTOR NEUROSIS OF THE EXTREMITIES,[1] AND ON THE MALADIES WITH WHICH IT MAY BE CONFOUNDED*

By S. Weir Mitchell, M.D., of Philadelphia, Member of the National
Academy of Sciences

A few years ago I published in the *Philadelphia Med. Times* (1872, pp. 81 and 113) a brief paper upon certain painful affections of the feet, and drew attention to a form of foot-disorder which I was unable to find fully described elsewhere. This paper attracted little attention; and I now find myself called upon, by a larger and more fertile knowledge, to review the subject, and again to call to the attention of physicians a somewhat rare, and yet most interesting, form of disease.

I have called it a rare disease, because, in a large experience, I have seen but few cases; yet it is likely that, when once recognized, it may be found to be more common than I now conceive it to be.

In dealing with this subject, I shall first draw a picture of the malady as I have seen it in its various degrees of severity; I shall then relate cases from the mildest to the most severe; and end by discussing them from such points of view as they may suggest.

The patient, nearly always a man, after some constitutional disease, like a low fever, or after prolonged physical exertion afoot, begins to suffer with pain in the foot or feet; usually it comes in the ball of the foot, or of the great toes, or in the heel; and from these parts it extends so as to involve a large

portion or all of the sole, and to reach the dorsum, and even the leg. More often it is felt finally in a limited region of one or both soles, and does not extend beyond these areas. At first it is felt only towards night, and is eased by the night's rest; but, soon or late, it comes nearer and nearer to the hour of rising from bed. In like manner, while at first it is made to increase only by excessive exertion afoot, by and by it comes on, whenever the upright posture is assumed, or even when the foot is allowed to hang down. Since, however, the disease is not necessarily progressive, there are instances in which the pain never passes a definite limit. One case may for years have the trouble only in the evening; a second may reach and remain at the point where only a long walk in summer causes it; a third may still, as it were, in a far more advanced stage of the malady, and, though suffering horrible pain, become no worse; while in the gravest cases, more familiar signs of organic disease of the spinal cord may arise to shed light upon the pathology of the minor forms of the trouble.

In rare cases, the first pain is said to be an ache of the foot; but in the mass of instances, and soon or late in nearly all, the pain is of a burning character. "It is the pain of a burn"; "the pain of mustard"; "of intense sun-burn"; at least these are the phrases used to describe it, and certainly the character of the suffering is so well marked as to be clinically distinctive. In the milder cases it may come and go, or be present daily at

---

[1] The foot and hand disorder I am about to describe may be conveniently labeled Erythromelalgia; ἐρυθρός, red; μέλος, 2 member; ἄλγος, pain.
* *Am. J. M. Sc.*, 1878, LXXVI, 1-36.

some time, as upon exertion, and yet be but trifling in its intensity; while in severer cases the burning reaches the extreme of torture. The sufferer, when placed on his feet, rocks as if unsteady; and if his eyes be closed, may deceive the observer into the belief that he has before him a case of locomotor ataxia. Yet a vigorous effort of will is fully competent to preserve the balance; and this unstable equilibrium is not seen until, owing to the upright posture having been preserved for some minutes, the pain has risen to a maximum of anguish.

In later stages of the disease the pain is throbbing, aching, and burning, owing, I suppose, to the vasal disorders, which are seen in some cases throughout, and always in the graver examples.

In every case and at all stages, the pain is relieved or arrested by the horizontal position, and by cold. It is brought on and made worse by standing or walking; and, in bad cases, by allowing the feet to hang down; while warmth, and, of course, heavy feet-covers, act in like manner. Summer is usually, not always, the season of greatest annoyance; winter a time of comparative ease. The sufferer sleeps with uncovered feet, and goes about without stockings in his house; and finds, even in winter, a light slipper or a low shoe comfortable.

The next striking peculiarity of this disorder is the flushing of the part upon exertion. This symptom, which is usually absent in the very early stages, is a notable feature of the worst of the prolonged cases, and in some mild instances can always be brought on by great exertion afoot. In the graver examples, the area of greatest pain in the soles or hands is distinctly and permanently marked by a dull, dusky, mottled redness, as if the smaller vessels were always over-distended. In these and in some of the less severe cases, the region of pain is in places tender, and firm pressure by the finger or hand will bring on increased pain, and even cause the whole foot or hand, or a part of it, to become red, just as it does when the man stands up.

The pain in these cases is also entirely inhibitory of walking, and if this action be persisted in, gives rise to intense redness, swelling from dilatation of vessels, and finally to blistering of the soles.

Where flushing is a part of the phenomena of this interesting malady, it comes on during the erect position slowly in milder cases, and almost at once in others, and involves both veins and arteries. The foot gets redder and redder, the veins stand out in a few moments as if a ligature had been tied around the limb, and the arteries throb violently for a time, until at length the extremity becomes a dark-purplish tint.

In the worst cases, when the patient is at rest, the limbs are cold, and even pale. The flushing, which, at first, seems to be an active condition, accompanied with rise of temperature, in a few minutes becomes passive; that is, the arteries cease to throb, the heat lessens, and there is evidence of less oxidation.

The less severe examples manage to get along by rest at intervals, but the worst cases are unable to stand for more than a moment, and the sufferer crawls on his hands and knees, keeping his feet off the floor, or is obliged to be carried about.

I have seen lately two examples in which the disease seemed to have been progressive, and to have been associated in the later stages with distinctive evidence of spinal disease, such as atrophic states, the pain-belt (douleur en ceinture), partial losses of power. and other phenomena, which vary in the two cases alluded to. Also in one of them all the singular features which in the early stages were seen in the feet, were at a later stage exhibited in equal fulness in the hands, or rather in the hand, since one had been lost by amputation.

One other peculiarity is common to all of them. They are rarely amendable to treatment. They are aided for a time by cold and by rest, but either they remain unchanged for years, or else in rare instances become gradually worse.

As to diagnosis, I am aware of no other malady with which the bad cases of this malady can be confounded; but there are certain other more or less painful affections of the feet, with which the lighter forms might be confused; and I shall, therefore, make some brief allusions, at the close of these pages, to the maladies of the feet, from which it is needful to distinguish the disease I am describing.

V. DISEASES OF THE BLOOD

The outstanding modern contributions to the subject of diseases of the blood, date from the employment of the microscope and the refinement of laboratory technique. It is noteworthy however, that chlorosis, pernicious anemia, purpura, and hemophilia were recognized without the aid of either the microscope or the laboratory. While the physicians of antiquity, notably Hippocrates, are thought by some to have described chlorosis, many authorities reject this view. Their accounts at best are uncertain, while Lange presents an easily recognizable picture. Pernicious anemia was described by Combe before Addison, although Combe's description did not attract enough attention to merit its mention in his obituary notice. This disease, whose course the physicians were unable to check for three generations, can now be controlled, as a result of the discovery of Minot and Murphy. Vaquez first clearly described polycythemia, although Osler's account is so excellent that many authorities call this malady the Vaquez-Osler disease. Bennett and Virchow described leukemia at almost the same time, although Virchow's explanation was correct and that of Bennett erroneous. Purpura was described by Amatus Lusitanus and Lazarus Riverius but was first clearly defined by Werlhof, whose priority is recognized by the term *morbus maculosis Werlhofii*. Hemophilia, known to the ancient Hebrews, became a definite clinical entity after Otto had drawn attention to its familial tendency and to its mode of transmission.

CHLOROSIS
Johannes Lange

Johannes Lange, one of the most highly esteemed physicians of the sixteenth century, was born in Löwenberg, Silesia, in 1485. Lange studied at Leipsic, where he received his master's degree in 1514, and then proceeded to Italy to study medicine. He went first to Ferrara, where he studied with the celebrated Nicolo Leoniceno, then to Bologna, and finally to Pisa, where he received the degree of M.D. in 1522. Upon his return to Germany he was appointed physician to the Elector of the Palatinate and held this position for more than forty years, serving under four Electors. He accompanied the Electors upon their journeys throughout Europe and on two occasions accompanied the Elector's Army against the Turks under Suleiman. He died in Heidelberg in 1565 at the age of eighty.

Lange's chief medical work was his *Epistolae medicinales*, which was first published at Basle in 1554. This work contains his well-known description of chlorosis, which is apparently the earliest published account of this disease.

DE MORBO VIRGINEO*

EPISTOLA XXI

You will have complained to me, your faithful companion, that your first born daughter, Anno, & now sad, is desired in marriage by many suitors, of great excellency and illustrious birth, and also with an abundance of wealth, descended by ancestry from your forebears not from your inferiors; whom you are compelled to refuse because of the weakness of your daughter. Neither is this as obnoxious to you, as that thus far none of the Doctors have been able to explain the internal cause & essence of her disease, and at the same time prescribe the treatment. For one says it is cardalgia, another throbbing of the heart, this one indeed dyspnoea, that one suffocation of the womb: nor are those wanting, who suspect a loathing of the stomach from disease of the liver, the differing judgment of them concerning the illness of your daughter, you say proves that you are quite perplexed, nor are you able to tell what indeed should be done.

The cause and accidents of the disease of virgins — Since you demand this opinion of the disease of the girl, and dependable advice concerning marriage, because of our old friendship, and at the same time you rightly ask with what kind of disease is she afflicted: since the qualities of her face, which in the past year was distinguished by rosiness of cheeks and redness of lips, is some how as if exsanguinated, sadly paled, the heart trembles with every movement of her body, and the arteries of her temples pulsate, & she is seized with dyspnoea in dancing or climbing the stairs, her stomach loathes food and particularly meat, & the legs, especially at the ankles, become edematous at night. From these accidents indeed, & from the pathognomonic signs of the disease, which betray the cause & nature of the disease, point out its treatment, I marvel that old physicians do not know the cause & nature of the disease. Although indeed they have not mentioned its name, which moreover contributes nothing to its treatment, that is nothing of importance.

There are many illnesses in the catalogue of diseases, lacking a name & not a treatment. Nor has this disease a proper name, as much as it is peculiar to virgins, might indeed

be called "virgineus," which it is the custom of the matrons of Brabant to call white fever, or pale face & the fever of love: since every lover becomes pale, & this color is proper for a lover, although a fever very rarely is present. But this disease frequently attacks virgins, when now mature they pass from youth to virility. For at this time, by nature, the menstrual blood flows from the liver to the small spaces & veins of the womb: which when from the narrow mouths, which are not yet distended, also obstructed by thick & crude humors, & finally from the thickness of the blood, cannot escape: then carried backwards through the vena cava and the large arteries flows to the heart, liver, diaphragm & veins of the diaphragm: also a good part is distributed to the head, & grave accidents appear in the viscera, dyspnoea, a tremulous throbbing of the heart, inflation of the liver, nausea of the stomach, cardalgia: not rarely epilepsy with loss of senses, & delirium.

Although Hippocrates in the book on diseases of Virgins declares: Virgins, he says, to whom the time of marriage comes, and are now mature, are afflicted with imaginary terrors of spectres, especially when the menses appear, for before this, they are not at all badly affected, afterwards indeed the blood in the small spaces of the womb, as it were escaping, drips and falls, since the obstructed mouths were the places of egress, and the blood abundant from the foods & the growth of the body, collected there, is present in large quantity and whence it flows distending the opening of the veins, the heart beyond its power moves up to the septum transversum & diaphragm, the heart itself does not hold out & becomes torpid, then from this torpidity the patient becomes foolish and delirious. It is certainly no wonder since the liver is not cleansed of the filthy blood of the menses, & by it the veins of the diaphragm are stopped up, the viscera of the abdomen swell, & the diaphragm is contracted (as in hydrops), then a difficulty in breathing appears, as Galen points out in his third book on Dyspnoea, where he says in general: If an internal tumor or pain has existed in the abdomen, then respiration is shallow & rapid.

After this the heart, stomach & liver, the veins & arteries of which are connected by juice & branches, as by a common bond,

*Lange, Johann, *Medicinalium epistolarum miscellanea*, Basle, Wechelus, 1554, p. 74.

these filled & obstructed indeed by the gross blood, crammed with spirits and vapors, so that the heart casts these out & expells them, that it may not be choked by the great numbers of arteries & struggles with the movement of contraction & trembles all over. . . .

Finally, whether your daughter ill with this

they recover, if indeed they be not attacked by this disease in puberty, then it attacks a little later unless they have been married. Moreover indeed of the married, very many are sterile. With this most wholesome advice of the divine Hippocrates, if medicines produce menses and loosening up obstructions, if

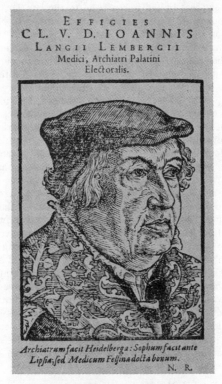

JOHANNES LANGE (1485-1565)
Frontispiece to Lange's *Epistolarum medicinalium*,
Frankfort, 1589

affection ought to marry, & what should be the treatment of it, see I shall communicate the trusty advice from the rich store of the medicine of Hippocrates, who says in his book on diseases of Virgins: the cure of this disease is venesection if nothing hinders. I therefore say, I instruct virgins afflicted with this disease, that as soon as possible they live with men & copulate, if they conceive

you produce a thinning of the thick blood, you can discover & devise nothing more powerful than this. In the treatment of this disease of virgins I have never been deceived or my hopes frustrated. Wherefore, be of good courage, you shall give away your daughter: also I shall be present at the nuptials with pleasure.

PERNICIOUS ANEMIA
James Scarth Combe

Another veteran medical practitioner has passed from among us, whose erect, gentle-manly figure and handsome, genial countenance must have been well known to most citizens of Edinburgh. For some years Dr. Combe had virtually retired from active life, but up till this winter he might often be seen walking leisurely along Queen Street, from his house at 36 York Place, to pay his almost daily visit to his widowed daughter in Glenfinlas Street. About twenty years ago she was united in marriage to the late Dr. James Simson, another well-known member of our profession, who was slightly senior to her father. She was left a few years ago, with a son and daughter.

Dr. Combe was born in Leith on the fifth of January, 1796, and so was in his eighty-seventh year when he died. He was connected by blood, although not very closely, with George and Andrew Combe, the eminent phrenologists. Having entered upon the study of medicine, he obtained his diploma as surgeon in 1814, while barely nineteen years of age, a thing possible in those days, and in the following year prepared to take his degree at the University. He told the writer of this that he was undergoing one of his examinations— probably in the house of Dr. Andrew Duncan, senior, who then resided in Adam Square— when the castle guns announced the crowning victory over Napoleon at Waterloo. This cessa-tion of war put an end to a purpose which he had formed of becoming a military surgeon. However, still being very young, he went to India for a short time, and extended his profes-sional knowledge very considerably, which afterwards stood much in his favor on his return home. He practised with marked success in his native town until 1847, when circumstances induced him to remove to Edinburgh. He had become a fellow of the Royal College of Sur-geons in 1823, and continued to serve the corporation in various ways until he filled the presidential chair in 1851-52. He acted as an examiner for many years, and latterly as an assessor of the examining board. Dr. Combe pursued the even tenor of his way, during all these years, as a respected and busy practitioner, until the pressure of advancing years entitled him to the *otium cum dignitate*. He was an honourable man, whom his brethren could safely confide in, and all who knew him felt that his quiet exterior and reasonable opinions, which always tended to what was liberal and hopeful, were associated with a latent potentiality, which had never thoroughly asserted itself. On several occasions, of late years, he had suffered from inflammatory affections of the chest, and we understand that one of these carried him off after an illness of a few days. His partner in life died a few years ago—an event which he felt very severely. He has left behind him, besides Mrs. Simpson, two sons, the elder of whom is Dr. Mathew Combe, Surgeon-Major of the Royal Artillery.*

* Obituary Notice in *Edinburgh Medical Journal*, 1883, XVII, 862.

DR. COMBE ON ANAEMIA
HISTORY OF A CASE OF ANAEMIA

By J. S. Combe, M.D., Fellow of the Royal College of Surgeons, Edinburgh
(Read 1st May 1822)*

The following case has been already brought under the notice of the Society by my distinguished preceptor and friend Dr. Kellie, in his paper on the Pathology of the Brain, as affording a striking corroboration of his views regarding the circulation within the head in health and disease. It appears to me entitled to still further attention, and to a more minute detail, as exhibiting a well marked instance of a very peculiar disease which has excited little attention among medi-cal men, and which has been altogether over-looked by any English author with whose writings I am acquainted. Unfortunately, however, such is the allowable diversity of opinion on most medical subjects, that it is very possible the following case may be viewed in different lights, and receive differ-ent appellations; and while some may be dis-posed to regard the peculiar characteristic

* *Tr. Med. Chir. Soc., Edin.*, 1824, I, 193-198.

from which it derives its denomination of Anaemia, as constituting a morbid state *sui generis*, others may consider the defect of the red circulating mass as an accidental and occasional circumstance, denoting some peculiar change in the assimilative powers, the primary stages of which we have been unable to detect. Doubtful myself which of these opinions may be the most correct, I shall do little more than state correctly the phenomena of the case, and minutely the appearances presented on dissection. One remark only I may at present offer, that if any train of symptoms may be allowed to constitute Anaemia a generic disease, the following may be considered an example of it in its most idiopathic form.

It was in the month of July 1821, that I was first consulted by Alexander Haynes, the subject of this case, on the nature of his complaints. Even at that time I was much struck by his peculiar appearance. He exactly resembled a person just recovering from an attack of syncope; his face, lips and the whole extent of the surface, were of a deadly pale colour; the albuginea of the eye bluish: his motions and speech were languid; he complained much of weakness; his respiration, free when at rest, became hurried on the slightest exertion; pulse 80, and feeble; tongue covered with a dry fur; the inner part of the lips and fauces were nearly as colourless as the surface. He says that his bowels are very irregular, generally lax, and that his stools are very dark and foetid; urine reported to be copius and pale; appetite impaired; of late his stomach has rejected almost every sort of food; has constant thirst; he has no pain referable to any part, and a minute examination could not detect any structural derangement of any organ. He is forty-seven years of age; was born and has spent the greater part of his life in the country, engaged in agricultural employments; for a few years has been servant to a corn-merchant, where his duties are neither laborious nor unhealthy. He is married, and has no family; leads a regular and temperate life; has enjoyed perfect health since childhood, and has never been blooded. He was advised to use some medicine to correct the state of his bowels, to confine himself to a light diet, and to take gentle exercise.

I saw him again in a few days, and found him nearly in the same state. His stools were consistent, dark and very foetid; urine pale and copious, depositing scarcely and sediment. His wife tells me that it is about two months since he began to complain, but not until his friends had observed his altered complexion: he then lost strength, and said his head troubled him. Of this last symptom, however, he has no distinct recollection; his feet became edematous, and his appetite failed him. My attention was again drawn towards the skin, which was of the same waxen colour, soft and delicate, the cellular texture about the eyes and breast being slightly distended with watery effusion. The pulse was feeble, and easily excited by any motion. The veins on the arm and neck were delicate, and could be felt on making pressure, but the colour of the blood did not appear through the skin. It was evident that the patient laboured under great debility, probably from a defective and languid circulation. Some tonic medicines, a mild nutritious diet, with wine, were prescribed, and I was inclined to hope for a favourable termination to the case.

About a fortnight after this he was evidently better, was stronger, and able occasionally to attend to his duty; but I was not at any time confident that there was any change in his complexion. He perspired freely on any exertion, but neither the face nor lips ever acquired any additional tinge. At one time, from the state of his stools and urine, I was led to suspect an affection of the liver; at another, from the thirst, great flow of urine (exceeding the liquid ingesta), and peculiar state of the skin, I was apprehensive of diabetes; but none of these indications remained long stationary.

In September, and occasionally afterwards. he was visited by Dr. Kellie, and Dr. R. Hamilton, from whose able advise I trusted he would derive much benefit. A very minute examination of the case, and a careful consideration of its history, however, scarcely solved the nature of the affection, and its long continuance and inveteracy rendered our prognosis more doubtful.

Towards the end of September, he tried the effects of a sea voyage, and afterwards drank the waters of a chalybeate spring. He returned in the middle of October with a loss of flesh and strength, his legs were much swollen, his skin had the same exsanguine appearance, secretion of urine copious, bowels lax, and appetite greatly impaired; he was still in good spirits, made no complaints excepting of debility, and looked forward to a speedy recovery.

It seems unnecessary to detail at great length the history of this case; for two months after this, it presented no peculiar features in addition to those already enumerated; all the symptoms, however, were aggravated, and the constitution began to sink under their pressure. About the middle of January 1822, the oedema had extended over his face and upper extremities, and evident marks of effusion into the chest presented themselves. He died in a few weeeks with all the symptoms usually attendant on hydrothorax.

George Richards Minot

George Richards Minot was born in Boston, Massachusetts, in 1885. He comes from a long line of forbears distinguished in the medical annals of

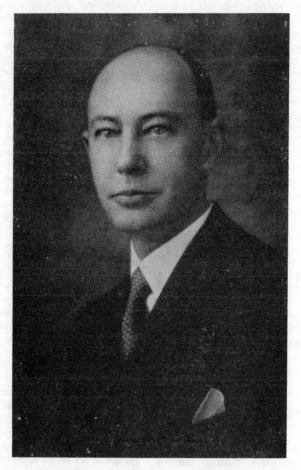

GEORGE RICHARDS MINOT (1885-   )
Photograph by Alfred Brown, Brookline, Massachusetts

New England. His great-grandfather, James Jackson, was one of the founders of the Massachusetts General Hospital; his great-uncle, Francis Minot, was one of the early physicians to this hospital; his cousin, Charles Sedgwich Minot, was one of the most outstanding anatomists America has produced, and his father, James Jackson Minot, a very distinguished physician of Boston.

Minot was educated at Harvard, taking his A.B. in 1908 and his M.D. *cum laude* in 1912. After his internship at the Massachusetts General Hospital, he went to Baltimore as assistant resident physician at the Johns Hopkins Hospital, and later he returned to Boston, where he became like James Jackson, Francis Minot, and James S. Minot, physician to the Massachusetts General Hospital. In 1923 he became chief of the medical service of the Collis P. Huntington Memorial Hospital and in 1928 became professor at Harvard Medical School, and the same year received the honorary degree of S.D. from Harvard. Minot was early interested in the study of diseases of the blood and published many important studies in this field. His investigations led to the discovery, in collaboration with William P. Murphy, of the beneficial effects of liver in pernicious anemia. This epochal discovery, first announced in 1926, soon received confirmation in various parts of the world and has saved the lives of hundreds of thousands of patients. It ranks among the greatest contributions the New World has made to the science of medicine. Every physician feels what the venerable Dr. George M. Kober expressed when he said on presenting the Kober Medal to Dr. Minot, "There follows the sincere hope that your years of usefulness to humanity may still be many, and that it may be given to you and your co-workers to add fresh laurels to your fair renown and thus uphold the glory of American Medicine, of which you are an exemplary product."

OBSERVATIONS OF PATIENTS WITH PERNICIOUS ANEMIA PARTAKING OF A SPECIAL DIET*

(A) CLINICAL ASPECTS

By George R. Minot, M.D., and William P. Murphy, M.D. (by invitation), Boston, Massachusetts

The dietetic treatment of pernicious anemia may be of more importance than hitherto generally recognized.

Forty-five patients with pernicious anemia have continued to take a diet for from six weeks to two years composed especially of foods rich in complete proteins—particularly liver (120 to 240 gm. a day). The diet also contains for each day at least 120 gm. of muscle meat and an abundance of fresh vegetables and fruits, a normal amount of starch foods and is relatively low in fat. The cases were seen essentially consecutively.

Following the diet, all of the patients showed a prompt, rapid and distinct remission of their anemia coincident with at least

* Read before the Association of American Physicians, May 4, 1926.

rather marked symptomatic improvement, except for marked disorders due to spinal-cord degeneration. Improvement was often striking, so that where the red blood cell count averaged for all before starting the diet 1,470,000 per cubic millimeter, about one month afterward it averaged 3,400,000 per cubic millimeter; and for the 27 cases observed four to six months after the diet was begun the average count was 4,500,000 per cubic millimeter.

Patients having had two or more relapses showed on the average slightly lower red blood corpuscle-counts about one and two months after commencing the diet than did those who had started it in their first or second relapse.

Data are not yet available to indicate

whether the remission will last any longer than in other cases, because most of the patients have taken the diet for less than seven months. All of the patients have remained to date in a good state of health except 3, who discontinued their diet: 2 of these rapidly improved upon resuming it, while the other has only just begun to take liver again.

(B) PHYSIOLOGICAL ASPECTS

By William P. Murphy, M.D. (by invitation), Reginald Fitz, M.D., and
Robert D. Monroe, M.D. (by invitation)

Special studies concerning changes which have occurred in the blood following the beginning of the dietary régime have been carried out in 11 of the 45 cases referred to above.

Within a few days after starting the diet there occurred in the 11 cases, and also in 5 others, a temporary greater output of young red blood cells from the marrow, lasting about ten days, as indicated by an increase of the reticulocytes in the peripheral blood from usually less than about 1 per cent to an average of about 8 per cent. The peak of their rise occurred in from four to ten days.

This early manifestation of improvement in blood formation was accompanied by a decrease of the bile pigments in the blood-serum. The icterus index began to drop quite promptly after the diet was begun, generally reaching normal or below in two or three weeks.

The corpuscular protein content increased in a fashion closely parallel to the increasing hemoglobin concentration, while the plasma protein nitrogen readings remained nearly constant. The nonprotein nitrogen of the blood was not affected during the patients' improvement.

As in other pernicious anemia cases, regenerating blood, coincident with the rise in hemoglobin percentage and red blood cell-count, there occurred a steady rise in the corpuscular volume. This was demonstrated by measurements of the blood and plasma volume by the Congo red method, which showed that although the total volume increased but slightly, the volume of corpuscles often was trebled in a period of a few weeks, from which it may be interpreted that a marked growth of blood tissue was observed.

SICKLE-CELL ANEMIA

PECULIAR ELONGATED AND SICKLE-SHAPED RED BLOOD CORPUSCLES IN A CASE OF SEVERE ANEMIA*

James B. Herrick, M.D., Chicago

This case is reported because of the unusual blood findings, no duplicate of which I have ever seen described. Whether the blood picture represents merely a freakish poikilocytosis or is dependent on some peculiar physical or chemical condition of the blood, or is characteristic of some particular disease, I cannot at present answer. I report some details that may seem non-essential, thinking that if a similar blood condition is found in some other case a comparison of clinical conditions may help in solving the problem.

History.—The patient was an intelligent negro of 20, who had been in the United States three months, during which time he was a student in one of the professional schools in Chicago. His former residence had been Grenada, West Indies, where he had been born and brought up, one of a family of four children, all living and all well with the exception of himself. His mother was living and in good health; his father had died of accident. At the age of 10 the patient had had yaws. This was a common disease in the locality where he lived. The lesions, as he described them, had been pustular, with formation of ulcers and scabs. On healing, scars, many of which he pointed out, were left. Some of the ulcers had been as large as a silver quarter of a dollar. The disease lasted about one year and during this time he had felt weak and indisposed. Most of the ulcers had been on the legs and the patient himself had thought that this location of the lesions might have been due to the bruises and

* *Arch. Int. Med.*, 1910, vi, 517.

scratches that were frequently produced as he ran about, a barefoot boy, through the streets and the brush. He was sure he had never had ground-itch, though he said it was not uncommon in Grenada. He had attended school up to the age of 17. Since leaving school, that is, for the past three years, he had felt a disinclination to take exercise. For about a year he had noticed some palpitation and shortness of breath which he had attributed to excessive smoking. There had been times when he thought he was bilious and when the whites of the eyes had been tinged with yellow. At such times he had not had any pain, chill or fever. Three years previous he had had a purulent discharge from the right ear lasting six months. He had had no diarrheas and no hemorrhages at any time. He denied syphilis and gonorrhea. There was never any rheumatism or other joint trouble. On landing in New York September, 1904, he had a sore on one ankle for which he consulted a physician. Tincture of iodin was applied and in a week the sore had healed, leaving a scar similar to the others on the limbs. For the past five weeks, he had been coughing. Two days prior to examination he had "taken cold," his cough had grown worse and he had had a slight fever. It was this cough and fever for which he wished treatment at the hospital, and of which he chiefly complained, though he mentioned also that he felt weak and dizzy, had headache and catarrh of the nose.

Physical Examination.—This showed him to be a young man of typical negro facies, with black, curly hair. He was fairly well developed physically and was bright and intelligent. There was a tinge of yellow in the sclerae and the visible mucous membranes were pale. The eyes were normal; the pupils showed prompt reaction to light and in accommodation. The hearing was good; there was no discharge from the ear. The nose showed chronic and acute rhinitis. The tongue was coated, the pharynx slightly reddened; no scars or other lesions were found here. The cervical glands were definitely enlarged, hard and not painful. The axillary, inguinal and epitrochlear glands were also enlarged, some in the axilla being the size of almonds. Over the chest and abdomen were several good-sized leukodermatous patches, the intervening skin being rather deeply pigmented. The scars to which he had referred were nearly all located on the legs and thighs,

some in the former location being as much as 3 cm. in diameter. There were perhaps twenty scars in all. They were rounded or oval, sometimes of irregular contour, the edges clean-cut; some were like tissue paper on thin parchment to the touch and were lighter in color than the surrounding skin. They were strikingly like scars often seen as the result of syphilis. The chest was well formed. There was fair expansion. Numerous râles, mostly of the moist variety, were heard scattered throughout the chest, especially posteriorly. There was a slight relative dulness over the base of either lung behind. The heart was enlarged to the left, the apex impulse, being in the sixth interspace one inch to the left of the left mammillary line. There was but a slight increase in the dulness to the right. A soft systolic murmur, not well transmitted in any direction, was heard over the base of the heart. A faint systolic murmur, or perhaps it would be better to call it an impure first tone—was heard at the apex. The heart's action reminded one of a heart under strong stimulation, though no history of ingestion of a stimulant of any kind was obtainable. Basedow's findings were not to be made out. The pulse was of good quality and of fair volume. The abdomen was not distended nor was it tender. Neither spleen nor liver could be palpated. There was no tenderness over the gallbladder region. The genitalia were normal. The patellar reflexes were sluggish. There was no ataxia and there were no sensory disturbances.

The temperature on admission was 101 F. It varied between 99 and 101 for four days, then gradually subsided, though for the next three weeks it was often found between 99 and 100 F., though with no regularity. The pulse varied from 64 to 104, averaging about 80. There was never any rapid breathing.

Urine and sputum.—The urine was amber in color, specific gravity 1.010 to 1.014, slightly increased in amount—2,000 c.c.— acid, contained a distinct trace of serum-albumin, a few granular and hyaline casts. This represents the average of several examinations. The urine on admission had a trace of bile. December 28, urinary examinations for hemoglobin and hematorporphylin were made and none found. Tests were made for paramidophenol, but none was found.

No tubercle bacilli were discovered in the sputum.

Blood Examination.—The blood count on

Dec. 26, 1904, was: red corpuscles, 2,570,000; white corpuscles, 40,000; hemoglobin (Dare), 40 per cent; color index, 0.78. December 31, the count was as follows: erythrocytes, 2,880.000; leukocytes, 15,250; hemoglobin, 50 per cent (Dare).

The red corpuscles varied much in size, many microcytes being seen and some macrocytes. Polychromatophilia was present. Nucleated reds were numerous, 74 being seen in a count of 200 leukocytes, there being about 5,000 to the c.mm. The shape of the reds was very irregular, but what especially attracted attention was the large number of thin, sickle-shaped and crescent-shaped forms. These were seen in fresh specimens, no matter in what way the blood was spread on the slide and they were seen also in specimens fixed by heat, by alcohol and ether, and stained with the Ehrlich tri-acid stain as well as with control stains. They were not seen in specimens of blood taken at the same time from other individuals and prepared under exactly similar conditions. They were surely not artefacts, nor were they any form of parasite. In staining reactions they were exactly like their neighbors, the ordinary red corpuscles, though many took the stain heavily. In a few of the elongated forms a nucleus was seen. In the fresh specimen where there was slight current in the blood before it had become entirely quiet, all of the red corpuscles, the elongated forms as well as those of ordinary form, seemed to be unusually pliable and flexible, bending and twisting in a remarkable manner as they bumped against each other or crowded through a narrow space and seeming almost rubber-like in their elastic resumption of the former shape. One received the impression that the flattened red discs might by reason of unusual pliability be rolled up as it were into a long narrow bundle. Once or twice I saw a corpuscle of ordinary form turn in such a way as to be seen on edge, when its appearance was suggestive of these peculiar forms.

The white corpuscles were made up of polymorphonuclear neutrophils, 72 per cent, small mononuclear lymphocytes, 15 per cent, large mononuclear forms, 7 per cent, polymorphonuclear eosinophils, 5 per cent, myeloctes (?), 1 per cent. Many polymorphonuclear cells and some mononuclear forms contained basophilic granules (Neusser's perinuclear basophils?). In overheated specimens especially, a number of cells with

shadowy outlines and staining but slightly were seen. These resembled white cells.

Stools.—The stools were examined not only as a matter of routine, but because of the possibility of detecting the presence of some parasite that might explain the eosinophilia, leukocytosis and anemia, a possibility not at all unlikely in one coming from the tropics and who had lived where ground-itch was a common occurrence. Many stools were thoroughly studied. Considerable mucus was found in some of the stools passed soon after admission, and some of the mucus was blood-stained. No blood was found in the interior of the fecal masses. On two occasions preceding the giving of the thymol, a body found resembling almost typically the egg of *Ankylostoma duodenale*. Portions of the stools were incubated, but no embryos were to be made out. Thymol was given, but neither eggs nor embryos could be found in the stools, following its administration.

Treatment and Course of Disease.—Under treatment, consisting of rest, nourishing food and syrup of the iodid of iron, the fever and râles disappeared, the glands become smaller, the blood improved in quality and the patient left the hospital after a four-weeks' stay, declaring that he felt well. The possible therapeutic influence of the thymol must not be overlooked. The blood at this time showed 3,900,000 red corpuscles, 15,000 white, 58 per cent hemoglobin. There was still to be seen a tendency to the peculiar crescent-shape in the red corpuscles though this was by no means so noticeable as before. Nucleated reds were present, though in smaller numbers. Eosinophils were found as before, making up about 5 per cent of the total number of leukocytes.

We were at a loss to account for this peculiar complexus of symptoms, a condition evidently chronic as revealed by the history of the past three years, with yaws and suppurating otitis as predecessors, yet with acute exacerbations, a condition not clearly explained on the basis of an organic lesion in any one organ, yet showing cardiac enlargement, albuminuria and cylindruria, general adenopathy, icterus, with a secondary anemia not remarkable for the great reduction in red corpuscles or hemoglobin, but strikingly atypical in the large number of nucleated red corpuscles of the normoblastic type and in the tendency of the erythrocytes to assume a slender sickle-like shape. The leukocytosis with a rather high eosinophil count was also to be noted.

* * *

COMMENT

No conclusions can be drawn from this case. Not even a definite diagnosis can be made. Syphilis is suggested by many of the facts, such as adenopathy and the condition of the heart and kidneys; it might explain the anemia, the arthritis and perhaps also the temperature, cough and attacks of pain resembling hepatic or gallbladder disease, for as is well known, visceral syphilis may furnish a most bizarre group of symptoms. The Wassermann test was not in use at this time. The scars said to have been due to yaws were like those left by syphilis.

The patient coming from the tropics, one thought of intestinal parasites such as uncinaria as a possible explanation of the anemia and the eosinophilia. What were thought to be eggs were found on one occasion only, and after thymol there was temporary improvement.

The odd blood picture made one examine for possible toxic effects of the coal-tar preparations, but neither from the history nor from the examination of the urine was there any evidence that such drugs were habitually taken. We are at this time particularly interested in the subject of chronic acetanilid intoxication as well as in uncinariasis, having just had a case of each of these interesting conditions under observation, so that we were on the lookout for such out-of-the-way diseases.

The question of diagnosis must remain an open one unless reports of other similar cases with the same peculiar blood-picture shall clear up this feature.

POLYCYTHEMIA

Louis Henri Vaquez

Louis Henry Vaquez was born in Paris in 1860 and, at the time of his death in 1936, was one of the outstanding French physicians. A favorite pupil of Potain's, he became interested early in the diseases of the circulatory system and devoted his entire life to their study. His masterful *Maladies du Coeur,* for a great many years the favorite work on the subject for those who read French, was translated into English in 1924 and immediately became one of the most widely read and most highly prized books on this subject in America. Vaquez's name became well known throughout the medical world from his description in 1892 of cyanotic polycythemia. Vaquez was a member of the *Académie de médicine,* physician to the *Hôpital de la Pitié,* and professor in the faculty of medicine in Paris.

CONCERNING A SPECIAL FORM OF CYANOSIS ACCOMPANIED BY AN EXCESSIVE AND PERSISTENT POLYCYTHAEMIA*

By M. H. Vaquez

Investigations pursued during the last few years concerning the modification of the blood in certain diseases have dealt almost exclusively with cellular alterations, the changes in appearances of the morphological elements, the constitution of the serum, etc.; different conditions have been noted capable of producing diminution in the number of the red cells or increases in that of the white cells, but hardly anyone has noted the possibility of an increase of the red cells.

There are moreover certain conditions where the number of red cells can be considerably increased and, because of this increase, a group of symptoms appear which it is interesting to study.

*Compt. rend, Soc. de biol., 1892, IV, 384.

From the physiological point of view certain authors have already noted that the number of red cells can be definitely increased following meals,[1] and by a stay at high altitudes. M Viault[2] has shown that under these conditions the number of red cells can at the end of a few days and varying with the individual person, reach 7,500,000 to 7,900,000. From the viewpoint non of the increase in the number of the red cells, the writers have suggested that it is either the simple effect of the concentration of the blood by the loss of serum or an exaggerated production of red cells by physiological or pathological hyperactivity of the hematopoietic tissue.

The first hypothesis has been verified in certain conditions, the second rests without

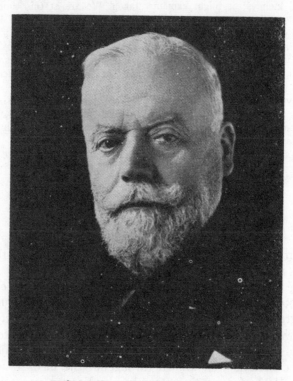

LOUIS HENRI VAQUEZ (1860-1936)

of pathology it has been shown for a long time that the rapid loss of large quantities of fluid in the organism, such as happens, for example, in cholera, can produce such concentration of the blood that the number of red cells is considerably increased.

M. Malassez, who is a great authority in such matters, has stated in his lectures that persistent cyanosis in cardiac patients is accompanied by an increase in the number of cells.

In order to explain this curious phenomenon of pathology it has been shown for a long a definite demonstration. As far as the symptoms produced by polycythemia either physiological or pathological are concerned, the writers remain nearly all silent on this matter. It should however be noted that the different observations made upon this subject insist upon two important points: the sensation of vertigo accompanied or not accompanied by vomiting and a tendency to hemorrhages.

I would say also in closing, that up to the present, polycythemia has been considered as a transitory phenomenon, or at any rate, its persistence has not been noted. For that reason it seems interesting to us to call atten-

[1] *Inaug. Dissert.*, Erlangen, 1881.
[2] *Comptes rendus de l'Académie des sciences,* 15 décembre 1890.

tion to-day to some cases of persistent polycythemia accompanying or determining perhaps the chronic cyanosis and producing a group of symptoms which appear to repeat themselves quite faithfully in the different observations which have dealt with this subject.

The case to which we refer is that of a patient admitted on several occasions on the service of our chief, Professor Potain, and which we have been able to study for two years. This patient, aged 40 years, has never noted any disease, any distress in waking, any shortness of breath, any palpitation, until ten years ago. In 1870, he took part in the campaign, was made prisoner in Germany and endured all the hardship and fatigue of captivity without noticing anything abnormal in his health. Ten years ago, when he was not subjected to any excessive work, he noticed that his extremities became progressively blue, that his veins were filled throughout his entire body, and then followed slowly shortness of breath and palpitations of the heart. At the same time, the functions of his stomach became feeble, dyspeptic phenomena appeared with distress in the right hypochondrium; the patient caught cold more easily and could scarcely get rid of a persistent bronchial catarrh. He remained in this condition until three years ago. At this time, attacks of vertigo commenced to appear, corresponding exactly to the vertigo of Menière, with buzzing, then whistling in the right ear, a sensation of suffering with turning of objects and vomiting, without loss of consciousness. This time also the gums of the patient were tumefied, became fungoid, bleeding at the slightest contact. When we examine him we find that we are dealing with a man afflicted with a chronic cyanosis, without a trace of edema, with considerable dilatation of the veins, with an intense redness of the face, marked injection of the conjunctiva, the whole caused probably in the absence of any other plausible hypothesis, by a congenital lesion of the heart which in any event does not give any certain sign on auscultation. Examination of the blood made by us at this time showed the surprising figure of 8,900,000 red cells, that of the white cells remaining practically normal for this proportion.

This patient having returned a few months later on our service, we repeated this examination and we perceive that the dizzy attacks

show a paroxysmal character, that they are accompanied by very severe lumbar pains and are terminated by a discharge of red cells through the kidneys, which lasts from four to six days.

Another phenomenon already appreciable for two years, but much plainer at the present moment, strikes us; this was the marked increase in volume of the liver (about 20 cm on the mammary line) and of the spleen (24 cm.). We will say to conclude that the quantity of urine voided equals usually 3 liters per day, the quantity being approximately equivalent to that of the ingested fluid. As to the examination of the blood, here is what he showed at present (the 5th of April):[1] the number of red cells equals 8,450,000 (blood of the vein at the elbow). The proportion of white cells is 1 to 300, the density equals 1080, finally the hemoglobin value measured by the hemoglobinometer of Malassez is 165. Dr. Drouin, chief of the chemical laboratory of the Charité, found in the blood of this patient a very evident hyperalkalinity. In conclusion then, we are dealing with a real polycythemia effecting all the blood of the body with a proportional increase in all of its normal qualities.

If we search among authors for a case similar to that which we have just reported, we find only one observation of Krehl[2] in which polycythemia was also noted and, a curious thing, the properties of the blood were almost identical to those observed in our case. Indeed the examination of the blood obtained by bleeding showed:

R.B.C. 8,104,000
Hb. 130% (apparatus of Fleischl)
Density 1071

The clinical observation is unfortunately incomplete and we know only that the patient affected with chronic cyanosis carried a congenital lesion of the pulmonary artery which was verified at autopsy. On the other hand, MM. Cuffer & Sollier published in 1889 in the *Revue de Medecine*, two observations of a generalized venous congestion which corresponds exactly in its clinical symptoms to the case which we report to-day. We find here the same exaggerated dilatation of the veins with the redness of the face and conjunctiva,

[1] On the 16th of April the count showed the figures of 9,130,000 red cells; the objective signs of cyanosis were not accentuated.
[2] *Deut. Arch. für klin. Med.*, 1889, p 426.

fungoid state of the gums, frequent vertigos without loss of consciousness and a tendency to hemorrhages. In one of these patients, the liver and the spleen were hypertrophied and one noted diffused pains in the bones. Unfortunately a count of the blood cells was not made; we sought out the patients to complete the observation on this subject but they had died recently.

What should one conclude from the facts which we have just presented? There is, among the different chronic cyanoses in which differentiation has not been made as yet, one class entirely apart, characterized by a predominant symptom, excessive polycythemia and one can attribute to this polycythemia an entire series of troubles which one could scarce explain otherwise. These troubles consist of, to repeat them briefly: the venous system in such a state of filling that one never sees a stream of blood of such energy until one carries out venesection on these patients; in crises of vertigo originating in the ear without true lesions of the ear, accompanied by vomitings which often end in hemorrhages. In these patients we note habitually a very definite and at times marked increase in the volume of the liver and of the spleen.

As far as the pathogenicity of the polycythemic cyanosis is concerned we can now do nothing but advance hypotheses. It does not seem to us that a peripheral stasis alone could explain it. We have carried out blood counts on patients with asystole as M. Malassez has done who suffered for a long time from a cyanosis particularly persistent.

The highest count never exceeded 6,000,000 cells. On the other hand it is difficult to record the loss of serum as the exclusive cause, for with our patient the liquid excreted equaled the liquid taken in and the polyuria which was noted (3 liters) corresponds to the thirst.

For our part we would be inclined to believe that there was a functional hyperactivity of the hematopoietic organs, as the excessive size of the liver and spleen proves. This hyperactivity is not present in all patients suffering from chronic cyanosis. We have in this particular, thanks to the kindness of Dr. Legroux, carried out blood counts on two small patients suffering from the blue disease caused by congenital lesion of the heart. In one case the count showed 4,550,000 red cells and in the other 7,200,000 red cells. In the last case the spleen was enlarged.

We think then that it is not correct to consider chronic cyanosis as the result of causes entirely mechanical and that one should in a goodly number of cases, keep in mind the possible alternation of the hematopoietic organs. It has been known for a long time that in some congenital lesions of the heart, the cyanoses appear at very variable periods, frequently when the subject is not subjected to any overwork and, we know that there are, as they say, late cyanoses. It is possible that the idea of polycythemia will account for, one day or the other, these different forms which up to the present have not been explained.

* * *

Sir William Osler

William Osler was born at Bond Head, Ontario, Canada, in 1849, the son of the Reverend Featherstone Lake Osler, who had settled in Canada in 1837. William Osler's early education was obtained at the Weston School, and in 1867 he entered Trinity College, Toronto, with a leaning towards theology. After a short time, however, he abandoned theology and entered the Toronto Medical School. Two years later he entered McGill University, where he graduated in 1872.

After two years in Europe, Osler was professor of the Institutes of Medicine at McGill for ten years, then Professor of Medicine at the University of Pennsylvania for five years and, in 1889, was called as professor of medicine in the newly founded Johns Hopkins Medical School. In 1904 he was called to Oxford as Regius Professor of Medicine and in 1911 was created a baronet. He died in 1919.

No physician exercised a greater influence upon the English-speaking medical world of his time than did Osler. A master clinician, an inspiring teacher, a forceful speaker and fascinating writer, he was a true leader of men. Endowed by Nature with charm of personality, buoyancy of spirit, a heart full

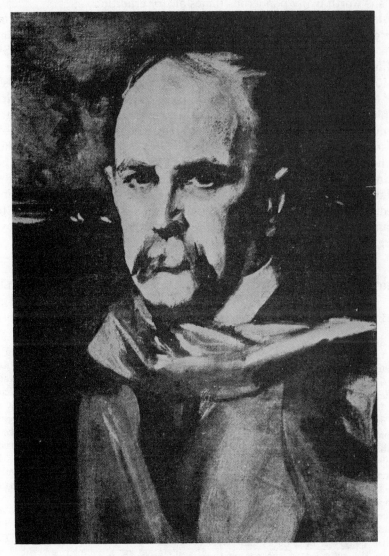

Sir William Osler (1849-1919)

The head of Osler from Sargent's famous painting *The Four Doctors* in the Welch Library of the Johns Hopkins University

of kindness and charity, and a total stranger to envy and malice, he was the ideal of what a great and good physician should be. Living his last years in the shadow of the World War, which cost him his only child, one of his first public activities after the establishment of peace was to assist in sending food supplies to the starving population of Vienna.

Osler's interests were manifold and, apart from his technical writings, he made numerous contributions of permanent value to medical history. Osler's historical writings, which were sound in scholarship and written in a chaste and charming style, called forth the remark of Sudhoff that "An essay of Osler's is worth many ponderous tomes of dry erudition."

Osler's *Principles and Practice of Medicine,* which first appeared in 1892, is the greatest textbook on the subject in our time. It went through nine revisions during his lifetime and was translated into French, German, Spanish, and Chinese. Osler was the editor of *Modern Medicine,* which appeared first in 1910, and was the founder of the *Quarterly Journal of Medicine.* Osler was one of the earliest investigators of blood-platelets, studied erythema multiforme, multiple telangiectasis, and, in 1903, described chronic cyanosis with polycythemia and enlarged spleen. The latter disease is sometimes referred to as the Vaquez-Osler disease or Osler's disease, but Osler himself wrote concerning it, "The priority of description rests with Vaquez and if a name is to be associated with the disease it should be that of our distinguished French colleague."

Harvey Cushing's *"Life of Sir William Osler,* which appeared in 1925, immediately became a classic and ranks as one of the greatest of medical biographies in the English language. A brief but charming biography by Edith Gittings Reid, *The Great Physician,* appeared in 1921.

CHRONIC CYANOSIS, WITH POLYCYTHAEMIA AND ENLARGED SPLEEN: A NEW CLINICAL ENTITY*

By William Osler, M.D., Professor of Medicine in Johns Hopkins University

* * *

ANALYSIS OF THE CASES

Six of the patients were males and three females. All were in the middle period of life, the youngest thirty-five years and the oldest fifty-three years. There was nothing in the occupation or in the station of life of any moment. The features may be considered in detail.

CYANOSIS. Naturally this attracted most attention and has been the feature which has led to further investigation. As is usual in all forms of cyanosis, it is most marked about the face and hands, but in Dr. Lowman's case and in both of my patients the skin of the entire body was of a dusky blue. When first seen the suffusion of the conjunctivae and the prominence of the eyes, as in Case I., may add to the startling appearance of the patient. The cyanosis is more intense in cold weather, and is aggravated by any existing bronchial catarrh. On bright, clear days, with but little moisture in the air, it may lessen greatly as in Case I. The period

Am. J. M. Sc., 1903, CXXVI, pp. 196-201.

over which the cyanosis has been noticed varies from ten years (Case V.) to three or four years (Case I.). While constant, as a rule, it may vary greatly in intensity. In Case II. the patient usually came in very deeply cyanosed, the condition aggravated, no doubt, by the vomiting and the loss of liquids, but after a few days, when the bowels were moved, the color became less intense; but I saw this patient only the other day, some six weeks after the attack of nausea and vomiting and he was intensely cyanosed. There is no respiratory distress with the cyanosis. While the skin looks full and tense and the face and hands bloated, yet marked dilatation of the larger superficial veins is not noted. On close examination of the skin, many fine, dilated venules are seen.

BLOOD. The viscidity is greatly increased. All observers have remarked not only upon the unusually dark, but upon the thick and sticky character of the blood drop. An extraordinary polycythemia is a special feature of the affection. The maximum blood count was 12,000,000 per c.mm. in Cabot's second case. In eight of the cases the count was above 9,000,000 per c.mm., and in the ninth (Case IV.) it was 8,250,000 per c.mm. There have been no measurements of the red blood corpuscles. The statement is made that in the polycythemia of congenital heart disease the red blood corpuscles are smaller than in that of high altitudes. The percentage of hemoglobin has been high, ranging to (in Case V.) 165. Usually the range has been from 120 to 150. In Case IV. it is stated to have been above the scale. The specific gravity of the blood in Case V. was 1080, and in Case II. it ranged from 1067 to 1083. In eight of the cases the leucocyte count ranged from 4000 in Case I. to 20,000 in Case VI. As a rule, in the majority of the cases it has been below 10,000 per c.mm. In Case II. on one admission the count reached 30,000 per c.mm.

SPLEEN. In seven of the nine cases the spleen was enlarged. In four of these the enlargement may be termed great, reaching nearly to the navel. In Case VI. there was no note. In Case II. it was not enlarged.

The liver was enlarged in Case V.

URINE. In seven of the cases a trace of albumin was noticed, with hyaline, sometimes granular, casts. In Cases V. and VII. there was no note on the urine. The specific gravity was usually low.

PIGMENTATION OF THE SKIN. As might be expected from the prolonged existence of the cyanosis, the skin was noted to be pigmented in several of the cases (II., III., IV., VII., IX.).

SYMPTOMS. The symptoms have been very varied. Most of the patients have complained of headache, weakness and prostration. Headache was a prominent symptom in four cases, vertigo in four, constipation in four, pains in back and abdomen in three cases. Attacks of nausea and vomiting were a special feature in Case II., and are mentioned as present in one case. Fever was not noticed in any of the cases. The pulse was noticed to be of high tension and the vessels sclerotic. There was no oedema of the skin. The torpor, mental and physical; the sensation of fulness in the head, with headache, vertigo, and in some cases nausea and vomiting, remind us of the symptoms to which mountain climbers and aeronauts are subject. Three of the cases were fatal. In Case IV. the patient died in collapse after a few hours of drowsiness. In Case VI. the patient died comatose, with cerebral hemorrhage. In Case IX. the patient

became drowsy and died in coma. The autopsy in Case IV. showed the heart to be about normal, moderate emphysema of the lungs, with cyanosis and oedema and moderately enlarged spleen. In Case VI. there was passive congestion of all the viscera and hemorrhage from the middle meningeal artery. In Case IX. there was hypertrophy of the left ventricle, with congestion of the brain.

REMARKS. *Chronic cyanosis,* a common enough feature in clinical work, is met with:

1. In organic disease of the heart, particularly in congenital malformation, in chronic myocardial and tricuspid lesions in children and adults, and in cases of adherent pericardium.

2. In certain diseases of the lungs, particularly emphysema, and in long-standing pulmonary tuberculosis of the fibroid type. Practically there are only two conditions in which patients walk into the hospital or into our consulting-rooms with extreme cyanosis, congenital heart disease and emphysema.

3. In the methaemoglobinaemia of chronic poisoning with coal-tar products, as antipyrin and acetanilid, etc. In this condition, too, the patient may startle one by the markedly cyanotic appearance.[1]

There are a good many people whose normal condition is one of great fulness of the blood vessels of the skin, so that in cold weather there may be marked cyanosis of the ears and of the face. We all know the stout, hearty, full-blooded man with rubicund face —the type which has been well described by Clifford Allbutt in his *Lane Lectures*—a common one among draymen and in men of that class, who live much in the open air and who drink freely. In them cyanosis, though not necessarily present, may be very marked in the face and hands when the temperature is low. As a rule, the peripheral circulation is active and the normal condition is a vivid hyperaemia of the skin associated with dilatation of numerous small venules.

Cyanosis, local or general, indicates one

[1] I am sorry I have not got a blood count in a case of this sort. As a rule, there is anaemia; in a remarkable case which I saw with Dr. T. R. Brown, the haemoglobin was only 50 per cent. Unfortunately no count was made of the red blood corpuscles. In the case of a physician with extreme cyanosis from long-continued use of antipyrin, a blood count was made, and I remember that the red corpuscles were not above normal, but I have not the actual figures.

fact—diminished oxygenation of the blood corpuscles. In the deepest cyanosis of the ear or of the finger-tip the blood count may not be above 5,000,000 per c.mm. Only recently Dr. Futcher examined for me the blood of a red-faced, short-breathed Englishman, whose skin seemed fairly bursting with blood and whose fingers and ears were quite cyanosed. The red blood corpuscles were only just above 5,000,000 per c.mm. In the local cyanosis of Raynaud's disease the blood count may be very little above the normal. I have a patient at present in the wards in whom the blood count from the cyanosed foot ranges from 4,500,000 to 6,500,000; the count from the ears about 5,500,000 (Dr. Briggs). A few weeks ago, in Dr. Brayton Ball's wards of the New York Hospital, I saw an interesting case of coma (which turned out to be due to a fracture of the skull) with the most intense localized cyanosis in the fingers of one hand active, vivid red hyperaemia of the fingers of the other hand, and normal-looking blood distribution in the ears. The count, very kindly made for me by Dr. N. B. Foster, was practically normal and the same in all three situations. Contrariwise, the anomaly may be present (though I must say it is rare of a red face and general superficial hyper-aemia with a very low blood count. During this session there has been under my care in Ward E a patient with what we have termed anaemia rubra. With a blood count of about 2,000,000 per c.mm. from ear-tip or finger-tip, he was as red as a beet, and it was not until his blood had fallen to nearly 1,200,000 that he began to present a typical picture of pernicious anaemia. On admission, with his blood at a little above 2,000,000, and look-ing the healthiest patient in the ward, he had nucleated red blood corpuscles. In the cyanosis of emphysema and the ordinary forms of heart disease, the number of red blood corpuscles per cubic millimetre is not, as a rule, much increased, and rarely reaches the limit of polycythaemia, which, as sug-gested by Cabot, may well be placed at 7,000,000. Occasionally most extraordinary cyanosis occurs in adherent pericardium, as in a case reported by me (*Archives of Pediatrics,* 1896) and in the case reported by Lorrain Smith and McKisack (*Transactions Pathological Society,* London, 1902). In the latter the blood count was 6,000,000.

Polycythaemia. There are two classes of polyglobulism—*relative,* in which the condi-tion is due to a diminution in the quantity of the plasma of the blood, and *true,* in which there is an actual increase in the number of blood corpuscles. Much work has been done of late years on the subject. Relative poly-cythaemia is very common. It may be caused by a deficient amount of fluids in-gested, which possibly may be the cause of polycythaemia of the newborn; more fre-quently it is caused by loss of liquids, either by (*a*) sweat; (*b*) diarrhoea (by far the most common); (*c*) increased dieuresis. (*d*) In another group of cases there is loss of liquids by secretion or transudation, as in narrowing of the pyloris with dilatation of the stomach, and in the constant loss of liquids from the blood in recurring ascites. It is interesting to note that in some of these cases the poly-cythaemia is of a high grade and may persist for months or even for years. It is not neces-sarily associated with cyanosis, as in cases of dilated stomach and in diarrhoea. There is also a toxic polycythaemia described in poisoning by phosphorus and carbon mon-oxide, which, too, is probably relative. The polycythaemia of vasomotor disturbances, such as has been determined by Becker, Thayer, and others after the cold bath and after violent exercise, also comes in this class. Where the much-discussed polycythaemia of high altitudes should be placed is by no means certain. While a number of observers hold that there is new-formation, the lack of oxygen acting as a stimulus, others believe that it is relative, and due to increased elimination of fluids from the body, or that it is entirely due to a large number of cor-puscles in the peripheral circulation. Others, again, think it is entirely due to the effects of decreased atmospheric pressure. The microcytes, poikilocytes, and nucleated red blood corpuscles point to new-formation, but the question is still under discussion.

True Polycythaemia. Vaquez and his pupil, Quiserne (*Thèse,* Paris, 1902), limit to this class the condition in which with an increased formation there is a continued increase in the number of red blood corpuscles in the cir-culating blood. It is met with where there is difficulty in proper aeration of the blood, as in high altitudes, or in heart disease, con-genital and otherwise; and also in the obscure cases of the form here under consideration. The polyglobulism is regarded as a mode of adaptation to the new conditions and a sort of functional reaction of the organism. Belonging to this group is the polycythaemia so readily studied in congenital heart disease, and described by Krehl, Gibson and others. The figures often reach as high as 8,000,000 or 9,000,000, rarely so high as in the form discussed in this paper.

It is by no means easy to offer a satisfactory explanation of the polycythaemia with cyanosis here under consideration. It does not seen possible to connect it in any way with the moderate grade of enlargement of the spleen, and yet there are one or two observations in the literature which are of great interest in this connection. Rendu and Widal (*Bull. et mem. Soc. med. des hôpitaux*, 1899, 3 s. xvi, 528) report the case of a policeman who had an attack of vomiting without apparent cause, with dyspnoea. The temperature was normal. Red blood corpuscles, 6,200,000; leucocytes, 6000. This count gradually diminished. On examination, skin subicteric; cyanosis of face and hands marked, to a less degree all over the body. A tumor, evidently the spleen, reaching from diaphragm to iliac crest. Eventually ulcers developed on tongue and the liver became enlarged. Autopsy: Spleen adherent to diaphragm, fibrous on section, and filled with caseous masses.

Moutard-Martin and Lefas (*Société des hôpitaux*, 1899) have also reported a case of a woman, aged forty-nine years, with pain in the left hypochondriac region, emaciation, no ascites, no cyanosis, with enlarged spleen, slight albuminuria. The red blood corpuscles were 8,200,000, the leucocytes, 31,428. At the autopsy the spleen weighed 750 grammes and contained large caseating nodules.

With our imperfect knowledge of the physiology of polycythaemia it would be premature to discuss at any length the pathology of this remarkable group of cases. We need:

1. A careful study of all forms of chronic cyanosis with polycythaemia, particularly those associated with heart disease and emphysema. (It is to be noted that the cases here reported have the highest blood count on record, much higher than the average in congenital heart disease or in dwellers at great altitudes.)

2. A more accurate study of the blood in this class of cases—the volume, the viscosity, the state of the plasma and the serum, the amount of haemoglobin, the specific gravity, and the diameter of the corpuscles. As increased viscosity of the blood, with resulting difficulty of flow, seems the most plausible explanation of cyanosis, it is especially important to test the viscosity by accurate physical methods and to determine the relation of the number of corpuscles to the viscosity of the blood.

3. The relation of the splenomegaly to the cyanosis and polyglobulism should be carefully observed. It may not be anything more than the effect of the chronic passive congestion.

Future investigation will determine whether we have here in reality a new disease. The clinical picture is certainly very distinctive; the symptoms, however, are somewhat indefinite, and the pathology quite obscure.

LEUKEMIA

John Hughes Bennett

John Hughes Bennett was born in London in 1812 and received his early education at Exeter. He began the study of medicine in 1829 as an articled pupil to Mr. Sedgwick, a surgeon of Maidstone, but in 1833 went to Edinburgh to pursue his medical studies. While still a student of medicine he published two papers, and in 1837 received the degree of M.D. with highest honors. He then spent two years in France and two years in Germany making microscopic studies and following clinical instruction. In 1841, he returned to Edinburgh and began to teach at the University. At Edinburgh, Bennett taught first histology and later pathology, becoming pathologist to the Royal Infirmary. In 1848 he was unanimously elected Professor of the Institutes of Medicine. He was a candidate for the Chair of Practice of Physic in 1855 but was unsuccessful. He died at Norwich in 1875.

Bennett had a remarkably clear and penetrating mind and was a very forceful and polished speaker. His histrionic abilities were of the highest order. Although unusually brilliant in *extempore* speaking, he always wrote out his lectures to avoid becoming diffuse. He insisted upon practical teaching, upon the routine use of the microscope, upon method and precision in studying patients. He was bent upon reforming medical teaching and was very outspoken in both his praises and his criticisms.

Bennett published several works on medicine and physiology and more than one hundred papers on medical subjects. In 1845 he published his best-known paper on a *Case of Hypertrophy of the Spleen and Liver in which Death took place from Suppuration of the Blood*. This was a case of leucocythemia or leukemia, one of the earliest recorded, although he did not at that time discern its true character.

TWO CASES OF DISEASE AND ENLARGEMENT OF THE SPLEEN IN WHICH DEATH TOOK PLACE FROM THE PRESENCE OF PURULENT MATTER IN THE BLOOD*

Case 2.—Case of Hypertrophy of the Spleen and Liver, in Which Death Took Place from Suppuration of the Blood

By John Hughes Bennett, M.D., F.R.S.E., Lecturer on the Practice of Physics, and on Clinical Medicine, Pathologist to the Royal Infirmary, &c.

The very remarkable case about to be related derives unusual interest from its similitude in almost every respect to the one just recorded by Dr. Craigie. Although the most evident lesion during life was enlargement of the spleen, I agree with him in thinking that the immediate cause of death was owing to the presence of purulent matter in the blood, notwithstanding the absence of any recent inflammation, or collection of pus in the tissues.

Numerous authors have asserted† that they have found purulent matter in the blood, independent of any local inflammation, or abscess from which it could have been derived. Hitherto all such statements have been very vague, because no measures were taken to ascertain whether this purulent-looking matter was really pus. We frequently meet with animal fluids, which, to the naked eye, resemble pus, although when more minutely examined, they are found deficient in the peculiar cells that characterize that morbid product. Gulliver more especially has pointed out that the colorless coagula which form in the heart and large vessels break down mechanically or by maceration into a pulpy mass of liquid. The purulent collections in

the heart and blood-vessels described by Goodsir and Andral are considered by him to be fibrin softened in this manner. Again, we know that the blood in a state of health contains a number of colourless corpuscles, which closely resemble those of pus. Hence has latterly arisen the opinion, that the isolated pus corpuscles described by some authors were only the normal structures of the blood, and that, where after death large intra-vascular collections of purulent-looking matter were discovered, they were caused by softened colourless coagula.

In the present state of our knowledge, then, as regards this subject, the following case seems to me particularly valuable, as it will serve to demonstrate the existence of true pus, formed universally within the vascular system, independent of any local purulent collection from which it could be derived. The individual entered the clinical ward of the Infirmary under Dr. Christison, to whom I am indebted for the history of the case. The *post mortem* examination, and microscopic investigation were conducted with the greatest care by myself, and my assistant Mr. Morris.

John Menteith, aged 28, a slater, married, admitted into the clinical ward of the Royal Infirmary, February 27, 1845. He is of dark complexion, usually healthy and temperate;

* *Edinburgh M. & S. J.*, 1845, LXIV, 413-423.
† Bichat, Ribles, Gendrin, Andral, Bouillaud, Carswell. &c. &c.

states that twenty months ago he was affected with great listlessness on exertion, which has continued to this time. In June last he noticed a tumour in the left side of the abdomen, which has gradually increased in size till four months since, when it became stationary.

It was never painful till last week, after the application of three blisters to it; since then several other small tumours have appeared in his neck, axillae, and groins, at first attended with a sharp pain, which has now, however, disappeared from all of them. Before he noticed the tumour he had frequently vomited in the morning. The bowels are usually constipated, appetite good, is not subject to indigestion, has had no vomiting since he noticed the tumour. Has used chiefly purgative medicines, especially croton oil, has employed friction with a liniment, and had the tumour blistered.

At present there appears a large tumor, extending from the ribs to the groin, and from the spinal column to the umbilicus, lying on the left side. It is painful on pressure near its upper part only. Percussion is dull over the tumour; pulse 90; states that for three months past he has not lost in strength. There is slight oedema. To have two pills of iodide of iron morning and evening.

March 15. Died suddenly in the morning.

Sectio Cadaveris. March 19th, (four days after death.)—Externally the body presented a considerable prominence of the ensiform cartilage and false ribs on both sides. The abdomen was contracted; considerable dulness on percussion on left side, which had previously been marked out by a line formed with nitrate of silver.

No ascites or oedema of the limbs.

Blood.—The blood throughout the body much changed. In the right cavities of the heart, pulmonary artery, *venae cavae, vena azygos* external and internal iliac veins, and many of the smaller veins leading into them, it was firmly coagulated, and formed a mold of their size and form internally. In the cavities of the heart and *vena cava* the blood when removed was seen to have separated into a red or inferior, and a yellow or superior portion. The red portion was of a brick-red colour; it did not present the dark purple smooth and glossy appearance of a healthy coagulum, but was dull and somewhat granular on section, and when squeezed readily broke down into a grumous pulp. The yellow

portion was of a light yellow colour, opaque and dull, in no way resembling the gelatinous appearance of a healthy decolorized clot. When squeezed out of the veins as was sometimes accidentally done where they were divided, it resembled thick creamy pus. In some portions of the veins the clot was wholly formed of red coagulum. In others it was divided into red and yellow. In a few places the yellow formed only a streak or superficial layer upon the red, or covered the latter with spots of various sizes. Whether this coagulum existed in all the veins could only have been ascertained by a complete dissection of the body. It was seen, however, that the femoral veins, after passing under Poupart's ligament, were empty and perfectly healthy as far down as the Sartorious muscle.

The external and internal iliac veins were full and distended. The azygos, both axillary and jugular, veins, were full, also the longitudinal, the lateral, and other sinuses at the base of the cranium and veins ramifying on the surface of the brain.

In this last situation some of the veins appeared as if full of pus, whilst others were gorged with a dark coagulum. In the aorta and external arteries were a few small clots resembling those found in the veins. These vessels, however, were comparatively empty. The basilar artery at the base of the brain was distended with a yellow clot.

Vessels.—The arteries and veins themselves were perfectly healthy. Although carefully looked for, in no place could thickening or increased vascularity be observed. Nowhere was the clot adherent to the vessels, but, on the contrary, readily split out when an accidental puncture was made in them.

The *spleen* was also enormously enlarged with simple hypertrophy. It was of a spindle shape, largest in the centre, tapering towards extremities. It weighed seven pounds twelve ounces. It measured in length fourteen inches; in breadth, at its widest part, seven inches; and in thickness, four and a-half inches. Toward its anterior surface was a yellow firm exudation, about an inch deep, and three inches long. The peritoneum, also covering a portion of its anterior surface, was thickened, opaque, and dense over a portion about the size of the hand.

* * *

The *lymphatic glands* were everywhere much enlarged. In the groin they formed a large cluster, some being nearly the size of a small hen's egg, and several being that of a walnut. The axillary glands were similarly affected. The bronchial glands were not only enlarged, but of a dark purple colour, and in some places black from pigmentary deposit. The mesenteric glands were of a whitish colour, some as large as an almond nut. A cluster of these surrounded and pressed upon the *ductus communis chole-dochus.* The lumbar glands were of a greenish yellow colour, also enlarged, forming a chain on each side, and in front of the abdominal aorta, more especially at its bifurcation into the iliacs.

Microscopic Examination.—The yellow coagulum of the blood was composed of coagulated fibrin filaments, intermixed with numerous pus corpuscles, which could be readily squeezed out from it when pressed between glasses. Where the yellow coagulum was unusually soft, the corpuscles were more numerous and the fibrin was broken down into a diffluent mass, partly molecular and granular, partly composed of the debris of the filaments broken into pieces of various lengths. The corpuscles varied in size from the 1/80th to the 1/120th of a mill. in diameter; they were round, their cell-wall granular, and presented all the appearance of pus corpuscles. That they really were such was proved by the action of water and of acetic acid, the former of which caused them to swell and lose their granular appearance, whilst the latter dissolved the cell-wall and caused a distinct nucleus to appear.

* * *

3. The next question is, how were these corpuscles formed? Pus has long been considered as one, if not the most characteristic proofs of preceding acute inflammation.

But in the case before us, what part was recently inflamed? There was none. Piorry and others have spoken of an inflammation of the blood, a true hematitis; and certainly if we can imagine such a lesion, the present must be an instance of it. But it would require no laboured argument to show, that such a view is entirely opposed to all we know of the phenomena of inflammation. Without entering into this discussion, however, I shall assume it to have been satisfactorily demonstrated that we can form no idea of this process, without the occurrence of exudation from the blood-vessels, and that, consequently, the expression inflammation of the blood is an error in terms.* A moment's reflection will make it evident that all our ideas of, and facts connected with inflammations are associated with some local change in the economy. The constitutional disturbances connected with it we invariably ascribe to phlegmasia or fever, which pathologists hitherto have always separated. Unless, therefore, it could be shown that inflammation and fever were like processes, we must conclude that the alteration of the blood in this case was independent of inflammation properly so called.

But can we explain the production of pus independent of inflammation? We reply in the affirmative. The corpuscles of pus arise in a blastema formed of *liquor sanguinis.* This fluid, when exuded through the blood-vessels, does not thereby in itself undergo any change. If any circumstances, therefore, should arise by means of which it could be separated from the red corpuscles within the vessels, there is no reason why these pus cells should not be formed in it. Facts point out that this coagulation happens not unfrequently.

* See the writer's *Treatise on Inflammation,* p. 52.

Rudolf Ludwig Karl Virchow

Rudolf Virchow was born at Schievelbein, Pomerania, in 1821, and attended the gymnasium at Koslin. In 1839 he began the study of medicine at the Kaiser Wilhelm Akademie, a training school for army surgeons, and in 1843 received his degree at the University of Berlin. He became at once an assistant at the Charité Hospital and two years later became Prosector of Anatomy and Assistant in Froriep's clinic. In 1847 he became Privatdozent in Pathology and entered upon the great work of his life. From this period onward, Virchow seems to have been interested in only two things—the study of pathology and the study of economic and social problems.

In 1848 Virchow was sent to investigate an epidemic of typhus in Silesia. His report contained not only a severe criticism of the hygienic regulations in that province, but also a harsh indictment of the prevalent social injustices. Virchow's report and his continued agitation for reforms caused trouble with the Prussian government and he was dismissed from his position at Berlin. His fame as a pathologist, however, was already established, and he was imme-

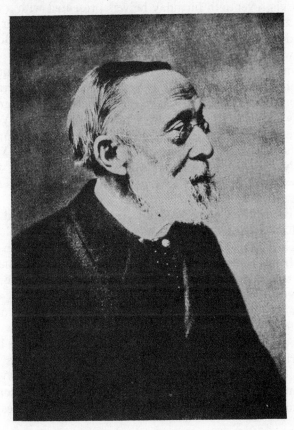

RULOLF LUDWIG VIRCHOW (1821-1902)

diately called to Würzburg as Professor of Pathology and director of their newly founded pathological institute. Virchow remained at Würzburg seven years and while there completed the work which formed the basis of his cellular theory.

In 1858, after the death of Professor Hemsbach, the faculty of the University of Berlin petitioned the government to offer the chair of pathology to Virchow. In spite of bitter political antagonism, the position was offered to him and he accepted on condition that the government build him a new pathological institute. Soon after his return to Berlin the first edition of his *Cellular-pathologie* appeared, in which he laid down his famous dictum, *Omnis cellula a cellula*. No other book on pathology, not excepting Morgagni's *de sedibus,* has exerted such a profound influence on medical thought.

In Berlin Virchow's life was one of unparalleled activity. He collected an amazing museum of pathology, was very active in teaching and research, and found time to enter political life, serving in the Reichstag for thirteen years. Here he was the leader of the Radical party and an active, outspoken, and persistent opponent of Bismarck. Students flocked from all over the world to attend his lectures and every year brought new honors and fresh testimonials of esteem. On his seventieth birthday he was presented with a gold medal by the Emperor and his eightieth birthday took on the character of a national holiday, with delegates from all over the world assembling in Berlin to do him honor. Virchow died the following year, 1902.

Virchow's name, which was of Slavic origin, was very frequently mispronounced by his contemporaries, as it is by succeeding generations. At the banquet in honor of Virchow's eightieth birthday, Lister greeted him as "Wirtchow," while Bacceli addressed him as "Wirtscho." When Professor Harnack addressed him as "Professor Fircho," the "f" being pronounced soft as in "fair," the "ch" like "k" but with the German guttural, Virchow smiled very pleasantly and turning to a colleague who was nearest to him at the table, said it was the first time he ever remembering hearing his name properly pronounced at a public function.

Virchow's conceptions of pathology were not only profound but extensive. In Berlin he had unrivaled opportunities for observing pathological material and the pathologist of today sees few pathological conditions unknown to Virchow. One of his many interesting original observations is that of leukemia, which he first correctly interpreted. This observation was made the same year as that of Bennett, which led to a discussion of priority in the discovery. Virchow wrote as follows on the discussion: "It is incorrect, as some recent authors state, to divide the discovery between Bennett and me, as simultaneous. Neither Bennett nor I observed the first case of leukemia. We both, however, had the opportunity almost simultaneously to observe such a case. Bennett considered his case one of pus formation in the blood (pyemia) and six years after I had immediately described mine as white blood (leukemia) and only after I had gradually developed this doctrine in a series of articles, did he accept this doctrine."

WHITE BLOOD*

Among the older authors we find here and there observations concerning blood, which had so completely lost its color that it was compared to milk, chyle, mucus (pituita) or pus (Haller, *Elem. physiol.* 1760, Tom. II, p. 14-16). The description of the following case will confirm this apparently fabulous report.

History of Illness (Extract from the history of the ward.) Marie Straide, cook, 50 years old, was admitted on March 1st into

* *Neue Notizen a. d. Geb. d. Nat. und Heilk.* Weimar, 1845, XXXVI, 151.

the Charité. According to her story, she noted one year ago a great loss of weight, a marked swelling of the lower extremities and some of the lower portion of the abdomen, severe coughing with copious mucous expectoration and pains in the abdomen. During the following summer the cough disappeared, but in autumn it returned worse than before, accompanied by an extraordinarily severe diarrhoea, which exhausted her very much. The latter then improved while the cough increased anew without however being accompanied by pain in the chest. Finally during the last 8 days frequent and at times bloody stools appeared.

On admission there was a slight edema of the lower extremities, abdomen full, distended, fluctuating, marked enlargement and moderate tenderness of the spleen; frequent persistent cough with copious rolled up *spulis*, râles over the chest; appetite and tongue good; pulse 17; urine scanty; great exhaustion (Infusio Colombo c. tinct. Cascarill. et. Tinct. theb.). In a few days her condition was improved; the diarrhoea decreased until finally constipation appeared (Inf. Rhei. c. Mell. Tarax.). Fresh diarrhoea (Emuls. comm. c. Aq. Amygd. amar.). Then followed from time to time epistaxis, which gradually became worse; the pulse scarcely exceeds 70 beats in the minute (Acid. sulphur.).

In April edema of the sacral region, urine scanty and dark (Inf. Calami et Scillae c. Extr. Absinth. et Spir. Nitr. aeth.). No increase in diuresis, epistaxis slight, condition good except for a recurring tendency to diarrhoea (Scilla discontinued). In May more severe pains in the splenic area; constipation (Baths Elect, lenit.).

Suddenly in the night from the 7th to the 8th of June, very severe epistaxis. (Ice cold compresses over the forehead, injections with alum solution, drinks containing sulphuric acid. On the 14th of June again a light bleeding, which soon subsides. From this time the condition is satisfactory except for a furuncular eruption on the nose and between the thumb and index finger of the right hand.

On the 6th of July fresh severe epistaxis, which lasted until the 8th in spite of cold compresses and drinks containing sulphuric acid. Then great exhaustion, marked edema of the lower extremities, inability to walk. On the 15th of July reddening and painful swelling of the skin in several places on the palmar surface of both hands, upon which small blisters formed, filled at first with a clear fluid then with a purulent fluid, which opened themselves after the use of poultices. An incision made on July 21st and much discolored pus evacuated. A few days later similar eruptions between the fingers (Cataplasm, soap baths). On the 29th of July suddenly fresh severe diarrhoea (Inf. Ipecac. c. Tinct. theb.). Rapid loss of strength. Death on the morning of July 31st.

Section, twenty-eight hours after death. On the palmar surfaces of both hands, incisions with a discolored blackish appearance which lead to superficial collections of pus which do not penetrate the fascia, and contain a reddish, fairly firm pus. The adjacent lymphatics and blood-vessels normal. In the muscular tissue of the flexors some old cysticercus cysts. In the veins above, some discolored blood, scarcely red, poorly clotted. As I examine the further course of the blood-vessels; there was everywhere in them a pus-like mass. The heart which was somewhat enlarged, was completely filled with large, loosely adherent, greenish, yellowish white coagula, which crumbled under the fingers, could be easily smeared about, not at all adherent to the walls and which looked exactly like firm pus. The same mass was also present in the aorta and in the larger arteries, in the veins of the body cavities and in the veins of the lower extremities. The veins with thin walls presented the picture of canals filled with pus, and the surface of the heart and of the meninges, whose veins were markedly dilated by their pus-like contents, seemed to be covered with solid yellowish white cords. Everywhere this material lay free in the vessels, whose walls appeared in no way changed. —All organs very pale. The lungs normal except for a slight bronchial catarrh. The intestinal tract was normal except for a succulent appearance of the mucosa. Liver not essentially changed. Spleen enormously hypertrophied, nearly a foot long, very heavy, dark brownish red, with a board-like firmness, crumbling, on cross-section pale and apparently composed of a homogenous tissue, the cut section slightly shiny, wax-like thus resembling a large ague cake. Kidneys normal, only in the calices and pelvis a large mass of uric acid stones, which were partly small particles the size of hemp-seeds, partly in masses the size of cherry-stones covering the papillae and partially filling the upper portion of the ureter. Genitalia normal.

The yellowish white almost greenish mass which the vessels contained and which was collected from the heart and the great vessels, weighed nearly 2 pounds. When removed with some care, it had the appearance of a loose coagulum; but when placed on an uneven surface it fell apart from its own weight and the microscope showed no adherent masses of fibrin. Except for a very few red blood corpuscles, the greater part was composed of colorless or white corpuscles, which also occur in normal blood, namely, small, somewhat irregular protein molecules, larger, nucleated, fatty capsules without nuclei and granular cells with a round, horseshoe-shaped or clover-like nuclei or with several bowl-shaped, distinct nuclei. The larger of these cells had a slightly yellowish appearance. The relationship between the pigmented and colorless blood corpuscles seemed to be reversed here from that of normal blood, for the white corpuscles seemed to be the rule and the red corpuscles a kind of exception. When I therefore speak of *white blood*, so I mean in fact a blood, in which the proportion between the red and white blood corpuscles is reversed, without noting any mixture of strange chemical or morphological elements.

Considerations.—It would be premature to draw sweeping conclusions from a single case, so unusual, since the relationships are not so clear and the history of the disease contains so many gaps. The older accounts of white blood are quite useless because a microscopic examination is lacking. They relate mostly to loss of blood by hemorrhage, fasting, etc.* Now it is further known since *Hippocrates*, that the diseases of the spleen rather frequently produce nose-bleed. In the present case we can construct the following etiological succession: splenic tumor, nose-bleed, white blood. The cough and the diarrhoea whose persistence was due to no local lesions, as well as the hydropic infiltration, the nose-bleed, the furuncular and pustular eruption, are all to be considered as signs of the increasing dissolution of the blood. The excessive formation of white blood cells (lymph corpuscles) cannot be explained by increased flow of chyle, since chylification is not especially active in the presence of diarrhoea, but this all speaks for an increased formation of the cells in the blood, which suggests a great mass of small molecules (primary nuclei). Also it should not be overlooked that the cough, diarrhoea and edema were present before the nose-bleed, and that the remarkable change of the red blood into white blood could have taken place only quite recently, because the blood from the epistaxis was always red.

I have presented these observations only

with the purpose of showing that such a remarkable and unusual case may have so many relationships with further investigations and so many suggestions for explaining other questions, but it remains a rather uncertain subject for positive proof and conclusion so long as it itself remains unexplained. A case very similar and very well described, has appeared in the recent literature but unfortunately the history of the patient's illness is lacking.

Lautner (Report of the Proceedings of the Pathological Institute of the Vienna General Hospital, directed by Prof. Rokitansky in the *Zeitschr. der. k.k. Ges. der Ärzte zu Wien 1845* Ba. IS 488) describes the following: general pyema in a locksmith aged 33. Decubitus over the sacral area, which extends into the subcutaneous tissue. The skin of the lower abdomen, back and posterior portions of the thighs covered with small abscesses varying in size from a pea to a groschen and filled with pus. The pleura at the base of the right lung covered with a delicate membraneous coagulated exudate. In most of the pulmonary vessels, large and small, there were yellowish-green *tough* coagula, in the posterior lower portion of the right lung there were two consolidated areas, large as walnuts. In the cavities and great vessels greenish yellow coagula. The liver is three times its normal size, weighs 6 pounds 4 ounces, pale, fatty, very anemic and dampened with a cloudy pus-like fluid; the spleen 5 pounds 14 ounces, heavy, course, and on the upper third of the convex surface shows a deposit the size of a walnut, partly pale yellow, partly dark red reticulated and fibrinous: the rest of the parenchyma brownish red, infiltrated like bacon. The lymph glands around the pancreas are swollen to the size of a pigeon's egg, pale reddish and infiltrated with a sticky greenish yellow pus-like fluid. Both kidneys pale, infiltrated with a cloudy discolored fluid.

It does not seem to me demonstrated that this case should be included under the term pyemia, although the purulent infiltration of the different parts seems to speak for this. The complete identity of the colorless blood corpuscles (lymph corpuscles) with pus, makes a conclusion uncertain even when the microscope is employed, as the case I described shows. The usual composition of the blood in pyemia is entirely different, not because of the presence of pus in the blood but

---

* The most convincing citation is in Haller (l.c.) : *De scorbutica post plurimam jacturam albus sanguis exiit.* As authority Matini is cited, *dé aneurysm.* p. 33 : I have however searched in vain for the citation in *Ant. Matani de aneurysmaticis praecordium morbis,* Francof. et Lips., 1766.

because it is characterized by a liquefaction and destruction of the blood components and by a tendency to the production of exudates with purulent metamorphosis. It seems to me clear that in this case there is not a purulent infiltration into the tissues but a purulent change in the exudate which has taken place through a stasis of the blood in various places. The course of the hepatized places in the lung and spleen seem to prove this; the abscesses of hands probably had a similar origin as well as the purulent eruption on the nose and hands. In the case from Vienna there were apparently no hemorrhages and yet there was white blood and a splenic tumor. Recent observers (*Donné*) has ascribed to the spleen an especial rôle in the transformation of red corpuscles into white. According to observations made repeatedly the loss of the spleen produces no similar condition: could a diseased spleen have such an effect? Is nose-bleed in splenic disease caused by a similar blood disease? Perhaps my report will cause one of the Viennese physicians to publish the history of the patient's disease in greater detail: I should consider myself lucky to have aided science with a new, and it seems to me, not unimportant fact.

Dr. Virchow

PURPURA

Amatus Lusitanus

Amatus Lusitanus, who described himself as Johannes Rodericus Castelli albi Lusitanus, was born in 1511 at Castel Branco, near Coimbra in Portugal.

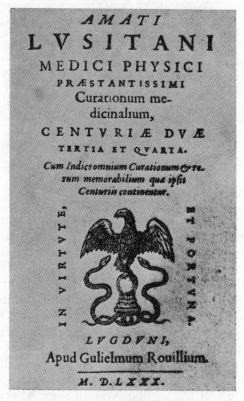

Title page of the Curationum medicinalium of
Amatus Lusitanus (Lyons, 1580)

His parents were Jews who had been forcibly converted to Christianity and
there is evidence that he was baptized in this faith. He studied medicine at
Salamanca and, after graduation, practiced in various parts of Portugal, but
left Portugal in 1535 because of religious persecution and went to Antwerp.
Six years later he was called as professor of medicine to Ferrara. Later he
removed to Ancona, but while there came under the suspicion of the authorities, his property was confiscated, and he sought safety in flight. In 1558 he
moved to Saloniki where he placed himself under the protection of a Turkish
Sultan and openly avowed his adherence to the Jewish faith. The date of his
death is uncertain but he was known to be alive in the year 1561.

Amatus Lusitanus is best remembered for his commentary on the works
of Dioscorides. His *Curatonum medicinalium centuriae septem* went through
many editions and in this work we find one of the earliest descriptions of
purpura under the title of *Morbus Pulicaris Absque Febre.*

* * *

THE SEVENTIETH CURE WHICH HAS TO DO WITH EXANTHEMATA WITH A DISEASE CALLED FLEA-LIKE WITHOUT FEVER APPEARING IN A BOY.*

A boy referred to me without fever, completely covered with spots which were similar to flea bites and which moreover were
quite black. So that it was quite astonishing
that such a disease should be without fever,
or without anxiety of mind or should break
out on the skin with injury to the boy himself. But we know nothing to be difficult
with a firm courage so that he pass by mouth
the material forming an abscess, as Galen

* Lusitanus, Amatus, *Curationum medicinalium
Centuriae duae tertia et quarta,* Lyons, Rouillium,
1580, p. 254.

mentions in his seventh book of Aphorisms,
in exposition fifty-five, so we need not be
surprised. Besides with two days of evacuations this boy passed much blood, black,
fetid, foul smelling and escaped sound and
free. But we saw other lads feverish with
the legs broken out or who were marked
with a disseminated eruption which moreover appeared suddenly and soon they became sound, or when malign pestilential fevers raged, as may be seen from what has
been said.

Lazarus Riverius

Lazare Rivière, better known as Lazarus Riverius, was born in 1589 in
Montpellier, received his doctor's title there in 1611, and in 1622 became professor of medicine, holding his chair until his death in 1655. Although the name
of Rivière does not occur in Garrison's *Introduction to the History of Medicine*
and references to him are rather sparse in medical literature, yet he enjoyed
a tremendous reputation in his time. While professor at Montpellier, he refused
calls to the Universities of Toulouse and Bologna, and was famous throughout
all Europe as a great physician and teacher. He was the first professor to introduce the study of chemistry into the medical school of Montpellier, and
was noteworthy for his insistence that certain metallic salts be used in the
treatment of disease. The works of Riverius enjoyed a great vogue in England,
largely perhaps because of the popularity given them by the English translations of Nicholas Culpeper.

Nicholas Culpeper, whose translation follows, was one of the interesting
physicians of his time and is usually described as a physician, astrologer, and

quack. He was born in 1616, son of a Sussex clergyman and a scion of the
famous house of Culpeper. At the age of eighteen, he went to Cambridge, where
he squandered most of his patrimony but acquired a good knowledge of Greek
and Latin. Originally intended for the church, he refused to become a clergyman and studied medicine instead, although his persistence in this course led

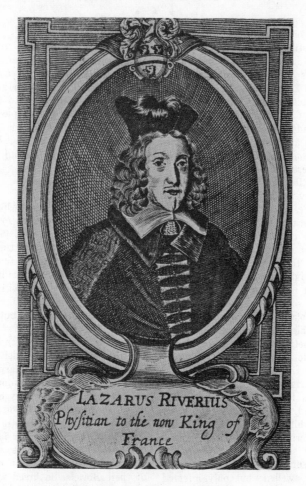

LAZARUS RIVERIUS (1589-1655)
Frontispiece to the *Practice of Physick, translated by*
Nicholas Culpepper 1668

his grandfather to disinherit him. In 1640 he set up as astrologer and physician
in great Red Lion Street, Spitalfields. He soon had a large practice in the East
End of London, was beloved by his poor neighbors, and was engaged in constant controversies with those who accused him of quackery and plagiarism. In
the midst of these activities he also found time to write numerous books, seventeen being published during his lifetime, while, according to his wife, he left
seventy-nine unpublished works at the time of his death. One of his books, *The
English Physician,* was the first book on medicine published in the American
Colonies. He died of phthisis at the age of thirty-eight. On his deathbed he
said to his wife, "I did by all persons as I would they should do by me. I never

gave a patient two medicines when one would serve. Farewell dearest, I am spent."

SECTION III*
OF PESTILENTIAL FEAVERS

* * *

But there is one Symptome proper and peculiar to a pestilential Feaver, which doth not happen in other Feavers; *viz* Purple Specks or Spots on the whole Body, but especially in the Loins, the breast and back, like unto Flea-bitings for the most part; which the Italian Physitians name *Peticulae* or *Petechiae;* and these Feavers which have these symptoms are commonly named *Purpuratae* or *Petechiales,* Purple or Spotted Feavers. For these Purple Spots do not appear in all Pestilential Feavers; but when they appear, they are a most certain Sign of a Pestilential Feaver: Now we call them Purple Spots, because they are for the most part of a Purple colour. Yet they are many times of a violet colour, Green, Blewish or Black, and then they are far worse, and do signifie greater Malignity. And although these Spots are for the most part like Flea-bitings: yet they appear somewhat greater: So as to represent those black and blew marks which remain after whipping, and then they are worse. And sometimes they are very large, and possess whole Members, and a great part of the Body, *viz.* the Arms, Thighs and Back, and then the parts appear tainted with redness; which in a few hours oftentimes vanisheth away, and then returns again, as it were by Fits, whilest the Feaver undergoes its Fits or Exacerbations, wherein the blood boiling doth not send forth its thinner Exhalations to the surface of the Skin, by which the Skin is not swelled; but only infected with a red color. Oftentimes notwithstanding, by these Ebullitions the Skin is in divers parts puffed up with a certain redness: and makes certain broad and soft Tumors in the Skin, which in a few hours vanish away, and are commonly called Ebullitions of the blood. In these and the aforesaid, there is always some Malignity, but so light, that it threatens no danger; unless in the progress of the Disease it prove more intense. Now the Spots

* Lazarus Riverius, *The Practice of Physick, in Seventeen several Books,* Translated by Nicholas Culpeper, London, Streator, 1668, p. 613.

aforesaid like Flea-bitings do differ from those Pushes, which are wont also somtimes to appear in these Feavers, and are mentioned by *Hypocrates* in *Epidemeis,* which have an Head, and are a kind of Tumors, which come sometimes to Suppuration or Exulceration. But the Purple Spots, have (as was said) no eminence or Head, and were unknown to the Antients, being described only by latter Physitians of after ages.

* * *

Finally, Purple spots like Flea-bitings, called by latter Physitians *Peticulae* or *Petechiae,* are the proper and peculiar Signs of a Malignant Feaver. For they are found in no other kind of Feaver; forasmuch as they do arise from a vitious quality of the Blood or other Humors, joyned with Malignity. Yet there do appear in other Diseases, spots very like unto those aforesaid, but springing from a far different Cause; *viz.* From the over thinness of the Blood, which being exagitated by the heat or the expulsive faculty, does sprout forth of the Capillary Veins into the Skin. These spots, are wont for the most part to appear in such as have some Flux of Blood, because the Blood in such is more thin and watery: and also in Splenetick persons, in such as have the Jaundice and old obstructions of the Bowels, and (in a word) in all such, who by reason of the weakness of their Bowels, do breed watry blood and are apt to fall into a Cachexy. For in such persons, the Blood being made thinner than ordinary, sometimes flows out at the Nose, sometimes at some other part, and sometimes it comes out of the Capillary Veins into the Skin; where being retained, it looseth its own colour, and becomes either blewish or black or light red, and causeth great variety of spots; which notwithstanding are very far different from the spots of Pestilential Feavers, and do argue nothing but the watry thinness of the Blood and weakness of the Liver.

Paul Gottlieb Werlhof

Paul Gottlieb Werlhof was born at Helmstedt in 1699, the son of the professor of law at the University. He was a very precocious youth, much interested in languages and natural science, and entered the University of Helmstedt as a student of medicine in 1716 at the age of seventeen. At the University he was a favorite pupil of Meibohm and Heister and through their influence became especially interested in anatomical and pathological studies.

Werlhof began practice in a small town, Peine bei Hiedesheim, and after several years of practice received his doctor's degree at Helmstedt in 1723. Two years later he removed to Hanover and in 1760 he became first physician

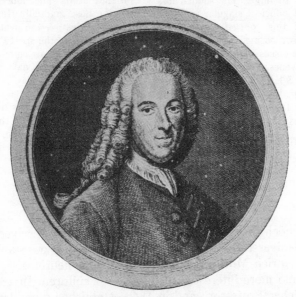

PAUL GOTTLIEB WERLHOF (1699-1767)
From Werlhof's *Opera omnia* (Hanover, 1775)

to the court. He remained in Hanover the rest of his life and declined several appointments to chairs in various German universities. He died in 1767.

Werlhof was one of the most highly respected physicians of his time. "His clientele extended from Moscow to Rome," and the respect in which he was universally held is shown by his election to membership in the Royal Society of London and in many other scientific societies. He was a master of Latin and of most of the European languages, mastering the Swedish language at the age of sixty-four. He also composed poetry and hymns, one of the latter being for many years frequently sung in German churches. He was an intimate friend of Albrecht von Haller, whose dual interest in science and poetry drew the two men together.

Werlhof in 1735 described quite accurately purpura haemorrhagica, since known as morbus maculosus Werlhofii. The following translation is from his *Opera omnia* published at Hanover in 1775.

XLVIII
MORBUS MACULOSUS HAEMORRHAGICUS*

An adult girl, robust, without manifest cause, was attacked recently, towards the period of her menses with a sudden severe hemorrhage from the nose, with bright but foul blood escaping together with a bloody vomiting of a very thick extremely black blood. Immediately there appeared about the neck & on the arms, spots partly black, partly violaceus or purple, such as are often seen in malignant smallpox. The sudden loss of strength, & the sufficient singular sufficient characteristics of this *spotted hemorrhagic disease* being known to me, of which indeed there is only little discussion in medical writings, we forbade venesection. I gave the first day acid remedies & largely nitric, which while they did not help, but enduring continually both hemorrhages from the nose & indeed by vomiting, weakness & chilliness of the ex-

tremities, with a small & most rapid pulse, a more efficient aid was needed; moreover the number of the spots increasing & surrounding completely both of the eyes, the back of the nose & the skin around the mouth & chin, with a livid black color, like marked from bruises. I gave twice hourly in any mixture desired half a drachm of Peruvian bark, adding alternately liquid laudanum of Seydenham four drops. The same day the bleeding from the nose gradually stopped, the vomiting became less, & the next day ceased; no lesions recurred; the spots daily, at the same time with a livid appearance assumed first a very ruddy then a pale color, and disappeared the seventh day, so that also the pulse now recovered the normal character of its beat, her strength was nearly restored to its normal state, although the menses do not appear at the proper time, which is by no means unusual following hemorrhages.

*Werlhof, Paul Gottlieb, *Opera omnia,* Hanover, Helwing, 1775, p. 748.

Eduard Henoch

Eduard Henoch was born in Berlin in 1820 and received his doctor's degree at the University of Berlin in 1843. He became assistant in the clinic of his uncle, Heinrich Moritz Romberg, the famous neurologist, but gradually became more and more interested in diseases of children. In 1858 he became "ausserordentlicher Professor" and in 1860 established a children's clinic and began to devote himself exclusively to the study of the diseases of children. The publication of his *Clinic of Abdominal Diseases* (1852), *Essays on Children's Diseases* (1861), and his *Lectures on Pediatrics* gave him a great reputation. His description of *Henoch's Purpura* was published in 1874.

Henoch was for a generation the acknowledged leader of German pediatricians. He resigned from his chair in Berlin in 1893, lived first at Meran, and then at Dresden, where he died in 1910 at the advanced age of ninety.

Henoch's *Lectures on Pediatrics* is one of the classic textbooks in that specialty. He was not only a clever writer but a gifted teacher. Personally he was a very charming man, a brilliant conversationalist, charitable and kind. Schlossmann, who was an intimate friend for many years, says "I have never heard from his mouth an unkind word or a derogatory opinion regarding anyone, he showed an active interest in every honest effort, he followed attentively and critically every advance in pediatrics, but his decision was always cautious and mild."

CONCERNING A PECULIAR FORM OF PURPURA
(From a Lecture before the Berlin Medical Society the 18th of November, 1874)
By Prof. Henoch*

Gentlemen: Six years ago I called your attention through the description of a case, to a peculiar symptom complex which we will consider to-day. This case was published in the Transactions of our Society for the 14th of October, 1868. Since this forms only the starting point of my communication to-day

sleep, and were accompanied with great sensitiveness of the abdomen in the region of the transverse colon, which was markedly distended and gave on percussion a light tympanic tone. Moderate fever was present, which never exceeded 38.6 C. After 5 days this symptom disappeared, but after an in-

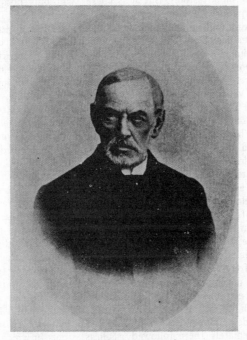

Courtesy of the "Münchener Medizinische Wochenschrift"

EDUARD HENOCH (1820-1910)

and as this society has changed since that time, I cannot assume that those present have all read of this case, so please allow me to refer to it again briefly. It concerns a 15 year old boy who, as the result of indigestion, developed a gastroduodenal catarrh with a slight icterus. A few days later, pain developed in the finger joints of both hands without any swelling. After a few days an extensive purpura appeared on the abdomen and on the skin of the thighs, and very soon several intestinal symptoms appeared, intense colic, vomiting and very black stools. The pains were exceedingly severe, prevented

* *Berl. Klin. Wchnschr*, 1874, XI, 641-643.

terval of 3 days, a relapse occurred, which took its course in the same manner, again extensive purpura, the green vomitus, severe colic, fever, and, after a week, again convalescence. In the same manner the symptoms reappeared in the following weeks 3 times; the stools were during this time constantly bloody, either quite black, as in melaena, or orange-colored, mixed with blood clots of various sizes. In all, 5 attacks took place, which with the intervals, occupied a period of 7 weeks. Concerning the therapy which we used at that time, I know only that preparations of opium were the most efficient, while purgatives seemed to be harmful; they intensified the pain and caused an increased blood content in the stools. The boy, moreover, became entirely healthy and developed into a strong young man.

Two years passed before I succeeded in observing again a similar case. Now, however, I have 4 cases, including the first one. The *second,* which was in the practice of my Colleague *Bergius,* I observed in March 1869. The patient, a 4 year old boy, showed dysenteric symptoms, pain in the abdomen, tenesmus, scanty, often bloody stools. But at the same time a purpura with large spots appeared on both elbows and on the thighs. Three days later, after castor oil and calomel had been given, improvement followed, but new purpuric spots developed on the scrotum and praepuce. A few days later diarrhoea reappeared with streaks of blood and severe colic, then followed constipation and then everything disappeared except later crops of purpura. Whether there were in this case also signs in the joints, I cannot say. This case lasted in all three weeks.

The 3rd case appeared to me in February 1873 and concerned a 12 year old, quite healthy girl. It was related to me that for 8 days pains like those of rheumatism appeared in the extremities, soon then pains and swellings, especially in the joints of the hands and the feet, accompanied by a slight fever, while the heart was free. A few days later an extensive purpura developed on the abdomen and the lower extremities. A terrible colic developed, which prevented the child from sleeping and made necessary the use of chloral hydrate. Immediately there followed repeated vomiting and numerous diarrhoeic stools, which contained a bloody admixture but no pure blood. This case was distinctive, in that the entire complex of symptoms disappeared about 5 or 6 days and then again a recurrence of the same symptoms followed. This continued for 4 weeks, during which four such attacks followed, until a final recovery appeared. There was no therapy. During convalescence, a disturbing occurrence took place in which through an error in the apothecary shop, the mixture of chloral hydrate and morphine which was ordered contained too large a dose of morphine and, as a result, there was an 18 hour morphine poisoning with convulsions and stupor, which, however, did not cause a reappearance of the disease.

The 4th case finally appeared to me in the summer of 1873 and concerned the 13 year old daughter of one of our most esteemed colleagues, which, in the absence of the father, I treated, with Dr. *Menzel.* This girl was formerly absolutely healthy, except that she showed constantly the peculiarity that her heart beat irregularly, without one being able to find anything abnormal in it. In the summer of 1872, rheumatic pains appeared in both feet of this girl, later in the right hip. These symptoms disappeared soon and the heart remained free. The first attack of our disease appeared in July 1873, a year after these pains. When I came, the disease had already lasted 5 weeks; at first there were pains of a rhumatoid nature in the joints of the hands and the joints of the feet, but without any swelling, soon afterwards purpura in the lower extremities, and moderate fever, and immediately also the intestinal symptoms, anorexia, vomitus, colic; the stools were normally formed masses, but heavily mixed with blood; urine normal. There were then in these 5 weeks, 3 attacks, followed by intervals of 8 or 9 days. The third and last attack was without fever, while in the first one there was a little fever present. We allowed an ice bag to lie upon the abdomen, which helped the child very much; the symptoms soon disappeared, the purpura faded. Suddenly the pains again appeared in the left arm and right elbow joint and on the night following (from the 23rd to the 24th of July) the child had a terrible colic, vomited a green material twice and had 4 orange colored stools in which there were numerous blood clots. The pulse seemed to me on the following day quite regular—104, temperature normal, tongue clean. We applied again the ice bag and gave an emulsion of the oil of sweet almond in ice cold milk. The 25th there was a dark, thin stool; the pulse became irregular and registered only 60. Until the 30th, complete health, then there were several spots of purpura appeared and the disease seemed ended until September, when the 5th attack occurred, so the father wrote me, and more severe. Since then, as far as I know, no new attack has been observed.

If one compares these 4 cases, it is seen that they agree remarkably. Characteristic for all, is the combination of *purpura* and the striking intestinal symptoms, which are present in the form of *colic, tenderness of the abdomen, vomiting* (often a green mass), and in *hemorrhages.* Also the *rheumatoid* pains, and, in one case, the swelling, which was absent in the second case. Characteristic, furthermore, is the appearance of these symptoms in *attacks,* with an interval of 8 days or more, so that in the usual cases 3 to 7 weeks passed before the process cleared up; in the last case, indeed, more than 3 months. The rheumatoid pains in the joints which have already been described, practically always preceded these attacks, which may be in the joints of the finger, the hand, the foot, sometimes also in the swelling, which however is not associated with a marked loss of movement as in rheumatism. So far as the purpura is concerned, this forms sometimes large ecchymoses (in two cases) and in the other two (1st and 3rd), they had only characteristic form of circumscribed, small, light red spots like those of an exanthema, which were not above the level of the skin, and did not disappear on pressure. These spots occurred particularly on the abdomen, on the region of the genitalia and in the lower extremities; I have never observed them in the face. As far as the intestinal symptoms are concerned, we have here in all cases repeated vomiting; then the colic, preventing sleep and causing the child to scream; and distention of the abdomen; in one case indeed tenesmus; further, the stools are either pure blood or streaked with blood. The fever was always quite moderate (not above 38.6 C.), sometimes was entirely absent and always showed a remarkable irregularity.

HEMOPHILIA

John C. Otto

John C. Otto was born in 1774 near Woodbury, New Jersey, the son, grandson, and great-grandson of physicians. His grandfather had emigrated from Germany in 1752 and served as a medical officer in the American Army during the Revolutionary War. John C. Otto graduated at the College of New Jersey (Princeton) in 1792, and received his M.D. degree from the University of Pennsylvania in 1796. As a student he worked in the office of Benjamin Rush, becoming the favorite pupil and friend of this eminent physician. On the death of Dr. Rush, in 1813, Otto succeeded him as Physician to the Pennsylvania Hospital.

Otto had experience in several epidemics of yellow fever and, in 1798, suffered, himself, from the disease. In 1832 he was chosen chairman of a committee to take measures against the yellow fever epidemic in Philadelphia. After the epidemic, the city presented him with a handsome silver pitcher in recognition of his services. He died in 1844.

Otto's account of hemophilia, written in his twenty-ninth year, contains a description of all the essential clinical features of this disease. Otto noted that the disease is transmitted in families and that males are subject to it and females are not, although the latter transmit it to their male children. The name hemophilia was given to this disease by Schönlein, but it was Otto who brought it to the attention of the medical world.

ARTICLE I
AN ACCOUNT OF AN HEMORRHAGIC DISPOSITION EXISTING IN CERTAIN FAMILIES

By John C. Otto, M.D., of Philadelphia*

About seventy or eighty years ago, a woman by the name of Smith, settled in the vicinity of Plymouth, New Hampshire. and transmitted the following idiosyncrasy to her descendants. It is one, she ob·erved. to which

a kind disposition to heal; and, in others, cicatrization has almost been perfect, when, generally about a week from the injury, an hemorrhage takes place from the whole surface of the wound, and continues several

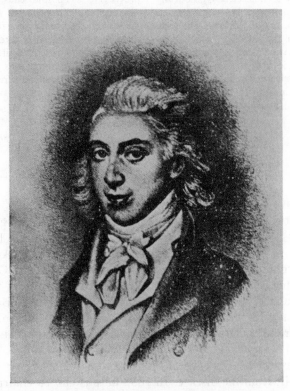

Courtesy of the "Bulletin of Johns Hopkins Hospital"

JOHN C. OTTO (1774-1844)
From lithograph in College of Physicians, Philadelphia

her family is unfortunately subject. and has been the source not only of great solicitude. but frequently the cause of death. If the least scratch is made on the skin of some of them, as mortal a hemorrhage will eventually ensue as if the largest wound is inflicted. The divided parts, in some instances, have had the appearance of uniting, and have shown

* *The Medical Repository,* 1803, Vol. VI, No. 1, pp. 1-4.

days, and is then succeeded by effusions of serous fluid; the strength and spirits of the person become rapidly prostrate; the countenance assumes a pale and ghastly appearance; the pulse loses its force, and is increased in frequency; and death, from mere debility, then soon closes the scene. Dr. Rogers attended a lad, who had a slight cut on his foot, whose pulse "was full and frequent" in the commencement of the complaint, and whose blood "seemed to be in a high state of effervescence." So assured are the members of this family of the terrible consequences of the least wound, that they will not suffer themselves to be bled on any consideration, having lost a relation by not being able to stop the discharge occasioned by his operation.

Various remedies have been employed to restrain the hemorrhages—the bark, astringents used topically and internally, strong styptics, opiates, and, in fact, all those means that experience has found serviceable, have been tried in vain. Physicians of acknowledged merit have been consulted, but have not been able to direct anything of utility. Those families that are subject to certain complaints are occasionaly relieved by medicines that are inefficacious when applied to others; and family receipts are often of greater advantage in restoring them, than all the drugs the materia medica offers for that purpose. A few years since the sulphate of soda was accidentally found to be completely curative of the hemorrhages I have described. An ordinary purging dose, administered two or three days in succession, generally stops them; and, by a more frequent repetition, is certain of producing this effect. The cases in which the most powerful, and apparently the most appropriate remedies have been used in vain, and those in which this mode of treatment has been attended with success, are so numerous, that no doubt can exist of the efficacy of this prescription. The persons who are subject to this hemorrhagic idiosyncrasy, speak of it with the greatest confidence. Deceptions may take place from accidental coincidence; but when a complaint has often occurred, and been almost uniformly fatal without the administration of a certain medicine, and has constantly yielded when it has been given, scepticism should be silent with regard to its utility. Nor should our inability to account for the fact, upon the theory and principles we have adopted, be conceived a sufficient reason for disbelieving it. An attempt to explain the mode of operation of this valuable remedy might give birth to much speculation. As the affection has been attended with mortality, and there is generally a disposition to give relief as early as possible. experiments have not been made with the other neutral salts to learn their comparative effect; nor have medi-

cines been tried whose operation might be supposed to be similar. The prescription being known to the whole family, application is rarely made to a physician, and when it is, it is rather with a view of directing him how to proceed, than of permitting him to make a series of trials and observations which might be at the hazard of the life of the patient. The utility of the sulphate of soda cannot arise from its debilitating effects, since it has been found serviceable when the previous depletion has been great, the strength much exhausted, and the system has evidenced symptoms of direct debility. Perhaps time will elucidate its mode of operation, and some general principles may be developed that may be applied to advantage in restraining ordinary hemorrhages; but reasoning upon what has been discovered to be useful in idiosyncracies, and applying it to the general constitution of human nature, must certainly be vague and productive of occasional evil. In every case, however, a doubtful remedy is preferable to leaving the patient to his fate. The sulphate of soda has constantly succeeded when administered; but the prescription being in the possession of the Shepard family the descendants of Smith, and the cases that have been attended by physicians not being very numerous, it is impossible to ascertain the various states of the system in which it has been given, or to form any correct conclusions respecting its manner of acting. No experiments have been made on the blood to discover if any or what changes take place in it.

It is a surprising circumstance that the males only are subject to this strange affection, and that all of them are not liable to it. Some persons, who are curious, suppose they can distinguish the bleeders (for this is the name given to them) even in infancy; but as yet the characteristic marks are not ascertained sufficiently definite. Although the females are exempt, they are still capable of transmitting it to their male children, as is evidenced by its introduction, and other instances, an account of which I have received from the Hon. Judge Livermore, who was polite enough to communicate to me many particulars about this subject. This fact is confirmed by Drs. Rogers and Porter, gentlemen of character residing in the neighbourhood, to whom I am indebted for some information upon this curious disposition.

When the cases shall become more numerous, it may perhaps be found that the female sex is not entirely exempt, but, as far as my knowledge extends, there has not been an instance of their being attacked.

The persons subject to this hemorrhagic disposition are remarkably healthy, and, when indisposed, they do not differ in their complaints, except in this particular, from their neighbours. No age is exempt, nor does anyone appear to be particularly liable to it. The situation of their residence is not favourable to scorbutic affections or disease in general. They live, like the inhabitants of the country, upon solid and nutritious food, and when arrived to manhood, are athletic, of florid complexions, and extremely irascible.

Dr. Rush has informed me, he has been consulted twice in the course of his practice upon this disease. The first time, by a family in York, and the second, by one in Northampton county, in this state. He likewise favoured me with the following account, which he received some years since from Mr. Boardley, of a family in Maryland, afflicted with this idiosyncrasy.

"A. B. of the State of Maryland, has had six children, four of whom have died of a loss of blood from the most trifling scratches or bruises. A small pebble fell on the nail of a forefinger of the last of them, when at play, being a year or two old: in a short time, the blood issued from the end of that finger, until he bled to death. The physicians could not stop the bleeding. Two of the brothers still living are going in the same way; they bleed greatly upon the slightest scratch, and the father looks every day for an accident which will destroy them. Their surviving sister shows not the least disposition to that threatening disorder, although scratched and wounded. The father gave me this account two days since, but I was not inquisitive enough for particulars."

VI. KIDNEY DISEASES

Salicetti, the great Italian surgeon of the thirteenth century, in his dissections observed chronic nephritis as his description of dropsy with contracted kidneys ("durities in renibus") clearly shows. There follows a long silence unbroken for five hundred years until Dekkers and Cotugno in the eighteenth century noted albuminuria without, however, fully appreciating its significance. Their observations were followed by the remarkable studies of Wells and of Blackall, both of whom noted the association of dropsy, albuminuria, and contracted kidneys and by their accounts paved the way for later investigators. It was, however, the masterly observations of Bright who studied this association with such painstaking accuracy and delineated it with such compelling

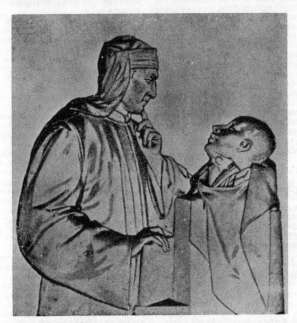

WILLIAM DE SALICETO (1210-1280)
From the bas-relief of Ferranini at Piacenza

fidelity, that painted the picture of a new disease to which, by universal consent, the term of Bright's disease has been applied. Little has been added to Bright's masterly portrayal of the clinical picture of this malady although the studies of a century have greatly enriched our knowledge of this disease.

William de Saliceto

William de Saliceto, also called Salicet and Guglielmo Salicetti, was born about 1210 at Piacenza and was sometimes referred to as Magister Placentinus, after his birthplace. Very few details of his life are known. He was probably a

Vlcera uesice ⁊ renũ

Siue post apata cũ ꝑuertuũt ad saniē: aut ex materia acura vlcerãte: aut pꝛusione ⁊ casu ⁊ suũt i vesica ⁊ emũctoꝛiꝭ in renibus.

Signa vlceꝛ i loeꝭ illis dictꝭ sũt emissio sanguinis vel saniei. sꝫ distinguiꞇ. Si aũt vlcꝰ fuerit i vesica sanies egrediꞇ añ vriñã et sentiꞇ doloꝛ circa veficam et femur et vrina cũ difficultate emittꞇ. Si aũt vlcꝰ suerit i emũctoꝛiꝭ vel renibꝰ sanies emittꞇ mixta cũ vriña: sꝫ siuenerit a renibꝰ sentiꞇ doloꝛ in gñto nodo spine versus caudã ⁊ i doꝛso. Si aũt suerit i emũctoꝛiꝭ erit doloꝛ circa parte i ꝗ ē vlcus. Est ⁊ aliꝯ distinctio vel differẽtia vlceꝛ renũ ⁊ vesice: qꝛ qꝺ egrediꞇ ex vlceribꝯ renũ est frustꝯ carnis paruũ: sꝫ ex vlcere vesice egrediũꞇ coꝛtices vel squame ⁊ doloꝛ vesice ē foꝛtioꝛ ꝗꝫ ē i renibꝯ ⁊ i ambobus la teribꝯ renuꝭ ē grauitas. Quãdo vero vlcꝰ ē i mea tu mꝰ inter veficã ⁊ renes distingueꞇ ꝑ doloꝛ loci vel punctoẽꝭ vel coꝛpoñeꝭ signoꝛ dictoꝛ i vlcere renum ⁊ vesice.

Cura vlceꝛ renuꝭ ⁊ viaꝭ vriñaliuꝭ ⁊ vesice ē eadē ⁊ cũ eisdē sit medicinꝯ Mundificeꞇ locꝯ saniosus aut exconaꞇ cũ aꝗ mellis: aut cũ aꝗ mellis decoctõꝭ se. endiuie lactucaꝭ ⁊ cicoꝛee: cipi ⁊ ciceris sacerdotalꝭ ⁊ se. altce vl mal ue iꝗ dissoluanꞇ trocisci alkekẽgi vice vna: ⁊ vice alio siañt troeisco ꝯsolidatiois ꝺ bolo ꝗ sic fiũt. R. boli armeni carabe añ. ʒ. v. acaꝛie b.kaustic: gũmi arabici iꝑoꝗstidꝭ añ. ʒ. i. ꝝ se. apij iusquã añ. ʒ. i. fiat trocisei cũ succo berberis vel mirtiloꝛ: ⁊ sit pꝺus vniuseuiusꝗ. ʒ. ij. daꝭ cũ aqua decoctiõꝭ mirtiloꝛ vel berberis aut sumat: ⁊ scias ꝙ trocisci alkekẽgi ꝯsolidãt ⁊ icarnaꞇ cũ istis.ꝭꝭ quos iuen eꝭ bono mõ i antidotario.

Si aũt vlcꝰ fuerit i vesica vel sanies iniciaꞇ cũ lacte ꝑ siringã coliriũ albũ qꝺ sic fit. R. ceruse sar cocole thuꝛꝭ gũmi: amilij opij sanguinis dꝛaconis añ. ʒ. i. fiat coliria cũ mucillagic al tee: ⁊ facta ꝑmo mudificatoẽ cũ aꝗ mellis itroinissa ivesicã cũ firingã: ⁊ inimicaꞇ ēt cũ siringa itra vesicã sepe cũ mun dificatõis aꝗ sicuũ vel mellis. Scias hic ꝙ ea ꝗ iniciuntur cum siringa in vesicam magis valent in vlceribꝯ vesice ꝗꝫ ea que sumuntur per os: ⁊ ea que sumuntur per os magis valẽt i vlceribꝯ re nũ ⁊ meatuũ. Unganꞇ loca extrinseca ꝗ suut sup vulnera cũ vngẽtis dissolutiuis qꝛ multũ adiuuãt sicut vnguetũ de cerusa aut vnguetũ fuscũ ⁊ epla stra ēt multũ ꝑseruunt. Bibat vinuꝭ stipticum ru beũ cũ aqua mellis limpbatũ vel cũ aqua sicuꝛ. Comedat lac cũ melle vel rizũ coctu cũ lacte: aut farꝭ cũ lacte aut fabã vel panicuꝭ. Comedat cũ carnes arietis vel castrati aut edi: ꝑducuꝭ ⁊ similium ꝯditas cũ lacte ⁊ puluere mirtiloꝛ ⁊ cardamo mi ⁊ cũꝰ rob aut vitellꝰ ouoꝛ. Comedat festicos auelanas ⁊ pineas mũdatas ⁊ filia.

Capltm. cxliij. de minctu saniei ⁊ sanguinis.

Ec egritudo fiꞇ aut

post casuꝭ ⁊ pcussionē aut ex comirtio ne cibi acuti sicut aleꝭ sinapis nasturtij ⁊ siliuм aut ex bumoꝛe acuto vel salso currẽte ad renes vel vias vriñaliũ. ꝓuenit aliꝗa aliꝗã a renibꝯ ⁊ partibꝯ illiꝭ. Et scias ꝙ mi ctꝰ saniei seꝗ ad minctũ sanguinis ⁊ apata rupta ⁊ vlcera: ⁊ ad excoꝛiationeꝭ viaꝭ vriñe vt dictũ ē.

Signa minctꝰ sanguinis ⁊ saniei ma nifesta sunt ex visu: sꝫ refert i distinctõe ꝑ signa vtꝛ a renibꝯ vel vesica: nã san guis ꝗ venit a renibꝯ vel chili subito venit: ⁊ mu

---

rkuum quod fit ex maluauisco ⁊ farina fenugreci ⁊ se. lini: ⁊ pinguedine poꝛci vel butiro: vel fiat em plastꝛ cũ farina fenugreci se. lini ⁊ oꝛdei ⁊ frumẽ ti mirtis ⁊ ꝓditis ⁊ coctis cũ oleo camomellino ⁊ anetino ⁊ de se. lini. Mudificeꞇ sepe cũ aqua de coctõis mãne cassie fi. ⁊ reubarbari ⁊ se. lactucaꝭ ⁊ cicoꝛee ⁊ filiuꝭ. Cũꝫ sed.iꞇ doloꝛ totꝭ ⁊ remanet grauitas tũc ꝑcipe iñrmo vt saltet sup pedes ⁊ de scedat ꝑ gradus scalaꝭ ⁊ moue doꝛsuꝭ renũ vbi ē grauitas leuiter coꝛprimedo ēt fortiter si saniē nõ inceperit mingere.

Si aũt saniē mingere iceperit: eris excusatus a fricatoꝛibꝯ ⁊ coꝛꝑessionibꝯ foꝛtibꝯ ⁊ leuibꝯ ⁊ tũc cũ minterit saniē da ei i potu mundificatiuũ vice vna ⁊ ꝯsolidatiuũ vice alia ⁊ fiat sic ꝓtinue donec facta fit ꝯsolidatio ⁊ mundificatio: sicut mudificatiuꝯ qꝺ fit ex aquã mell'in quo poniꞇ semē apij ⁊ lactucaꝭ ⁊ ciceris sacerdotalis ⁊ gũmi arabicũ qꝺ daꞇ cũ trocisꝯ. atꝩ ekẽgi ⁊ ꝯsolidatiuũ sicut electua riaꝭ de thure vel trociscos de bolo ꝗ dantur post mũdificatoẽꝭ ⁊ cũ ꝯsolidatõis ⁊ etũ alia mundifica tiua ⁊ ꝯsolidatiua ꝗ faciẽt.ꝭ.c. de vlcere renũ ⁊ ve sice. Bibat vinuꝭ limphatũ albuꝭ cũ aqua deco ctõis mellis ro. ⁊ gũmi ara. ⁊ milij folis ⁊ ameos ⁊ ciperi ⁊ ciceris sacerdotalis. Comedat carnes aia liũ ⁊ auiũ coctas ⁊ ꝯditas cum cucurbitis lactucis poꝛtulacis: aut cũ feniculo petroselino ⁊ boragi ne vel spinachijs: ⁊ ꝓdianꞇ cũ puluere specieꝭ ⁊ rob: vel cũ sinapi melle ⁊ rob. Ut taꞇ sepe lacte sto maco ieiuno i quo ponaꞇ mel vel zuchaꝭ. Ut taꞇr rizꝯ ⁊ farro ⁊ farina oꝛdei ꝓditis cum lacte amig. vel lacte capꝛino sup renes ⁊ extrinseco ponaꞇ em plastruꝭ qꝺ sic fit. R. boli armeni: mirre: mumie: thuris masticis: pulueris nucis cipꝛessi ⁊ mirtiloꝛ añ. ʒ. s. dꝛagãti gũmi arabici sang. dꝛaconis añ. ʒ iij. misceanꞇ cũ oleo de mastice ⁊ cera ⁊ extendiꞇ tur sup coꝛiuꝭ et postea cohopianꞇ ex pãno subtili valde et sumaꞇ cũ coꝛio bñ et firmiter.

Captm. cxl. de duritie in renibus.

Durities in renibus

fit aut post apa a quo resoluiꞇ subtile aut ꝙ icipit ex se: et fit ex materia gip sea: vel melãcolica vel coꝛposita ex biꝯ: ⁊ b egriꞇudo ē vterioꝛ: aliꝯ: qꝛ aut male curaꞇ: aut nullomõ curatur.

Signa duritiei i renibꝯ sunt ꝙ mino raꞇ quãtitas vriñe: ⁊ ꝙ ē gra uitas renũ ⁊ spine cũ aliquo doloꝛe: ⁊ icipit veꞇr i flari post ꞇbꝯ ⁊ fit idropicꝯ. ꝝm dies: ⁊ vt plurimũ fit talis durities post apa calidũ in renibus ⁊ post febꝛem eius.

Cura duritiei i renibus ⁊ vt fiat empla stꝛ de maluauisco dicto i.c. ante rioꝛi sup renes ⁊ doꝛsuꝭ ⁊ fiat inuctio cũ vnguẽto facto ex adipe anseris anatis ⁊ galinaꝭ ⁊ adipe re nũ yrci vel edi vel arietis liꝗ factis ⁊ mirtis cũ ce ra ⁊ oleo de camomilla: aut fiat iunctio sup renes ⁊ doꝛsuꝭ cũ medulla ossis cruꝛꝭ tauri vl'vitulli aut cerui. Bibat busi i die añ pꝛãdiuꝭ ⁊ añ cenã oꝛimel coꝛpofitũ qꝺ fit aqua decoctionꝭ ⁊ mellis vel se. maluauisci ⁊ mell'. ⁊ b ē melioꝛ. Mundificeꞇ semel i ebdomada cũ aqua decoctõis reubarbari se. mal ꝭe ⁊ altee ⁊ apij ⁊ dulcoreꞇ cũ syrupo de nenufare vel syrupo vio. Regaꞇ cũ dieta ⁊ potu vt dictũ ē i.c. supꝛaꝛi i cura apatis calidi tpe quo feb. minuiꞇ vel remouetur.

aplm. cxlj. de vlceribuꝭ in istrumẽtis. s. intra virgam. renes ⁊ emunctoꝛia.

priest, was professor at Bologna from 1269 to 1274, and later became city physician at Verona. He died in 1280.

Saliceto's books on surgery and medicine are landmarks in medical history. He wrote careful case histories of his patients, restored the use of the knife in surgery, described alcoholic tremors and kidney abscess, and pointed out the differential diagnosis between kidney stone and colic of intestinal origin. His best-known contribution, however, is his description of dropsy due to contracted kidneys, which is probably the earliest account of chronic nephritis. The following translation of this chapter on "durities in renibus" (sclerosis of the kidneys) is from the *Liber Magistri Guglielmi placentini de Saliceto In scientia medicinali*, Venice 1490.

HARDNESS IN THE KIDNEYS is produced either after an abscess from which it is gradually scattered or it begins of itself: and it is formed either from calcareous material: or from black bile or composed of both: and this illness is worse than the others: for it is either not well cured or cured by no means.

THE SIGNS of hardness in the kidneys are that the quantity of the urine is diminished, that there is heaviness of the kidneys, and of the spine with some pain: and the belly begins to swell up after a time and dropsy is produced the second day: and thus such hardness is produced after a warm abscess in the kidneys and after fever of them.

THE CURE of hardness in the kidneys is that there be made a paster of mistletoe described in the preceding chapter apply over the kidneys and back and make an inunction with an ointment made from the fat of goose, duck and hen and fat of the kidneys of a bear or of a kid or of a ram liquefied and mixed with wax and oil of camomile: or make an inunction over the kidneys and back with the bone-marrow of the leg of a bull or of a calf or of a deer. Drink twice daily before meals and before dinner a drink of vinegar and honey mixed with an aqueous concoction of barley and honey or of mistletoe berries and honey: and this is better. Purge once in the week with an aqueous decoction of rhubarb, mallow seeds, and althea and parsley and sweeten with syrup of water lily or syrup of violets. Conduct the diet and drink as described in the chapter above in the cure of hot abscess at the time when the fever is diminished or removed.

Frederik Dekkers

Frederik Dekkers was born in 1648 at s'Hertogenbrosch, Holland, and studied at Leyden under Sylvius. He graduated in 1668 and, the following year, wrote a commentary on the *Praxis* of Barbette. In 1673, he published his well-known *Exercitationes practicae circa methodum medendi* (Practical exercises in methods of treatment), and, in 1694, became professor of medicine at Leyden. Dekkers died in 1720.

Dekkers' *Exercitationes* is a curious work in which the chapters are arranged, not according to disease, but according to the remedies employed. The frontispiece of this work shows the physician with his healing wand passing among the sick, many of whose ailments the artist has depicted with startling accuracy.* Dekkers' description of albumin in the urine is found in Chapter v, "De medicamentis purgantibus," and the following translation was made from the edition of 1695 published at Leyden.

* See Frontispiece.

THE URINE IS CLEAR AND LIMPID IN CONSUMPTIVES†

I cannot pass by that the urines in phthisics and those affected with consumption are limpid & clear, especially if not boiled. Indeed I have observed these placed over a flame too soon become milky, indeed to smell like milk and to have the savor of sweet milk, indeed if a drop or so of acetic acid be

† Dekkers, Frederik, *Exercitationes practicae circa medendi methodum*, Leyden, Boutesteyn, 1695, p. 338.

added and it is exposed to the cold air, soon a white coagulum falls to the bottom without doubt cheesy particles, & oily, or buttery particles swim on the top, and now deprived of the said particles all but resembles serum & which all observers agree with me: wherefore we should conclude it to be not so much urine as chyle or limpid chyme finely dissolved or aqueous & usually too on that account to grant the men a brief life.

Domenico Cotugno

Domenico Cotugno was born at Ruvo in the province of Bari in 1736 and studied medicine at Naples. He was a diligent student of anatomy and at the age of twenty-five described the aqueduct of Cotugno and shortly afterwards the nasopalatine nerve. He also gave a description of the intestinal lesion of typhoid fever and the skin lesions of smallpox. He became professor of anatomy at Naples, achieved great fame as a physician, and became physician to the royal household. He died in 1822 at the advanced age of eighty-seven.

Cotugno's best-known work was his *De ischiade nervosa commentarius,* which was first published at Naples in 1765. In this work he attributed sciatica to a dropsy of the dural sheaths of the roots of the sciatic nerve. He studied the properties of the cerebrospinal fluid and showed that it produced no coagulum on heating. The urine of certain patients, however, he found showed a coagulum on boiling. This observation apparently is the second after that of Dekkers in which the coagulability of the urine was demonstrated.

Thus* I shall show that all the humors of the body which, when secreted naturally from the blood, are not coagulable, frequently become coagulable from serious disturbances. I shall begin with urine, which everyone knows is not coagulable but which was seen to coagulate in those experiments of our which I am about to describe.

XVII. A soldier, twenty-eight years old, was stationed for many years at mild and very damp Baiae. About the end of August he was seized with an intermittent quotidian fever, which strangely broke out in dropsy in five days. At the beginning of September he was brought to my Sanatorium and intrusted to my care. He was suffering at this

* Cotugno, Domenico, *De ischiade Nervosa commentarius,* Naples and Bologna, St. Thomas Aquina, 1775, p. 27. Translated by William Dock in *Annals of Medical History,* New York: Paul B. Hoeber Co., Inc., 1922, IV, 288.

time with immense watery swellings of his whole body, and overwhelmed by the hitherto daily attacks of fever; the dropsy seemed to increase daily, shortly before the paroxysms. The excreta were dry, there was but little urine and he was wholly cast down in mind.

* * *

But the urine flowed much less and finally the dropsical swelling seemed to grow. . . . In this case it seemed best to use cream of tartar, whose effect in provoking urine, without accelerating the pulse, I have shown in other experiments. By this remedy the output of urine was increased so that the sick man passed ten or twelve pints of concentrated urine in a night. However, since the sick man himself admitted that his drinking had been very slight, it was certain that the enormous quantities of urine were being drawn especially from water collected in the dropsy.

Although this was shown by the decrease in the distention of the body, it seemed best to settle this question by a definite experiment, heating the urine. For I had often conclusively shown that the fluid collected beneath the skin of such dropsical cadavers contained material capable of coagulation and I hoped that if the sick man passed such fluid by way of the urine, coagulation would be seen if the material which flowed out were heated; which, as I had anticipated, was proved by experiment. For with two pints of this urine exposed to the fire, when scarcely half evaporated, the remainder made a white mass, already loosely coagulated like egg albumen. Thus it was shown for the first time that urine, which no one had shown to be coagulable if from healthy people, can at some time contain a coagulable substance.

William Charles Wells

XVII. ON THE PRESENCE OF THE RED MATTER AND SERUM OF BLOOD IN THE URINE OF DROPSY, WHICH HAS NOT ORIGINATED FROM SCARLET FEVER*

By William Charles Wells, M.D., &c.

Read June 4, 1811

In the paper which I presented to this society, several years ago, on the dropsy after scarlet fever, I mentioned that the urine in that disease contains almost always the serous, and sometimes the red, matter of blood. I shall now communicate several observations, which I have made upon similar states of urine in dropsy arising from other causes.

* * *

I have examined by means of one, or other, or both, of the tests which have been mentioned, the urine of one hundred and thirty persons, affected with dropsy from other causes than scarlet fever, of whom ninety-five were males, and thirty-five females; and have found serum in that of seventy-eight, sixty of whom were males and eighteen females.

In about a third of the cases in which serum was detected in the urine, its quantity was small, the bulk of the coagulum produced by heat and nitrous acid, after remaining undisturbed twenty-four hours, being only from one-tenth to one-fortieth of that of the urine, which contained it. On the other hand, the urine, after being exposed to the heat of boiling water, in five cases, became firmly solid, and in seven became a soft solid, which separated, from the sides of the glass vial in which it had been formed, when the bottom of the vial was placed uppermost. In one of these cases the urine became solid at every trial during six weeks; in the other eleven, it was sometimes rendered only considerably turbid. In the remaining cases with serous urine, amounting to about a half of the whole number, all the distinguishable intermediate quantities of coagulated matter were formed in that fluid by heat and nitrous acid.

Urine in dropsy, when it contains serum, is often more abundant than in health. It is sometimes discharged, though not for any long time, in the quantity of six pints daily; in one person the daily quantity was for a short time ten pints. It must be mentioned, however, that a great part of my information upon this subject has been derived from the reports of the patients themselves, and their nurses in St. Thomas's Hospital.

* * *

No conclusion is to be drawn from these numbers, in regard to the comparative frequency of dropsy in the different sexes; for the whole number of male patients admitted into St. Thomas's Hospital, where by far the greater part of the cases were seen by me, is much greater than that of the female.

* * *

Urine containing a considerable quantity of serum is sometimes not distinguishable, by its appearance, from that which is healthy. Sometimes, however, it is very pale, and though abundant, and without sediment, slightly opake when cold, having a resem-

---

* Wells, William Charles, *Tr. Soc. Improve. Med. and Chir. Knowledge* London, 1812, III, 194.

blance of whey, or to water with which a little milk has been mixed. When it is scanty, and gives a sediment upon cooling. this is almost always white, cream coloured, or grey. Now and then the sediment looks like powdered chalk, or like very light curds of milk.

* * *

I have never hitherto obtained permission to examine, after death, the body of any dropsical person, whose urine had been made solid, or nearly solid, by heat. I have described, however, in the first part of this paper, the appearances which were observed, on opening the body of an old sailor, who had died dropsical after passing urine, in which there was a considerable quantity of serum; and I shall now mention what was seen in the body of another person, a soldier, forty-seven years old, who had likewise died dropsical, and in whose urine a considerable quantity of serum had been present. He had also, shortly before his death, laboured under an inflammatory affection of his chest.

The inferior lobe of the right lung was greatly inflamed, and its air cells were much compressed by effused coagulable lymph. mixed with some blood. The upper part of the diaphragm was also much inflamed. There was about a pint of watery fluid in the cavity of the chest. The kidneys were much harder than they usually are. Their cortical part was thickened and changed in its structure, from the deposition of coagulable lymph, and there was a small quantity of pus in the pelvis of one of them. I do not conclude, however, from these appearances, and those which were found in the former case, that the kidnies are always diseased, when the urine in dropsy contains much serum. The morbid appearances in the kidneys might be altogether unconnected with the morbid secretion, and if they were not, a diseased action of the secreting vessels, which was in those cases induced by an organic disease of the glands, may probably arise from various other causes.

* * *

Soon after this paper was read to the Society, an elderly man died in St. Thomas's Hospital, who had become ascitical, after labouring some time under a disease in his chest, and dropsy of the skin, and whose urine had contained a considerable quantity of serum. On opening his body, all the parts. which are naturally red, were found to be much paler than such parts usually are. The kidnies were larger and softer than if in a healthy state, and on the outside of both were several vesicles, partly embedded in their cortical substance, and containing an amber-coloured fluid. The greatest of them was of the size of a hazelnut. Both ureters were enlarged at their commencement. The liver was larger and indurated; the colour of its surface and of that of the spleen was blue. The lungs adhered very generally to the ribs, and when they were cut, a fluid oozed from them which seemed to contain pus. The quantity of water under the skin was much less than it had been several weeks before his death. There were about fifteen pints of water in the abdomen, about one pint in the chest, about half an ounce in the ventricles of the brain, and a little between the pia mater and tunica arachnoides. Samples of all these fluids, except the last, which was lost, were exposed to heat, and the coagulum formed by it in the three first was very great; but I possessed no means of judging, whether it was greater than that produced by a similar treatment of water, taken from the same parts of dropsical persons, whose urine had been without serum. The water from the ventricles of the brain gave a coagulum, which, after being at rest twenty-four hours, was equal in bulk to a third of the original fluid. Whytt says, that no coagulum is produced by heat in the water contained in the ventricles of the brain in children, who have died of hydrocephalus; but Dr. Baille found, that the water in the ventricles of the brain, in the hydrocephalus of children, sometimes contains a considerable quantity of coagulable matter.

John Blackall

John Blackall was born at Exeter in 1771, the sixth son of the Reverend Theophilus Blackall, a prebendary of Exeter Cathedral. He was educated at Exeter Grammar School and Balliol College, Oxford, receiving his B.A. in

1793 and his M.D. in 1797. He also received an M.D. degree from St. Bartholomew's Hospital in 1801.

Blackall settled first at Exeter, moved later to Totness, and in 1807 returned to Exeter, where he was eminently successful and regarded as the outstanding physician in that part of England. He retired from practice at the age of eighty and died nine years later.

Blackall's *Observations on the Nature and Cure of Dropsies* appeared first in 1813. In it he made the notable observation that dropsy is often associated with albuminuria and at times with diseased kidneys. The following selections from this work are taken from the third edition, published at London in 1818.

CHAPTER VI

OF THE ANASARCA AND GENERAL DROPSY, IN WHICH THE URINE IS COAGULABLE BY HEAT*

The dropsy diffused through the cellular membrane, and in its progress usually involving the large cavitities likewise, is a very common form of the disease. Its exciting causes are sometimes sufficiently remarkable, and where they can be readily ascertained, constitute a natural and useful distinction, of which I have availed myself in arranging the cases contained in this chapter.

One of these causes is scarlatina, which operates to a great extent in certain seasons; another is courses of mercury imprudently conducted, and perhaps aided by cold; a third the drinking of cold water, when heated; and

Observations on the Nature and Cure of Dropsies, and particularly on The Presence of the Coagulable Part of the Blood in Dropsical Urine; To which is added on Appendix, containing Several Cases of Angina Pectoris, with Dissections, &c. By John Blackall, M.D. London, Longman, Hurst, Rees, Orm and Brown, 1818, pp. 83-89, 193.

I have reserved a fourth section for those cases, in which the exciting cause was not very obvious nor precise, but appeared connected with different circumstances of fatigue, cold, the use of strong liquors, visceral disease, or the injudicious employment of tonics.

In the histories themselves the general character of the urine is given, and the extent of its coagulation by heat. The occasional experiments, which I have tried with other chemical tests, are to prevent the necessity of repetition, placed together. I lament, undoubtedly, that they are so few and so limited, because the discharge of albumen by this unusual channel might probably be much illustrated, by ascertaining whether any saline matters were present, that particularly favoured its solution. The complicated nature of that fluid, at all times, but especially in disease, seems to surround the subject with difficulties.

SECTION I

CASES OF ANASARCA, &c AFTER SCARLATINA, WITH A DISSECTION.—REMARKS

CASE I

E. Hammet, ætat. 42, Hospital, June, 1798, had been confined by scarlatina five months since, and three weeks afterwards had become dropsical. At the time of her admission she had an ascites, very universal anasarca, great feebleness and frequency of pulse, with general weakness and a bad appetite.

The urine was nearly natural in colour and quantity. On being subjected to heat the

whole fluid was rendered uniformly opaque at 160°, and soon deposited a considerable coagulum.

Squills, the bitter alkaline infusion, crystals of tartar, and many other diuretics and purgatives, were exhibited without effect. Her apparent loss of tone induced me to try bark and steel, both with and without evacuants; but they aggravated the symptoms. At length scarifications of the legs were employed, and there was much discharge from the wounds. This fluid gave no precipitate even at boiling heat, and very little by the addition of nitrous acid. The oedema was not permanently lessened by these means; but in two or three weeks a severe erysipelas of the lower extremities followed, and gangrenous spots, with a total failure of strength. In this dangerous state it was necessary to give bark and port wine very largely. These not only succeeded in stopping the erysipelas, but encouraged such a flow of urine and discharge from the legs, as speedily unloaded her. The urine in this increased quantity contained a less proportion of serum; the greater heat was required for its precipitation. Discontinuing the bark too soon, she became again somewhat oedematous, the urine altering in the same proportion; and it was only by returning to a long and regular course of that medicine that she perfectly recovered.

Case II

R.D., ætat. 10, just recovered from an attack of scarlatina, so slight, that he had been hardly kept one day from school, complained of pain on the outside of the right leg, somewhat above the ankle. The part was very hot, difficult to be moved, slightly swelled as if from rheumatism, and did not retain the impression of the finger. This seemed to be the complaint, which his friends noticed most. I observed besides a quick and feverish pulse, with a bloated abdomen, pale purple lips, languor and shortness of breathing. The night before, he had been awakened by some spasm on his chest, and cough. His urine on examination proved to be scanty, and very serous.

A few mild purges reduced his fever, and brought him into a state in which he bore the cinchona well. The urine then cleared, and he recovered.

Case III

M. J., ætat. 10, anasarca; ascites; palpitations of the heart, dyspnoea, excessive languor; urine pale, not scanty, not depositing any sediment, but greatly loaded with serum.

These symptoms had succeeded a mild scarlatina about ten days before. Bark had produced a tightness of the chest; and under the use of calomel, squill, and other diuretics, there was a rapid increase of all the bad signs. Particularly, the exhibition of two grains of calomel, every night, had been followed by a great debility and frequent retching.

I directed two drachms of the infusion digitalis every day, which restored her speedily.

Case IV

J. E., ætat. 12, had recovered from scarlatina about three weeks, when he became suddenly dropsical. There was an ascites and very universal anasarca, the scrotum particularly being very enormously distended. I found his urine so overloaded, as to resemble serum of the blood three or four times diluted with water. It was high-coloured, and contained a bloody sediment.

Two drachms of the infusum of digitalis, every eight hours, soon removed his swellings, whilst the urine immediately became more diluted, and in a short time quite natural. Let me add once for all, that in the instance of cure by digitalis, this improvement of the urinary discharge is simultaneous with a relief of the other symptoms, is certainly not subsequent to them, but always amongst the earliest good signs. This child, however, continued feeble, and although the dropsy did not return, yet on again applying the test of heat to the urine, whilst he was continuing that remedy, it became quite opaque at boiling point.

The Peruvian bark soon corrected this appearance; and he regained strength rapidly.

* * *

CHAPTER XII
RECAPITULATION

From the foregoing cases it is evident, that the urine of dropsy assumes very different, and even opposite, appearances; and that though it often errs, as indeed we might expect it always would, by an excess of colour, sediment, and extractive matter; yet that sometimes it verges towards the opposite extreme, is apparently little animalized and crude, does not seem to possess the appropriate characters of urine, and is, I suppose, particularly deficient in what the chemists have lately called urea. I consider the former of these to indicate a strength of constitution, but an internal obstruction, and to require both active diuretics and deobstruents;* the latter to denote a feeble and impoverished habit, either simply, or combined with great disease and with an entirely broken state of health.†

In the midst of these extremes it need not surprise us that, if the constitution is not greatly shocked, or the extravasation be small, this secretion should occasionally differ but little from the healthy state.‡

In addition to those characters which are discoverable by mere inspection, there is another infinitely more important, its property of coagulation by heat.§ This property is not connected exclusively with any particular situation of the accumulated fluid, nor with the affection of any particular organ. It very generally, although not uniformly, attends what may be called original dropsy, and frequently is superadded to great visceral unsoundness; and there cannot be a more fruitful source of error in practice, than to consider it as an evidence of mere debility, a term so incorrectly applied to several different species of disordered action. In short, it occurs under a great variety of circumstances, and where, from a resemblance of other symptoms, it has been most expected, is sometimes absent. The laws that regulate its appearance, what it denotes, and what it requires, have been hitherto almost equally unnoticed.

But is it possible, that such facts can be indifferent? Or, will any one flatter himself that he understands an individual dropsical case, whilst he overlooks this important feature of it? The neglect, which it has received from practitioners in general, makes me almost mistrust myself, when I estimate it so highly; and I should be unwilling to strain any consideration in medicine, as is too often done, beyond its reasonable and proper value. But it really does appear to me, that a more correct application of diuretic remedies is one only amongst the many advantages which may be derived from this distinction; and that it will hereafter be found capable of explaining many doubts of reconciling many apparent anomalies, and of affording an insight hitherto rather desired than expected into the state of the blood and the secretions. I shall therefore dedicate the remaining pages to a more complete investigation of its nature, founded in a great measure on the preceding cases, partly on others which it is unnecessary to detail.

Of the encysted dropsies I have designedly omitted to speak; because, as the very term implies, consisting of accumulations not diffused through the natural cavities, but confined to cysts usually either hydatids or an enlarged viscus, they admit neither of the same explanation nor the same relief that is applied to the disorders of serous membranes.

The ovarian dropsy, the most common of these, can be viewed only in the light of an enlarged viscus; and I have not found the urine to be distinguished by any very remarkable qualities.

IX. Case (for which see the postcript) of a young man, in whom the disease, a general anasarca, was apparently brought on by cold and exposure to rain, and proved rapidly fatal by the spreading of an erysipelas on the integuments of the chest and abdomen. The pleurae inflamed and covered almost universally with an adventitious lymphy membrane; cellular membrane loaded with water, and with a soft, gelatinous, imperfectly coagulated effusion, interspersed with spots of blood, opposite to the inflamed surface of the skin. Viscera nearly sound.

The lymphatic vessels are found unusually thickened and distended in dropsical bodies; so that such subjects are much preferred for anatomical preparations. This appears to be a state similar to the dilatation and thickening of varicose veins, indicating inactivity and consequent accumulation.

The serum of the cavities in this disease possesses various degrees of dilution; the fluid drawn off by tapping in the ascites, has resembled soapy water, and that not once only, but after repeated operations;* and what is discharged by scarifications is almost aqueous.

The following remarks occur to me from the preceding statement:—

1st. That the urinary organs are often free from any appearance of unsound structure, notwithstanding the great fault in their secretion.

2nd. That in two mercurial cases, the kid-

* Chapter iv.
† Chapter ii.
‡ Chapter iii.
§ Chapter v.

* Page 122.

neys were firmer than ordinary, in one of them very strikingly so, approaching to scirrhus; but whether this is merely accidental, or the effect of such a course, and what relation it bears to the discharge of serum, must be left for future observation.†

† In a dissection related by Dr. Wells, for which see the postscript, the kidneys were found thickened and confused in their structure.

Richard Bright

Richard Bright was born in Briston, England, in 1789, the son of a wealthy banker. His father gave him an excellent education and enabled him to travel

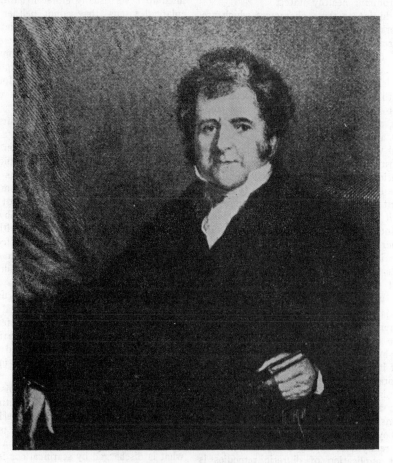

SIR RICHARD BRIGHT (1789-1858)
A portrait by T. R. Say

extensively. He graduated in medicine at Edinburgh in 1813. In 1820 he began practice in London and became assistant physician at Guy's Hospital, where he became associated with Addison and Hodgkin. These three great men of Guy's—Bright, Addison, and Hodgkin—each have the distinction of having a disease named after them.

Bright's rise to fame was slow and gradual. At Guy's Hospital he was noted for diligent attendance in the wards and postmortem room. His *Report of Medical Cases,* which appeared in 1827, contained the epochal account of renal disease. Bright not only pointed out the association between dropsy, albuminuria, and hardened kidneys, but also found that there was an excess of urea in the blood of these patients.

Bright was a very favored man, handsome, cheerful, courteous, even-tempered, highly respected by his colleagues, and deeply loved by his friends. He had a remarkably keen, analytical mind and made the most careful and minute notes on his patients, often illustrating them by beautiful drawings, for he was a very skillful draughtsman. He died in 1858 from arterio-sclerotic aortic disease and at the time of his death was the most widely-known British physician.

Bright was little interested in theories and had no doctrines, but, as Sir Samuel Wilks, his colleague wrote, "he could see and we are struck with astonishment at his powers of observation, as he photographed pictures of disease for the study of posterity." Wilks, who was associated with Guy's Hospital all his life, was its loyal historian and his writings "really gave the diseases called after Bright, Addison, and Hodgkin their place in English medicine." (Garrison)

SELECT REPORTS OF MEDICAL CASES

CASES ILLUSTRATIVE OF SOME OF THE APPEARANCES OBSERVABLE ON THE EXAMINATION OF DISEASES TERMINATING IN DROPSICAL EFFUSION*

The morbid appearances which present themselves on the examination of those who have died with dropsical effusion, either into the large cavities of the body or into the cellular membrane, are exceedingly various: and it often becomes a matter of doubt how far these organic changes are to be regarded as originally causing or subsequently aiding the production of the effusion, and how far they are to be considered merely as the consequence either of the effusion or of some more general unhealthy state of the system. If it were possible to arrive at a perfect solution of these questions, we might hope to obtain the highest reward which can repay our labours,—an increased knowledge of the nature of the disease, and improvement in the means of its treatment.

One great cause of dropsical effusion appears to be obstructed circulation; and whatever either generally or locally prevents the

* Bright, Richard, *Reports of Medical Cases selected with a View of Illustrating the Symptoms and Cure of Diseases by a Reference to Morbid Anatomy,* London, Longman, 1827, Vol. 1, p. 1.

return of the blood through the venous system, gives rise to effusion of serum more or less extensive. Thus, diseases of the heart which delay the passage of the blood in the venous system, give rise to general effusion, both into the cavities and into the cellular tissue. Obstructions of the circulation through the liver, by causing a delay in the passage of the blood through the veins connected with the vena portae, give rise to ascites. The pressure of tumours within the abdomen preventing the free passage of blood through the vena cava, gives rise to dropsical effusion into the cellular tissue of the lower extremities: and not unfrequently, the obliteration of particular veins from accidental pressure is the source of most obstinate anasarcous accumulation.

These great and tangible causes of hydropic swellings betray themselves obviously after death, and are often easily detected during life; yet they include so great a variety of diseases, that they still present a very wide field for the observation of the Pathologist. The different diseases of the heart and of the lungs on which dropsy depends, and the various changes to which the liver is subject rendering it a cause of impediment to the circulation, are still open to much investigation. In fatal cases of dropsy we likewise find the peritoneum greatly diseased in various ways; frequently covered with an adventitious membrane more or less opake, and capable of being stripped from the peritoneum, which is then left with its natural shining and glossy appearance. At other times the peritoneum is itself altered in structure, or is affected with tubercular or other diseases, presenting an accumulation of morbid growth.

There are other appearances to which I think too little attention has hitherto been paid. They are those evidences of organic change which occasionally present themselves in the structure of the *kidney;* and which, whether they are to be considered as the cause of the dropsical effusion or as the consequence of some other disease, cannot be unimportant. Where those conditions of the kidney to which I allude have occurred, I have often found the dropsy connected with the secretion of albuminous urine, more or less coagulable on the application of heat. I have in general found that the liver has not in these cases betrayed any considerable marks of disease, either during life or on examination after death, though occasionally incipient disorganization of a peculiar kind has been traced in that organ. On the other hand, I have found that where the dropsy has depended on organic change in liver, even in the most aggravated state of such change no diseased structure has generally been discovered in the kidneys, and the urine has not coagulated by heat. I have never yet examined the body of a patient dying with dropsy attended with coagulable urine, in whom some obvious derangement was not discovered in the kidneys.

Whether the morbid structure by which my attention was first directed to this subject, is to be considered as having in its incipient state given rise to an alteration in the secreting power, or whether the organic change be the consequence of a long continued morbid action, may admit of doubt: the more probable solution appears to be, that the altered action of the kidney is the result of the various hurtful causes influencing it through the medium of the stomach and the skin, thus deranging the healthy balance of

the circulation, or producing a decidedly inflammatory state of the kidney itself: that when this continues long, the structure of the kidney becomes permanently changed, either in accordance with, and in furtherance of, that morbid action; or by a deposit which is the consequence of the morbid action, but has no share in that arrangement of the vessels on which the morbid action depends.

The observations which I have made respecting the condition of the urine in dropsy, are in a great degree in accordance with what has been laid down by Dr. Blackall in his most valued treatise.

Where anasarca has come on from exposure to cold, or from some accidental excess, I have in general found the urine to be coagulable by heat. The coagulation is in different degrees: it likewise differs somewhat in its character: most commonly when the urine has been exposed to the heat of a candle in a spoon, before it rises quite to the boiling point it becomes clouded, sometimes simply opalescent, at other times almost milky, beginning at the edges of the spoon and quickly meeting in the middle. In a short time the coagulating particles break up into a flocculent or a curdled form, and the quantity of this flocculent matter varies from a quantity scarcely perceptible floating in the fluid, to so much as converts the whole matter into the appearance of curdled milk. Sometimes it rises to the surface in the form of a fine scum, which still remains after the boiled fluid has completely cooled. There is another form of coagulable urine, which in my experience has been much more rare; when the urine on being exposed to heat assumes a gelatinous appearance, as if a certain quantity of isinglass had been dissolved in water. I have indeed met with this in one or two cases only.

During some part of the progress of these cases of anasarca, I have in almost all instances found a great tendency to throw off the red particles of blood by the kidneys, betrayed by various degrees of haematuria from the simple dingy colour of the urine, which is easily recognized; or the slight brown deposit; to the completely bloody urine, when the whole appears to be little but blood, and when not unfrequently a thick ropy deposit is found at the bottom of the vessel.

Besides these cases of sudden anasarcous swelling being generally accompanied by coagulable urine, I have found another and apparently a very opposite state of the system prone to a secretion of the same character; namely, in persons who have been long the subjects of anasarca recurring again and again, worn out and cachetic in their whole frame and appearance, and usually persons addicted to an irregular life and to the use of spirituous liquors. In these cases the albuminous matter has coagulated, in the more ordinary way, in flakes and little curdled clots; but instead of rendering the whole milky, the flocculi often incline to a brown colour, looking like the finest particles of bran more or less thickly disseminated throughout the heated urine. Occasionally in these cases the urine has been much loaded with saline ingredients becoming turbid by standing, but rendered quite clear by the application of a much lower degree of heat, than is necessary to coagulate the albumen.

In all the cases in which I have observed the albuminous urine, it has appeared to me that the kidney has itself acted a more important part, and has been more deranged both functionally and organically than has generally been imagined. In the latter class of cases I have alway found the kidney decidedly disorganized. In the former, when very recent, I have found the kidney gorged with blood. And in mixed cases, where the attack was recent, although apparently the foundation has been laid for it in a course of intemperance, I have found the kidney likewise disorganized.

It is now nearly twelve years since I first observed the altered structure of the kidney in a patient who had died dropsical; and I have still the slight drawing which I then made. It was not however till within the last two years that I had an opportunity of connecting these appearances with any particular symptoms, and since that time I have added several observations. I shall now detail a few Cases, beginning with the two first, in which I had an opportunity of connecting the fact of the coagulation of the urine with the disorganized state of the kidneys.

* * *

Case XXIII

William Hunter, aet. 47, was admitted into Guy's Hospital March 7, 1827, labouring under general anasarcous swelling. On the 14th my attention was first drawn to him when he was greatly swollen, more particularly his legs, and lay with difficulty on his left side. His face was puffy and pallid, his urine scanty, very dingy in colour and *coagulable* by heat. By trade he was a tailor; and although he said that he had always been temperate, and had indeed refrained from drinking because he had observed for the last two years that his water was often very scanty, and therefore feared some bad consequences from drinking much, yet he acknowledged that he had frequently taken a pot of porter and two or three glasses of rum in a day, and that occasionally he took gin instead of rum, with a view of promoting the flow of urine. He said he had occasionally experienced pain in his loins, and his bowels were habitually costive, but he had never observed anything peculiar in his evacuations, nor had he been in the least jaundiced. He was first taken ill two days after Christmas, having been in difficulties in his business about that time and exposed much to wet. The first symptom he observed was the swelling of his legs, which increased so much that he was unable to walk or bend his knees; his hands, and more particularly his left hand, swelled very much. He had taken medicine before his admission, and said that for about a fortnight his gums were rendered sore by the medicine he took; he had derived no benefit from the treatment adopted. When he came into the Hospital, it was understood that he had suffered from a fit, which had left one side much weaker than the other; and after he had been in the house about three weeks he had two fits somewhat of an epileptic character, which greatly impaired his mental powers. Blisters being applied between his shoulders, and a seton inserted in his neck, his reason returned after some days. The chief remedies employed with a view to his dropsical affection were mercurials, the action of which was maintained till his death. The swelling was decidedly reduced, and the urine for the few last days of his life was so little coagulable, that nothing of the kind was traced except in the frothy scum which was produced by boiling and remained after cooling; but he seemed to decline under the influence of mercury, and died on the 20th of April.

Sectio Cadaveris.—April 21st, 1827

In the cavity of the chest, a very considerable quantity of serum was effused,—at least four or five points, of a light straw colour. The right lung adhered by rather long and not very recent adhesions to the pleura costalis. On the surface of the upper lobe several puckered parts were observed, beneath which, in one or two parts a gritty earthy deposit was found. In the lower lobe an abscess had formed with defined parietes, as from a single suppurating tubercle; yet the pus which it contained was of a greener colour than generally seen in tubercles, and in other respects seemed to differ from it. The whole substance of the lung was compressed by the effused fluid. The left lung was attached by slighter adhesions to the pleura costalis; in its substance not diseased, but in some parts considerably compressed by the fluid in the cavity, in other parts very oedematous. The heart firm in its structure; the left ventricle particularly thick and firm, and the columnae carnae thick and hard. The valves perfectly healthy. The aorta large. The quantity of serum in the pericardium was not precisely ascertained, owing to its making its escape; but there was evidently more than natural; the cellular substance towards the apex of the heart was filled with oedematous effusion, and the whole of both portions of the pericardium covered with a thin coating of coagulable matter, forming a villous membrane easily detached. The liver in its first appearance healthy, except from some part of the peritoneum being thickened by old inflammation: on narrow inspection it became obvious that the whole organ was composed of acini rather larger and more pale than natural, held together by the red connecting substance. The gall-bladder was moderately full of a very imperfect bile, of a turbid orange or saffron color. The intestines appeared healthy; the bladder was full of urine of a light straw colour, which did not coagulate by heat; but when boiled in a spoon formed a permanent scum upon the surface. The *kidneys* were both of them decidedly diseased, the whole cortical part presenting the granulated structure of which I have so often spoken; it was by no means in its most advanced state. The kidneys were of a natural size, rather flaccid, but tough to the feel, the granulated texture was not strongly, yet quite distinctly, marked on their surface. In the pelvis of the right kidney, which was considerably the smaller of the two, a great number, not less than a couple of hundred of exceedingly minute calculi like millet seeds, of a yellow colour, were found. The brain

was unusually free from vascularity, looking externally blanched, and this appearance was very remakable at the base. The ventricles rather distended with fluid; and the membrane lining the ventricles, more particularly the right, was rendered rough by very minute villi, as from some process of inflammation, not unlike what occurs on the pericardium.

* * *

In this case we again observe an illustration of many circumstances attending anasarca with coagulable urine:—the slight derangement of the liver, the marked disease of the kidneys, and the tendency to insidious inflammatory affection of the serous membranes, betrayed not only in the pericardium but in the lining membrane of the ventricles of the brain.

CASE XIV

Leonard Evans, a Welshman of remarkably stout frame: about ten or twelve years ago said to have been the strongest man out of 1400 in Deptford dockyard; has enjoyed health till about two years ago, when he had the syphilitic disease; but this was completley subdued. His occupation of late has been one which has exposed him very much to alternations of heat and cold, being a journeyman currier; in some part of which business he has often been exposed to cold, when in a state of most profuse perspiration; but his habits have been very sober and steady throughout life. The day before his attack, about ten days before his admission into Guy's Hospital, he had been employed in washing skins; his feet were very wet; he found the swelling coming on about six o'clock the same evening, and he continued to swell until the time of his coming into the Hospital, under my care, Nov. 15th. He was at that time labouring under general anasarca to a great extent. Urine very scanty. He had taken very little medicine.

Sumat Extract. Elaterii gr. fs sexta quaque hora.

18th. The swelling rather diminishes.

Extract. Elaterii gr. j bis quotidie.

19th. The pills have purged him very often, with much pain before they act, and much sickness. Pulse 80, full. Urine rather increased: today he first observed the dark-brown tinge in the urine, which is now very obvious, being a mixture of the red particles; *coagulates by heat.*

Rep. Extractum Elaterii mane quotidie.

20th. Urine three pints and a half in twelve hours, which is nearly six times as much as he had passed before; slightly coagulable; turbid, with red particles: feels altogether much relieved: one very copious watery and faeculent dejection.

Sumat Infus. Spartii scoparii lbij quotidie.

Habeat pulverem ex Jalapae Radice et Potassae Supertart. alternis auroris.

21st. Swelling a good deal reduced; urine in sixteen hours six pints and a half, of a high brandy colour; does not coagulate.

Repetantur Medicamenta.

24th. Urine six pints from 8 o'clock last night to 8 o'clock this morning, lighter-coloured; scarcely coagulates.

27th. Urine contains some red particles, and is copious, but does not coagulate; swellings diminish daily.

Extr. Conii gr. v, ter die.

Repetantur Medicamenta.

Dec. 1st. Complains of a pain under his jaw, but the oedematous swellings are nearly gone, except a little on the instep. Urine four pints, coagulates, and contains much blood, looking quite red; three stools yesterday from the powder. Pulse 84, of good strength.

Mittatur sanguis ad f℥x. Rep. Infusum et Pulvis.

2nd. Blood not buffed, but a firm and large coagulum, quite elastic, like a mould of jelly, and of florid colour. Urine about four pints, very red, with a great quantity of ropy mucus deposited at the bottom. Oedema much subsided. Bowels not yet opened by the powder.

Mittatur sanguis ad f℥x.

℞ Antimonii tartarizati gr. ½,

Opii purificati gr. ij,

Theriacae q.s.

Fiant Pilulae ij, quarum sumat unam bis quotidie.

Omitt. Infus. Spartii; habeat Haustum Sennae pro re nata.

3rd. Blood with thin buff; complains of a sore throat; reports the urine which has been thrown away to be of same colour as yesterday. He is walking about, and appears much improved upon the whole.

Liniment. Ammoniae gutturi infricandum.

Repetantur Medicamenta.

4th. Urine decidedly less red, but less copious; about two pints, mucous matter at the bottom diminished; it coagulates much more sparingly: throat relieved; he looks rather pallid; tongue moist and clear; pulse moderate.

5th. The whole of yesterday afternoon he seemed well, was walking about the ward, and seemed comfortable: he slept soundly, but this morning at seven o'clock suddenly complained of a great difficulty of swallowing and breathing, and constriction at his throat and chest. Fourteen ounces of blood were taken from his arm, sixteen leeches were applied to his throat, and an emetic was administered; but all was unavailing, and at about eleven o'clock he expired: the blood was highly buffed. I was informed that the urine passed since I saw him was somewhat further improved in appearance.

As I felt sure that this was a case in which neither the general circulation through disease of the heart, nor the biliary secretion through disease of the liver had any direct influence in the production of Anasarca, but could not doubt that the kidney was more immediately the seat of the derangement, I was very desirous of obtaining an examination, to ascertain whether any change had taken place in that organ, which could betray itself to the eye; and this was at length granted, at the late residence of the patient, about sixty hours after death.

Sectio Cadaveris

No sign of effusion of serum into the cellular membrane of the integuments; muscles of the body unusually strong; limbs rigid. Lungs rather gorged with blood; otherwise in structure quite healthy. Heart and pericardium quite healthy. In the cavity of the chest on each side about four ounces of fluid; in the right cavity the serum of a red colour, the lung adhering by old adhesion on the front part, and there was great congestion of blood in the back part by subsidence after death.

The liver rather gorged with blood, but perfectly healthy in structure. Spleen so soft that when the tunic was lacerated, the substance of the viscus flowed out of a chocolate colour. Stomach and intestines healthy; no effusion of serum into the cavity. The bladder contained about three-quarters of a pint of clear and yellow urine, which was not coagulable, or at least yielded only the slightest flaky coagulum; but some mucus had subsided to the bottom. The *kidneys* presented a very curious appearance; they were easily slipped out of their investing membrane, were large, and less firm than they often are, of the darkest chocolate colour, interspersed with a few white points, and a great number nearly black; and this, with a little tinge of red in parts, gave the appearance of a polished fine-grained porphyry or greenstone. On cutting longitudinally into the kidney, this structure and these colours were found to pervade the whole cortical part; but the natural striated appearance was not lost, and the external part of each mass of tubuli was peculiarly dark; the whole mamillary processes were also of a dark colour. On being cut through and left for some time, a very considerable quantity of blood oozed from the kidney, showing a most unusual accumulation in the organ; and indeed it seemed to be from this cause that the peculiar appearance and colour arose; the very dark spots being the effect of blood either extravasated or in vessels greatly gorged. I had an opportunity of procuring very faithful drawings of the kidney (Plate v). We next examined the epiglottis; and this we found to be thickened by an oedematous effusion beneath the membrane on its upper side: it was bent into the form of a penthouse with a sharp angle; and the lower surface was also thickened, and presented a doubtful appearance of superficial ulceration. When the epiglottis was cut into, a considerable quantity of serous fluid was easily squeezed out; and on the whole the opening was much contracted, and the epiglottis completely disqualified for performing its natural valvular functions.

There could then be no doubt of the nature of the attack under which the patient sank so rapidly: inflammation of the epiglottis had been followed by oedema of that part which had produced suffocation.

In this case we have the most unequivocal proof of the derangement of the kidney being connected with the extensive and sudden occurrence of anasarca:—there could indeed be no doubt of this, from the first moment that I had an opportunity of seeing the patient. The coagulable urine,—and that urine already containing the red particles of the blood in large abundance,—led me from the beginning to form my opinion as to the seat of the disease. Moreover, dissection showed no other adequate cause for the dropsical affection: and as during life no suspicion could be entertained that either the liver, the intestines, the heart, or the lungs were diseased, so the examination showed all these organs to be in a state of perfect health. I feel that it may be a matter of doubt how far the employment of diuretics during such diseased tendency may have been instrumental in producing the peculiar appearance of the kidneys; but it is to be remembered that the particular symptom, the haematuria, which appears so immediately connected with this morbid state, has been observed to occur in a greater or less degree under all modes of treatment, and even before any treatment has been adopted in the sudden anasarca, and therefore we cannot in fairness ascribe the morbid appearance of the kidney to the remedies,—or at all events we must admit a certain high degree of disease to have existed in that organ from the commencement of the symptoms; but whether to the extent discovered in this case after death or not, we can never determine. The symptom of haematuria was evidently on its decline when the accident occurred which led to a fatal termination; and it was my intention in this case, as in the case of *Fish,* (to be related hereafter), to have had recourse to local bleeding by cupping from the loins, as soon as the excessive general action had been sufficiently subdued: and very possibly if the sudden affection of the epiglottis had not come on, the disease in this case would for a time at least have completely yielded, as the symptoms of anasarca had already totally disappeared, under the treatment adopted.

PAROXYSMAL HEMOGLOBINURIA

Johannis Actuarius

Johannis Actuarius, the son of Zacharias, was a court physician at Constantinople during the latter part of the thirteenth century. The name Actuarius was a title corresponding to court-physician but has since been employed to designate this particular physician. His medical writings prove him to have been a consistent and rigid Galenist. His best known work was his *De urinis,* which

Sprengel considered the best treatise on this subject which antiquity has produced. Vierordt refers to him as the first physician to describe paroxysmal hemoglobinuria. The following translation is from the edition of *De urinis,* translated by Ambrosio Leone Nolono and published by Andreas Cratander at Basle in 1529.

CONCERNING THE SIGNS OF AZURE & LIVID AS WELL AS BLACK URINE. CHAPTER XX*

The urine may be tinged with the same color, azure & livid as well as black, which in thickness as well as in thinness of the earlier an azure blue in malignity, but later the same appears blackish blue. Black is by no means allowed to be a bad color itself,

surrounding humors, are found in different varieties as well as with different names; so that we should study their signification in various different diseases. Therefore it is

since the door of the rich is distinguished by the gloominess of this color. Besides there are colors which can occur concerning which we have just spoken, and which will be discussed a little later. An azure color appears when one suffers a moderate mixing of the melancholy humor, or a more severe chilling,

* Johannis Actuarius, Filius Zachariae, *De urinis. De iudiciis urinarum,* Basle, Cratander, 1529, p. 97.

or when some mortification is encountered. Indeed a livid color is seen in the urine, produced in the same manner, moreover it surely suggests injuries or blows inflicted upon a man. On the other hand an azure urine which seems very thin, is generated on the surface of a thin, melancholic humor, which indeed inclines to thickness, this happens because of much coldness. However this azure color may appear from loss of strength, although there was no sign of mixing earlier, but it was changed from bad colors to worse ones. Thou mayest judge by the same reasons the significant livid urine by saying the same. Which indeed appears livid on account of injuries & blows, the bruises and marks of the body will point this out to thee as well as other signs which thou mayest be able to obtain.

Yea indeed an extremely black urine, moreover is a sign of heat advanced to an extreme degree, especially where the urine shall have been green, or something approaching this. Moreover it signifies extreme chilliness. And thus thou shalt know this to be due to this cause. Moreover if the livid & azure urine was present before, it signifies chilliness. . . . Nevertheless not in all or in part may we see the bad black colors of the urine demonstrated, it is to be understood by the same reason. Since indeed it is found that black urine in men to be salutary in preceding diseases, which betray their origin from black humours: now also kinds of melancholia, when a quartan fever terminates, produce a black urine which appears very rapidly.

A CASE OF INTERMITTENT ALBUMINURIA AND CHROMATURIA
By Dr. Dressler in Würzburg*

N.N., 10½ years old, was retarded in bodily and also mental development, with genitalia undeveloped and small for his age (the left testicle is atrophic, the right undescended), and in earlier years he suffered several times from severe inflammation of the eyes (*Syphilis congenital?*). During the latter part of December of last year, he suffered from several attacks coming on between 10 and 11 A.M., which were characterized by chilliness, cold extremities, rapid small pulse, greyish face with blue nose and blue ears. The boy felt ill and went to bed. About 4 P.M. the attack slowly passed away completely without any fever. His appearance, aside from the attacks, was pale and sickly, the pulse somewhat increase and small, his appetite usually good, and especially after the attacks, he sleeps quietly at night. I prescribed quinine and milk sugar with meat diet.

In spite of this treatment the attacks continued, and often there was a stage of feverishness following the stage of chilliness, and towards the end of December attacks of vomiting appeared.

About this time (December 30) I noted that the urine which the patient passed immediately before the attack was small in amount (circa 1 ounce) and characterized by a dark brown color and a still darker

cloudy precipitate. It showed a nearly neutral reaction (very weakly acid), formed with nitric acid a flaky dark precipitate (albumin and pigment) and showed under the microscope much amorphous, granular, dirty brown pigment, some desquamated cells, but no blood corpuscles.

Also, on the 30th shortly after the attack. as well as on the 31st after the onset of the attack, the urine voided showed the same characteristics.

The rectal examination on the 31st showed no enlargement of the prostate. During the attack, the spleen showed no enlargement on percussion.

The urine passed on the 31st, shortly after the attack was clear, contained a light mucous cloud but no albumin.

There was an attack on January 1st, 10 A.M. without any noticeable shivering and characterized only by a grayish color of the face, weakness and pain in both feet; the urine passed at midday was dark, showed no precipitate and contained pigment but no albumin. The urine passed in the evening showed a deep but not exactly dark color, a small amount of mucous sediment, no albumin.

The urine passed early in the morning of January 2nd was light in color, had a slightly cloudy sediment, no albumin.

A specimen of the urine passed in my presence at the beginning of the attack was light

*Arch. f. path Anat., Virchow, 1854, VI, 264.

colored and showed on standing an abundant red sediment composed of ammonium urate. The specimen passed in the afternoon was of dark color with an abundant heavy precipitate, contained much pigment and a small quantity of albumin.

In regard to treatment it should be noted that in addition to the use of quinine an infusion of China root was given.

The amount of urine passed has recently become much greater.

The urine passed in the forenoon of January the 3rd, was of a light color and on standing, formed a whitish sediment which was covered with a thin blood red layer, but contained no albumin. The urine passed in the afternoon was light, had an abundant rose red sediment and contained ammonium urate but no albumin.

The attacks of fever changed at this time in such a manner that no chilly attack appeared, the sunkenness of the face was less but the boy complained of severe pain in his feet.

The urine passed on the morning of January the 4th was light and clear; that passed in the afternoon showed a dark brown sediment.

The urine passed in the morning of January the 5th was light brown with a light brown cloudy sediment; at midday it was jumentous with a reddish sediment; in the evening, light and clear.

On the 6th morning a clear urine was passed. At midday the urine was cloudy, appeared a dirty red and contained albumin in considerable quantity, ammonium urate, granular pigments, desquamated cells and a few soft tubules.

The urine of the afternoon of the 6th day and the morning of the 7th day was clear. The urine passed in the evening of the 7th day was dark with a little brown sediment.

The urine of the morning of the 8th day was clear; urine passed in the evening, which was accidentally thrown away, was said to be dark.

The urine on the morning of the 9th day was cloudy and on standing formed a dirty white, rough sediment containing a trace of albumin, much debris, pigment and soft tubules of different lengths in considerable amounts. The boy had on this day at 10 o'clock, again a severe attack of shivering. The urine passed on the evening of the 9th and on the morning of the 10th was light and clear.

The urine passed on the morning of the 11th was cloudy; dirty brown and formed an abundance of dirty brown sediments containing much albumin.

The urine on the evening of the same day as well as that passed on the morning of the 12th was again light and clear.

The recent attacks are more characterized by pain in the joints of the feet.

The boy received daily a little red wine, quinine and infusions of China bark were continued.

From this time on the urine remained clear, passed in normal amounts and showed only now and then a stronger concentrated color. The attacks, that is those pains accompanying the earlier attacks of fever, gradually became less frequent and by January 17th had entirely disappeared. The appearance of the child improved and by the end of January his former relatively good health returned.

George Harley

George Harley was born at Haddington, in East Lothian, Scotland, in 1829. He studied medicine at Edinburgh and while still an undergraduate student, performed single handed and with no preparation, an emergency Caesarian section upon a pregnant woman who had died suddenly from heart disease. The child lived and Harley had the satisfaction later of seeing him grow up and become the father of a family.

Harley took his M.D. degree at Edinburgh in 1850 and after serving in the Edinburgh Royal Infirmary, proceeded to Paris where he worked in the physiological laboratory of the College de France under Magendie and Claude Bernard. After two years in Paris, Harley went to Germany where he spent two years working with Liebig, Scherer, Virchow, Kölliker, and Bunsen. Upon his return to London, Harley was appointed lecturer on physiology and histology at University College. In 1856, Harley started in practice, but at the end of twelve months, having had but two patients and collected only a few pounds, he decided to remove his doorplate until he had more reputation.

George Harley was appointed professor of medical jurisprudence at University College in 1859 and in a few years had a very large consulting practice.

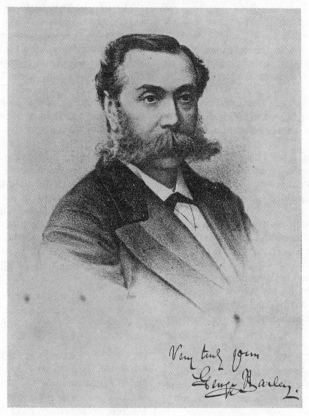

GEORGE HARLEY (1829-1896)
Courtesy of Surgeon General's Library, Washington

He was elected to membership in the Royal Society and in the Royal College of Physicians and subsequently became physician to the University Hospital. He died in 1896.

The numerous scientific papers of Harley show a most active and alert mind, interested in every phase of medicine. While a student in France, Harley carried out important experiments on the metabolism of diabetes and discovered the urinary pigment, urohaematin, which he proved contained iron. While in Paris, he was elected president of the Paris Medical Society. In Würzburg where he worked with Scherer, Kölliker, and Virchow, his investigations on urinary pigments created such interest that he was elected a member of the Academy of Würzburg. In Heidelberg, Harley worked with Bunsen, from whom he learned methods of gas analysis, which he later employed in his studies of respiration. Harley's pharmacological studies were extensive and of great merit. Harley contributed many interesting papers on clinical subjects, among them his interesting account of paroxysmal hemoglobinuria.

MEDICAL SOCIETIES

ROYAL MEDICAL AND CHIRURGICAL SOCIETY*
Tuesday, May 9, 1865
Dr. Alderson, F.R.S., President

NOTES OF TWO CASES OF INTERMITTENT HAEMATURIA; WITH REMARKS UPON THEIR PATHOLOGY AND TREATMENT

By George Harley, M.D., Professor in University College, and Assistant-Physician to University College Hospital

The chief peculiarity presented in the cases described in this communication was that the urine passed at one period of the day varied from a dark chocolate colour to an almost purple blackness, whereas at all other times the secretion was to all intents and purposes normal. One of the patients was a medical gentleman who had for many years been resident in a warm climate, where he had contracted malarial fever; the other was a Londoner who had never suffered any true aguish attack, but in whose case the bloody urine was passed whenever he was exposed to cold. Indeed, according to the patient's own statement, during the last two winters his urine invariably became bloody about an hour after his suffering from cold hands or feet. Both patients appeared to suffer from hepatic derangement, the one whose attack could be traced to malaria being slightly jaundiced at the time the urinary symptom manifested itself. The other, although not suffering from true jaundice, had an exceedingly sallow, bilious appearance.

As regards the pathology of these specimens of urine, the author remarked that had the morning's urine only been brought under the notice of the physician, he could never have dreamt of the existence of any urinary infection; whereas had the midday specimen alone been subjected to his inspection, he could not have failed to suspect the existence

* *Lancet,* 1865, I, 568.

of grave organic changes in the renal organs. Neither of these opinions could possibly be correct; the varying condition of the renal secretion clearly pointing to intense congestion of the chylopoietic viscera of a transient and periodic character.

Professor Harley further pointed out the difference between the affection here described and the other form of disease with which it is apt to be confounded—namely, ordinary haematuria. The easiest way of establishing a correct differential diagnosis was, he said, that in ordinary haematuria the urine is not only coagulable by heat and nitric acid, but contains blood-corpuscles, which gradually become deposited on standing, and leave a clear, pale-coloured supernatant liquid. In this form of intermitting haematuria, as also in some cases of the non-intermittent variety, the urine, although coagulable by heat and nitric acid, contains few or no blood-corpuscles, and the colouring matter is not deposited on standing, but remains uniformly distributed throughout the liquid. Besides this, the urine contains numerous granular tube casts, and has an increased per-centage of urea.

Lastly, as regards treatment, it was shown that while the usual remedies employed in the treatment of haematuria failed to make the slightest impression on this form of disease, the employment of mercurials and quinine caused it rapidly to disappear.

William H. Dickinson

William Howship Dickinson was born at Brighton in 1832 and entered the Medical School of St. George's Hospital in 1851. He later entered Gonville and Caius College, Cambridge. He took the degree of M.B. in 1859 and, returning to London, became successively assistant physician, physician and consulting physician to St. George's Hospital. Upon his retirement, he removed to Tintagel in North Cornwall, where he wrote a book on *King Arthur in Cornwall*. He died in 1913.

Dickinson, Sir Humphry Rolleston writes, "was a fearless supporter of what have mainly turned out to be lost causes." Sir Humphry continues:

"Old Dick," as he was reverently called, was a great character, a kind of medical Samuel Johnson, a student of Addisonian English which he wrote with great effect, and the maker of epigrammatic phrases, such as "he wrote because he had something to say, not because he had to say something"; in proposing the health of his contemporary, Sir Jonathan Hutchinson (1828-1913), at a dinner of the Cambridge Graduates' Medical Club, soon after his own Lumleian lectures at the Royal College of Physicians of London in 1888 on *The Tongue as an Indicator of Disease* he said that it was appropriate that "Dickinson's tongue should praise Hutchinson's teeth." *Places and Commonplaces in Renal Disease* was the title he gave to a paper of his own on the climatic treatment of renal disease.

"His wit ensured him a good following in the wards, where he was a masterful diagnostician, and was not pleased if his house physician anticipated him, and indeed would for that reason sometimes take a different view."

NOTES OF FOUR CASES OF INTERMITTENT HAEMATURIA*

By Wm. H. Dickinson, M.D., Cantab., Curator of the Museum of St. George's Hospital, Assistant-Physician to the Hospital for Sick Children

The case most fully reported was that of a man who had frequently been in St. George's Hospital. In the autumn of 1859 he was first attacked with his present complaint. One morning he was seized with shivering, nausea, and pain in the loins; and when he passed urine, he found it was black and apparently bloody. From that time to the present he had often been under observation at St. George's Hospital, and he had been in the hands of all the physicians of that establishment, latterly under the care of Dr. Fuller. He had no constant ailment, but his health was broken by short attacks of haematuria. From the beginning of the disorder these had always been of the same character. They owned no other cause but exposure to cold. He usually got up and went to his work apparently well. In

cold weather he was liable to be attacked with shivering, retching, and dull pain in the loins, at the same time yawning and feeling disposed to stretch himself. The testicles were retracted, and he had pain passing down the thighs. When he passed urine, it was black and turbid, and was found to be highly albuminous, of great specific gravity, and containing an excess of urea; the microscope showed numbers of dark granular casts, and a dark molecular deposit; no blood-globules had ever been found. The urine retained these characters for two or three urinations. When he got warm it recovered its natural characters; and next day he was well, excepting that he was somewhat reduced by the attack. In continuous cold weather these attacks had come on for several successive days, but they had never lasted through the night. He had never had an attack in the summer; though

* *Lancet*, 1865, I, 568.

once, in comparatively warm weather, it was brought on by washing windows with cold water. Movement had no tendency to produce it; he was always better when taking exercise, as it kept him warm. The man had an anaemic and cachectic appearance. No organic disease could be discovered. While in the hospital many plans of treatment had been tried, but none had appeared to prevent the recurrence of the complaint. Quinine proved inefficacious; mercurials were apparently injurious. While taking blue-pill, he had, for the first time in his life, an attack while in-doors. During the time he was under this treatment he had an attack of pneumonia, which was followed by peculiar symptoms of prostration, which it was thought must have proved fatal, but from which he eventually recovered.

Three similar cases were briefly reported, two of which had occurred in the practice of Dr. George Johnson, and one in that of Dr. F. Cock, which gentlemen had communicated the facts to the author.

In conclusion, Dr. Dickinson maintained that the disorder was essentially due to an alteration in the blood, a similar state of urine having been found during typhus, and also in man and animals after the inhalation of arseniuretted hydrogen. The points which the disorder has in common with ague were adverted to, but the absence of any periodical tendency and the inefficacy of quine as a remedy were cited as essential differences. As to treatment, it was considered that as yet the disorder was beyond our reach; the most we could do was to palliate the effects of the loss of blood. Quinine was believed to be useless except in this respect; while the administration of mercurials, both on general principles and on the experience afforded by the above case, was believed to be detrimental.

Dr. Greenhow believed that the second case mentioned in the paper had been under his care in the Middlesex Hospital, and had been treated in every possible way, and with mercury and quinine amongst other remedies.

He could not understand how the remedies employed by Dr. Harley of a similar kind had been so successful as to effect a cure in forty-eight hours. The boy who was the subject of this case was affected with haematuria at irregular intervals, cold being the chief exciting cause. The attacks were less frequent in summer than winter.

Dr. Fuller said that in his case he could not attribute any effects to the drugs or the modes of treatment employed. The patient did as well when no means of cure were resorted to; simply lying in bed was sufficient. The complaint recurred at irregular intervals, no cause, except cold, appearing to influence their occurrence.

Dr. C. J. B. Williams said that we could only arrive at the cause of these attacks from post-mortem evidence. The peculiarity of these cases was the severity of the attacks and their total cessation without apparent cause. In cases of intermittent fever, blood and albumen were occasionally found in the urine, arising from congestion of the internal organs during the paroxysms. It was interesting thus to see symptoms of Bright's disease in an early stage, and then pass off. It was also remarkable that the symptoms recurred sometimes with cold, sometimes without. It would seem as if there were some structural change of the kidneys which was unable to resist the influence of an influx of blood upon them, and their secretion became thus modified. Hemorrhage from the nose it was known occurred from cold. In aguish countries the cold stage of intermittent fever sometimes produced epistaxis. Remedies did not seem to be of much avail in recurrent haematuria, as patients appeared to get well without treatment.

Dr. Harley explained that in the case alluded by Dr. Greenhow, the treatment consisted in the administration of a good dose of calomel, followed by a large dose of quinine.

Dr. Dickinson having replied, the Society adjourned.

VII. RESPIRATORY DISEASES

The section on diseases of the respiratory tract contains selections by some of the best-known characters and most outstanding figures in the history of medicine. While diseases of the lungs and pleura were described by physicians from the time of Hippocrates down yet it was not until the discoveries of Aurenbrugger and of Laënnec that precision and accuracy in the diagnosis began. Cheyne-Stokes' respiration and mountain sickness, we now know, are not respiratory diseases, but have been included here because the respiratory symptoms in each are very prominent. Asthma, which may be more properly considered as an allergic disease, is included here because the outstanding symptoms as well as lesions are in the respiratory tract.

CHEYNE-STOKES' RESPIRATION

Hippocrates

13. FOURTEEN CASES OF DISEASE*

CASE I.—Philiscus, who lived by the wall, took to bed on the first day of acute fever; he sweated; towards night was uneasy. On the second day, all the symptoms were exacerbated; late in the evening had a proper stool from a small clyster; the night quiet. On the third day, early in the morning and until noon he appeard to be free from fever; towards evening, acute fever, with sweating, thirst, tongue parched; passed black urine; night uncomfortable, no sleep; he was delirious on all subjects. On the fourth, all the symptoms exacerbated, urine black; night more comfortable, urine of a better color.

* *The Genuine Works of Hippocrates,* translated by Francis Adams, New York, Wm. Wood. Vol. I, p. 308.

On the fifth, about mid-day, had a slight trickling of pure blood from the nose; urine varied in character, having floating in it round bodies, resembling semen, and scattered, but which did not fall to the bottom; a suppository having been applied, some scanty flatulent matters were passed; night uncomfortable, little sleep, talking incoherently; extremities altogether cold, and could not be warmed; urine black; slept a little towards day; loss of speech, cold sweats; extremities livid; about the middle of the sixth day he died. The respiration throughout like that of man recollecting himself, and rare, and large, and spleen was swelled upon in a round tumor, the sweats cold throughout the paroxysms on the even days.

John Cheyne

John Cheyne was born in Leith, Scotland, in 1777, the son of John Cheyne, a surgeon of that city. He should not be confused with the famous English physician, George Cheyne, whose *Essay of Health and Long Life* was so widely read and quoted, a man of enormous bulk who reduced himself by dieting from 448 pounds to normal proportions.

John Cheyne was educated first at the Grammar School of Leith and at the age of ten years was sent to the High School of Edinburgh. In his thirteenth year, he began to attend his father's poor patients "to ascertain that they were supplied with medicine, to bleed them, dress their wounds and report upon their condition." In his fifteenth year, he began the study of medicine at the University of Edinburgh and obtained his medical degree in 1795 at the age of eighteen. He entered the British Army the same year and served as an army surgeon for four years, returning to Leith in 1799.

He acted as assistant to his father for several years and during this period formed a friendship with Charles Bell, who awakened his interest in the study of pathology. In 1809, he went to Dublin and in 1811 was appointed physician to Meath Hospital. In 1820, he was appointed Physician-General to the Army in Ireland, a position which conferred upon its possessor the highest medical

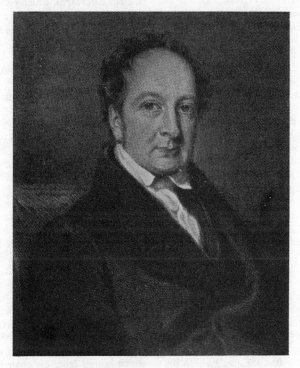

Kindness of George Blumer

JOHN CHEYNE (1777-1836)

rank in Ireland. Cheyne wrote in his *Autobiography*, "As my practice yielded £5000, which was about its annual average during the next ten years, I felt that I had fully attained the object of my ambition." In 1831, Cheyne, feeling that his large medical practice was proving an intolerable burden and being in bad health, left Dublin and settled down in Sherington, a small village in Buckinghamshire, England. Here he lived a comparatively quiet life, looked after the health of the villagers and wrote medical articles and essays. He died in 1836.

Cheyne was universally beloved and respected by his patients and by the medical profession. He was the founder of the Irish school which included such names as Colles, Adams, Corrigan, Graves, and Stokes, and is remembered by the medical historian for his description of Cheyne-Stokes' respiration in 1818.

A CASE OF APOPLEXY IN WHICH THE FLESHY PART OF THE HEART WAS CONVERTED INTO FAT*

By J. Cheyne, M.D., &c.

Doubts have been entertained of the conversion of the fleshy part of the heart into fat, and only one dissection,† in as far as I know, having been published illustrative of that very curious morbid alteration, the following case and dissection have been thought of sufficient importance to meet the public eye.

In this dissection, although no chemical experiment was made in proof of the matter into which the heart was converted being fatty, I have no doubt that it was so. Placed along side of the fat which lay over the ribs. I could perceive no difference, save that it was softer and more easily torn, and rather of a deeper yellow; the substance in question communicated a greasy stain to paper, and the animal oil in viscous drops adhered to the knife used in dissecting the heart. I was not at the time of dissection, aware that the morbid change was so uncommon, or that the specimen which lay before me was perhaps the most complete exemplification ever witnessed of the conversion of the flesh of the heart into fat.

The patient certainly died of apoplexy; and apoplexy in this case must have depended upon increased action of the vessels of the head. The heart itself was apparently incapable of communicating much impetus to the circulating mass.

Certainly the dissection would have been more complete had the liver been examined: at the time I may observe that although the function of the liver had frequently been disordered during the last ten years of the patient's life, I should not have been surprised had that viscus been found apparently sound. I am persuaded that diseases of the liver, which do not end in structural changes, often produce the greatest disturbance of the constitution, laying the foundation of fatal diseases of distant organs.

A. B., sixty years of age, of a sanguine temperament, circular chest, and full habit of body, for years had lived a very sedentary

life, while he indulged habitually in the luxuries of the table.

This gentleman having had several attacks of the gout in his feet, began a course of magnesia in the year 1813, after which he had only one regular attack of the gout. For many years he had been subject to severe attacks of catarrh, which ended without much expectoration. He had long been subject to oedema of the ankles in the evening; for two or three years before his death (the time could not be ascertained) he had remarked an occasional intermission in the pulse of his heart.

In the latter end of January 1816, he consulted me for a pain in his right side under the false ribs, for which he took calomel at bedtime, and salts in the morning, repeating these once or twice; but he neglected my directions with regard to diet; nay, his appetite being remarkably keen, he ate more than usual, and took at least a pint of port wine or Madiera daily, as was his habit, and this notwithstanding a hard frequent cough, which came on after I was consulted by him.

On the third of February he had walked a good many miles, and came home exhausted, with a fluttering or palpitation of his heart, for he could not well say which, in a degree he had not felt before. He ate as usual and drank six or seven glasses of wine, which he thought relieved the fluttering. He was sitting at tea about nine o'clock, when he was attacked with a severe fit of coughing, during which he fell from his chair insensible. I saw him in three or four minutes after his fall, and found him with a contusion on the upper and left side of the frontal bone. He was confused and unable to recollect himself; he was conscious that some accident had befallen him, the exact nature of which he declared himself incapable of understanding. His pulse was extremely irregular and unequal. It bounded quickly for several pulsations, then it paused and went on more quickly, but with less force. He was pale but none of the muscles were affected with palsy. I lost no time in having blood drawn from his arm to the amount of nearly a pound. He gradually became more collected, but his pulse continued irregular and unequal; his countenance

---

* *Dublin Hosp. Rep.*, 1818, II, p. 216.

† See a dissection, illustrative of the morbid change, in an elaborate paper on inflammation of the heart, by Dr. Duncan, jun. See *Edin. Med. and Surgical Journal*, Jan., 1816.

became flushed, the cough occurred in suffocative fits, and he complained of pain on either side of the tuberosity of the occipital bone. Twelve ounces more of blood were drawn about an hour after the blood-letting, after which the pulse, though it continued equally irregular, was much softer. He complained of the contusion, and of considerable pain behind his ears. He was removed to bed, the heat of the extremities was restored, and fifteen leechs were applied over the contusion, and he took two pills consisting of two grains of James's powder, three of calomel and four of compound extract of colocynth.

On the 4th of February he had several large bilious stools; his understanding was unimpaired, his recollection restored, and he seemed to comprehend the nature of his illness, and he had a sense of fullness in his head, which led me to order him to lose a few more ounces of blood. It would be tedious and unprofitable to particularize the medicines which were ordered from day to day for this patient; they consisted of a mild mercurial every second or third day, and squills with ammoniacum, &c. These were indicated by the loaded tongue, scanty high coloured urine and dry cough. The expectoration being restored, the squills were laid aside on the 15th of February, as they produced nausea and extreme depression of spirits, and bitter infusion with tincture of cardamoms and soda prescribed. On the nineteenth a horseradish bath was ordered in consequence of some slight demonstration of gout. On the 21st he had some smart pain, with slight inflammation in the ball of the left great toe. About this period he submitted with so much dissatisfaction to a reduced diet, and declared himself so much better after food, that we were induced to allow him a couple of glasses of wine, and to encourage him to take carriage exercise. The irregularity of his pulse never ceased. On the first of March, he had a return of the suffocating cough and flushing, with some wheezing, which again seemed to demand blood-letting, which was practiced with immediate relief. At this period a blister was applied over the region of the heart, which had become the seat of considerable increase in pain, and a discharge was maintained from the blistered surface, by means of ointment of savine and cantharides; about the 4th of March, the sputa became free and concocted. His tongue

at this period was for many days furred and a dark brown colour, as if it had been sprinkled with ground coffee; it was expanded and its edge was moist. On the 25th of March he began to complain of wheezing, more particularly after exertion, but it sometimes attacked him when he was at perfect rest; his legs and ankles became oedematous, the urine very scanty, much loaded, but without being coagulable by heat. At no period of illness did his pulse beat more than twelve or fifteen strokes in regular succession. Various diuretics were given; the digitalis was proposed, but he refused to take it. Crystals of tartar, the extractum lactucae virosae, nitrous aether, &c. were tried without any benefit.

The symptoms of dropsy rapidly increasing, on the ninth of April, he took a draught of infusion of senna, tincture of jalap and Rochelle salts, which operated largely. On the 10th of April he was found in bed flushed, speechless, and hemiplegiac. How long he had been in that state could not be ascertained, as he had peremptorily ordered his servant not to remain in the chamber with him, and not to come to him in the morning until called. All attempts to relieve him were unavailing; his right side continued powerless, and his attempts to articulate were vain. The only peculiarity in the last period of his illness, which lasted eight or nine days, was in the state of the respiration. For several days his breathing was irregular; it would entirely cease for a quarter of a minute, then it would become perceptible, though very low, then by degrees it became heaving and quick, and then it would gradually cease again. This revolution in the state of his breathing occupied about a minute, during which there were about thirty acts of respiration.*

* * *

The Dissection was made by Dr. Crampton, the Surgeon General, and witnessed by Mr. John Moore and myself.

There was nothing remarkable in the configuration of the body but the great depth of the chest; the anasarcous swelling of the inferior extremities was considerable.

* The same description of breathing was observed by me in a relative of the subject of this case, who also died of a disease of the heart, the exact nature of which however I am ignorant of, not having been permitted to examine the body after death.

The scalp was bloodless. The arachnoid membrane was slightly opaque; there was some fluid between it and the pia matter, and the vascularity of the latter increased, more particularly over the middle and posterior lobes of the cerebrum of the left side, where, in a large patch, it was thickened and of a deep red colour. The brain was firm, its cortical substance of a pale drab colour. There were between three and four ounces of fluid in the ventricles.

There were not more than two ounces of fluid in the pericardium. The heart was about three times its natural size. The lower part of the right ventricle was converted into a soft fatty substance; the upper part was remarkably thin, and it gradually degenerated into this soft fatty substance. The cavity of the left ventricle was greatly enlarged. The whole substance of the left ventricle, with the exception of the internal reticulated structure and carneae columnae, was converted into fat. The valves were sound. The aorta was studded with steatomatous and earthly concretions.

William Stokes

SYMPTOMS REFERRIBLE TO THE RESPIRATORY FUNCTION*

There is no evidence that the existence of this disease, even in an aggravated form, is an exciting cause of any organic affection of the lung. On the other hand, the researches of Ormerod, Quain, and others, have demonstrated the frequent combination of fatty heart with pulmonary disease; but in such cases we may hold that the conditions of the lung and heart have little, if any, mutual relation; they are rather to be considered as the secondary accidents of a general morbid state.

But there is a symptom which appears to belong to a weakened state of the heart, and which, therefore, may be looked for in many cases of the fatty degeneration. I have never seen it except in examples of that disease. The symptom in question was observed by Dr. Cheyne, although he did not connect it with the special lesion of the heart. It consists in the occurrence of a series of inspirations, increasing to a maximum, and then declining in force and length, until a state of apparent apnoea is established. In this condition the patient may remain for such a length of time as to make his attendants believe that he is dead, when a low inspiration, followed by one more decided, marks the commencement of a new ascending and then descending series of inspirations. This symptom, as occurring in its highest degree, I have only seen during a few weeks previous to the death of the patient. I do not know any more remarkable or characteristic phenomena than those presented in this condition, whether we view the long-continued cessation of breathing, yet without any suffering on the part of the patient, or the maximum point of the series of inspirations, when the head is thrown back, the shoulders raised, and every muscle of inspiration thrown into the most violent action; yet all this without râle or any sign of mechanical obstruction. The vesicular murmur becomes gradually louder, and at the height of the paroxysm is intensely puerile.

The decline in the length and force of the respirations is as regular and remarkable as their progressive increase. The inspirations become each one less deep than the preceding, until they are all but imperceptible, and then the state of apparent apnoea occurs. This is at last broken by the faintest possible inspiration; the next effort is a little stronger, until, so to speak, the paroxysm of breathing is at its height, again to subside by a descending scale.

* * *

25. That the respiratory symptoms are divisible into three classes:—

a. Attacks of dyspnoea on exertion, similar to those observed in other cardiac diseases.

b. Gradually increasing difficulty of breathing, amounting to orthopnoea, and coming on spontaneously.

c. A form of respiratory distress, peculiar to this affection, consisting of a period of apparently perfect apnoea, succeeded by

* The Diseases of the Heart and the Aorta, by William Stokes, Dublin, Hodges and Smith, 1854, pp. 323-324, 336. This description was first published in the Dublin Quarterly Journal of Medical Science in 1846.

feeble and short inspirations, which gradually increase in strength and depth until the respiratory act is carried to the highest pitch of which it seems capable, when the respirations, pursuing a descending scale, regularly diminish until the commencement of another apnoeal period. During the height of the paroxysm the vesicular murmur becomes intensely puerile.

26. That although this affection may exist without valvular disease, yet the coexistence of a certain amount of alteration of the aortic valves is common; so that the combination of a slow pulse, a feeble impulse, and a diminished first sound over the left ventricle, attended with a single murmur, while the second sound remains clear, will be sufficient.

27. But that in cases where no such murmur exists, we may also diagnose the disease when we observe,—in connection with a slow and regular, or rapid, but irregular and unequal, pulse,—the occurrence of the pseudo-apoplectic symptoms, with or without the special character of apnoeal intervals and the ascending and descending respirations.

MOUNTAIN SICKNESS
Joseph Acosta
LIB. 3, CHAP. 9*

Wherefore it is a matter certaine, & tried, that the aire of the sea, doth commonly cause this effect in such as newly go to sea. I thought good to speake this, to shew a strange effect, which happens in some partes of the Indies, where the ayre & the wind that rains make men dazie, not lesse, but more then at sea. Some hold it for a fable, others say it is an addition: for my part I will speake what I have tried. There is in Peru, a high mountaine which they call pariacaca, and having heard speake of the alteration it bred, I went as well prepared as I could according to the instructions which was given me, by such as they call Vaguianos or expert men; but notwithstanding all my provision, when I came to mount the degrees, as they call them, which is the top of this mountaine, I was suddenly surprized with so mortall and strange a payn, that I was ready to fall from the top to the ground: and although we were many in company, yet every one made haste (without any tarrying for his companion,) to free himself speedily from this ill passage. Being then alone with one Indian, whom I intreated to helpe to stay me, I was surprised with such pangs of straining & casting, as I thought to cast up my heart too; for having cast up meate, fleugme, & choller, both yellow and greene; in the end I cast up blood, with the straining of my stomacke. To conclude, if this had continued, I should undoubtedly have died; but this lasted not above three or foure houres, that we were come into a more convenient and naturale temperature, where all our companions (being fourteene or fifteene) were much wearied. Some in the passage demaunded confession, thinking verily to die; others left the ladders and went to the ground, beeing overcome with casting, and going to the stoole: and it was tolde me, that some have lost their lives there with this accident. I beheld one that did beate himself against the earth, crying out for the rage and griefe which this passage of Pariacaca hadde caused. But commonly it dooth no important harme, onely this, paine and troublesome distaste while it endures: and not onely the passage of Pariacaca hath this propertie, but also all this ridge of the mountaine, which runnes above five hundred leagues long, and in what place soever you passe, you shall find strange intemperatures, yet more in some partes then in others, and rather to those which mount from the sea, than from the plaines. Besides Pariacaca, I have passed it by Lucanas and Soras; in an other place, by Colleguas, and by Cavanas. Finally, by foure different places, going and comming and alwaies in this passage I have felt this alteration, although in no place so strongly, as at the furst in Pariacaca, which hath beene tried by all such as have passed it. And no doubt but the wind is the cause of this intemperature and strange alteration, or the aire that raignes there. For the best remedy (and all they finde) is to stoppe their noses, their ears, and their

* Acosta, Joseph, *The Naturall and Morall Historie of the East and West Indies*, London, V. Sims for E. Blount and W. Asplay, 1604. Kindness of F. H. Garrison.

mouthes, as much as may be, and to cover themselves with cloathes, especially the stomacke, for that the ayre is subtile and piercing, going into the entrailes, and not onely men feele this alteration, but also beasts that sometimes stay there, so as there is no spurre can make them goe forward. For my part I holde this place to be one of the highest parts of land in the worlde; for we mount wonderfull space. And in my opinion, the mountaine Nevada of Spaine, the Pirenees, and the Alpes of Italie, are as ordinarie houses, in regarde to hie towers. I therefore perswade my selfe that the element of the aire is there so subtile and delicate, as it is not proportionable with the breathing of man, which requires a more grosse and temperate aire, and I beleeve it is the cause that doth so much alter the stomacke, & trouble all the disposition. The passages of the mountaines, Nevada and others of Europe, which I have seene, although the aire be colde there, and doth force men to weare more clothes, yet this colde doth not take away the appetite from meate, but contrariwise it provokes; neyther doth it cause any casting of the stomacke, but onely some pain in the feete and handes. Finally, their operation is outward. But that of the Indies, whereof I speake (without molesting of foote or hand, or any outward parte) troubles all the entrailes within: and that which is more admirable, when the funne is hot, which maketh me imagine, that the griefs wee feele comes from the qualitie of the aire which wee breathe: therefore that is most subtile and delicate, whose colde is not so sensible, as piercing. All this ridge of mountaines is, for the most part, desart, without any villages or habitations for men, so as you shall scarce finde any small cotages to lodge such as do passe by night: there are no beasts, good or bad, but some Vicunos, which are their countrey muttons, and have a strange and wonderful property, as I shall shew in his place. The grasse is often burnt, and all black with the aire and this desart runnes five and twenty or thirty leagues overthwart, and in length about five hundred leagues. There are other deserts or places uninhabited, which at Peru they call Punas (speaking of the second poynt we promised) where the quallitie of the ayre cutteth off mans life without feeling. In former time the Spaniards went from Peru, to the realme of Chille by this mountaine, but at this day they do passe commonly by sea, and somtimes alongst the side of it. And though that way be laborious and troublesome, yet is there not so great danger as by the mountaine, where there are Plaines, on the which many men have perished and died, and sometimes have scaped by great happs, whereof some have remained lame. There runs a small breath, which is not very strong nor violent, but proceedes in such sorte, that men fall downe dead, in a manner without feeling, or at the least, they loose their feete and handes: the which may seeme fabulous, yet is it most true.

I have knowne and frequented long the Gennerall Jerome Costilla, the auntient peopler of Cusco, who had lost three or four toes, which fell off in passing the desart of Chille, being perished with this aire, and when he came to looke on them they were dead, and fell off without any paine, even as a rotten Apple falleth from the tree. This Captaine reported, that of a good army which he had conducted by that place, in the former yeeres, since the discoverie of this kingdome by Almagro the great part of the men remained dead there, whose bodies he found lying in the desart, without any stink or corruption; adding therunto one thing very strange, that they found a yong boy alive, and being examined how he had lived in that place, hee saide, that hee laie hidden in a small cave, whence he came to cutte the flesh of a dead horse with a little knife, and thus had he nourished himself a long time, with I know not how many companions that lived in that fort, but now they were all dead, one dying this day, and another tomorrow, saying that hee desired nothing more than to die there with the rest, seeing that he found not in himselfe any disposition to goe to any other place, nor to take any taste in anything. I have understoode the like of others, and particularly of one that was of our company, who being then a Secular man, had passed by these desarts: and it is a strange thing, the qualitie of this colde aire, which killes, and also preserves the dead bodies without corruption. I have also understoode it of a reverend religious man, of the Order of Saint Dominike, and Prelate thereof, who hadde seen it passing by the desarts: and which is strange, hee reported, that traveling that way by night, was forced to defend himself against that deadly winde which blowes there (having no other meanes but to gather together a great number of those dead bodies that lay there, and made thereof, as it were, a rampire and bolster for his head: in this manner did he sleepe, the dead bodies giving him life. Without doubt this is a kinde of cold so piercing, that it quencheth the vitall heate, cutting off his influence; and being so exceedingly colde, yet doth not corrupt nor give any putrifaction to the dead bodies, for that putrifaction groweth from heate and moystness. As for the other kinde of ayre which thunders under the earth, and causeth earthquakes, more at the Indies, then in any other Regions, I will speake thereof in treating the qualities of the land at the Indies. We will content our selves now with what wee have spoken of the wind and aire, and passe to that which is to be spoken of the water.

BRONCHIAL CAST

Nicholas Tulp

CHAPTER XIII

AN ENTIRE VEIN CAST UP FROM THE LUNGS*

A ship's captain of Amsterdam, who lived a long time on the sea, acquired, a long time since, from a chronic catarrh, a cough more troublesome on land than on sea. This cough, for two years, tormenting his feeble lungs he finally cleared out this organ, which had been greatly harassed and he cast forth, unexpectedly, not so much blood, but besides two remarkable branches of veins; each equal in extent to the size of the hand. Moreover they stood out separately from the rest of the tissue showing quite distinctly the finest details: when patient anatomist removed the tissue about which obscured it.

In truth from the apparent evidence, the whole lung was injured and hence by no means a wonder since these young branches were excreted, and cast out, with the life

blood itself. And indeed the physicians were astonished at such a dissolution of tissue without previous pus. This itself by chance will also be the greatest marvel to succeeding generations: for a similar case has neither been seen nor written about in any records of physicians. But as the deepest rivers flow with the least sound, thus the greatest misfortunes happen to a man immediately; without noisy warnings.

Now these veins were dissected, this unheard of wonder, indeed, I saw myself, and it was examined publicly by my Preceptor Peter Paaw, showing the same form, as the artist showed them by his skill: in this table which I have added to this work. This was given to me by the official Egbert Bodaeus, who made the medicine for this patient, and that gentleman, of profound erudition, Sebastian Egbert Burgomaster of Amsterdam.

* Tulp, Nicholas, *Observationes Medicae*, Book II, Chapter XIII (Leyden, du Vivie, 1716), p. 116.

Richard Warren

Richard Warren was born in 1731 at Cavendish in Suffolkshire, England, the son of the Reverend Richard Warren, archdeacon of Suffolk. He was educated at the grammar school at Bury St. Edmunds and in 1748 entered Jesus College, Cambridge. After obtaining his bachelor's degree in 1752, Warren was undecided whether to enter the church or to study law. While in this state of indecision, Dr. Peter Shaw, an eminent London physician, placed his son in Jesus College under Warren's tuition. Dr. Shaw became much interested in young Warren, urged him to study medicine and later gave him the hand of his daughter Elizabeth in marriage.

Warren received the degree of M.D. in 1762 and became a member of the Royal College of Physicians the same year. His progress as a physician was

unusually rapid. He soon obtained a large practice, became physician to
Princess Amelia, daughter of King George II, and in 1763, one year after receiving his M.D., became physician to George III. Warren died in 1797. He
is said to have realized 9000 pounds a year from the time of the regency, and

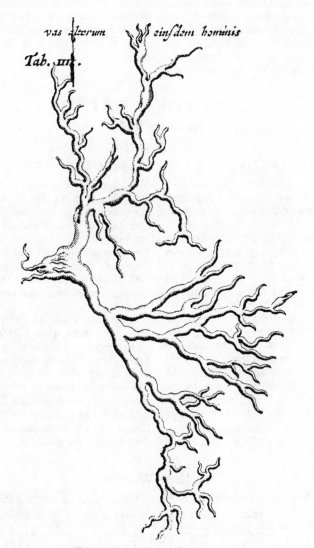

Tulp's illustration of bronchial cast

to have bequeathed to his family above 150,000 pounds. Munk remarks, "If
posterity should ask what works Dr. Warren left behind him worthy of the
great reputation he enjoyed during his lifetime, it must be answered that such
was his constant occupation in practice among all classes of people, from the
highest to the lowest, that he had no leisure for writing, with the exception of a
very few papers published in the College Transactions."

XVI. OF THE BRONCHIAL POLYPUS: BY R. WARREN, M.D., FELLOW OF THE COLLEGE OF PHYSICIANS, AND OF THE ROYAL SOCIETY; AND PHYSICIAN IN ORDINARY TO HIS MAJESTY*

Read at the College, August 11, 1767

Polypous concretions, in different parts of the body, have been described by various anatomical and medical writers; but that species of *polypus* called the bronchial, formed in the ramifications of the *aspera*

from complaint the next morning. About six weeks after this, I found her more oppressed than she was described to me to have been before; her pulse was too quick to be counted with accuracy; her tongue was white and

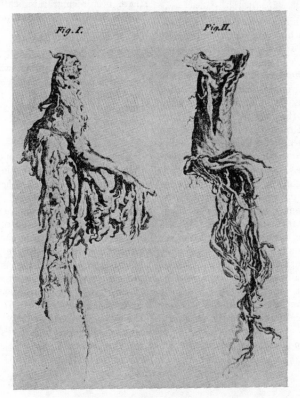

Warren's illustration of bronchial cast

arteria, has escaped the observation of the greater number of them, and has almost always been mistaken for something else by the few who have seen it.

In the spring of the year 1764, a young lady, eight years old, of a strumous habit, was seized with a difficulty of breathing, attended with a short, dry and almost incessant cough; but without any pain in her sides or breast. During the course of the day, the difficulty of breathing and cough lessened; she rested tolerably well at night, and was free

moist, her head was clear; her bowels were costive; and she was perfectly free from all painful sensations, except that of weight on the chest. Five ounces of blood were taken away, a blister was applied to her back; and an opening draught was directed. Soon after the bleeding, the difficulty of breathing began to lessen; and after the opening draught had operated, it was still more relieved.

The next morning her breathing continuing oppressed, and her pulse beating about an hundred and twenty times a minute, it was determined to purge her still more, upon a supposition that worms, in so young a

* *Med. Tr. Coll. Phy.*, London, 1772, I, 407.

subject, might probably be the cause of these complaints: no worms, however came away; but after two or three copious stools, her breathing was considerably relieved. During the six following days, her pulse beat about an hundred times to a minute; and her breathing, when she was quite still, was tolerably easy; she eat heartily; coughed frequently, but without any expectoration; sweated profusely in the nights; and wasted very much. On the seventh day the extreme difficulty of breathing returned with a pulse as quick as before; but was much relieved by a dose of *exymel scilliticum,* which made her vomit two or three times. During the four following days, she took ten drops of *oxymel scilliticum* in an ounce and half of water every eighth hour. The difficulty of breathing decreased under this course; but the pulse continued to beat more than an hundred and twenty times in a minute. In the night of the twelfth day from the attack, she waked suddenly, and was almost choked in bringing up, by coughing, a large polypous concretion. It came up without either blood or *mucus;* and instantly gave her great relief. During the two following months, she seldom passed three days without coughing up some pieces, but none so large as the first. Her breathing continued to be much affected by motion in the room; but was tolerably easy when she was sitting still, or even when she was in motion in the open air. Though her pulse never beat less than an hundred and twenty times in a minute; from the time that she began to cough up the *polypi,* yet she had a good appetite; gained some strength and flesh, and entirely lost her sweats.

* * *

FIGURE

In figure they represent very exactly a branch of the *aspera arteria* with its smaller ramifications. At one end they are formed into a thick trunk, the extremity of which is brcken and ragged, and towards the other end there is a regular ramification into smaller, and at last almost evanescent twigs. Figs. I. II.

COLOUR

Their colour immediately, and for some days after they came up, was neither of the yellowish nor bluish cast, which is commonly observed in the *mucus* that is brought up by coughing; but of as bright and as opake too, as a curd of milk.

SUBSTANCE

Some of them are of a much firmer texture than others, and bear shaking in water without breaking to pieces. Others are so tender that a very gentle motion in water breaks off a great many of their smaller branches. They are solid, composed of *laminae,* which are easily separated from each other, and are manifestily of a texture less and less firm. as you approach the center or *axis,* which consists of a white pappy *mucus* as thick as cream. I observed one about the size of a quill, which was tubular. It seemed to consist of a few *lamellae* only; the inner part, making up at least two thirds of the cone, being shot out of it.

SKODAIC RESONANCE

Josef Skoda

One of the greatest physicians of the famous Vienna school of the early nineteenth century was Josef Skoda. He was born in Pilsen, Bohemia, in 1805, the son of a poor blacksmith. He grew up in a poverty stricken home and because of his poor health and the poverty at home he decided to become a priest. An older brother, Franz, was a student at Vienna and was tutor in the family of a wealthy manufacturer. The wife of this manufacturer while on a journey met young Josef in Pilsen and was much attracted by the youth. On hearing that he wished to study medicine but because of poverty was planning to enter the Church, she invited him to come to Vienna and live at her home. Josef accepted her invitation and in 1825, when twenty years of age, he walked to Vienna—a six days' journey by foot—and began his studies.

In Vienna he worked hard at his medical studies and also found time to study physics and mathematics. He showed such unusual ability in his mathematical studies that his professor, the celebrated Baumgartner, urged him to abandon medicine and devote himself entirely to mathematics. He did not however follow this advice, but continued his medical studies, and received his doctor's degree in 1831. He spent a year in Bohemia studying cholera and then returned to Vienna, where he became an assistant physician at the Allgemeines

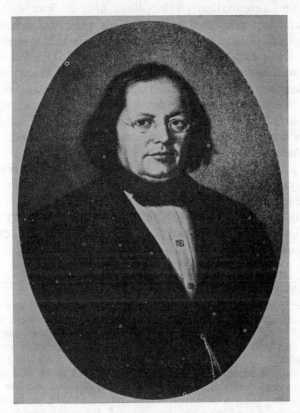

JOSEPH SKODA (1805-1881)
From Sternberg's "Josef Skoda" Vienna 1924

Krankenhaus and began to give courses in physical diagnosis. He devoted himself particularly to the study of diseases of the chest and his skill in diagnosis attracted the attention of Rokitansky who became his close friend. A striking circumstance brought out his remarkable ability in diagnosis and started him upon the road to fame.

The Duke de Blacas, French minister to Austria, was very ill and Doctors Malfatti, Türckheim, and Wirer, the first physicians in Vienna, diagnosed a disease of the liver and ordered him to Carlsbad. Skoda was called into consultation, made a diagnosis of aneurysm of the abdominal aorta, and said the patient would die in a very short time. Skoda's prediction was soon fulfilled and the autopsy confirmed his diagnosis. Skoda's diagnosis and its verification created a sensation and Türckheim remarked, "wenn ich jünger wäre, würde ich bei Ihnen lernen" (if I were younger, I would go to school to you). Türckheim became his champion and, through his influence, young Skoda was later advanced to the rank of physician in the Allgemeines Krankenhaus, with a service of his own.

Skoda was one of the first to recognize the importance of Semmelweiss' work on puerperal fever. He is best remembered however for his treatise on percussion and auscultation (*Abhandlung über Perkussion und Auskultation*), which was first published in 1839. This work still remains one of the best books on physical diagnosis and is noteworthy in that it stresses the underlying physical basis of auscultation and percussion. The following selection describes the well-known Skodaic resonance, "a permanent part of modern diagnosis" (Garrison). This sign seems, however, to have been known to Auenbrugger. "Verùm si media pars aquâ repleta fuerit, evocabitur resonantia major in illâ parte, quam aquosus humor non occupaverit." (But if it is only half filled with water, an increased resonance is produced in that part, which the fluid does not fill.)

Skoda was a bachelor and a man of few words. He was generally considered hard and cold, yet he was devoted to his patients, was a great lover of animals, and was so considerate, we are told, that he wore queer clothes for years because he disliked to offend his tailor. He suffered from gout for many years and his funeral in 1881 was an imposing and striking testimony of the respect and love that all classes of society had for this remarkable man.

---

*THIRD CLASS:—PERCUSSION SOUNDS. TYMPANITIC. NON-TYMPANITIC

The tympanitic percussion sound passes gradually into the non-tympanitic, just as the full into the empty, and the clear into the dull; no distinct line of demarkation can be drawn between them.

The non-tympanitic is represented by the sound which percussion produces at those parts of the thorax, beneath which lies healthy lung, normally distended by air. An abnormally distended lung, as in vesicular emphysema, gives us at one time a tympanitic, at another, a non-tympanitic sound. A partial emphysema in the midst of lung deprived of air (as happens in pneumonia, where not unfrequently the tissue around the hepatized portion and especially at the borders of the lung, is emphysematous) generally produces a tympanitic sound; but if the whole of the lung is emphysematous, the sound is seldom distinctly tympanitic. If the lung contains less than its normal quantity of air, it yields a sound which approaches the tympanitic, or is distinctly tympanitic. The sound is, moreover, in many cases remarkably tympanitic, even when the diminution of the quantity of air in the lung is the effect of an increase in its fluid or solid constituents; and this, too, whether the lung retains its normal volume, or becomes larger than natural. When the lung is much reduced in volume by compression, but still contains air, its sound is invariably tympanitic.

* * *

That the lungs partially deprived of air, should yield a tympanitic, and when the quantity of air in them is increased, a non-tympanitic sound appears opposed to the laws of physics. The fact however is certain, and is corroborated both by experiments on the dead body (which will presently be referred to,) and also by this constant phenomenon, viz.: that when the lower portion of a lung is entirely compressed by any pleuritic effusion, and its upper portion reduced in volume, the percussion-sound at the upper part of the thorax is distinctly tympanitic.

* From *Auscultation and Percussion*, by Dr. Joseph Skoda. Translated from the Fourth Edition by W. O. Markham, M.D., Philadelphia, Lindsay and Blakiston, 1854, p. 46.

When the walls of the thorax are thin and yielding, the percussion-sound may remain tympanitic, even though the quantity of air in the lung be very small: this fact we occasionally observe in cases of pneumonia and tubercular infiltration. The condensed portions of the lung, beneath the thoracic walls thus thin and yielding, give, in some cases, a distinctly tympanitic, though very empty, and not very loud sound. The percussion-sound is seldom tympanitic when the walls of the thorax are dense and unyielding.

LOBAR PNEUMONIA

Hippocrates*

REGIMEN IN ACUTE DISEASES

11. Peripneumonia, and pleuritic affections, are to be thus observed: If the fever be acute, and if there be pains on either side, or in both, and if expiration be attended with pain, if cough be present, and the sputa expectorated be of a blond or livid color, or likewise thin, frothy, and florid, or having any other character different from the common, in such a case, the physician should proceed thus: if the pain pass upward to the clavicle, or the breast, or the arm, the inner vein in the arm should be opened on the side affected, and the blood abstracted according to the habit, age, and color of the patient, and the season of the year, and that largely and boldly, if the pain be acute, so as to bring on deliquium animi, and afterwards a clyster is to be given But if the pain be below the chest, and if very intense, purge the bowels gently in such an attack of pleurisy, and during the act of purging give nothing; but after the purging give oxymel. The medicine is to be administered on the fourth day; on the first three days after the commencement, a clyster should be given, and if it does not relieve the patient, he should then be gently purged, but he is to be watched until the fever goes off, and till the seventh day; then if he appear to be free from danger, give him some unstrained ptisan, in a small quantity, and thin at first, mixing it with honey. If the expectoration be easy, and the breathing free, if his sides be free of pain, and if the fever be gone, he may take the ptisan thicker, and in larger quantity, twice a day. But if he do not progress favorably, he must get less of the drink, and of the draught, which should be thin, and only given once a day, at whatever is judged to be the most favorable hour; this you will ascertain from the urine. The draught is not to be given to persons after fever, until you see that the urine and sputa are concocted, (if, indeed, after the administration of the medicine he be purged frequently, it may be necessary to give it, but it should be given in smaller quantities and thinner than usual, for from inanition he will be unable to sleep, or digest properly, or wait the crisis;) but when the melting down of crude matters has taken place, and his system has cast off what is offensive, there will then be no objection. The sputa are concocted when they resemble pus, and the urine when it has a reddish sediment like tares. But there is nothing to prevent fomentations and cerates being applied for the other pains of the sides; and the legs and loins may be rubbed with hot oil, or annointed with fat; linseed, too, in the form of a cataplasm, may be applied to the hypochondrium and as far up as the breasts. When pneumonia is at its height, the case is beyond remedy if he be not purged, and it is bad if he has dyspnoea, and the urine is thin and acrid, and if sweat comes out about the neck and head, for such sweats are bad, as proceeding from the suffocation, *râles*, and the violence of the disease which is obtaining the upper hand. unless there be a copious evacuation of thick urine, and the sputa be concocted; when either of these come on spontaneously, that will carry off the disease. A linctus for pneumonia: Galbanum and pine-fruit in Attic honey, and southernwood in oxymel; make a decoction of pepper and black hellebore, and give it in cases of pleurisy attended with violent pains at the commencement. It is also a good thing to boil opoponax in oxymel, and, having strained it, to give it to drink; it answers well, also, in diseases of the liver, and in severe pains proceeding from the dia-

* The Genuine Works of Hippocrates, translated by Francis Adams, LL.D. London, Sydenham Society, 1859, Vol. I, p. 324.

phragm, and in all cases in which it is beneficial to determine to the bowels or urinary organs, when given in wine and honey; when given to act upon the bowels, it should be drunk in larger quantity, along with a watery hydromel.

Aretaeus

CHAPTER I

ON PNEUMONIA*

Animals live by two principal things, food and breath (*spirit, pneuma*); of these by far the most important is the respiration, for if it be stopped, the man will not endure long, but immediately dies. The organs of it are many, the commencement being the nostrils; the passage, the trachea; the containing vessel, the lungs; the protection and receptacle of the lungs, the thorax. But the other parts, indeed, minister only as instruments to the animal; but the lungs also contain the cause of attraction, for in the midst of them is seated a hot organ, the heart, which is the origin of life and respiration. It imparts to the lungs the desire of drawing in cold air, for it raises a heat in them; but it is the heart which attracts, If, therefore, the heart suffer primarily, death is not far off.

But if the lungs be affected, from a slight cause there is difficulty of breathing; the patient lives miserably, and death is the issue, unless some one effects a cure. But in a great affection, such as inflammation, there is a sense of suffocation, loss of speech and of breathing, and a speedy death. This is what we call Peripneumonia, being an inflammation of the lungs, with acute fever, when they are attended with heaviness of the chest, freedom from pain, provided the lungs alone are inflamed; for they are naturally insensible, being of loose texture, like wool. But branches of the aspera arteria are spread through them, of a cartilaginous nature, and these, also, are insensible; muscles there are nowhere, and the nerves are small, slender, and minister to motion. This is the cause of the insensibility to pain. But if any of the membranes, by which it is connected with the chest, be inflamed, pain also is present; respiration bad, and hot; they wish to get up into an erect posture, as being the easiest of all postures for the respiration. Ruddy in countenance, but especially the cheeks; the

The Extant Works of Aretaeus the Cappadocian, edited and translated by Francis Adams, London Sydenham Society, 1856, p. 261.

white of the eyes very bright and fatty; the point of the nose flat; the veins in the temples and neck distended; loss of appetite; pulse, at first, large, empty, very frequent, as if forcibly accelerated; heat indeed, externally, feeble, and more humid than natural, but, internally, dry, and very hot, by means of which the breath is hot; there is thirst, dryness of the tongue, desire of cold air, aberration of mind; cough mostly dry, but if anything be brought up it is a frothy phlegm, or slightly tinged with bile, or with a very florid tinge of blood. The blood-stained is of all others the worst.

But if the disease tend to a fatal termination, there is insomnolency; sleep brief, heavy, of comatose nature; vain fancies; they are in a doting state of mind, but not violently delirious; they have no knowledge of their present sufferings. If you interrogate them respecting the disease, they will not acknowledge any formidable symptom; the extremities cold; the nails livid, and curved; the pulse small, very frequent, and failing, in which case death is near at hand, for they die mostly on the seventh day.

But if the disease abate and take a favourable turn, there is a copious hemorrhage from the nose, a discharge from the bowels of much bilious and frothy matters, such as might seem to be expelled from the lungs to the lower belley, provided it readily brings off much in a liquid state. Sometimes there is a determination to the urine. But they recover the most speedily in whose cases all these occur together.

In certain cases much pus is formed in the lungs, or there is a metastasis from the side, if a greater symptom of convalescence be at hand. But if, indeed, the matter be translated from the side to the intestine or bladder, the patients immediately recover from the peripneumony; but they have a chronic abscess in the side, which, however, gets better. But if the matter burst upon the lungs, some have thereby been suffocated, from the copious effusion and inability to bring it up. But such as escape suffocation from the bursting of the abscess, have a large ulceration in the lungs, and pass into phthisis; and from the abscess and phthisis old persons do not readily recover; but from the peripneumony, youths and adults.

Leopold Auenbrugger

Leopold Auenbrugger, the discoverer of percussion, was born in Gratz, Austria, in 1722. His father was an inn-keeper and according to an old tradition, young Leopold, having to find the level of the wine in his father's casks, later

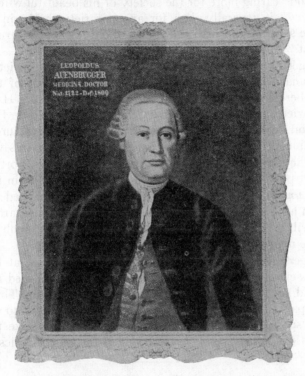

LEOPOLD AUENBRUGGER (1722-1809)
Painted in 1770. Artist unknown. Restored by
Kurt von Goldenstein

utilized this knowledge in the discovery of percussion. Indeed, Auenbrugger in his work on percussion remarks that "casks as long as they are empty are resonant everywhere, but when filled lose this resonance in proportion as the volume of air they contain is diminished."

Leopold Auenbrugger went to school in his native city and then entered the University of Vienna, where he studied medicine, receiving his doctor's degree in 1752. In 1751 he obtained an appointment as physician to the Spanish Military Hospital in Vienna, the largest and finest in the Austrian capital, and ten years later published his *Inventum novum ex percussione thoracis humani ut signo abstrusos interni pectoris morbus detegendi* (New invention, by means of percussing the human chest as a sign of detecting obscure diseases in the interior of the chest). This book apparently was not noticed by the medical profession but the neglect does not seem to have embittered Auenbrugger. He was dismissed from his position at the Spanish Military Hospital the year after the appearance of his book and began to devote himself entirely to his private practice. He became quite popular at the Court of Vienna, became an intimate friend of the Empress Marie Theresa, and was ennobled by the Emperor Joseph II with the title "Edler von Auenbrugg." He also wrote the libretto of an opera, *The Chimney-Sweep,* but seems to have refused requests to repeat the experiment, and "caring more for the society of his beautiful wife, good music, and *Gemüthlichkeit* generally than for any notoriety, he is, indeed, a noble example of the substantial worth and charm of old-fashioned German character at its very best." (Garrison)

Auenbrugger's *Inventum novum* was unnoticed by van Swieten, then professor in Vienna, who wrote a treatise in 1764 on hydrops of the chest and pulmonary tuberculosis making no mention of percussion. De Haen, who succeeded von Swieten, also ignored it, but Stoll, who followed de Haen, took up the method and demonstrated it to many students. Stoll's lectures on chronic diseases mentioned this method and Corvisart, on reading this work, became interested in the discovery and began to practice percussion. Forty-seven years later Corvisart published, in 1808, his well-known translation in French of the *Inventum novum* with his own commentaries. Corvisart praised the discovery most highly in his preface and his magnanimous conduct in regard to this book has been described elsewhere. This translation established Auenbrugger's fame and spread the news of the discovery throughout the world.

Auenbrugger died the year after Corvisart's translation, at the advanced age of eighty-seven. His *Inventum novum,* which he published at the age of thirty-nine, did not make him famous until he was eighty-six. This small book of ninety-five pages, written, as he says not "because of an itch to write or of an exuberance of speculations" but because of a desire "to recognize, prognosticate and cure affections of the chest," remains one of the great classics of medicine.

OBSERVATION X*

CONCERNING SCIRRHUS OF THE LUNGS AND ITS SIGNS

XXXXVIII—I say that scirrhus of the lung is present when the spongy substance of the lung has degenerated into a fleshy and indolent mass.

Scholium—A spongy particle of the lung immersed in water always floats; which indeed when indurated, changed into a fleshy mass, is observed to sink.

Great differences are observed in these indurations. I have seen the scirrhous lungs of cadavers to be different, not only in

* Auenbrugger, Leopold, *Inventum novum,* Vienna, Trattner, 1761, p. 61.

hardness, but also in color and in the nature of the contents.

Thus in inflammatory diseases of the chest (which are fatal the 5th, 7th, or 9th day) the lung is found so engorged with blood, that it seems very often not to differ much from the liver, neither in color, nor in consistency.

One thing is worthy of mention, that a purulent pseudo-membrane often surrounds it, when an acute pleurisy has given origin to a lethal peripneumonia.

Indeed the lungs are deceiving in their remarkable variations, which autopsy reveals in chronic diseases. For often sabaceous materials are scattered about resembling marble: often they show, under a cartilaginous consistency a fleshy mass: many times they are found indurated with a thick and black blood. This difference appears indeed to depend upon the variety of the morbid material.

XXXIX—Where this is present complete, and not yet is changed into liquid, these signs are observed.

The signs of scirrhus of the lungs—With the findings of the resonance impaired or totally suppressed in the affected parts of the thorax, the patients are more rarely afflicted with a cough.

They bring up no sputum or it is viscid. raw and scanty.

In the quiet patient nothing is noted in the pulse nor in the respiration, which in good faith could be suspected.

Only with more active movements suffocation attacks them: but after talking some they suffer pain and are fatigued.

It happens that at the same time they feel a dry harshness in the throat, and also the pulse which is moderately fast, now becomes rapid and irregular.

Respiration and speech are now interrupted and broken by sighs.

The face now presents signs worthy of note: for the temporal, sublingual and jugular veins on the affected side are more distended than usual: meanwhile the ill affected side of the chest appears less mobile on inspiration.

On the other hand the natural and animal functions proceed normally: and he can lie down easily on either side.

And these are the signs which indicate a hardening of the lungs. For these all become the more serious as it occupies a greater space in the side of the chest.

R.-T.-H. Laënnec

SECT. II—SIGNS AND SYMPTOMS OF PERIPNEUMONY*

This is one of the diseases most anciently known; and before pathological anatomy (which has been prosecuted with zeal in every part of Europe since the time of Morgagni) had investigated the true nature of diseases, it was generally regarded as one of the internal affections most readily recognized. This however, is far from being the case. It is not easily recognized except when it is uncomplicated, and has already attained a considerable degree of intensity. When complicated with another disease, and also in its very commencement, it remains latent because its most usual symptoms are either frequently wanting or are common to other diseases.

In the present section, I shall first notice the physical signs which characterize the disease in all cases, and from its onset; I shall then speak of the symptoms depending on the disorder of the functions of the lungs, and examine how far, and in what cases these may serve as signs; and finally I shall describe the general symptoms and progress of the disease.

* Laënnec, R-T-H., *A Treatise on the Diseases of the Chest and on Mediate Auscultation,* translated by John Forbes, M.D., New York, Samuel Wood & Sons, 1830, p. 211.

Physical signs. The crepitous rattle is the pathognomonic sign of the first stage of peripneumony. It is perceptible from the very invasion of the inflammation; at this time it conveys the notion of very small equalsized bubbles, and seems hardly to possess the character of humidity. These characters are more marked, according as the inflamed spot is near the surface of the lungs. The sound of respiration is still heard distinctly, combined with the crepitous rattle; and percussion affords the natural resonance. The extent over which the stethoscope detects the rattle, indicates the extent of the inflammation. This is frequently hardly greater than the diameter of the instrument. The further we remove the cylinder from the point affected, the rattle becomes more obscure, and ceases to be heard altogether at the distance of two or three inches. In proportion as the obstruction increases and verges towards hepatization, the rattle becomes moister, and its bubbles more unequal and less numerous; the sound of respiration, which accompanied it at first, gradually disappears; and at last, as hepatization takes place, the rattle itself ceases to be heard. At this period of the disease, the sound on percussion does not sensibly differ from that of health, unless the obstruction is very extensive and already verging on hepatization. In this latter case, it becomes somewhat more obscure. But when the obstruction is confined to a small portion of the lung, or when it exists in the form of isolated masses here and there, percussion affords no information. This is also frequently the case, even in an extensive engorgement of the lower part of the right lung, on account of the natural obscurity of the sound in that region from the presence of the liver.

Such are the physical signs of pneumonia in the first degree. Of these the most important is unquestionably the crepitous rattle; inasmuch as it is invariably present, and from the very invasion of the disease; and exists in no other case, except in oedema of the lungs and pulmonary apoplexy, two diseases which are easily distinguished from this, by their own peculiar signs and symptoms. M. Andral is mistaken in saying that the crepitous rattle sometimes exists in simple acute bronchitis (Cl. Med. tom. II. p. 333;) and I think this is evident from his own cases. From its constant presence in this disease, I regard it as the most practically useful of all the stethoscopic signs, inasmuch as it points out, in its very earliest stage, one of the most severe and most common diseases, and thereby enables the physician to apply his means with much more chance of success than he could have done even a few hours later.

When the inflammation has reached the degree of hepatization, we no longer perceive in the affected part, either the crepitous rattle or the respiratory sound; and the absence of these phenomena is frequently the only sign we have of hepatization having taken place. Bronchophonism exists near the roots of the lungs, or in the upper lobes, in which places the bronchial tubes are largest. When the pneumonia is central, bronchophonism either does not exist at all, or is very obscure; it becomes more and more manifest, as the inflammation approaches the surface of the lungs. By means of this sign I have frequently been able to indicate, previously to opening the chest, the precise point where a central peripneumony had reached the exterior of the organ. This is easily accounted for, by the fact that a hepatized lung is a better conductor of sound than a healthy one,—bronchophonism being nothing more

than the resonance of the voice within the bronchia of the inflamed part. A pleuritic effusion, if posterior to the hepatization, renders bronchophonism stronger, by compressing and condensing the superficial parts of the lungs not yet affected by the inflammation; but the reverse happens when the pleurisy precedes the peripneumony. It is more especially when existing near the roots of the lungs, that bronchophonism is rendered much stronger by the interposition of a small layer of fluid; and it is in this case that the co-existence of aegophonism gives rise to the mixed phenomena described in the Preliminary Essay. Bronchophonism is always less strongly marked and more diffused, in the lower parts of the lungs, owing to the lesser diameter of the bronchia there; and becomes quite imperceptible in this situation, if the corresponding parts of the pleura contain a fluid. The bronchial respiration and cough always accompany bronchophonism; and the former sometimes are very distinct when the latter is not so. In this case, an attentive examination enables us to discover that the bronchial respiration and cough have their seat in the interior of the lungs, and that the superficial parts are still permeable to the air, or simply obstructed. If a rattle exists in the bronchia at the same time, the hepatization renders it much stronger and more distinct. When the hepatization is near the surface, and involves within it bronchial tubes of a considerable size, as when it has its seat at the roots or in the top of the lungs, bronchophonism becomes then almost like pectoriloquism. In this case, it is frequently accompanied by the sensation of *blowing into the ear*, and if a thin portion of pulmonary substance, not yet hepatized, intervenes between the ear and the affected bronchia, the sensation denominated the *veiled puff*, is produced. As long as the inflammation increases, the crepitous rattle extends daily around the hepatized part, or arises in new points; it precedes the signs of hepatization, which commonly are found, on the following day, very distinct in those points where the crepitous rattle had existed the day before.

These are the physical signs of hepatization; which is always further accompanied by a dull sound on percussion, over the affected parts; except in the case where the pneumonia is central. In this case, and especially if the hepatization occupies the centre of the left inferior lobe, and the lower part of the right side be naturally imperfectly sonorous, as commonly happens, percussion will frequently furnish us with no useful result, or will at most lead us to suspect the affection of the left lower lobe. For the same reason, if the hepatization occupies the right inferior lobe, percussion will only then enable us to recognize its presence, where we had previously ascertained the natural sonorousness of this part; since there are many persons in whom the right side of the chest, as high as the fourth or fifth rib, is naturally destitute of sound. In almost all cases, where the points hepatized are of small extent, percussion gives us no assistance.

Signs of suppuration. The infiltration of pus within the pulmonary tissue furnishes no new sign as long as the pus remains concrete. When this begins to soften, we preceive in the bronchia a more or less distinct mucous rattle, occasioned either by the introduction of the pus into them, or by the more copious mucous secretion which then takes place, sympathetic of the suppurative process going on within the pulmonary substance.

Signs of abscess. When the pus is not absorbed or expectorated in proportion as it becomes softened, but collects into one spot, a very strong mucous or cavernous rattle, with large bubbles, is perceived over the site of the abscess. The bronchophonism is converted into pectoriloquism, and the respiration and cough change from bronchial to cavernous. If the abscess is near the surface, the respiration and cough yield the *puffing respiration*, and according to circumstances, the *veiled puff.* These signs are almost always easily distinguished from the analogous phenomena which exist in hepatization, viz. bronchophonism, bronchial cough and respiration, and bronchial mucous rattle. A little experience will enable us to discriminate the *bronchial* from the *cavernous* phenomena. The latter always are distinctly circumscribed, and appear to have their site in a space larger than any bronchial trunk. The intensity of the rattle when the abscess is only half-full, the stuttering sound of the pectoriloquism in the same case, and the small extent of the peripneumonic affection (which had either been partial from the be-

ginning or is now become so by the resolution of the remaining parts) are additional signs which in most cases leave no room for doubt. On the other hand, the bronchial phenomena are remarkable by their diffused character; bronchophonism when most like pectoriloquism, always differs from it in this respect: moreover, in bronchophonism the voice rarely traverses the whole extent of the cylinder: it is also *pure* in this case, or if accompanied by a mucous rattle, which is not common, this has never the exact circumscription, and rarely has the intensity, of the cavernous rattle.

Signs or resolution. When resolution takes place before hepatization has supervened, the crepitous rattle becomes daily less perceptible, while the natural sound of respiration becomes gradually more distinct and at last is alone heard. When hepatization has taken place, its resolution is invariably announced by the return of the crepitous rattle. I have never seen this sign wanting in any case which I have been able to examine daily: I commonly denominate it—*the renewed crepitous rattle (rhonchus crepitans redux).* M. Andral has noticed in it most of his examples of pneumonia cured. (Obs. XI, XII, XIII, XV, XVI, XXXVIII, XXXIX.) To the crepitous rattle is gradually joined the natural sound of respiration which becomes daily more distinct and at last exists alone. The crepitous rattle equally announces the resolution of the pneumonia when it has arrived at the stage of suppuration; but in this case, it is usually preceded by a mucous or submucous rattle, indicating the softening of a part of the pus. In this case, the natural sound of respiration returns much more slowly than in the preceding instances. At the expiration of a few days, or even sometimes of a few hours, the crepitous rattle becomes subcrepitous, indicating the supervention of oedema which usually attends the resolution of this stage of peripneumony. The same thing is observed when oedema accompanies the resolution of the other two stages of the inflammation. When the disease has extended to the greater part of the lungs, the extreme points and the parts most recently attacked, are usually those in which resolution commences: the contrary, however, is sometimes the case.

PLEURISY AND EMPYEMA

The following account of the procedure known as Hippocratic succussion is found in the treatise *de morbis*. The authenticity of this treatise is doubtful and many authorities reject it as the work of Hippocrates. The translation is from Fuchs' edition.*

Hippocrates

If as a result of the treatments of the pus does not break through, one should not be surprised, for often it breaks into the body, and the patient seems to be better, because the pus has passed from a narrow space to a larger one. As time goes on, the fever becomes more severe, coughing begins, the side begins to pain, the patient can not lie any more on the healthy side but on the diseased side, the feet and the eyes swell. When the fifteenth day after the rupture has appeared, prepare a warm bath, set him upon a stool, which is not wobbly, someone should hold his hands, then shake him by the shoulders and listen to see on which side a noise is heard. And right at this place—preferably on the left—make an incision, then it produces death more rarely.

* * *

ON THE PROGNOSTICS†

17. Empyema may be recognized in all cases by the following symptoms: In the first place, the fever does not go off, but is slight during the day, and increases at night, and copious sweats intervene, there is a desire to cough, and the patients expectorate nothing worth mentioning, the eyes became hollow, the cheeks have red spots on them, the nails of the hand are bent, the fingers are hot, especially their extremities, there are swellings in the feet, they have no desire for food, and small blisters (phlyctaenae) occur over the body. These symptoms attend chronic empyemata, and may be much trusted to; and such as are of short standing are indicated by the same, provided they be accompanied by those signs which occur at the commencement, and if at the same time the patient has some difficulty of breathing. Whether they will break earlier or later may be determined by these symptoms; or there be pain at the commencement, and if the dsypnoea, cough, and ptyalism be severe, the rupture may be expected in the course of twenty days or still earlier; but if the pain be more mild, and all the other symptoms in proportion, you may expect from these the rupture to be later; but pain, dyspnoea, and ptyalism, must take place before the rupture of the abscess. Those patients recover must readily whom the fever leaves the same day, that the abscess bursts—when they recover their appetite speedily, and are freed from thirst —when the alvine discharges are small and consistent, the matter white, smooth, uniform in color, and free of phlegm, and if brought up without pain or strong coughing. Those die whom the fever does not leave, or when appearing to leave them it returns with an exacerbation; when they have thirst, but no desire of food, and there are watery discharges from the bowels; when the expectoration is green or livid, or pituitous and frothy; if all these occur they die, but if certain of these symptoms supervene, and others not, some patients die and some recover, after a long interval. But from all the symptoms taken together one should form a judgment, and so in all other cases.

* * *

REGIMEN IN ACUTE DISEASES*

30. *For persons affected with empyema.* Having cut some bulbs of squill, boil in water, and when well boiled, throw this away, and having poured in more water, boil until it appear to the touch soft and well-boiled; then triurate finely and mix roasted cumin, and white sesames, and young almonds

---

* Hippokrates, Sämmtliche Werke, *Ins Deutsche übersetzt und ausfürlich commentiert von Robert Fuchs,* München, Lüneberg. 1897-1900, II, 438.

† *The Genuine Works of Hippocrates,* translated from the Greek with a preliminary discourse and annotations by Francis Adams, LL.D. New York, Wm. Wood, n.d., I, p. 206.

* *The Genuine Works of Hippocrates,* translated from the Greek with a preliminary discourse and annotations by Francis Adams, LL.D., New York, Wm. Wood, n.d., II, p. 235, 236, 254, 266.

pounded in honey, form into an electuary and give; and afterwards sweet wine. In draughts, having pounded about a small acetabulum of the white poppy, moisten it with water in which summer wheat has been washed, add honey, and boil. Let him take frequently during the day. And then taking into account what are to happen, give him supper.

* * *

APHORISMS*

SECTION V

8. In pleuritic affections, when the disease is not purged off in fourteen days, it usually terminates in empyema.

15. Persons who become affected with empyema after pleurisy, if they get clear of it in forty days from the breaking of it, escape the disease; but if not, it passes into phthisis.

SECTION VI

27. Those cases of empyema or dropsy which are treated by incision or the cautery, if the water or pus flow rapidly all at once, certainly prove fatal.

44. When empyema is treated either by the cautery or incision, if pure and white pus flow from the wound, the patients recover, but if mixed with blood, slimy and fetid, they die.

FRICTION RUB†

Lung falling against the side: When the lung falls against the side, the patient has a cough and orthopnea; expectoration colorless; pain appears in the chest and in the back; the lung expands, rests upon the side; it seems to the patient as if he had a weight within his chest; acute pains torment him; a sound like that made by leather is heard, and respiration is halted. The patient can rest lying on the painful side, but he cannot on the healthy side, feeling that there is something heavy hanging from the side. One could say that he breathes by his chest. The patient should be bathed twice daily with a great deal of warm water and given melicrate to drink. After the bath he should take the following warm: Mix white wine and a little honey, pound the grain of daucus and centaury and cause them to digest. You should apply this against the side with warm water in a small leathern bottle or in a beef bladder.

You should support the chest with a bandage; then the patient will lie on the healthy side. He should take a decoction of barley, and, especially of wine diluted with water. If this disease follows as a result of a wound or of an incision for empyema (this happens sometimes), one should attach a cannula to a bladder, one should fill the bladder with air, and inject the air into the interior. One should insert a solid sound of tin and push it in first. It is by this treatment especially that you will succeed.

* * *

* *Ibid.*
† *Oeuvres Completes D'Hippocrate, traduction* par E. Litre, Paris, Baillière, 1851, vii, p. 93.

Aretaeus
CHAPTER X
ON PLEURISY†

Under the ribs, the spine, and the internal part of the thorax as far as the clavicles, there is stretched a thin strong membrane, adhering to the bones, which is named *succingens*. When inflammation occurs in it, and there is heat with cough and parti-coloured sputa, the affection is named Pleurisy. But all these symptoms must harmonize and conspire together as all springing from one

† *The Extant Works of Aretaeus, the Cappadocian,* Edited and translated by Francis Adams, LL.D. London, Sydenham Society, 1856, p. 255.

cause; for such of them as occur separately from different causes, even if they all occur together, are not called pleurisy. It is accompanied by acute pain of the clavicles; heat acrid; *decubitus* on the inflamed side easy, for thus the membrane (*pleura*) remains in its proper seat, but on the opposite side painful; for by its weight, the inflammation and suspension of the membrane, the pain stretches to all its adhesions at the shoulders and clavicles; and in certain cases even to the back and shoulder blade; the ancients called this affection Dorsal pleurisy. It is attended with dyspnoea, insomnolency, anorexia, florid redness of the cheeks, dry cough, difficult expectoration of phlegm, or bilious, or deeply tinged with blood, or yellowish; and these symptoms observe no order, but come and go irregularly; but, worst of all, if the bloody sputa cease, and the patients become delirious; and sometimes they become comatose, and in their somnolency the mind wavers.

But if the disease take a bad turn, all the symptoms getting worse, they die within the seventh day by falling into syncope; or, if the commencement of the expectoration, and the more intense symptoms occurred with the second hebdomad, they die on the fourteenth day. It sometimes happens that in the intermediate period there is a transference of all the symptoms to the lungs; for the lung attracts to itself, being both porous and hot, and being moved for the attraction of the substances around, when the patient is suddenly suffocated by metasis of the affection. But if the patient pass this period, and does not die within the twentieth day, he becomes affected with empyema. These, then, are the symptoms if the disease get into a bad state.

But if it take a favourable turn, there is a profuse hemorrhage by the nostrils, when the disease is suddenly resolved; then follow sleep and expectoration of phlegm, and afterwards of thin, bilious matters; then of still thinner, and again of bloody, thick, and flesh-like; and if, with the bloody, the bile return, and with it the phlegm, the patient's convalescence is secure; and these symptoms, if they should commence on the third day, with an easy expectoration of smooth, consistent, liquid, and (not) rounded sputa, the resolution takes place on the seventh day, when after bilious discharges from the bowels, there is freedom of respiration, the mind settled, fever diminishing, and return of appetite. But if these symptoms commence with the second week, the resolution occurs on the fourteenth day.

But if not so, it is converted into Empyema, as indicated by rigors, pungent pains, the desire of sitting erect, and the respiration becoming worse. It is then to be dreaded, lest, the lungs suddenly attracting the pus, the patient should be thereby suffocated, after having escaped the first and greater evils. But if the abscess creep in between the ribs and separate them, and point outwardly; or, if it burst into an intestine, for the most part the patient recovers.

Among the seasons of the year winter most especially engenders the disease; next, autumn; spring, less frequently; but summer most rarely. With regard to age, old men are most apt to suffer, and most readily escape from an attack; for neither is there apt to be a great inflammation in an arid frame; nor is there a metasis to the lungs, for old age is more frigid than any other age, and the respiration small, and the attraction of all things deficient. Young men and adults are not, indeed, very apt to suffer attacks; but neither, also, do they readily recover, for from a slight cause they would not experience even a slight attack of inflammation, and from great attacks there is greater danger. Children are least of all liable to pleurisy, and in their case it is less frequently fatal; for their bodies are rare, secretions copious, perspiration and exhalation abundant; hence neither is a great inflammation formed. This is the felicity of their period of life in the present affection.

Ambroise Paré

Chap. X

Of the Pleurisie*

What it is — The Pleurisie is an inflammation of the membrane, investing the ribs, caused by subtile and cholerick blood, springing upwards with great violence from the hollow vein into the *Azygos,* and thence

The Workes of that famous Chirurgion Ambrose Parey, Translated . . . by Tho. Johnson, London, Cotes, 1649, p. 234.

into the intercostall veins, and is Of a Pleurisie coming to suppuration at length powred forth into the emptie spaces of the intercostall muscles, and the metioned membrane. Being contained there, if it tend to suppuration, it commonly infers a pricking pain, a Feaver and difficulty of breathing. This suppurated blood is purged and evacuated one while by the mouth; the Lungs sucking it, and so casting it into the Weazon, and so into the mouth, otherwhiles by urine, and sometimes by stool.

Of the change thereof into an *Empyema*

But if nature being too weak. cannot expectorate the purulent blood, poured forth into the capacity of the chest, the disease is turned into an *Empyema,* wherefore the Chirurgeon must then be called, who beginning to reckon from below upwards, may make a vent between the third and fourth true and legitimate ribs; and that must be done either with an actual or potentiall cautery, or with a sharpe knife drawn upwards, towards the back, but

Of the aperition of the side in an *Empyema*

not downwards, less the vessels should be violated which are disseminated under the rib. This apertion may be safely and easily performed by this actual cautery; it is perforated with four holes, through one whereof there is a pin put higher or lower according to the depth and manner of your incision; then the point thereof is thrust through a plate of Iron perforated also in the midst, into the part designed by the Physitian, lest the wavering hand might peradventure touch, and so hurt the other parts not to be meddled withall. This same plate must be somewhat hollowed, that so it might be more easily fitted to the gibbous side, and bound by the corners on the contrary side with four strings. Wherefore I have thought good here to express the figures thereof.

But if the patient shall have a large body, Chest and ribs, you may divide and perforate the ribs themselves with a Trepan; howsoever the apertion be made, the *pus* or matter must be evacuated by little and little at severall times; and the capacity of the Chest cleansed from the purulent matter by a detergent inection of vj ounces of Barley water. and ʒij. hony of Roses, and other the like things mentioned at large in our cure of wounds.

Thomas Willis

SEC. I. CHAP IX*

OF A PLEURISIE

The diseases of a *Pluerisie* and *Peripneumonie* are akin

How great affinity there is between a Pleurisie and Peripneumonie, we have hinted before; *viz* although either distemper is..sometimes solitary, and exists separately from the other, yet they often happen together, or one while this, another while that, come one upon the other, or succeeds it. The foregoing cause is the same of both, *viz.* a disposition of the blood to be clammy and boyl up withall; also, the conjunct cause is the same, *viz.* an obstructing Phlegmon in some part of the lesser Vessels, by reason of such a disposition of blood. Moreover, the same method of Cure is prescribed by most modern Physicians for either disease: The chief reason of the difference whereby they are distinguished one from the other, is taken from the places affected, which their Names denote. For the blood predisposed to the enkindling in some place an enflaming ob-

How they differ betwixt themselves

struction, therefore often plants the nest of the disease in the breast, because here it burns out more hideously, by reason of the Hearth of vital fire; and also is not freed from the vaporous Effluviums and other Recrements which hinder Circulation. To all which there ensues, that in this Region, the mass of blood being shut up. and not able to pass through the more strait Conveyances; is not as in the bowels of the lower Belly, opened with any ferment, or new washt with any watery juice; wherefore, if perhaps the blood, carried through the vertebral Arteries into the membrane encompassing the ribs, shall stick in its passage, about the narrowness of the Vessels or interspaces, the Distemper of which we now treat succeeds; in like manner, if an obstruction happens within the passages of the Lungs, a Peripneumonie will ensue, as we have declared before. Wherefore, according to the Pathologie of this disease before delivered, those things which belong to the Theory of a Pleurisie, as well as the Curatory method, may with final labour be designed.

---

* Willis, Thomas, *Pharmaceutice Rationalis,* London, Dring, Harper and Leigh, 1679, Second Part, p. 67.

Both the sense of pain, as well *The seat of a Pleurisie* as Anatomical Observations taken from the Patients dead of a Pleurisie do painly attest, the seat of this Disease (as often as it exists primarily and solitarily) consists in the Pleura or Membrane environing the inside of the ribs. And a true and singular Pleurisie is an inflammation of the Pleura it self, from the abundant flowing in of inflamed blood, growing clammy withall, taking its motion through the vertebral Arteries, with a continual and acute Feaver, a pricking pain of the side, a Cough and difficulty of breathing.

The next Cause is the blood ob- *The next cause of it* structed by reason of its clamminess in the lesser vessels and interspaces of that membrane (in like manner as it is in a Peripneumonie) or being extravasated, being heaped in the same place more plentifully, by reason of the swelling up, for that cause exciting an inflammation. An acute pain ariseth upon this, by a wound in a part highly sensible; also there ariseth a Cough by reason of a provocation giving impression to the intercostal muscles; moreover a difficult breathing by reason of the muscular fibers being hurt as to their action; which because they cannot perform long and strong contractions, they are constrained to undergo weak although more frequent Contractions: otherwise than in a Peripneumonie, in which that symptome ariseth from a Lung too much fill'd and stuffed. The Feaver is caus'd from effervescence of blood, and is for the most part rather the associate than the effect of a Pleurisie. For the blood from what cause soever driven into a feverish turgescency, if it be bound up together in its mass, will be apt to grow clammy, which together with the Feaver most often induces a Pleurisie or a Peripneumonie, or both of them. From hence we may observe this disease doth frequently vary its kind, and change its place, *viz.* from a Pleurisie into a Peripneumonie, and on the contrary; afterwards it passes from both or either into a Frenzy or a Squinancy: for that the blood while it is boyling throws off its viscous recrements one while in this part, another while in that, another while in more together, and lastly it reassumes them again, and variously transferrs them.

The more remote causes of a Pleurisie are the same as of a Peripneumonie, *viz.* what-soever stirs up the blood, predisposed to grow clammy and also to boyl *The more remote causes of this Disease* up, and provokes a feaverish turgescency. Hither appertains excess of a heat and cold, a sudden constipation of the pores, surfeit, drinking of Wines or Strong waters, immoderate exercise; sometimes the malignant constitution of the Air brings this disease almost on every body, and renders it Epidemical: whereto may be added, that this disease is very familiar to some from their constitution or custome; so that a distemperature of blood, induced almost by any occasion, immediately passes into a Pleurisie.

From what we have already said, the signs of this disease do appear manifest enough, by which it is well known as to its Essence, and is distinguished from other diseases and especially from a Bastard Pleurisie and a Peripneumonie. But it is to be observed that a pain in the side arises sometimes very troublesome, which while it counterfeits a Pleurisie, is sometimes taken for it, although falsly. For in some persons obnoxious to the Scurvy, and the affects of the nervous kinde, sometimes it happens that a sharp humour, and very painful descends into the Pleura or intercostal Muscles, and being fixt there produces most fierce tortures; which distemper is yet discriminated from the Pleurisie, inasmuch as it is void both of Feaver and Thirst, the Pulse always abides moderate and laudable, frequently the appetite and strength endure; moreover the pain is not long fixed or limited to one place, but sensibly creeps hither and thither into the neighbouring parts as the matter slides down through the passages of the fibres, out of one place into another.

We meet not with many dif- *The differences of it* ferences of this disease, notwithstanding it is used to be distinguished, *viz.* to be either true and exquisite even as we have now described, or spurious, which having its seat in the intercostal muscles, or their interspaces, proceeds from winde, or a serous and sharp humour heaped up in the same place, and raised a pain, less sharp, without so much as an inflammation or feaver: And whereas the grief is planted externally, the Patient for the most part lyes better on the opposite side, otherwise than in a true Pleurisie. Secondly, a Pleurisie is either single or complicated with a peripneumonie or some other distemper, and so it is either primary, or secondary, or join'd with some other affection.

The Prognosticks As to the Prognosticks of this disease, *Hippocrates* hath observed many certain tokens whereby a good or evil event is signified to patients sick of the Pleurisie. To run through each of these, and to unfold them with Commentaries added to them, we have neither leisure, nor does it seem worth our endeavours. The chief thing of all in a Pleurisie, is, that the disease be presently dispatch'd, partly with a free and frequent bleeding, and partly by a Critical Sweat, arising about the fourth day, or before the eighth; or these things not duely succeeding, it will be prolonged, and then most frequently a Peripneumonie or Empyema, or a collection of corrupt matter between the Breasts and Lungs, or both distempers do arise upon this disease; from which there follows a solution of the disease but slow and incertain, and most frequently full of dangerous chances.

A peripneumonie coming upon a Pleurisie not presently cured (as it is often wont to be) all our hope is placed in digesting maturely the Spittle and quick Expectoration thereof: for if this be laudable and plentiful, and easily and hastily thrown off, it doth often finish both diseases intirely. Notwithstanding, it is not therefore a consequent that the matter of a Pleurisie is derived from the side into the Lungs by I know not what blinde passages, or that the same being sweat out of the Pleura into the cavity of the breast is imbibed by the Lungs, and at length drawn upwards through the passages, and excern'd forth. But when a Peripneumonie arises on a Pleurisie, and the matter impacted in the Lungs begins to be evacuated by Spittle, so that the affected places of the Lungs are continually emptyed; the blood resumes the other matter fixed in the Pleura, and carryes it to the Lungs where the places of conveyance are open, to be ejected by Spitting. But if the Pleurisie be cured neither by it self, nor associating with a Peripneumonie, then at length either by an Imposthume made in the Pleura or in the Lungs, an Empyema or corruption between the Breast and Lungs succeeds; or all the matter being brought into the Lungs and there putrified, loosning the unity of the Viscera, it propagates a mortal or scarce curable Consumption.

Leopold Auenbrugger
OBSERVATION XII*
CONCERNING HYDROPS OF THE CHEST
§XLV.

When fluid has collected in the cavity of the chest between the pleura and the lungs, we say that there exists a hydrops of the chest: Two types of this are observed; for the fluid occupies either one side of the chest, or both sides.

Scholium.—The percussion of the chest determines this in living persons; moreover the anatomical inspection in cadavers demonstrated this to be true.

The general signs of hydrops of the chest. The general signs of this are principally:

1. Difficult and suffocative respiration.

2. A dry cough, sputum is produced, thin, watery, at times subviscid.

3. A contracted pulse, rather hard, rapid and unequal, often intermitting.

4. Dyspnoea and a sense of suffocation at the slightest movement.

5. An increasing distaste for warm foods.

6. Perpetual anxiety about the epigastrium.

7. A great pressure of the chest, and distension of the stomach during digestion.

8. A murmur in the hypochondrium, and the frequent eructation of gas above (with momentary relief).

9. Thirst practically absent.

10. Urine very scanty, red, rarely excreted, with a brickish sediment.

11. Swelling of the abdomen, principally confined to the epigastric region which is especially felt on lying down, from the great weight of the fluid.

12. A sublivid swelling of the extremities and especially of the feet and cold to the touch.

13. Edematous swelling of the lower lids.

* Auenbrugger, Leopold, *Inventum novum*, Vienna, Trettner, 1761, p. 81.

14. Pallor, often according to the nature of the disease, a slight lividity of the cheeks, lips and tongue.

15. Anxious nights, lying down uncomfortable, stuporous often without sleep.

But these things vary greatly because of the course of the disease.

The signs of hydrops of the chest on one side of the thorax—Besides these general signs which I have just presented, the affected side (if it is entirely filled with fluid), is weakened, and is perceived to be less movable in inspiration.

Moreover on percussion, there is no resonance in any part.

But if it is half filled with fluid, a greater resonance is obtained in that part which is not filled with fluid.

R.-T.-H. Laënnec
SECT. IV.—OF THE SIGNS AND SYMPTOMS OF ACUTE PLEURISY†

Physical Signs. As soon as the effusion takes place, the natural sound of the chest, on percussion, fails over the whole space occupied by the fluid. From this result simply, we could not indeed be certain whether the disease is pleurisy or peripneumony, although the common symptoms, general and local, must assist us in making the distinction. Under the circumstances, I have seen physicians endeavour to obtain a mark of distinction between the two diseases, by placing the patient in different positions; and I have myself made a like experiment, but without any satisfactory result. This might be expected, since the chest is always full; and fluids change place by position, only in a vessel that is more or less empty: in the chest the extravasated fluid can only change its position by compressing the lung. It is true, that when the effusion is inconsiderable, it tends to the posterior or inferior parts of the chest, (when the patient lies on the back) on account of its being heavier than the lungs; but if it exists in considerable quantity, it diffuses itself over the whole surface of the lungs, except in the points where old adhesions exist. To these natural impediments to change of position of the extravasated fluids may be added, the increased fixedness of the lungs from the compression of their substance by the effusion, and from the presence of old adhesions; besides, even if this motion of the fluids were practicable, the frequent co-existence of peripneumony would often render the result of percussion of no value, as a mark of discrimination. The great extent of surface over which the sound is wanting, is, however, a much more certain and practical indication: in the case of pleurisy, it frequently happens, that, in the course of a few hours from the attack, the dull sound, exists over the whole affected side, or, at least, over its lower half,—a thing which is never, or almost never, observed in peripneumony. But mediate auscultation furnishes us with much more certain means of discriminating these two diseases, and enables us to ascertain with precision, not merely the existence of the effusion, but its quantity. The signs by which the cylinder affects this, are, 1st, the total absence, or great diminution, of the respiratory sound; and 2nd, the appearance, disappearance, and return of *Ægophonism*. When, as is often the case, the pleuritic effusion is very copious from its very commencement, the sound of respiration is then totally absent through the whole of the side affected, except in the space of three fingers' breadth along the vertebral column, where it is still heard, though less strongly than on the other side. This complete disappearance of respiration after the existence of disease for a few hours, is quite pathognomonic of pleurisy with copious effusion, whether there exists pain in the side or not. In peripneumony, the disappearance of the respiration is gradual, and is perceived to be unequal in different parts of the chest; it is scarcely ever quite wanting below the clavicle; and when this takes place, it is not till after some days or even weeks. It is, further, preceded for twenty-four or thirty-six hours, by the crepitous rattle, which is quite characteristic. In pleurisy with copious effusion, on the contrary, the loss of the respiratory murmur is sudden, equable, uniform, and so complete, that no effort of inspiration can render it perceptible. The

† Laënnec, R.-T.-H., *A Treatise on the Diseases of the Chest and on Mediate Auscultation,* translated by John Forbes, M.D., New York, Samuel Wood & Sons, 1830, p. 443.

continuance of the respiration along the spinal column is an equally constant sign. This exists equally in the chronic disease, attended with the most copious effusion; and even in the cases wherein, on examination after death, the lungs are found so much compressed, as to be discovered with some difficulty. The thing is explained by the compression of the lungs backwards towards their roots. In many cases, the respiration still continues to be perceived immediately under the clavicle, when all the other signs announce the existence of a large effusion; a circumstance which is explained, in such cases, by the presence of old adhesions in that spot. But when the same thing is observed when the extravasation is moderate, we can only infer, either that the fluid does not reach so high, or covers the upper lobe with a very thin layer. In these cases of sudden and complete cessation of the sound of respiration, we must not imagine that, although extensive, the extravasation is so abundant as it is in many cases of chronic pleurisy, in which we find the lungs completely flattened against the mediastinum. In the instances now under notice, it would seem, that the lung is suddenly chocked, as it were, and ceases to admit the air in respiration, although it has hardly yet lost one fourth of its volume, and is only slightly compressed. And it frequently happens, after the lapse of a few days, that the lung, becoming habituated to the pressure, recommences its functions; so that we again can hear the sound of respiration in some places, although the effusion continues undiminished, or even is somewhat increased. This fact I have more than once proved by dissection, and by the comparison of the signs of auscultation and *mensuration* of the chest, of which last I shall presently have occasion to speak. These copious and sudden effusions occur chiefly in old persons, or in adults of weak and cachetic habits, and in the haemorrhagic pleurisy. The sudden and complete cessation of the respiration in such cases, must, therefore, be considered as affording a very bad prognostic; as we may be assured that the conversion of the false membranes into cellular substance, and the absorption of the effusion, will take place either not at all, or imperfectly, and the disease will soon pass into the chronic state. In children and persons of a good constitution, the effusion be-

comes scarcely ever so suddenly abundant. After some hours, or even days, the respiration is still perceptible over the whole affected side; and even more distinctly than we might be led to expect from the imperfection of the sound on percussion. It is, however, much less than on the healthy side; and is without any rattle, except in the rare case of a catarrhal complication. If the effusion increases, the respiratory sound becomes less; it then appears to be heard more remotely, and finally disappears entirely, except at the root of the lungs, where it always is more or less perceptible. The decrease of the resonance from percussion, does not by any means preserve this regular progression; the sound being usually as dull at the period when the respiratory murmur is merely diminished, as when it has entirely ceased. When the pleuritic effusion is at all considerable, the respiration usually becomes *puerile* on the sound side. It even sometimes happens that this puerile respiration is transmitted through the diffused fluid, and is perceived over the whole extent of the diseased side. To prevent this being mistaken for respiration existing in the affected parts, we must explore the whole of these, and we shall then find that the sound becomes louder the nearer we approach the other side. Besides, the quality of the sound, its distance and its clearness, indicate its real site; and this may sometimes be further demonstrated by a momentary compression of the healthy side, which will cause it to cease. But exclusively of these, the other signs afforded by aegophonism, percussion, and mensuration, prevent any misconception, respecting the effusion. This particular case is, moreover, uncommon, and only occurs in the chronic disease. (M. Cayol pointed out to me a case in which a similar transmission of sound took place through a copious collection of air in the chest.) When the effusion begins to diminish, by absorption, this is first observable by the augmented intensity of the respiratory sound along the side of the spine, where it had never quite disappeared. Shortly after it is perceptible on the anterior-superior part of the chest, and top of the shoulder; and in a few days it returns below the scapula, and at last gradually re-appears, successively, on the side, and the lower part of the chest before and behind. Wherever there are adhesions between the lungs and pleura, of any considerable extent, the respiration continues audible over them, in a greater or less degree, throughout the whole period of the effusion; and the commencement of the absorption is perceived by the augmented intensity of sound in these places, and in the summit and anterior border of the lung, which parts had been but little affected. The return of the respiratory sound is much more slow in pleurisy than peripneumony. Sometimes, and particularly in cachetic subjects, it is weeks and even months, after the re-appearance of it near clavicle, before it is perceptible in the inferior parts of the chest; and often for months after the convalescence of a patient, it is only one half so distinct in the affected side as in the sound one. This is owing, I conceive, partly to the very slow process by which the false membranes are converted into cellular substance, and partly to the diminution of the inherent action of the lung, on account of the long compression which it had undergone. The resonance of the chest is still longer in being restored, and, indeed, in many cases, it never returns to the natural condition, in consequence of the contraction of the chest, which succeeds the absorption of the fluid. In examples of this kind, percussion yields a completely dull sound long after the re-appearance of the respiration under the stethoscope.

The successive increase and diminution of the quantity of the extravasation, are also indicated by another sign, which, although much less evident, less constant, and less certain than the preceding, is nevertheless, frequently of use: I mean *mensuration of the chest*. If we uncover the chest of a person affected with pleurisy with abundant effusion, we shall, in most cases, easily perceive that the affected side is larger than the sound one. This dilatation of the affected side has been noticed by all writers on empyema since the time of Hippocrates; but I have ascer-

tained that the same thing takes place in the effusions of a recent pleurisy. I have often found it very distinct after two days' illness. It is, of course, much more evident in lean than fat persons; and it is very indistinct in women with large mammae. On measuring the affected side with a piece of ribbon, we find it enlarged, but never so much as it appears to the eye. An increase of half an inch on the circumference is very obvious to the sight. In proportion as the effusion diminishes, the dilatation of the chest insensibly disappears; and sometimes, as we shall see more particularly hereafter, the affected side becomes narrower than before the disease.

To these signs we must add another, also formerly noticed, *Aegophonism;* a sign which is quite pathognomonic when it exists, and which always indicates a moderate degree of effusion. I shall not here repeat what I stated formerly, but will merely remind the reader— 1. that aegophonism appears about the period when the effusion begins to be somewhat considerable, when the sound, on percussion becomes dull, and the respiratory murmur fails in the affected side; 2. that it disappears when the extravasation becomes very abundant; 3. that it may continue during several months, when the quantity of fluid remains stationary; 4. that after having disappeared, it re-appears upon the quantity of the extravasation being lessened; 5. that it goes off entirely when the fluid is altogether or nearly absorbed. I would also repeat, that the site of this phenomenon appears to be the upper or thinnest part of the layer of effused fluid; that where it is present, we frequently observe also bronchial respiration and bronchophonism; and, finally, that when it is perceived over the whole or greater part of one side, it indicated a moderate quantity and equable diffusion of fluid over the whole surface of the lung.

ASTHMA
Aretaeus
CHAPTER XI
ON ASTHMA*

If from running, gymnastic exercises, or any other work, the breathing become diffi-

* *The Extant Works of Aretaeus, the Cappadocian,* Edited by Francis Adams, LL.D., London, Sydenham Society, 1856, p. 316.

cult, it is called *Asthma* (ἄσθμα); and the disease *Orthopnoea* (ὀρθόπνοια) is also called Asthma, for in the paroxysms the patients also pant for breath. The disease is called *Orthopnoea*, because it is only when in an erect position (ὀρθίῳσχήματι) that they breathe freely; for when reclined there is a sense of suffocation. From the confinement in the breathing, the name *Orthopnoea* is derived. For the patient sits erect on account of the breathing; and, if reclined, there is danger of being suffocated.

The lungs suffer, and the parts which assist in respiration, namely the diaphragm and thorax, sympathise with them. But if the heart be affected, the patient could not stand out long, for in it is the origin of respiration and of life.

The cause is a coldness and humidity of the spirit (*Pneuma*); but the *materiel* is a thick and viscid humour. Women are more subject to the disease than men because they are humid and cold. Children recover more readily than these, for nature in the increase is very powerful to heat. Men, if they do not readily suffer from the disease, died of it more speedily. There is a postponement of death to those in whom the lungs are warmed and heated in the exercise of their trade, from being wrapped in wool, such as the workers in gypsum, or braziers, or blacksmiths, or the heaters of baths.

The symptoms of its approach are heaviness of the chest; sluggishness to one's accustomed work, and to every other exertion; difficulty of breathing in running or on a steep road; they are hoarse and troubled with cough; flatulence and extraordinary evacuations in the hypochondriac region, restlessness; heat at night small and imperceptible; nose sharp and ready for respiration.

But if the evil gradually get worse, the cheeks are ruddy; eyes protuberant, as if from strangulation; a *râle* during the waking state, but the evil much worse in sleep; voice liquid and without resonance; a desire of much and of cold air; they eagerly go into the open air, since no house sufficeth for their respiration; they breathe standing, as if desiring to draw in all the air which they possibly can inhale; and, in their want of air, they also open the mouth as if thus to enjoy the more of it; pale in the countenance, except the cheeks, which are ruddy; sweat about the forehead and clavicles; cough incessant and laborious; expectoration small, thin, cold, resembling the efflorescence of foam; neck swells with the inflation of the breath (*pneuma*); the praecordia retracted; pulse small, dense, compressed; legs slender: and if these symptoms increase, they sometimes produce suffocation, after the form of epilepsy.

But if it takes a favourable turn, cough more protracted and rarer; a more copious expectoration of more fluid matters; discharges from the bowels plentiful and watery; secretion of urine copious, although unattended with sediment; voice louder; sleep sufficient; relaxation of the praecordia; sometimes a pain comes into the back during the remission; panting rare, soft, hoarse. Thus they escape a fatal termination. But, during the remissions, although they may walk about erect, they bear the traces of the affection.

Thomas Willis
SECT. I. CHAP. XII
OF AN ASTHMA*

Among the Diseases whereby the Region of the breath is wont to be infested, if you regard their tyranny and cruelty, an Asthma (which is sometimes by reason of a peculiar symptome denominated likewise an Orthopnoea) doth not deserve the last place; for there is scarce any thing more sharp and terrible than the fits thereof; the organs of breathing, and the precordia themselves, which are the foundations and Pillars

An Asthma a most terrible disease

of Life, are shaken by this disease, as by an Earthquake, and so totter, that nothing less than the ruine of the whole animal Fabrick seems to be threatned; for breathing, whereby we chiefly live, is very much hindred by the assault of this disease, and is in danger, or runs the risque of being quite taken away.

As Asthma is demoninated from ἀσθμαίνην (which is to breath pursie, or difficultly) and may have this description, that it is a difficult, frequent, and pursie breathing with a great shaking of the breast, and for the most part without any Feaver.

The act of breathing depends as well on

* Willis, Thomas, *Pharmaceutice Rationalis*, London, Dring, Harper and Leigh, 1679, Second Part, p. 82.

moving the Lungs, the Structure whereof ought to be that sort that its passages, and all the pores may perpetually be open, for the free sucking in and letting out air; as from the parts or organs moving them, which by alternate turns of Systole and Diastole, do cause the hollowness of the breast, and consequently the Lungs themselves to be dilated, and contracted: whereas therefore there are many and divers reasons of disturbance, whereby respiration is prejudiced, for the most part they may all be reduced to these two heads; *viz.* that there is a fault either in moving the Lungs, or in the parts or instruments that ought to move them, and from hence the differences and kinds of this disease are best of all design'd; for according to the various nature and position of the morbific cause, it is called an Asthma, either meerly pneumonick, proceeding altogether from the passages bringing in aire being obstructed, or not enough open; or it is meerly convulsive, which only arises by reason of a defect or fault in the motive organs; or mixt, when either parts conspire in the fault, which origine every great and inveterate Asthma is wont to have; of each of these we will treat in order.

The causes of respiration hurt

1. The ancient Physicians, and for the most part hitherto the Moderns have only acknowledged the first kind of Asthma, judging the next cause, and almost the only cause of this Disease, to be the straitness of the Broncia, *viz.* inasmuch as the spaces of those passages, being either straitned together by obstruction, or compression, as often as the use of breathing is required, do not admit of plenty enough of Aire, wherefore, for the more free inspiration of aire, as shall be needfull, the organs of breathing do most difficultly labour, with throes most frequently repeated. But that some are found obnoxious to fits of an Asthma, without manifest taint of the Lungs, it was wont to be ascribed to vapours from the Spleen, Womb, Mesentery, or some other bowel, undeservedly enough; but surely that passion, without the straitness of the Bronchia, or fault of those bowels we have in another place sufficiently evidenced to arise from Cramps of the moving parts, and shall be presently clearly made out. But in the

The Ancients allowed the cause of it only from the Bronchia Obstructed

Of vapours from the Spleen or Womb but erroneously

mean time by what means it may arise also from the passages of the Trachea obstructed, or compressed, it lyes upon me to declare.

The straitness of the Bronchia, inducing the first kind of an Asthma, is supposed to come to pass by an obstruction, as often as either thick humours and viscous, or purulent matter or blood extravasated, are forced in upon them; or that little swellings, or Schirrus's, or little Stones, stop up their passages; or finally that a Catarrh of a serous humour suddenly distills upon them. Moreover the same distemper is thought to be raised by compression, as often as matter of that kind (and of every kind of them) shall cleve to the passages of the pneumonic Arterie or vein. Surely, an asthmatical disposition depends upon these various causes and manners of disturbance: but all invasions of the disease, or at least the greater fits are usually provoked by reason of some accidents or occasions. For while the stream of blood sliding and running down gently can be content with a small breathing it passes through the precordia without great labour either of Lungs or Breast. But being boyling and passing through the Lungs more impetuously, it requires a more full inspiration of aire; for the freer admittance of this through strait passages presently all the organs are alarmed into most frequent throes. Whatsoever therefore makes the blood to boyl, or raises it into an effervescence, as violent motion of the body or minde, excess of extern cold or heat, the drinking of Wine, Venery, yea sometimes mere heat of the Bed doth cause asthmatical assaults to such as are predisposed. It is usual that those who are obnoxious to this disease oftentimes dare not enter into a Bed, only sleep in a Chair, or on a bed, being covered with garments. The reason whereof is that the body covered and heated with bed-cloathes, the blood being a little raised into a more quick motion, and grown hot, requires a more plentifull sucking in of air than may be supplyed from the passages of the Trachea being straitned: for more blood passes the Lungs each Sysotle and Diastole, by so much, for the enkindling and eventilation thereof, the air ought to be more plentifully

After what manner the straitness of the Bronchia arises

Whatever causes an effervescence of the blood is the evident cause of an Asthma

Why Asthmatical Persons are worse in bed

and quickly brought in and sent forth: to which task (when by reason of impediments it is not easily dispatched) yet in some manner to be performed, the ultimate endeavors of all the parts appointed for breathing are made use of with a great contention of the whole breast. Moreover the blood being stirr'd is not only an occasion, but also in some part a cause in those that are asthmatically predisposed; for the vessels bringing blood being thereby more fill'd and distended within the lungs, compress the Tracheal passages being already very strait, and render them much more close.

A convulsive Asthma 11. A convulsive Asthma (which we judged to be the second kind of this disease, and to be raised without any great obstruction or compression of the Bronchia, from the mere Cramps of the moving fibres) is not limited to one place or to any peculiar organ, but being a diffused energy, it is extended to almost all the parts employed in breathing (whereof one while this, another while that, or some other is in fault.) For a convulsive affection inciting an Asthmatical invasion, *Its Seat manifold and diffused* hath regard to the moving fibres of the vessels of the Lungs, to the Diaphragma, to the muscle of the breast, to the Nerves, which belong unto the Breast, or Lungs, nay to the origine of those Nerves planted within the Brain; and whilest the morbific matter dwells in every of these places, hindering or perverting the work of breathing, it brings on the fits of this Disease, as in another Tract we have somewhile since plainly demonstrated. For the animal Spirits destin'd to the function of breathing, if at any time they are very much molested and constrained into irregular motions, enter inordinately into the Fibres as well nervous as moving of the organs of breathing, and make them for that cause one while to be contracted, another while to be distended irregularly, as also their solemn and equal turns of Systole and Diastole to be variously disturbed or hindered.

The morbific cause or matter provoking the Spirits prepared for the pneumonic work, *The morbic matter consists in several places* as in divers places, so chiefly in these three, is wont to advance its force or power, *viz.* 1. Either in the muscular fibres themselves, or 2. In the branches or nervous slips, or lastly within the Brain by the origine of the Nerves.

1. As to the former, the heterogene matter being inimical to the Spirits is sometimes shaken off from the Brain into the trunks of the Nerves, and from thence by their passages and slips, if perhaps it shall *1. In the muscular fibres* be in a very little quantity, without very great or sensible hurt slides down to their lower ends. And when it falls in the nervous fibres, and being heaped up daily, shall at length sensibly increase unto a great quantity, it begins to trouble the inmate Spirits, and to provoke them into asthmatical Convulsions; which forthwith infest, and are encreased by reason of evident causes, neither do they utterly cease, untill the stock of matter so accumulated, be wholly dispers'd, and consumed; afterwards when it being renewed arises to a fulness, the fits of that disease return, and are for that cause most frequently periodical, as is manifest to common observation. According to this account we do deservedly suspect the cause of a convulsive asthma sometimes to lurk in the muscular coats of the pneumonick vessels, also sometimes in the fibres of the Diaphragma, or the Processes thereof towards the loyns. It is not very probable that the nest of this disease consists within the fibres of this or that pectoral muscle, although in Scobutical persons from these also possessed with a convulsive matter, we have known pains to have risen with breathing being hurt.

2. But truly (even as in another place we have not only demonstrated by reason, but *Within the Nerves and their unfoldings* by the observations, and Histories of the sick) a convulsive asthma is often incurred, as often as the morbific matter down into the pneumonic Nerves, sticks in some place within their passages, and especially about their foldings: whence as often as it is accumulated to a plenitude it begins to be mov'd and shaken; wherefore the spirits lying lurking, and flowing into the organs of breathing disturbed, are forced into irregularity, and those spirits presently affect other inmates of the fibres of the Lungs and breast, and provoke them into unequal and asthmatical convulsions. For this cause and the reason of the disturbance, we have declared that not only invasions of this disease, but also the precordia being disturbed thereby the Cardiack passions do arise.

3. We have clearly unfolded by anatomical observations that the cause of a convulsive

Asthma sometimes consists in the hinder part of the head near the origine of the nerves. Surely I have observ'd *3. Near the Origines of the Nerves* some patients, who when, lying sick of other desperate diseases, they were also asthmatick, found it necessary to be whether in bed or chair with their head always erect, or looking down, but lying on their back or leaning backwards incontinently they gaped for breath as if they were dying, and hardly breathed; the cause whereof (as apper'd by dissection after they were dead) was only a huge collection of sharp Serum which was gather'd within the cavities of the brain; which, if by reason of the head inclining backwards, it fell into the origine of the Nerves of the eighth pair, presently the precordia, and chiefly the breathing organs were affected with horrid cramps. Moreover sometimes for this very reason it seems that Orthopnoick persons cannot lie down in their bed without danger of choaking, but are constrained to sit up with an erect body.

III. Although an Asthma is sometimes simple from the beginning, *viz.* either merely pneumonical or convulsive, not-*3. A mixt Asthma or partly Pneumonic and partly Convulsive* withstanding after either disease hath for some time encreased, for the most part it gains the other to it self: hence it may be concluded every inveterate Asthma to be a mixt affection, stirr'd up by the default partly of the Lungs ill fram'd, and partly by default of the Nerves and nervous fibres appertaining to the breathing parts. For when the pneumonic passages being straitned or obstructed from some cause, do not admit of a free sucking in, and breathing out of the air, for that cause, also the blood, yea and nervous humour, being hindred in their courses, and compell'd to proceed slowly and to stagnate, do fasten their feculency and dregs upon the nervous parts; whence the passages of the spirits are obstructed, or perverted, and at length a convulsive taint accrues to them. Moreover the blood, being not duly inspir'd and eventilated within the precordia, at length being vitiated in its temperament supplies the brain and nervous stock but with a depraved juice, whose faults do chiefly punish the organs of respiration before hurt and debilitated. In like manner also the evil is reciprocrated on the contrary part, as oft as this disease begins by fault of the nervous stock; for as much as the motion of the Lungs is often stopt or hindered, by reason of Convulsions in the muscular fibres, both the blood and the nervous juice being restrain'd from their usual motions do heap up dregs and filths, fastening them to the parts containing them, by which not only viscous humours and obstructing the passages, but even Tumours and other more solid concretes vitiating the structure of the Lungs, are produced.

PNEUMOTHORAX

R.-T.-H. Laënnec

SECT. III—OF THE EXPLORATION OF PNEUMOTHORAX WITH LIQUID EFFUSION, BY MEANS OF FLUCTUATION*

When I first began to make use of the stethoscope, I was in hopes that this instrument might furnish some sign analogous to the rattle, and calculated to discover collections of serum or pus within the chest, by means of fluctuation. Two methods of effecting this exploration naturally presented themselves; one was to percuss the chest on one side, as in ascites, and apply the stethoscope to the opposite one; the other was to listen simply to the sounds occasioned by the agitation of the fluid from the natural action of the heart and lungs. A little reflection might have convinced me of the unlikelihood of my expectations; yet this conviction did not rise till after many vain attempts to obtain the obect I had in view. I ascertained that the instrument readily communicated the shock in the cases of ascites; but I never could obtain a similar result in the case of thoracic effusions: and the reason of this is obvious. On account of the solid and bony character of the walls of the chest, the percussion used to produce the fluctuation conveys more impulse and sound to the ear of the observer, than does the shock produced

*Laënnec, R.-T.-H., *A Treatise on the Diseases of the Chest and on Mediate Auscultation,* translated by John Forbes, M.D., New York, Samuel Wood & Sons, 1830, p. 509.

by the liquid, and consequently completely masks the latter. This result is a necessary consequence of the known principle that solids communicate impulse and sound better than fluids. In the case of ascites, the shock communicated to one side of the abdomen, is not transmitted by the abdominal parietes on account of their softness; and in aeriform collections in this cavity, the impulse is not conveyed by the air, on account of its being a worse conductor than fluid. Simple auscultation would seem, from reasoning, to be more capable of supplying some signs of the effusion of fluids into the pleura; but from causes hereafter to be detailed, it will appear evident, that this could only be the case when there existed at the same time a liquid and aeriform effusion, and when fluctuation was excited by means of a severe cough. The thing, however, does not seem altogether impossible, although I am doubtful if it ever yet was observed. I have already stated that we can sometimes distinctly hear fluctuation in tuberculous excavations of considerable size, when they are only half filled with a very liquid matter; and this is easily explained by the relative condition of the parts concerned in the production of this phenomenon. In this case the quantity of fluid to be moved is small, the communication with the bronchia is usually narrow, and the soft walls of the excavation are strongly impressed both by the mediate and immediate compressions produced by the cough. Air effused into the pleura, on the contrary, almost always communicates with the air in the larger bronchia, by means of a short and wide channel; and being confined between the bony walls of the chest and the lung bound down against the spinal column, it is very little susceptible of compression, much less of agitation, by the action of coughing. The fistulous opening is, moreover, rarely situated below the level of the fluid. For these reasons, then, I am of opinion, that the cough will hardly, in any case, occasion an audible fluctuation of a liquid contained in the pleura: and we may be assured that, whenever such fluctuation is heard, the cause of it is situated in an ulcerous excavation. We can have still less expectation of hearing any sounds of this kind by simple auscultation, independently of coughing. I have repeatedly endeavoured to do this, in cases wherein the co-existence of air and liquid was proved by other means, and always unsuccessfully. In cases of simple hydrothorax or empyema without any accompanying extravasation of air, the impossibility of doing this, is still more clearly demonstrated.

I ought to be the less surprised at these unsuccessful results of my attempts, as Hippocrates himself, as I have elsewhere shown, committed the same mistake. But if auscultation by itself cannot, as Hippocrates supposed, detect the presence of a fluid in the chest, we obtain, at least, from the writings of this great man, or those of his disciples, a sign very characteristic of this affection, in one particular form of it. This method of exploration, which perhaps has never been practised but by the Asclepiades, consists in shaking the patient's trunk, and at the same time listening to the sounds thereby produced. This process is described by the author of the treatise *De Morbis* (Lib. II. 45) in the following terms: "having placed the patient in a firm seat, cause his hands to be held by an assistant, and then shake him by the shoulder, in order to hear on which side the disease shall produce a sound." Although this method is described in a work which is not unanimously attributed to Hippocrates, we cannot doubt of its having been known to him, and of its having a common practice among his followers: many passages in the Hippocratic writings either speak of it formally, or by implication. On this point, as on several others, the Asclepiades have generalized too much on the facts observed by them: every where they mention this method as a sure means of recognising empyema; and yet there cannot be a doubt, as will be shewn hereafter, that the simple empyema was never so detected. It is no doubt owing to the fruitless attempts made in different times to discover the simple disease in this manner, to which we are to attribute the entire abandonment of the method in question. So complete, indeed, has been this abandonment, that in reading the Commentators of Hippocrates we do not find a single indication of the plan having been ever put in practice by any of them; and we even find that the cleverest of them do not seem to have always well understood the passages in which it is mentioned. Succeeding practitioners appear to have paid as little attention to it; although most of the systematic writers on surgery mention it, but doubtfully, and it would seem, merely out of respect to Hippocrates.

EMPHYSEMA
Matthew Baillie

Matthew Baillie, the nephew of William and John Hunter, was born in Lanarkshire, Scotland, in 1761. His father was professor of divinity in the University of Glasgow, where Matthew was sent at the age of thirteen. In 1779 at the age of eighteen he entered Balliol College, Oxford, and while a student there spent his vacations in the house of Dr. William Hunter in London. During these vacations he made preparations for Dr. Hunter's lectures, assisted in demon-

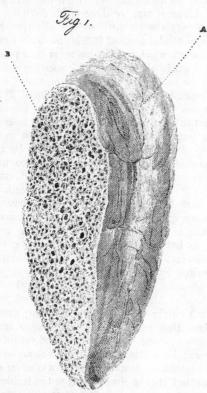

Fig. 1.

A plate from Matthew Baillie's *Morbid Anatomy** of a lung showing emphysema

PLATE VI

In this Plate are exhibited two very rare diseased appearances of the lungs, the one an enlargement of their cells, and the other an ossification of their substance.

FIG. I

Represents a section of one of the lungs, exhibiting the first kind of disease. In this section the air-cells are seen much enlarged beyond their natural size, so as to resemble the air cells of the lungs in amphibious animals.

A. The external surface of this section of the lungs.
B. Its cut edge, showing a large cellular structure. The very dark cavities, which are about ten in number, are the orifices of some divided branches of the pulmonary blood vessels and the trachea.

From the Author's Collection

* Baillie, Matthew, *The Morbid Anatomy of some of the most important parts of the Human Body,* London, Bulmer, 1812.

strations, and supervised the dissections by the students. Baillie received the degree of M.B. at Oxford in 1786 and shortly afterwards began practice in London.

Baillie was elected physician to St. George's Hospital in 1787 and became a fellow of the Royal College of Physicians in 1789. Upon the retirement of Pitcairn, Baillie succeeded to a great part of his practice and in a few years had the largest and most lucrative practice in London. He was called to see King George III during his illness and was appointed physician to the King. He was also offered a baronetcy in 1810 but declined the honor. He died in 1823 leaving a fortune in excess of 80,000 pounds, most of which had been earned by his professional labors.

Matthew Baillie's life is the subject of one of the sketches in that delightful volume of William Macmichael's, *The Gold Headed Cane*. The gold headed cane, the symbol of medical leadership in London, belonged first to Radcliffe and was passed on successively to the great doctors of the metropolis: Mead, Askew, Pitcairn, and finally to Baillie. On Baillie's death his widow presented it to the College of Physicians.

Baillie's success in practice was due to his good sense, affability, and particularly to his knowledge of pathological anatomy. He is best remembered for his *Morbid Anatomy of some of the most Important Parts of the Human Body*, which was first published in 1793. The materials for this work were furnished principally by the museum of his uncle, Dr. William Hunter. This atlas is illustrated by numerous steel engravings that are noteworthy for their accuracy of presentation and skill in execution. Among the pathological conditions described and illustrated are emphysema of the lung and cirrhosis of the liver. The specimen of emphysema of the lung has a further historical interest since it was the lung of Dr. Samuel Johnson, the lexicographer. (Singer)

R.-T.-H. Laënnec
CHAPTER III
OF EMPHYSEMA OF THE LUNGS*

Signs and symptoms. Both the local and general symptoms of pulmonary emphysema are rather equivocal. Dyspnoea being its principal feature, it is usually confounded under the name of *asthma*. The difficulty of breathing is constant, but is aggravated by paroxysms, which are irregular both in the period of their return and their duration; it is likewise increased by all the causes which usually increase dyspnoea, from whatever source arising; such as the action of digestion, flatulence in the stomach or bowels, anxiety, living in elevated situations, strong exercise, running or ascending a height, and above all, the supervention of an acute catarrh. There is no fever, and the pulse is generally regular. In slight cases the complexion and habit of the body are little altered; but when the affection is more considerable, the skin usually assumes a dull earthly hue, with a slight shade of blue here and there. The lips become violet, thick, and look swollen. In every case that I have met with, there existed an habitual cough. Sometimes this was infrequent, slight, and either dry or attended with a trifling expectoration of very viscid

grayish and transparent matter; at other times, it was more severe, returning in paroxysms, and accompanied by the usual mucous expectoration. In some instances the patients denied having either habitual cough or expectoration; but on watching them carefully it was found that they coughed slightly, at least once or twice daily, and expectorated every morning a little of the viscid bronchial mucus above mentioned.

This disease begins frequently in infancy, and may continue a great many years. It does not always prevent the subjects of it from attaining an advanced age; although it must be admitted that the influence it may have in unfavourably modifying other accidental diseases, must very considerably diminish the probabilities of life. The constant and frequently very great efforts which the patient is obliged to make during respiration, often, at last, give rise to hypertrophy or dilatation of the heart.

When the emphysema is confined to one lung, or is much greater in one than the other, the side most affected is perceptibly larger than the other; its intercostal spaces are wider; and it yields a clearer sound on percussion. If both sides are affected equally, the whole chest yields a very distinct sound, and instead of its natural compressed shape, it

* Laënnec, R.-T.-H., *A Treatise on the Diseases of the Chest and on Mediate Auscultation*, translated by John Forbes, M.D., New York, Samuel Wood & Sons, 1830, p. 161.

exhibits an almost round or globular outline, swelling out both before and behind. This conformation of the chest is sufficiently remarkable to have enabled me sometimes to announce the existence of emphysema from simple inspection.

The pathognomonic signs of this disease are furnished by a comparison of the indications derived from percussion and mediate auscultation. The respiratory sound is inaudible over the greater part of the chest, and is very feeble in the points where it is audible: at the same time, a very clear sound is produced by percussion. From time to time also, we perceive while exploring the respiration or cough, a slight sibilous rattle, or sound of the valve, as in the dry catarrh, occasioned by the displacement of the pearly sputa. So far, indeed, these signs are merely those formerly described as indicating the dry catarrh, to which, as we have already seen, this disease is almost always owing. In doubtful cases, the long continuance of the disorder, the severity of the habitual dyspnoea, and the asthmatic paroxysms occasionally occurring, will suffice to point out the existence of emphysema in some parts of the lungs. These indications will be strengthened by the existence of extreme indistinctness of the respiratory sound generally, and by its entire absence in certain points; characters which might be expected to be much more marked in this affection, than in the simple dry catarrh, owing to the compression of the neighbouring cells by those which are dilated. The clyindrical form of the chest, and the slight lividity of the skin, will also help the diagnosis. In the case of one lung being principally affected, the augmented sonorousness and increased size of this side, will discriminate the disease from all others, except pneumothorax, from which likewise, as will be shown when we come to treat of that disease, it can be readily distinguished. When existing in a high degree, this disease may in the last place, be recognized by a sign which is altogether pathognomonic, and which I have described in the preliminary essay under the name of *the crepitous rattle with large bubbles.* In this case, the sound during inspiration or coughing is like that which would be produced by blowing into half-dried cellular substance. It differs from the common crepitous rattle, in conveying the notion of dryness, and also as being connected with bubbles which are at once large and unequal, the other rattle having qualities exactly the reverse. This phenomenon is however not common, and when it exists, it is of very short duration, and is observed only in points of small extent. It is much more common and more permanent in the interlobular emphysema. In some instances the patients have been sensible of a crackling in the spot where this rattle was heard; and still more rarely I have perceived, in thin subjects, a crepitation in the same place, when pressing it externally with the finger.

VIII. DEFICIENCY DISEASES

Interest in deficiency diseases has increased with the development of our knowledge of vitamins. Many of the early accounts of these maladies were from the pens of adventurers or physicians who had left home and their accustomed diet behind and were exploring or waging war in new and strange lands. Scurvy raged among the armies of the Crusaders and was described by Jacques de Vitry at the siege of Damietta in the Fifth Crusade. Sieur de Joinville, the friend and companion of St. Louis, described the ravages of scurvy during the Seventh Crusade. One of the most interesting of all early accounts of this disease is the description of its appearance among sailors exploring the New World in the expedition of Cartier. His men learned from the Indians of a cure for the malady. Lind's monumental work on scurvy led to the routine use of lemon juice in the rations of the British sailor with the result that scurvy soon disappeared from the British navy. Lind further notes "in the first accounts given us of this disease . . . it is surprising to find, not only an accurate description of it, but an enumeration of almost all the truly antiscorbutic medicines that are known to the world even at this day." Rickets became a clearly recognized disease after the appearance of Glisson's book, although Still has pointed out that the disease was described first by Whistler. Ketelaer observed sprue before Hillary, but the latter's account remains the classic one. Nyctalopia was accurately described by that great clinician William Heberden. Heberden, of course, had no idea that night blindness is the result of vitamin A deficiency. This knowledge was reserved for a later generation.

SCURVY

Jacques de Vitry*

Jacques de Vitry, who has left us the first concise account of scurvy was born at Vitry near Paris, the exact date of his birth being unknown. He was educated for the priesthood, and in the year 1210, because of his eloquence as a priest, was called by Pope Innocent the Third to preach the Crusade against the Albigenses. He was later appointed bishop of St. Jean D'Acre, and spent several years in Palestine. He was presently relieved of his bishopric of St. Jean D'Acre and became bishop of Tusculum and later a cardinal. He died in Italy in the year 1244. During his stay in the Orient, he wrote his "Histoire des croisades," from which the following selection is taken:

"A large number of men in our army were attacked also by a certain pestilence, against which the doctors could not find any remedy in their art. A sudden pain seized the feet and legs; immediately afterwards the gums and teeth were attacked by a sort of gangrene, and the patient could not eat any more. Then the bones of the legs became horribly black, and so, after having suffered continued pain, during which they showed the greatest patience, a large number of Christians went to rest on the bosom of the Lord."

* M. Guizot: *Collection des Mémories relatifs a l'historie de France*, Paris, Brière, 1825, 351-352

Jean, Sire de Joinville

Jean, Sire de Joinville was one of the great writers of history in old French. He was born in the year 1224 and accompanied Louis the Ninth in the Seventh Crusade. He remained on terms of intimacy and friendship with the King after his return from the Crusade, but declined to accompany Louis on his last and fatal expedition. He was one of the witnesses in the matter of canonization of Louis, and in 1298 was present at the exhumation of the Saint's body.

Joinville's history of "Saint Louis" was written in his old age, and describes very vividly the events of his youth. The history is of great interest as an eye witness account. The original manuscript of this work has been lost and the first printed edition in 1547 was made from a fifteenth century copy. Later a fourteenth century copy was found in Brussels, and this is the standard authority of the text of Joinville.

Joinville died in 1319 at the advanced age of 95 years.

---

*In the name of Almighty God, I, John, Sire de Joinville, Seneschal of Champagne, cause to be written the life of our sainted Louis, what I saw and heard for the space of six years that I was in his company in the pilgrimage over the sea, and since we returned from it. And before I recount to you his great exploits and feats of arms, I will tell you what I saw and heard of his holy words and sage teachings, that they may be found in their order for the edification of those who shall hear them. This holy man loved God with all his heart, and imitated His works; which appeared in this that, as God died for the love He had for His people, he also several times imperilled his life for the love he had for his people when he could have done otherwise had he wished, as you will hear by-and-bye. The love he had for his people was shown in what he said to his eldest son during a sore sickness which he had at Fontainebleau.

* * *

We had no fish in the camp to eat during Lent except the karmout (a kind of eel), which preyed upon the dead bodies, for they are a gluttonous fish. And in consequence of this misfortune, and of the unhealthiness of the country, where never a drop of rain falls, we were attacked with the army sickness, which was such that our legs shrivelled up and became covered with black spots, and.

* The Sire de Joinville: *Saint Louis, King of France.* Translated by James Hutton, London, 1910, p. 3, 77, 81.

spots of the colour of earth, like an old boot; and in such of us as fell sick the gums became putrid with sores, and no man recovered of that sickness, but all had to die. It was a sure sign of death when the nose began to bleed: there was nothing left then but to die. About a fortnight afterwards the Turks, in order to starve us out (at which many of our people were astonished), took several of their galleys which were above our camp, dragged them overland to a good league below our camp, and placed them in the river by which supplies came from Damietta. These galleys brought famine upon us, for no one now ventured to come to us from Damietta to bring us provisions by ascending the stream. We knew nothing of all this until a small vessel of the count of Flanders, which fount its way past them, brought us the news, by which time the sultan's galleys had captured eighty of our galleys that were coming from Damietta, and killed all who were on board.

There thence arose such a scarcity in the camp that when Easter had arrived an ox was worth 80 livres, a sheep 30 livres, a pig 30 livres, an egg 12 deniers, and a 60-gallon measure of wine 10 livres.

* * *

The sickness became much more severe throughout the camp, and the proud flesh in our men's mouths grew to such excess that the barber-surgeons were obliged to cut it off, to give them a chance of chewing their food or swallowing anything. It was piteous to hear through the camp the shrieks of the people who were being operated for proud flesh, for they shrieked like women in childbirth.

Jacques Cartier

Jacques Cartier, the French navigator and explorer, was born at St. Malo, the principal seaport of Brittany, in 1491. In 1534, with two vessels of sixty tons each, he sailed from St. Malo, and a month later reached Newfoundland. After exploring the west coast of Newfoundland, he sighted Magdalen and Prince Edward Islands and then returned home. Two years later he again sailed for America. On this second voyage he discovered and navigated the Saint Lawrence River and pressed as far westward as the present site of Montreal. During this expedition, his men were attacked by scurvy, which is so graphically related in the following account.

This account is related by the famous Hakluyt and appears in the 1600 edition of his *The Principall Navigations*. Richard Hakluyt, one of the great men of England in the sixteenth century, saw clearly the opportunities that exploration in the Western Continent offered to England as a means of extending her power and dominion. His work did much to stimulate the English nation's taste for exploration.

Survy was known long before Cartier's experience with it, but his description of the miracle wrought by an infusion of the bark and leaves of the *Ameda* tree remains one of the most interesting and graphic accounts of this disease. Hakluyt's account refers to the *ameda* tree as sassafras, although James Lind, who studied Cartier's voyages with great care, states in the *Treatise of the Scurvy,* his belief that it was "the large, swampy *American* Spruce tree."

OF A STRANGE AND CRUELL DISEASE THAT CAME TO THE PEOPLE OF
STADACONA, WHEREWITH BECAUSE WE DID HAUNT THEIR
COMPANY, WE WERE SO INFECTED, THAT THERE
DIED 25 OF OUR COMPANY

CHAPTER 13

In the moneth of December, wee understood that the pestilence was come among the people of Stadacona, in such sort, that before we knew of it, according to their confession, there were dead above 50: whereupon we charged them neither to come neere our Fort, nor about our ships, or us. And albeit we had driven them from us, the said unkowen sicknesse began to spread itselfe amongst us after the strangest sort that ever was eyther heard of or seene, insomuch as some did lose all their strength, and could not stand on their feete, then did their legges swel, their sinnowes shrinke as black as any cole. Others also had all their skins spotted with spots of blood of a purple colour: then did it ascend up to their ankels, knees, thighes, shoulders, armes and necke: their mouth became stincking, their gummes so rotten, that all the flesh did fall off, even to the rootes of the teeth, which did also almost all fall out. With such infection did this sicknesse[1] spread itselfe in our three ships, that about the middle of February, of a hundreth and tenne persons that we were, there were not ten whole, so that one could not help the other, a most horrible and pitifull case, considering the place we were in, forsomuch as the people of the country would dayly come before our fort, and saw but few of us. There were alreadie eight dead, and more than fifty sicke, and as we thought, past all hope of recovery.

[1] The Scurvy.

Our Captaine seeing this our misery, and that the sicknesse was gone so farre, ordained and commanded, that every one should devoutly prepare himselfe to prayer, and in remembrance of Christ, caused his Image to be set upon a tree, about a flight shot from the fort amidst the yce and snow, giving all men to understand, that on the Sunday following, service should be said there, and that whosoever could goe, sicke or whole, should goe thither in Procession, singing the seven Psalmes of David, with other Letanies, praying most heartily that it would please the said our Christ to have compassion upon us. Service being done, and as well celebrated as we could, our Captaine there made a vow, that if it would please God to give him leave to return into France, he would go on Pilgrimage to our Ladie of Rocquemado. That day Philip Rougemont, borne in Amboise, died, being 22 yeeres olde, and because the sicknesse was to us unknowen, our Captaine caused him to be ripped to see if by any meanes possible we might know what it was, and so seeke meanes to save and preserve the rest of the company: he was found to have his heart white, but rotten, and more than a quart of red water about it: his liver was indifferent faire, but his lungs blacke and mortified, his blood was altogither shrunke about the heart, so that when he was opened great quantitie of rotten blood issued out from about his heart: his milt toward the backe was somewhat perished, rough as it had bene rubbed against a stone, Moreover, because one of his thighs was very blacke without, it was opened, but within it was whole and sound: that done, as well as we

could he was buried. In such sort did the sicknesse continue and increase, that there were not above three sound men in the ships, and none was able to goe under hatches or draw drinke for himselfe, nor his fellowes. Sometimes we were constrained to bury under the snow, because we were not able to digge any graves for them the ground was so hard frozen, and we so weake. Besides this, we did greatly feare that the people of the countrey would perceive our weaknesse and miserie, which to hide, our Captaine, whom it pleased God always to keepe in health, would go out with two or three of the company, some sicke and some whole, whom when he saw out of the Fort, he would throw stones at them and chide them, faigning that so soone as he came againe, he would beate them, and then with signes shewe the people of the countrey that he caused all his men to worke and labour in the ships, some in calking them, some in beating of chalke, some in one thing, and some in another, and that he would not have them come foorth till their worke was done. And to make his tale seeme true and likely, he would make all his men whole and sound to make a great noyse with knocking stickes, stones, hammers, and other things togither, at which time we were so oppressed and grieved with that sicknesse, that we had lost all hope ever to see France againe, if God in his infinite goodnesse and mercie had not with his pitifull eye looked upon us, and revealed a singular and excellent remedie against all diseases unto us, the best that ever was found upon earth, as hereafter shall follow.

* * *

HOW LONG WE STAYED IN THE PORT OF THE HOLY CROSSE AMIDST THE SNOW AND YCE, AND HOW MANY DIED OF THE SAID DISEASE, FROM THE BEGINNING OF IT TO THE MIDST OF MARCH

CHAP. 14

From the midst of November until the midst of March, we were kept in amidst the yce above two fathomes thicke, and snow above foure foot high and more, higher then the sides of our ships, which lasted till that time, in such sort, that all our drinkes were frozen in the Vessels, and the yce through all the ships was above a hand-breadth thicke, as well above hatches as beneath, and so much of the river as was fresh, even to

Hochelaga, was frozen, in which space there died five and twenty of our best and chiefest men, and all the rest were so sicke, that wee thought they should never recover againe, only three or foure excepted. Then it pleased God to cast his pitiful eye upon us, and sent us the knowledge of remedie of our healthes and recoverie, in such maner as in the next Chapter shall be shewed.

* * *

HOW BY THE GRACE OF GOD WE HAD NOTICE OF A CERTAINE TREE, WHEREBY WE ALL RECOVERED OUR HEALTH: AND THE MANER HOW TO USE IT

CHAP. 15

Our Captaine considering our estate (and how that sicknesse was encreased and hot amongst us) one day went foorth of the Forte, and walking upon the yce, hee saw a troupe of those Countreymen comming from Stadacona, among which was Domagaia, who not passing ten or twelve days afore, had been very sicke with that disease, and had his knees swolne as bigge as a childe of two yeres old, all his sinews shrunk together, his teeth spoyled, his gummes rotten, and stinking. Our Captaine seeing him whole and sound, was thereat marvellous glad, hoping to understand and know of him how he had healed himselfe, to the end he might ease and help his men. So soone as they were come neere him, he asked Domagaia how he had done to heale himselfe: he answered, that he had taken the juice and sappe of the leaves of a certain Tree, and therewith had healed himselfe: For it is a singular remedy against that disease. Then our Captaine asked him if any were to be had thereabout, desiring him to shew him, for to heale a servant of his, who whilest he was in Canada and Donnacona, was stricken with that disease: That he did because he would not shew the number of his sicke men. Domagaia straight sent two women to fetch some of it, which brought ten or twelve branches of it, and therewithall shewed the way how to use it, and that is thus, to take the barke and leaves of the sayd tree, and boile them togither, then to drinke of the sayd decoction every other day, and to put the dregs of it upon his legs that is sicke: moreover, they told us, that the vertue of that tree was, to heale any other disease: the tree is in their language called Ameda or Hanneda, this is thought to be the Sassafras tree. Our Captaine presently caused some of that drink to be made for his men to drink of it, but there was none durst tast of it, except one or two, who ventured the drinking of it, only to tast and prove it: the other seeing that did the like, and presently recovered their health, and were delivered of that sickenes, and what other disease soever, in such sorte, that there were some had bene diseased and troubled with the French Pockes foure or five yeres, and with this drink were cleane healed. After this medicine was found and proved to be true, there was such strife about it, who should be first to take it, that they were ready to kill one another, so that a tree as big as any Oake in France was spoiled and lopped bare, and occupied all in five or sixe daies, and it wrought so wel, that if all the phicicians of Mountpelier and Lovaine had bene there with all the drugs of Alexandria, they would not have done so much in one yere, as that tree did in sixe dayes, for it did so prevaile, that as many as used of it, by the grace of God recovered their health.

James Lind

James Lind was born in Edinburgh in 1716 and at the age of fifteen began his medical studies as an apprentice to George Langlands, a member of the Incorporation of Surgeons. At the age of twenty-three he entered the naval medical service, where he remained for nine years. During these years he saw service in the English channel and went on cruises to the Mediterranean, the Guinea Coast, and the West Indies. These voyages gave him an opportunity of studying tropical diseases and aroused his interest in naval hygiene. He saw also two severe outbreaks of scurvy in the Channel fleet, in one of which there were 80 cases out of a crew of 350.

He left the navy in 1748 and the same year received an M.D. from the University of Edinburgh. He immediately started practice in Edinburgh and two years later became a fellow of the Royal College of Physicians. In 1758 he left Edinburgh to become Physician to the Haslar Hospital—a naval hospital near Portsmouth—where he worked for twenty-five years, resigning in 1783 at the age of sixty-seven. He died in 1794.

Lind's reputation today rests upon his three epoch-making treatises on scurvy, on naval hygiene, and on tropical medicine. His work on scurvy, which was published in 1753, recommended the use of lemon juice in the prevention and cure of scurvy, a method of treatment which he later employed with great success in the Haslar Hospital, where he usually had 300 to 400 cases of scurvy

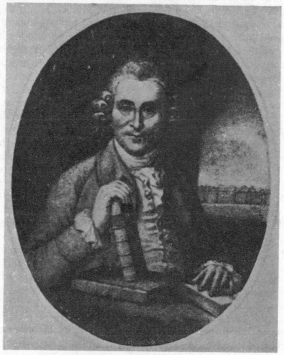

Courtesy of "Edinburgh Medical Journal"

JAMES LIND (1716-1794)
From a portrait by Sir George Chalmers

under his care and often 1000 at one time. Lind died forty-one years after the publication of his *Treatise of the Scurvy*, without seeing any of his suggestions officially adopted by the British Navy; for, as he wrote in 1762, "The Province has been mine to deliver Precepts; the Power is in others to execute." The year of his death, a small squadron sailing for the East Indies was supplied with an adequate supply of lemon juice and the squadron arrived at Madras twenty-three weeks later without a single case of scurvy on board. Two years later lemon juice was added to the rations of the sailors and scurvy soon disappeared from the British navy.

Lind's *Essay on the Jail Distemper*, which appeared in 1773 and is included in his essay *On the most Effectual Means of Preserving the Health of Seamen*, London, 1779, recommends the destruction of clothing and bedding of patients suffering from typhus fever. The measure was prompted by his conviction that the disease was transmitted by fomites. The transmission by lice had not yet been demonstrated, and his discussion of typhus fever appears earlier in these readings.

———

I COME* in the next place, to an additional and extremely powerful cause, observed at sea to occasion this disease, and which concurring with the former, in progress of time, seldom fails to breed it. And this is, the want of fresh vegetables and greens; either, as may be supposed, to counteract the bad effects of their before mentioned situation; or rather, and more truly, to correct the quality of such hard and dry food as they are obliged to make use of. Experience indeed sufficiently shews, that as greens or fresh vegetables, with ripe fruits, are the best remedies for it, so they prove the most effectual preservatives against it. And the difficulty of obtaining them at sea, together with a long continuance in the moist sea-air, are the true causes of its so general and fatal malignity upon that element.

The diet which people are necessarily obliged to live upon while at sea, was before assigned as the *occasional cause of the disease*;[f] as in a particular manner it determines the effects of the before mentioned predisposing causes to the production of it. And there will be no difficulty to conceive the propriety of this distinction, or understand how the most innocent and wholesome food, at times, and in peculiar situations, will with great certainty form a disease. Thus, if a man lives on a very slender diet, and drinks water, in the fens of *Lincolnshire*, he will almost infallibly fall into an ague.

All rules and precepts of diet, as well as the distinction of ailments into wholesome and unwholesome, are to be understood only as relative to the constitution or state of the body. We find a child and a grown person, a valetudinarian and a man of health, require aliment of different kinds; as does even the same person in the heat of summer and in the depth of winter, during a dry or rainy season. Betwixt the tropics, the natives live chiefly on fruits, seeds and vegetables; whereas northern nations find a flesh and solid diet more suitable to their climate. In like manner

it appears, I think, very plainly, that such hard dry food as ship's provisions, or the sea-diet, is extremely wholesome; and that no better nourishment could be well contrived for labouring people, or any person in perfect health, using proper exercise in a dry pure air; and that, in such circumstances, seamen will live upon it for several years, without any inconvenience. But where the constitution is predisposed to the scorbutic taint, by the causes before assigned, (the effects of which, as shall be shewn in a proper place,[g] are a weakening of the animal powers of digestion), the influence of such diet in bringing on this disease, sooner or later, according to the state and constitution of the body, becomes extremely visible. . . .

* * *

The first indication of the approach of this disease, is generally a change of colour in the face, from the natural and usual look, to a pale and bloated complexion; with a listlessness to action, or an aversion to any sort of exercise. When we examine narrowly the lips, or the caruncles of the eye, where the blood-vessels lie most exposed, they appear of a greenish cast. Mean while the person eats and drinks heartily, and seems in perfect health; except that his countenance and lazy inactive disposition, portend a future scurvy.

This change of colour in the face, although it does not always preceed the other symptoms, yet constantly attends them when advanced. Scorbutic people for the most part appear at first of a pale or yellowish hue, which becomes afterwards more darkish or livid.[a]

Their former aversion to motion degenerates soon into an universal lassitude, with a stiffness and feebleness of their knees upon using exercise; with which they are apt to be much fatigued, and upon that occasion subject to a breathlessness or panting. And this lassitude, with a breathlessness upon motion,

---

*Lind, James, *A Treatise of the Scurvy*, Edinburgh, Souds, Murray and Cochran, 1753, pp. 115-117, 148-151, 207, 209.
[f] P. 93.

[g] Chap. 6.
[a] *Mr. Murray's remark.*—They commonly appear of a meloncholy and sullen countenance; such also is their disposition of mind. So that dejection of spirits may justly be reckoned a cause as well as symptom of the future malady.

are observed to be among the most constant concomitants of the distemper.

Their gums soon after become itchy, swell, and are apt to bleed upon the gentlest friction. Their breath is then offensive; and upon looking into their mouth, the gums appear of an unusual livid redness, are soft and spongy, and become afterwards extremely putrid and fungous; the pathognomonic sign of the disease. They are subject not only to a bleeding from the gums, but prone to fall into hemorrhages from other parts of the body.

Their skin at this time feels dry, as it does through the whole course of the malady.[b] In many, especially if feverish, it is extremely rough; in some it has an anserine appearance; but most frequently it is smooth and shining. And, when examined, it is found covered with several reddish, bluish, or rather black and livid spots, equal with the surface of the skin, resembling an extravasation under it, as it were from a bruise.[c] These spots are of different sizes, from the bigness of a lentil to that of a handbreadth, and larger. But the last are more uncommon in the beginning of the distemper; they being usually then but small, and of an irregular roundish figure. They are to be seen chiefly on the legs and thighs; often on the arms, breast, and trunks of the body; but more rarely on the head and face.

Many have a swelling of their legs; which is first observed on their ancles towards the evening, and hardly to be seen next morning; but, after continuing a short time in this manner, it gradually advances up the leg, and the whole member becomes oedematous; with this difference only in some, that it

[b] Mr. Murray.—Except in the last stage, when a cold clammy moisture may be often observed on the skin, especially if the patient is subject to faintings.

[c] Mr. Murray.—The skin begins to look in spots with a yellow rim. From thence the deepness of the dye gradually increases, till it becomes of a deep purple, and sometimes quite black.

does not so easily yield to the finger, and preserves the impression of it longer afterwards than a true oedema.

* * *

Let the squeezed juice of these fruits be well cleared from the pulp, and depurated by standing for some time; then poured off from the gross sediment: or, to have it still purer, it may be filtrated. Let it then be put into any clean open earthen vessel, well glazed; which should be wider at the top than bottom, so that there may be the largest surface above to favour the evaporation. For this purpose a china bason or punch-bowl is proper; or a common earthen bason used for washing, if well glazed, will be sufficient, as it is generally made in the form required. Into this pour the purified juice; and put it into a pan of water, upon a clear fire. Let the water come almost to boil, and continue nearly in a state of boiling (with the bason containing the juice in the middle of it) for several hours, until the juice is found to be of the consistence of oil when warm, or of a syrup when cold. It is then to be corked up in a bottle for use. Two dozen of good oranges, weighing five pounds four ounces, will yield one pound nine ounces and a half of depurated juice; and when evaporated, there will remain about five ounces of the extract; which in bulk will be equal to less than three ounces of water. So that thus the acid, and virtues of twelve dozen of lemons or oranges, may be put into a quart bottle, and preserved for several years.

I have some of the extract of lemons now by me, which was made four years ago. And when this is mixed with water, or made into punch, few are able to distinguish it from the fresh squeezed juice mixed up in like manner; except when both are present, and their different tastes compared at the same time; when the fresh fruits discover a greater degree of smartness and fragrancy.

* * *

John Huxham

A METHOD FOR PRESERVING THE HEALTH OF SEAMEN IN LONG CRUISES AND VOYAGES*

* * *

I have known more than a thousand Men put

*Huxham, John, Plymouth, Sept. 30, 1747. Published with *An Essay on Fevers,* London, Hinton, 1757.

ashore sick out of one single Squadron, after a three Months Cruise, most of them highly scorbutic; besides many that died in the Voyage. The Fleet returns to its Port; fresh

Air, wholesome Liquor, fresh Provisions, especially proper Fruits and Herbage, soon purify the Blood and Juices of the Sick, and restore their Health. The fresh Air, Provisions, Fruits, and Garden-stuff, which the *English* and *Dutch* meet with at *St. Helena,* and the *Cape of Good Hope,* are of the highest Advantage to them in their *East-India* Voyages; without which they always become extreamly sickly.

Physicians well know, that the most effectual Method of correcting an alcalescent Acrimony of the Blood, and of preventing the further Advances of Putrefaction in the Humors, is by vegetable and mineral Acids; the former of which are much the safest, and may be given in Draughts, the other only by Drops.

That the State of the Blood, in the common Sea-scurvy, is of this Nature, appears from the stinking Breath of the Sick, their rotten corroded Gums, high-coloured foetid Urine, sordid Ulcerts, black, blue, and brown Spots, and Eruptions on the Skin, frequent feverish Heats, foul Tongues, bilious and bloody Dysenteries, which more or less always attend it. Now it is also well known, that a vegetable acescent Diet and Regimen, fresh Air, fresh Provisions, subacid and vinous Drinks, are its certain and speedy Cure, when not very far advanced. Apples, Oranges, and Lemons, alone, have been often known to do surprising Things in the Cure of very deplorable scorbutic Cases, that arose from bad Provisions, bad Water, &c. in long Voyages.

But what will cure will prevent. If therefore such a Diet and Regimen can be used at Sea, it will prove a Kind of a continual Antidote to the rank putrescent Qualities of the common Ships Provision, and correct, at least very much lessen, the ill Effects. And it is eventually found, that the Officers, who carry Wine, Cyder, Lemons, fresh Provisions, &c. are infinitely less affected with the Scurvy, than the poor common Sailors, who are not so provided.

It is practicable then to introduce such a general Regimen into the Navy? I think it is; and, from Reason and Experience, I recommend the following Method.

Let all Ships, that are to proceed on a long Cruise or Voyage, be supplied with a sufficient Quantity of sound generous Cyder; the rougher, provided it is perfectly sound,

the better. If Apples are found of such vast Service in the Scurvy, surely the Juice of them, when become a vinous Liquor, cannot but be very salutary; and seems exceedingly well adapted, as a common Drink, to correct by its Acidity the alcalescent putrefying Quality of bad, corrupt Provisions. This Cyder should be at least three Months old before it is served in, and quite fine. If it be too new, and foul, it is apt to give severe Colics: It should be racked off once at least from its gross Ley into good and sweet Vessels, which will contribute to its becoming fine, and prevent it from growing ropy, in which State it is good for nothing. But if some of it should turn to Vinegar, which may frequently happen, it will still be very serviceable; but it is found, when well managed, to keep good and sound even to the *Indies.*

Every Sailor should have at least a Pint of Cyder a Day, besides Beer and Water. And I would advise also a frequent and free Use of Vinegar in the Seamen's Diet; especially when the Provisions begin to grow rancid. Besides this, the Decks, &c. should be frequently washed or sprinkled with Vinegar; after having drawn the gross and foul Air out of the Ship by Mr. *Sutton's* Contrivance, or by Dr. *Hale's* Ventilators; which should be done once at least every Day.

In autumnal Cruises a Quantity of Apples might be also carried, which, when well chosen and well put up in dry tight Casks, will keep very good for two or three Months. Even Lemons and Oranges wrapt in Flannel (or something that will imbibe their exhaling Moisture) kept in close dry Vessels, and pretty cool, may be preserved a long while also. If this is not so feasible, a Mixture of Lemon Juice and Rum (Shrub as they call it) may be carried in any Quantity; as it will keep a long Time, and would prove infinitely more wholesome than the nasty fiery poisonous Spirits, which are dealt about so largely in the Navy and elsewhere. By the bye, nothing would more effectually correct the pernicious Qualities of these Spirits than Lemon Juice.

In the Case of stinking Water, Juice of Lemon, Elixir of Vitriol, or Vinegar, should be always mixed with it, which will render it much less unwholesome: The *Roman* Soldiers drank *Posca* (*viz.* Water and Vinegar) for their common Drink, and found it very healthy and useful.

RICKETS

Daniel Whistler

Although the name of Glisson is associated with the classic description of rickets, there is no question that others had preceded him in describing this affection. One of the earliest if not the first description is that of Daniel Whistler.

Daniel Whistler was born in 1619 and entered Merton College, Oxford, at the age of twenty. After taking his degree in arts he proceeded to Leyden,

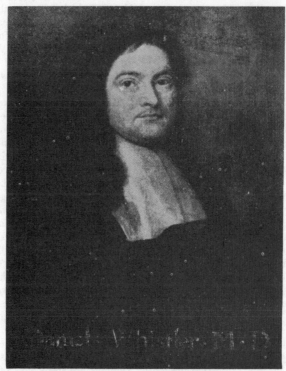

Courtesy of the Royal College of Physicians, London

DANIEL WHISTLER (1619-1684)
From a portrait in the Royal College of Physicians, London

where he studied medicine and took his medical degree in 1645. The title of his thesis was, *De morbo puerile Anglorum quem patrio idiomate indigenae vocant the Rickets,* the earliest published account of this disease. He then returned to Oxford, where he was incorporated Doctor of Physick in 1647. Whistler began practice soon afterwards in London and, as he was a good mathematician, was made professor of geometry in Gresham College in 1648. In 1652 he attended the seamen wounded during the war with Holland, and gradually became a very popular and successful physician. He was a friend of Samuel Pepys, who describes him as "good company and a very ingenious man." Pepys in his immortal *Diary* mentions Dr. Whistler no less than fourteen times.

Whistler became a Fellow of the Royal College of Physicians in 1649 and after holding various offices became its President in 1683. He was also one of the founders of the Royal Society and seems to have been upon intimate terms with all the great scientists of that day. As the years rolled on Whistler seems to have fallen upon evil days and to have gradually sunk deeper and deeper into debt. He died in 1684 after a very brief illness and he was buried secretly from fear that his creditors would pounce upon his body and seize it for his debts.

Whistler's thesis, written upon graduation at the age of twenty-five, was his only contribution to medical science, and important as it was, it attracted but little attention. Rickets first took its place in textbooks on pediatrics after the publication of Glisson's book.

Daniel Whistler's character was severely attacked by Munk, who states in his *Roll of the Royal College of Physicians* that Whistler defrauded the College. Still, his *History of Paediatrics* produces evidence indicating that the College's finances were in bad condition because of Whistler's carelessness and not on account of any intent to defraud. Whistler's will, drawn the day before his death, bequeaths all his books, collections, manuscripts, aand one-third of his estate to the College.

———

(1) Distension of the hypochondria or an undue fullness of the abdomen with some hardness especially on the right side below the region of the liver.*

(2) The epiphyses at the joints are massive and large out of proportion to the age (*exuberant mole supra aetatem*); in size too they are out of proportion to the growth of the other parts of the body, especially those of the arms and feet. It is from the presence of this symptom that some dignify the whole affection with the name Paedarthrocaces or Paedarthroncias.

(3) Knotty swellings also grow out on the sides (of the chest) where the cartilaginous parts join the bony.

(4) The whole bony system is in truth flexible like wax that is rather liquid (*cerae instar udioris flexile est*), so that the flabby and toneless legs scarcely sustain the weight of the superimposed body, so that the tibiae yield to the weight of the fabric pressing down upon them from above and become bent; and for the same reason the thighs above are curved and the back, through the bending of the spine, projects hump-fashion in the lumbar region: so that they are too feeble to sit up, much less to stand, when the disease is increasing. From this symptom some name this affection Paedosteocaces.

(5) These children have enlargement of the head, sometimes with hydrocephalus also, from which complication some writers wished to give the whole affection the not inappropriate name of Paedocephalarthroncias.

(6) In the softer tissues, e.g. skin, flesh, ligaments, &c., a flabbiness and softness unnatural for the age are noticed.

(7) The teeth are cut too late and with excessive trouble, and often when cut they decay.

(8) Other accompaniments are narrowness of the chest, prominence of the sternum, and asymmetry (*pectoris angustia, sterni acuminatio et inaequalis positio*) sometimes the whole sternum especially towards the ensiform cartilage (*micronatum cartilaginem*) is depressed, and is drawn inwards as far as the osseous ends of the ribs: this often happens at the beginning.

(9) Respiration is found difficult at last, sometimes with a little cough and wasting.

(10) A slow fever is also associated with this disease; irregular of no constant type, with erratic rises of temperature.

* Whistler, Daniel, *De morbo puerili Anglorum quem patrio idiomate idigenae vocant the Rickets . . . Leyden, 1645.* By permission from *The History of Paediatrics* by George Frederic Still, London, Oxford University Press, 1931.

(11) The pulse of the patient is uneven and feeble.

(12) The urine is often thicker than normal, often variable in colour and consistency as in scurvy.

(13) In the diarrhoea and vomiting which sometimes supervene the material evacuated is viscid and phlegmy.

opinions therefrom as to their living long: they take but little pleasure in fun, being serious above their years.

Those who have Hydocephalus with it, are duller because the brain is oppressed by much water or phlegm. They are not passionate or fretful children, they like quietness and are rather sluggish in movement (*minus*

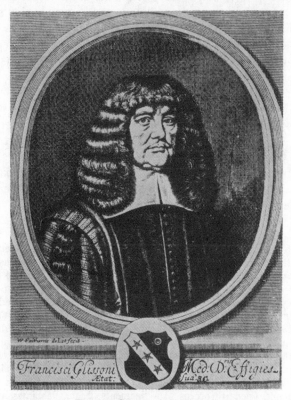

FRANCIS GLISSON (1597-1677)
Glisson at the age of thirty. From the drawing
by W. Faithorne

(14) Their appetite is either moderate or poor; they are not fond of sweet things, for instance sugary foods.

(15) They sleep tolerably, if not too much, unless something prevents.

(16) As to disposition they are usually bright and of precocious intelligence, so that superstitious parents may form unfavourable

iracundi sunt et queruli, quietem affectant, ad motum tardiores).

(17) There are sometimes pustules and blotches scattered on the face, chest, and limbs, suggestive of scurvy or venereal diseases, according as there is a suspicion of this or that in the parents or grandparents or great-grandparents.

Francis Glisson

Francis Glisson was born in Dorsetshire, England, in 1597 and went to Gonville and Caius College, Cambridge, where he took his B.A. in 1624 and his M.D. in 1634. The following year he was elected a member of the Royal College of Physicians and was made Regius Professor of Physic at Cambridge, a chair he held until his death.

Glisson is remembered chiefly for his anatomical study of the liver, which is still commemorated by the term "Glisson's capsule," and for his description of rickets. His book, *De Rachitide,* appeared in 1650 and, although somewhat verbose, as was the literary style of those days, contains a striking account of the disease. The frontispiece of the book shows some interesting pictures of patients. Glisson died in London, October 14, 1677.

We shall propound therefore:*

First, *the Signs which relate to the Animal actions.*

Secondly, *Those which have reference to the irregular Nutrition.*

Thirdly, *Those that concern the Respiration.*

Fourthly, *Those that appertain to the Vital Influx.*

Fiftly, *Certain vagabond and fugitive Signs reducible to no Classis.* Under each of which we shall subjoyn the value of the Signs.

First, the *Diagnostical* Signs relating to the Animal Actions, are these. *The looseness and softness of the parts. The debility and languidness. And finally, the slothfulness and stupifaction.*

First, A certain laxity and softness, if not a flaccidity of all first affected parts is usually observed in this affect. The Skin also is soft and smooth to the touch, the musculous flesh is less rigid and firm, the joynts are easily flexible, and many times unable to sustain the body. Whereupon the Body being erected it is bent forwards or backwards, or to the right side or to the left.

Secondly, A certain debility, weakness, and enervation befalleth all the parts subservient to motion. This weakness dependeth much up the laxity, softness, and litherness of the parts aforesaid: for which reason we have placed those Signs before this, as also this before the slothfulness and stupifaction in the next place to be enumerated, which owe much both to the looseness and softness. Moreover, this debility beginneth from the very first rudiments of the Disease. For if

* Glisson, Francis, *A Treatise of the Rickets, Being a Disease common to children.* Published in Latine by Francis Glisson, George Bate, and Abasuevus Regemorter. Translated by Phil. Armin, London, Streator, 1668, p. 231.

Children be infested within the first year of their age or thereabouts, they go upon their feet later by reason of that weakness, and for the most part they speak before they walk, which amongst us English men, is vulgarly held to be a bad *Omen.* But if they be afflicted with this Disease, after they have begun to walk, by degrees they stand more and more feebly upon their legs, and they often stagger as they are going, and stumble upon every slight occasion: neither are they able to sustain themselves long upon their legs without sitting, or to move and play up and down with usual alacrity, till they have rested. Lastly, upon a vehement increase of the Disease they totally lose the use of their feet; yea, they can scarce sit with an erected posture and the weak and feeble Neck doth scarcely, or not at all sustain the burthen of the Head.

Thirdly, A kind of slothfulness and numbness doth invade the Joynts presently after the beginning of the Disease, and by little and little is increased, so that dayly they are more and more avers from motion. The younger Children who are carried about in their Nurses arms, when they are delighted and pleased with any thing do not laugh so heartily, neither do they stir themselves with so much vigor, and shake and brandish their little Joynts, as if they were desirous to leap out of their Nurses hands, also when they are angred they do not kick so fiercely, neither do they cry with so much fierceness as those who are in health. Being grown greater, and committed to their feet, they run up and down with a wayward unchearfulness, they are soon weary, and they love to play rather sitting than standing, neither when they sit, do they erect their body with vigor, but they bend it sometimes forward, sometimes backward, and sometimes on either side, seeking some props to lean upon that may gratifie their slothfulness. They are not delighted like other Children with the agitation of their bodies, or any violent motion; yea, when the Disease prevaileth they are averse from all motion of their limbs, crying as they are at any play that is never so little vehement; and being pleased again with gentle usage and

tent and ruminating upon some serious matter.

These Signs being taken together (unless they result from some evident wariness, or proceed from some primary affect of the Brain, which indeed happeneth very seldom in this tenderness of age) do constitute a

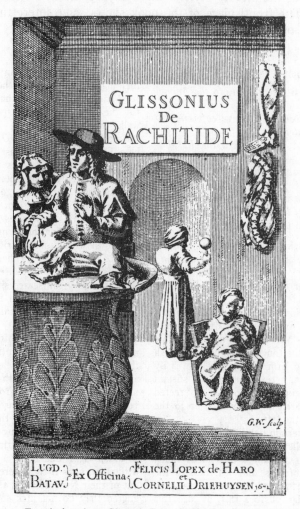

Frontispiece from Glisson's *De rachitide* (Leyden, 1671)

quiet rest. In the interim, unless some other disease, Symptom, or cause of sickness doth come between, they are moderate in sleeping and waking, they are ingenious, not stupid, but for the most part of forward wits, unless some other impediments arise, their countenances are much more composed and severe than their age requireth, as if they were in-

sufficient *Pathognomonical* Syndrom of the first kind, and where they are present together, they certainly witness the presence of the Disease, and when they are absent together they infallibly attest the Essence of this Disease. But if at any time a wearisomeness do bewray any Feaverish, or other like Signs, they may easily be distinguished from these, both because the reasons of the weariness have gone before, and also because the Signs from thence arising do suddenly break out, and as soon vanish. But in this affect the signs do invade by degrees, and persevere, or else they are daily more encreased. Now the primary Diseases of the Brain are distinguished by their proper Signs. And thus much of the Signs which relate to the Animal Actions.

The Signs Which Belong to the Disproportioned Nourishment of the Parts

Of how great moment the *Alogotophry*, or unequal Nourishment of the Parts in this affect, we have already shewed; we shall here therefore prosecute those signs which in some great measure depend upon it, and we shall present them as if they were to be beheld at one View.

First, there appeareth the unusual bigness of the Head, and the fulness and lively complexion of the Face, compared with the other parts of the body. But although this Sign may presuppose some motion of the Disease before it shine out, yet is the Disease so obscure before the appearance of it, that it is accounted in a manner unperceivable: Therefore commonly this Sign sheweth it self more or less from the first beginning, and continueth till the departure of the affect, unless (as we have noted before) the pining of those parts supervene from some other cause.

Secondly, The fleshy parts, especially those which are full of Muscles beneath the Head which we have listed among the first affected, in the progress of the Disease are daily more and more worn away, made thin and lean. This Sign doth not presently shew it self from the beginning of the Disease, because it pre-requireth some notable motion of the Disease before it evidently appeareth; yet in time most certainly is exposed to the senses, and accompanieth the Disease to the last step be it either to life or death; excellently demonstrating the motion and degree of the Disease by its encrease. Moreover this Sign being conjoyned with the former doth at least constitute a *Pathognomonical* Sign of the second kind, that is such an one as is proper to this Disease alone; and where they are present together they infallibly denote the presence of this Disease, although upon their absence they do not equally signifie the absence of the Disease.

Thirdly, Certain swellings and knotty excrescences, about some of the joynts are observed in this affect; these are chiefly conspicuous in the Wrists, and somewhat less in the Ankles. The like Tumors also are in the tops of the Ribs where they are conjoyned with gristles in the Breast. We have noted above in our Anatomical Observations that these tumors are not situated in the Parts, but in the very bones, although this consideration doth scarce belong to them as Signs, seeing that of themselves they are scarce conspicuous. This Sign doth also suppose some kind of motion of the Disease, neither is it emergent a *Principio principiante*, as the Philosophers phrase it, yet offers of it self as an object to the senses sooner than any considerable extenuation of the parts. But where it is present, it constitutes a *Pathognomonical* Sign of the Second kind, and without dispute witnesseth the Species of the Disease.

Fourthly, Some Bones wax crooked, especially the Bones called Shank-bone and the Fibula or the small Bone in the Leg, then afterwards the greater Shank-bone, and the undermost and lesser of the two long Bones of the Elbow, but not so much altogether nor so often; sometimes also the Thigh-bone and the Shoulder-bone. Again, there is sometimes observed a certain shortning of the Bones and a defective growth of them in respect of their longitude. This by chance was omitted above, where we gave the Reason of the Organical faults. Yet this affect doth seem to depend upon the same irregular nourishment; namely so far forth as the nourishment taken in encreaseth the Bones according to breadth and thickness more than length. From hence it comes to pass that some Children long afflicted with this Disease become Dwarfs. Hither perhaps may be referred that folding in the Wrists, the Skin it may be having better nourishment and more growth than the Bones of those parts, whereupon it must needs be contracted in the Wrists into a folding, or wrinkledness. Finally, to this place also may belong a certain sticking out of the Bones of the Head, especially of the Bone of the forehead forwards. For it concerneth the common kind of vitiated Figure and the *Alogotophry* of the Bones. Yet this in the Bone of the Forehead doth evidently seem to depend upon the free nourishment of that Bone in his circumference, wherewith it is coupled to the Bones of the fore part of the Head, and constitutes that seam called *Sutura Coronalis*, which lieth in the foremost part thereof. For hereupon it must needs be thrust forwards. And indeed in that place it is plentifully nourished without any difficulty, because this Bone in Children is cartilaginous towards that Seam. And this also was pretermitted above where we discoursed of the Organical faultiness, because we have but lately observed it.

Fifthly, The Teeth come forth both slowly and with trouble, they grow loose upon every slight occasion, sometimes they wax black and even fall out by pieces. In their stead new ones come again though late and with much pain. This kind of Sign, as also that which we noted in the former Article, may be referred to the *Synedremontal* Signs, because neither of these is either perpetually present, or if it be present, it doth not undoubtedly confirm the presence of the Disease.

Some have imagined that the Bones in this Disease are transfigurable like wax; But we have never seen it, neither have we received it from any eye witness who was not of suspected credit. Wherefore we reject this

Sign as altogether Fabulous.

Sixthly, The Breast in the higher progression of the Disease, becomes narrow on the sides, and sticking up foreright, so that it may not be unaptly compared to the Keel of a Ship inverted, or the Breast of a Hen or Capon. For on each side of the middle it riseth up into a point, the sides being as it were pressed down. If any demand whether this Sign be solely appropriated and peculiar to this affect; We answer, That the Breast may be a little encreased in an Atrophy or Phtisick, and less than the other parts of the Body, and so by consequence it may be narrower: But it can scarce so fall out according to the change of the Figure without an *Alogotrophy,* namely that which is proper to this Disease. Wherefore this Sign also when it it present, although the invasion of it be tardy must be reputed a *Pathognomonical* Sign of the second kind, because when it is present, it certainly denoteth the Species of the Disease, though not on the contrary. And thus much of the Signs which have reference to the unequal nourishment.

SPRUE

Aretaeus

Aretaeus, the Cappadocian, among his excellent descriptions of diseases has left us the first clearcut account of sprue.

CHAPTER VII*

ON THE COELIAC AFFECTION

The stomach being the digestive organ, labours in digestion, when diarrhoea seizes the patient. Diarrhoea consists in the discharge of undigested food in a fluid state; and if this does not proceed from a slight cause of only one or two days' duration; and if, in addition, the patient's general system be debilitated by atrophy of the body, the Coeliac disease of a chronic nature is formed, from atony of the heat which digests, and refrigeration of the stomach, when the food, indeed, is dissolved in the heat, but the heat does not digest it, nor convert it into its proper chyme, but leaves its work half finished, from inability to complete it; the food then being deprived of this operation, is changed to a state which is bad in colour, smell, and consistence. For its colour is white and without bile; it has an

offensive smell, and is flatulent; it is liquid, and wants consistence from not being completely elaborated, and from no part of the digestive process having been properly done except the commencement.

Wherefore they have flatulence of the stomach, continued eructations, of a bad smell; but if these pass downwards, the bowels rumble, evacuations are flatulent, thick, fluid, or clayey, along with the phantasy, as if a fluid were passing through them; heavy pain of the stomach now and then, as if from a puncture; the patient emaciated and atrophied, pale, feeble, incapable of performing any of his accustomed works. But if he attempt to walk, the limbs fail; the veins in the temples are prominent, for owing to wasting, the temples are hollow; but also over all the body the veins are enlarged, for not only does the disease not digest properly, but it does not even distribute that portion in which the

*The Extant Works of Aretaeus, the Cappadocian. Edited and Translated by Francis Adams, LL.D. London: Sydenham Society, 1856, p. 350.

digestion had commenced for the support of the body; it appears to me, therefore, to be an affection, not only of the digestion, but also of the distribution.

But if the disease be on the increase, it carries back the matters from the general system to the belly, when there is wasting of the constitution; the patients are parched in the mouth, surface dry and devoid of sweat, stomach sometimes as if burnt up with a coal, and sometimes as if congealed with ice. Sometimes also, along with the last scybala, there flows bright, pure, unmixed blood, so as to make it appear that the mouth of a vein has been opened; for the acrid discharge corrodes the veins. It is a very protracted and intractable illness; for, even when it would seem to have ceased, it relapses again without any obvious cause, and comes back upon even a slight mistake. Now, therefore, it returns periodically.

This illness is familiar to old persons, and to women rather than to men. Children are subject to continued diarrhoea, from an ephemeral intemperance of food; but in their case the disease is not seated in the cavity of the stomach. Summer engenders the disease more than any other of the seasons; autumn next; and the coldest season, winter, also, if the heat be almost extinguished. This affection, dysentery and lientery, sometimes are engendered by a chronic disease. But, likewise, a copious draught of cold water has sometimes given rise to this disease.

Vincent Ketelaer

Vincent Ketelaer was a Dutch physician of the seventeenth century who was rector of the gymnasium of Zierikzsee. He is remembered for his work, *De aaphthis nostratibus, seu Belgarum Sprouw* (Concerning native aphtha or sprue of the Belgians), which first appeared in 1669 and was reprinted several times. This work contains a clear description of sprue which antedates that of Hillary.

Why* the name of Aphtha was given in this disease, which is frequent and dangerous in the northern regions, we may well wonder. For those Aphthae described to us by the ancient founders of Medicine, are to us so diverse, that they differ in every climate. Hippocrates in his twenty fourth Aphorism section three, and in many other places describes these things among the diseases peculiar to the first years of infants, & superficial ulcers of the mouth, malign & serpent-like, he says these are possessed of a burning heat, which happens to infants recently born and delicate. Concerning this, Galen says, in little boys brought out into the light, Aphtha appears. So also they call the superficial ulcerations of the mouth, produced mainly by the flexibility of the Instruments, they can not bear either the touch or the nature of milk, although they contain quite a little serum. And moreover this is provided by nature with a drying quality, so that it is no wonder that, if in more tender persons it causes such ulcerations on the surface.

* * *

The Aphtha therefore, as it appears to us.

I describe more roughly and generally in this manner: the Blisters are whitish on the top and inside of the mouth & especially occurring in the vacinity of the organs of respiration and of swallowing, for the most part following upon a slow and imperfect crisis in fevers, common to these northern regions. The evidence of our eyes proves there is a diminution of sensation in the tubercles & blisters, not in the ulcer. Wherefore I ask is it thus with the ulcer? Here there is not a continuous dissolving, not a diminution but an increase in size. In like manner not by destroying do they form an eschar or crust for the delicate parts; but they either fall off unexpectedly when mature, or by healing the inner and not evident traces of it, they disappear from the mouth as if they never had been there. Although they glisten or whiten or approach the color of ashes especially if they are fatal, nevertheless they soften. You could hold that the redness & blackness of the fluid are figments of speculation rather than that they occur in practice. Anyhow so long as we are taught better things we deny these.

Moreover it is not likely that in the things themselves related & known, chance may play such a rôle, for the white may appear to

* Ketelaer, Vincent, Commentarius Medicus de Aphthis nostratibus Seu Belgarum Sprouw, Amsterdam, Bernard, 1715, p. 9.

us more than a thousand times while the shades of reds and blacks may never have appeared. These superficial blisters with glistening round tips begin most frequently on both sides of the uvula & whence progressing by the sloping parts of the palate they are contained sometimes within these limits. Now and then if they are more severe they are

Title page of Ketelaer's de Aphthis, 1672

scattered over the entire mouth: they are located on the Tongue, gums; the lips themselves whence they are spread out throughout the whole mouth. Often they do not stay within these limits but extend their bounds to the lower fauces, throat, Esophagus & which continuous with these is wont to be moistened with serum. The signs of this are either slight or few: For in addition those who are attacked by a difficulty in swallowing & drawing their breath, according to the experience of all, Aphtha, now when they become mature & are shed, such quantities are cast out certain days both by mouth & sometimes by rectum, that several basins or pots scarsely hold these accumulations.

You cannot mix with this the tough & sticky mucus which is the inseparable companion of these things, and seems to be able to increase these symptoms; moreover in whatever manner this is considered, so many

of the Aphthae always remain that neither the mouth nor any one of the neighboring organs alone suffers from their attack. Since without reason I may seem, because of certain stupidity, carried away by this opinion, yet in so many Aphthae, I have seen the stomach itself & the entire small intestine within is full of them. But concerning this thing the judgment of our native practitioners shall be: To hide their opinion was not just.

* * *

Whatever of this miasma then returns into the vessels (as from a recrudescence of the fever, with oppression of the heart, sometimes with a hurried discharge of the bowels) then it produces new material, which becomes obnoxious to it; & by the change of fermantation in its organs seizes anything which is at hand and ready. With this strife repeated, in which nature if not exhausted & supported by proper nourishment & assisting medicines, once again breaks forth and produces new Aphtha. Which usually are not different as if none had ever existed, fill a certain space, in which they mature and are cast off. This happens not once but sometimes six times, and seven times or more frequently, so that the cause of the Aphthae expelled, it attacks the body with dangerous symptoms. From these things it seems to be clear, that all Aphthae are produced in the nature of crises, which from the double & lasting struggles of nature & disease suffer longer, or shorter delays, so that one or the other is stronger in the numerous or infrequent battles they have carried on in this warfare.

Now there is discussion regarding the preceding & accompanying causes of Aphthae. The preceding are not of the same nature & quality, or this is one argument, although there may be sometimes very much regularity & mildness of that so that although the force wearies, subdued moreover & mitigated it produces no difficulty for the heart. However it attacks & infects others with a deadly madness, so whatever organs it attacks, it reddens the extremities with these lesions: if he is attacked in the heart, its heat, movement & any other powers from it are diffused in the entire body, to such a degree that he may not suffocate. If finally it attacks precipitately the abdomen, it brings on a phalanx of symptoms, & among these a most pernicious diarrhoea, which leaves behind scarcely any juice for his body & fuel for his strength.

William Hillary

William Hillary studied medicine at Leyden under Boerhaave and received the degree of M.D. in 1722. He began practice at Ripon but moved to Bath in 1734. In 1752 he went to Barbadoes, where he remained six years. After his return he settled in London, where he died in 1763.

Hillary was a systematic observer of the weather and its relationship to prevalent diseases. He began these observations at Ripon, discontinued them while at Bath, but resumed them at Barbadoes. His best-known work is his *Observations on the changes of the Air and the Concomitant Epidemical Diseases of the Island of Barbadoes*, first published at London in 1759. The work contains many interesting observations upon various diseases, particularly lead poisoning, which Hillary calls "the Dry Belly-Ache," and also gives the first description of sprue written by a physician. The following extract from Hillary's description of sprue is taken from the second edition of 1766.

OF CHRONICAL DISEASES*

Having treated on such *Acute Diseases* in the preceding Part, as are either peculiar to, or endemial in the West-India Islands, and such Countries as are situated within the Torrid Zone, and are not so frequently seen in most Parts of Europe; I shall here speak of such *Chronical Diseases* as are either indigenous or endemial, in the same warm Countries, and are unknown and never seen but in the hot Climates, except when they are carried by the Sick into the colder Countries.

And I shall begin with the Description of a Disease, which I think I may safely say is new, and has never yet been described by any Author, neither Ancient nor Modern, not even by any of the *Arabian Physicians;* most of whom lived and practised in the hot Countries of *Persia, Syria, Arabia* and *Ægypt;* but of late years is become endemial and frequent in Barbadoes, and the other West-India Islands.

From the best Accounts that I can obtain, this Malady has been some chance time seen in this Island, near these thirty Years, though but very seldom; and after I came there in 1747, I did but see one Person who had it, in the first four Years of my residing there; and three more in the next three Years; But within the four last years past, it is become so frequent that I have seen some Scores of Patients labouring under it, yet it seems not to be in the least infectious or contagious.

The Patient who labours under this Disease, usually first complains of an uneasy Sensation, or slight burning Heat about the Cardia, or upper Mouth of the Stomach; which comes slowly on, and gradually increases, and rises up the *Oesophagus* into the Mouth, without any Fever or the least feverish Heat, or much Pain attending it; most commonly without any observable Intemperance or Irregularity in living, or without any Surfeit, taking Cold, or any sort of Fever or other Disorder, which it can be attributed to, preceding it, or any manifest or immediate Cause, to which it can be ascribed.

Soon after this burning Heat, little small Pustulae, or Pimples, filled with a clear acrid Lymph, no bigger than a Pin's Head begin to rise; generally first on the End and Sides of the Tongue, which gradually increase in Number, not in Magnitude, and slowly spread under the Tongue, and sometimes to the Palate and Roof of the Mouth, and Inside of the Lips; and soon after the thin Skin which covers those Pustulae, slips off, and the Tongue looks red and a little inflamed, though not swelled, yet is almost raw like a Piece of raw Flesh, and is so tender and sore that the Patient can eat no Food but what is soft and smooth, nor drink anything that is vinous, spirituous, or the least pungent, without acute Pain; so that some suffer much from the want of proper Food. In some a Ptyalisime comes on, and continues a long time, which is so far from being of any Service, or giving any Relief to the Pa-

* Hillary, William, *Observations on the changes of the Air and the Concomitant Epidemical Diseases in the Island of Barbadoes*, II Ed., London, Lawes, Clarke and Collins, 1766, p. 276.

tient, that on the contrary it drains and exhausts the Fluids of the Body, and greatly wastes and sinks them.

In this State they continue several Days, or Weeks, and sometimes for Months, sometimes a little better, then worse again; and after a considerable time, sometimes longer, and sometimes shorter, the Pustulae will disappear and the Mouth grow well, without any Medicines or Applications, or any manifest Cause, and continue so for several Days or Weeks; but soon after this, the Patient finds a burning heat in the Oesaphagus and Stomach, attended with Ructuses and sometimes Vomittings, by which a clear acrid Lymph, or waterish Phlegm, which is very hot, and most commonly very acid, is brought up; though in some few it is not so acid: This generally continues but a little time before a Diarrhoea comes on, and continues a longer or shorter time in different Patients, and sometimes for a longer or shorter time in the same Person, and in some it continues for Weeks; and in all it greatly wastes their Flesh and Strength, and sinks their Spirits very much. The Diarrhoea after continuing a longer or shorter Time, sometimes stops without taking any Medicines, or doing anything to stay it, and the Patient thinks himself better for a short Time, and sometimes for a longer Time; but in general the acrid Humour soon returns to the Mouth again, with all the same Symptoms, but somewhat increased or aggravated; and after some stay there, it removes from thence to the Stomach and Bowels again, and thus a Metastasis of the Humour from the Mouth to the Bowels, and *vice versa,* is frequently, and sometimes suddenly made, without any manifest or perceptible Cause. Some chance time, though but seldom, after the Disease has continued a long time, it affects all the *Primæ Viæ* from the Lips to the Anus at the same time, and excoriates the last; and I have observed in one or two Cases, where the Pustulae appeared about the genital Parts, as we sometimes find the Aphthae do,

as *Hippocrates* observes;* and in one or two Cases I observed it to break out like an Impetigo, about the Mouth.

The Patients are all along without any Fever or feverish Heat, and their Pulse is all this Time rather small, lower, slower, and more languid than it was when they were in full Health; and their Body and Countenance rather paler and somewhat colder, especially in the extreme Parts, than when they were well: No Thirst, except what the Diarrhoea causes, when it continues long, and that generally moderate. The Patient's Skin is generally dry, all the Time of the Disease, and he perspires very little.

The frequent Metastases which this acrid Humour makes from the Mouth to the Stomach and Bowels, and from those of the Mouth again, greatly emaciate, weaken and consume the Patient. For when it is in the Mouth, both it and the Tongue are so excoriated, raw, tender and sore, that they can take no Nourishment, but such is very soft, smooth and mild, and in a liquid Form, without giving them exquisite Pain: and when it is in the Stomach, it gives a painful burning Sensation, and a frequent gulping up, or vomiting a little clear, acrid, acid Liquor, and their Food also; so that the Stomach can retain and digest nothing but what is very soft, smooth and light, and sometimes not even that. And when the Humour falls upon the Intestines, it produces a Diarrhoea with a Sense of Heat, and sometimes a Griping, (tho' the last not often) and sometimes with hot Stools and a Tenesmus; so that most of the nutricious Juices run off that Way, which greatly wastes and sinks the Patient. These circumstances continuing, and the Disease frequently changing from place to place, almost continualy deprives the Sick of their proper Nourishment, whence a true *Atrophy* is produced, which at the last, either sinks the Patient, or brings on a *Marasmus,* which soon ends in Death.

* Hippoc., *de Nat. Muliebr.* C. 61; *Epidem* Lib. 3, &c.

BERIBERI

Jacobus Bontius

Jacobus Bontius was born in 1592 in Leyden, the son of Geeraerdt de Bondt, professor of medicine at Leyden. He was the youngest of four sons. The eldest, Reinier, became subsequently professor of medicine and physician to Prince Maurice; the second, Jon, also a physician, was later municipal tax collector in Rotterdam; and the third, William, was professor of law at Leyden and later sheriff.

Jacobus Bontius received his M.D. at Leyden in 1614 and began practice witnessing two devastating epidemics of the plague in 1624 and 1625. Presently, as he wrote his brother William, becoming discouraged by the meager earnings of his practice because of the poor remuneration received and the competition of quacks, he decided to enter the service of the East India Company as a doctor. He sailed from Holland in 1627 and arrived in Batavia seven months later.

In Java, Bontius realized his inadequate knowledge of tropical diseases and began at once to study the new and strange diseases and jot down his observations. An ardent student of botany and natural history, he also made many observations on the flora and fauna of the East Indies. Bontius lived only four years after his arrival in Batavia and his scientific studies were soon interfered with by his official duties, since he was appointed Attorney-General of the colony the year after he arrived. He died in 1631 at the age of thirty-nine. Bontius wrote six books, four of which were published first in 1642 in Leyden, eleven years after his death, the edition being issued by his brother William under the title *"De Medicina Indorum Libri IV."* In 1658 the fifth book *"De Quadrupedibus, Aribus et Piscibus"* (concerning quadripeds, birds and fishes) and the sixth book *"De Plantis & Aromatibus"* (on plants and spices) both describing animals and plants observed in the East Indies, appeared in compilation of William Piso. The fourth book of *"De Medicina Indorum"* describes the diseases peculiar to the East Indies and contains the first European description of beriberi.

CHAPTER I

CONCERNING A CERTAIN TYPE OF PARALYSIS WHICH THE NATIVES CALL BERI-BERI*

A certain very troublesome affection, which attacks men, which is called by the inhabitants Beri-beri (which means sheep). I believe those, whom this same disease attacks, with their knees shaking, and their legs raised up, walk like sheep. It is a kind of paralysis, or rather Tremor: for it penetrates the motion and sensation of the hands and feet indeed sometimes of the whole body, and produces tremors.

The especial cause of this disease is the dense and sticky phlegmatic humor, which in the nocturnal time, particularly in the rainy season (for heavy rains fall from the beginning of November up to the beginning of May) corrupt the nerves, while truly the men fatigued by the heat during the day, by night without cover and throw the blankets off, from which most easily, this phlegmatic humor just mentioned generated especially

in the brain, attacks the nerves. Now the nights, in these places, by comparison with the heat of the day, can be called cold. In this condition the limbs are extended, not contracted, the phlegm insinuating itself between the joints, so that the nerves and ligaments are relaxed.

On the other hand this malady although commonly by steps and gradually attacks men, nevertheless sometimes is very sudden, while truly the men fatigued by the heat ingest a drink from the Palma Indica copiously and repeatedly; and just so in the country, we see sometimes done during dog days, or heated by some other violent motion they swallow excessively greedily a drink of beer and of pressed juice, also indeed often at the greatest risk of life, it certainly produces their death. From a distance the signs of this disease are obvious to the sight. Namely there is a spontaneous lassitude of the whole body; movement and sensation, particularly of the

* Bontius. Jacob., *De medicina Indorum libr. IV*, Leyden. Patuliet. 1745, p. 209.

hands and feet are depraved and they are weak; and in them is felt very often a tickling which is like that which in a cold country by wintry weather attacks hands and the toes of the feet, save that here much pain is not present.

Now the voice moreover is sometimes so affected that it is scarcely possible to speak distinctly: this happened to me myself, that the sound of the voice of sufferers from this disease, was so very weak for a whole mouth that sitting down very close to me they were scarcely intelligible. There appear, besides this, very often many signs, and symptoms, which all moreover smack of a tenacious and frigid humor but it suffices to discuss them particularly.

We are equipped for the cure consequently which often is prolonged a long time, for truly this humour, sticky and cold, is dispersed with difficulty: moreover in itself (at the utmost) it is not fatal: it invades neither the muscles of the heart or chest, &, by this manner blocks the air to the voice passages. But this in the first place is curable, not (if this can be done by any other method) by putting the afflicted recumbent on a couch: but indeed ambulant, or riding a horse, or by some other good method, known to all, you exercise him: to run however is impossible. Brisk rubbings too and painful are necessary here, such as commonly the Bengalese servants and Malay women make use of. Now our people are not accustomed to such exercises, nor to the baths, which are common here.

Fomentations and Applications are used here from the noble herb called Lagondi, the leaf of which indeed was known to the Persians and is of a pleasant and aromatic odor. Certainly we do not permit too much the use of Chamomile and Clover, for it produces, in my own judgment dispersion and weakness in the men; feet and hands moreover are annointed with oil of Cloves and Nutmeg; but a mixture of oil of roses, if applied alone is too caustic & easily erodes the skin. We have besides this the noble kind of Naphtha brought from the Kingdom of Sumatra, from the Kingdom of Java from a region in the adjoining territory. Which the Indians call Minjac Tannah, which signified oil of the earth, that indeed is known to us as Naphtha, which we call petroleum and runs from the earth; or it is cast down from the rocks, in the neighboring rivers. This oil in Barbary is held in such value, that the King Achinensis, which is the most powerful Tyrant of this island, prohibits its removal from that place under the penalty of death; so that the inhabitants, by stormy nights, if our own or English ships land on their shores, carry it away secretly to us. This oil, smeared on the affected parts, like a miracle alleviates the sick. Its odor is heavy, but nevertheless not disagreeable.

But since this disease is chronic, and of long duration, nothing does as much good, as decoctions from China-root, sarsaparilla, and Guaiacum; which by the soothing, and heat, pleasant to our bodies, disperse and eliminate those frigid and cross humours through sweats and the urine. Interposing moreover then the usual evacuations by the intestinal tract, among which principally is an Extract which we make from aloes (corruptly called among us gutta bamba) the description of which you will see below.

To bleed here is bad, for in this disease there is not plethora but loss of fluid: & anyone does not perceive the blood to be the source of heat and store-house of life?

The remnants of this disease furthermore properly are dispersed by Theriac, Mithridates, etc., sweats, and passing urine, and medicines strengthening the nerves. Suitable exercise and the mighty power of Nature heal the troublesome after-effects of this disease.

Nicholas Tulp

CHAPTER V

BERIBERI INDORUM*

Joost de Vogelaar, a youth fond of traveling, at that time in a particular part of the Orient, was however in the region of Chloromandel, where the Sun sometimes burned so hotly, that the natives sought to escape it, and they are compelled to pass the greater part of the day in cold baths, this youth to shun such consuming heat, yielded to his servants, put himself on deck every day, under the sky, and extended in the air, they bathed

* Tulp, Nicholas, *Observationes medicae*, Leyden, du Vivie, 1716, p. 286.

him with lots of cold water, and certainly the watering, and this kind of unseasonable bathing besides did him no good; for it rather injured him, on the contrary the youth became sick, he had no power to control by his mind, obstipation as well as fluid in the skin, and the inordinate cold, repercussing excessively in the nerves, produced that species of paralysis, which is called India Beriberi, or *ovem* (sheep), which disease has a small amount of danger, is however cured with difficulty, as this youth teaches by his example, because, returning to his home, he gave us opportunity of inquiring into the nature of the disease.

We have observed this to vary greatly. For it fits in with a partial paralysis, his body for instance certainly was drowsy, and languid, and his limbs inert, and inactive, however by no mean destitute of motion altogether, & albeit sick he was little by little restored to health, gradually to take food, not only to walk about, but he was permitted to sit in a chair to perform some slight movements, indeed in his dull limbs now and then a movement was detected, and then that wandering sense of tickling, which is accustomed to precede the flowing of animal spirits into the nerves, and at this very time the passage of the same through narrow openings which has been sought for.

Although the healing of the nerves was imperfect and furthermore the method of the treatment was somewhat unusual, the patient regained his health fortunately by the familiar remedies of his country and, since the treatment should have been by those very things, which is prescribed specially for this disease, which was from the Chief of the Indies to the Doctors, (Jacob Bontius, meth. medend. [methods of physicians, Chap. 1]) they are not indeed lacking with us, that precious oil of the earth, which is called Miniac Tennah Indis; & in the Island of Sumatra, which the King of Ashien rules, like the petroleum arips from rocks, a trial of this Indian oil is frequently made by us. now in chilly disorders, in the nerves and deep seated in the muscles, now moreover in strangulation of the uterus, in which it is aided not less by an oil, a kind of chyme, taken from the juice, that is the fluid of the evacuated phlegm (in which above all lies the cause of this disease) they do the work especially well, with convenient cathartics, then Guaiac wood, sassafras, and China root & externally an ointment partly from petroleum, partly indeed of castor oil, of wax, of the seeds of myristica, of cloves, of peppermint, and of rose-wood, and by the legitimate use of all these things, not however constantly, in this manner he was restored soon to a condition of perfect health.

PELLAGRA

Gaspar Casál and François Thiéry

Gaspar Casál was born, probably, in 1679. Several different places have been mentioned as his birthplace. His friend Thiéry states that he was born in Aragon and practiced medicine in various places in Castille. Jourdán describes Oviedo as his birthplace, while the historian Garcia maintained that he was born in Gerona, and other accounts describe him as "a native of Utrilla" and as "the son of a native of the city of Pavia in the state of Milan." Morejon, the Spanish medical historian, states, "We do not know for certain the place of his birth," and his biographer Canella, after discussing the various theories and bits of evidence, fails to arrive at any definite conclusion.

We have no information regarding Casál's medical studies. At the age of twenty-eight he was practising medicine in the villages of Alcarria. In 1709 he studied in Siguenza and in 1713, at the age of thirty-four, he received the degree of bachelor of arts. We have no exact information regarding his medical studies but he apparently went to Madrid after receiving his bachelor degree and in that city began the practice of medicine. In 1720, he was appointed city physician of Oviedo in the Asturias and soon enjoyed a very extensive practice. With the years his reputation increased and presently he became known as the

Asturian Hippocrates and, as his fame increased, and patients came from far and wide to consult him, he was called the Spanish Hippocrates.

In 1751, after practising more than thirty years in Oviedo, Casál returned to Madrid, where he was appointed physician to King Ferdinand and proto-medico of Castille. He died in 1759. Three years later his posthumous *Historia natural y medica de el principado de Asturias* was published by his colleague,

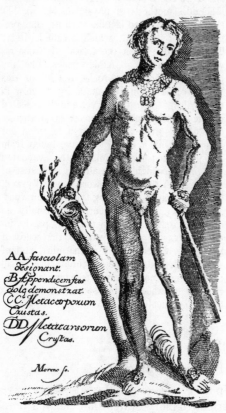

AA *fasciolam designant.*
B *Appendicem sæ dolg demonstrat.*
CC. *Hetacarpoxum Cuistas.*
DD *Hetatarsorum Cruftas.*

Moreno fo.

A patient suffering from pellagra
From Casal's *Historia natural y medica de el principado de Asturias* (Madrid, 1762)

Dr. Juan Jose Garcia Sevillano. This work, the result of thirty years' observation, describes the topography, climate, winds, waters, flora, fauna, minerals, metals, epidemics and diseases. In this work, the third section of which was written in Latin and not in Spanish as the preceding sections, the author describes the disease "Mal de la Rosa," now known as pellagra. The latter name dates from the description of Francesco Frapolli, an Italian physician, in 1771.

François Thiéry was born in Nancy and graduated at Paris in 1740. While physician to the French ambassador to Spain, he met Casál at Court, and hearing of this new and strange malady, sent a report of it to Paris, where it was published in 1755 in the *Journal de médecine, chirurgie et pharmacie*. Although Thiéry's publication antedates that of Casál, he states specifically that he obtained his account of the disease from his Spanish colleague. After a three years' stay in Spain he returned to Paris. He was the author of several books and his *Observations de physique et de médecine faites en différents lieux de l'Espagne*, published in Paris in 1791, gives a further account of the "Mal de la Rosa."

VIII. The following article on a disease peculiar to Asturias, is by M. Thiéry, Regent of the Faculty of Medicine of Paris, at present in Madrid with the Duc de Duras, Ambassador of France. He sent it to M. Chomel, Dean of the Faculty, to be read at an assembly called *Prima-mensis*, & to be inserted in the register where a journal is kept of the disease observed at Paris & in the Kingdom during the course of each month & of the remedies which have been employed with the greatest success. But as it is not customary to take notice of the diseases which prevail in foreign countries, the Dean has sent us this dissertation, to bring it to public notice by means of this Journal.

DESCRIPTION

OF A MALADY CALLED MAL DE LA ROSA*

VIII. Among a large number of complica-

* *Jour. de méd., chir. et pharm.,* Paris, 1755. pp. 337-346.

tions which accompany this disease, there is one which characterizes it & makes it very easy to distinguish. This is a horrible crust, dry, scabby, blackish, crossed with cracks, which causes much pain to the sufferer and throws off a very foetid odor. This crust may be upon the elbows, the arms, the head, the abdomen, &c. But the people of Asturia, where this disease is endemic, do not give it the name of *mal de la Rosa* unless it is located exactly on the metacarpals or metatarsals of the hands or of the feet; and following them in this restriction I am going to write in a few words the history of this disease.

It commences ordinarily towards the spring equinox, more rarely at other seasons. In the beginning it is nothing more than a simple redness accompanied by roughness. It degenerates later into true crusts such as we are going to describe. They dry up ordinarily during the summer, & the affected metacarpus or metatarsus is completely rid of its crusts or pustules. There remain red and shiny marks, very smooth, and denuded of hair, more sunken than the neighboring skin, resembling somewhat those scars which burns leave after they are cured. It is probably the red and glossy color of these marks which has given to this disease the name of *mal de la Rosa*. These scars, besides, in those who have been affected for a long time with this kind of illness, last their entire life; & every year at spring time they become recovered with new crusts which became more horrible from year to year. They do not always involve the two hands, sometimes one sees then on one hand alone & on one foot: sometime on two hands and on one foot. It happens also that they involve all at once both hands and both feet. They do not extend to the palms of the hands or the soles of the feet: they involve constantly the back, either extending thus over the entire metacarpals or metatarsals, or they cover a slight portion.

There is another very remarkable sign of this disease, which, in truth, is not essential to it, because it is not always present; but, as it is never observed in other diseases except this one of which we speak, we may regard it as an accompaniment. This symptom is another crust of an ashy & jaundiced color, which involves the anterior & inferior portion of the neck, extending out from here & along the clavicles & the superior extremity of the sternum, forming a band as wide as two fingers. It rarely covers the entire back of the neck; most often the middle portion of the trapezius muscle remains free, & prevents this collar from making a circuit of the neck, but, in revenge, it forms ordinarily on the sternum a lesion of the same kind & the same size which extends the length of this bone to the middle of the thorax. This malady does resemble the collar of an order, which renders the Asturian thus unfortunately affected, very easy to distinguish from all of his fellow citizens.

So singular a disease ought to be without doubt accompanied by peculiar symptoms. Independent of the horrible crusts of which we have just spoken, the patients are attacked by a perpetual shaking of the head & indeed of all the upper part of trunk. This trembling is often so marked that they can scarcely keep on their feet: We have seen a woman in the hospital whose head & trunk trembled so as to resemble a reed continually shaken by the wind. She could not hold herself upright without changing every moment the position of her feet, holding thus by instinct the equilibrium which this perpetual trembling caused her to lose. The patients have further a painful burning of the mouth, vesicles upon the lips & they have a dirty tongue. They complain of extreme feebleness of the stomach & of all of the body, principally the thighs & of a heaviness which takes away from them all activity. At night they feel a burning which often deprives them of slumber. The bed is then insupportable to them because of the heat, but they do not feel better with cold; the slightest degree of cold or of heat is equally insupportable to them. They are sad and melancholy: one sees them shedding tears and emitting cries without any object, although otherwise they seem to possess their reason. They claim that they are compelled to in spite of themselves by the nature of their illness. These symptoms besides are common to all. And here are a few of them in detail. Slight delirium, a certain stupidity, loss of certain senses, of taste & of touch principally, crusts, ulcers, erysipelas in different parts, irregular fevers, restless slumber, the skin entirely discolored & elephantiasis to a slight degree.

This disease is terminated most commonly by hydrops, by lymphatic or scrofulous tumors, & by marasmus. It has also another termination but it does not happen indifferently at every season. This is the mania into which these unhappy sufferers fall towards the summer solstice. This mania is not ordinarily severe but however it deranges the mind of the patients & forces them to leave their dwellings & to save themselves in solitude where the excess of ennui & of illness throws them sometimes into great depression. It should be remarked that this maniacal melancholia which follows at the height of summer in those who are affected by the *mal de la Rosa* are much more terrible, & more commonly mortal than those which have another origin. Without doubt because these are produced by metastasis to the brain of the acrid & malign humour which produced this malady. But what is its nature? If one wishes to describe with care the symptoms which we have described one would not be far from thinking that it is a mixture of leprosy; tetter & of scurvy which constitutes a disease of a peculiar and definite type which has its proper & constant symptoms. This malady has never been described as far as I know, and dones not exist perhaps elsewhere with as much violence as in Asturians, especially those of *Oviedo*: for the Asturians of *Santillana* are more healthy by the nature of the soil, by the quality of the air, & of the food. . . .

* * *

M. Casal, physician of the Court, who adds to a taste for observation all the frankness of the earlier times, who has practiced medicine in Asturias for 25 or 30 years & from whom I take the history which I have just read; this wise observer, I say, assures me that the mal de la Rosa has always resisted all remedies, & that he regards it as incurable. Moreover he cites the example of a woman of the people who during one of the melancholy deliriums so frequent in this disease, had a great desire to feed herself from cow's butter, for which she spent all of her property, and she was cured.*

I treated, myself, here in the autumn of 1753, a woman attacked by this malady from

* M. Chomel makes the remark that this observation is entirely in conformity with the most sensible practice. One does not know any curative method more efficacious for diseases of the skin, tetter, itch &c. & for certain kinds of scurvy, than the use of milk for all nourishment, & indeed as an external remedy, for bath, douche, &c. That the patient ate up her property in butter is not surprising in Spain. More butter is sold in Paris on one market day than is sold throughout the year at Madrid.

10 to 12 years, which always appeared on the occasion of a depression and of suppression of the menses. All of the remedies which she tried had been without success & the majority of the physicians assured me that they could not cure it. She had a frightful crust on one of the metacarpals and some others, smaller, on the forearm of the same side. But she did not have the collar of the order, nor any considerable complication. I made her take a mixture of mineral aethiops, of crude antimony, saffron of Mars, with some balsamic subsances, the whole mixed with some purgatives & aided by regime and proper ptisanes. She cured properly in the course of two months.

I did not know then what name to give to this malady, regarding it solely as a diminutive of leprosy. During the spring of 1754, there came on the site of the crusts a simple redness which disappeared in a short time & without any remedy. I do not yet know if this redness will reappear in the spring.

---

§ III

Concerning the Affection, which is Commonly called in this Region mal de la Rosa*

Since I have observed carefully, in the practice of many years all the symptoms common to this disease: and I saw among all the indigenous disease in this region none more horrible or refractory: I have decided it would not be out of place for me to write the history of it.

* * *

§ IV

Concerning the History of this Disease

As I have said, I have attempted for a long time, to examine with the greatest care, all the symptoms of this disease; but thinking that I could not obtain the information anywhere else than directly from the patients themselves, I began in the year 1735, to examine them and to write down everything that they answered to my questions, relevant or irrelevant. Here is the result.

1. The 26 of Mar. 1735, a certain individual of forty years, who complained of this disease, came to consult me, and in correct

* Casal, Don Gaspar, *Historia natural, y medica de el Principado de Asturias*, Madrid. Martin, 1762, p. 327, translated by Rafael Rivera y Miranda.

and elegant language related to me the following:

It has happened that he complains on occasions of certain fevers like the epherema. He did not lose his appetite entirely, but after dinner he immediately became sleepy, which lasted then for a time as if he were a stupid person, and especially in the month of March. A few times he was troubled with thirst, he felt continually a certain fatigue or better a weakness in his extremities, especially the lower extremities. When he walked around or took any other kind of violent exercise, suddenly he was confused and mixed up in his head in such a manner, that if he did not stop immediately he tottered and could not avoid falling; and it should be noted that this happened without losing his senses. He walked always carelessly and lazily. He was always bothered with a bitter taste in his mouth. He could not stand cold weather, it tormented him terribly. When he was still he had constantly his feet frozen, if he walked they felt like fire.

2. His wife had the same disease; in addition to the common symptoms which she herself confessed tormented her, there was one that tormented her above all, she could not endure heat, nor sun, nor fire because of the terrible headache these things caused her: neither could she endure cold, because she felt it penetrated her body in such a way, that it passed through her innermost organs. Every year, a little before the equinox of Spring, there appeared on the metacarpals and metatarsals of the hands and of the feet, horrible crusts, when the heat of the summer solstice came they separated and fell off, the scar remaining.

3. A few days afterwards Manuel Carreno, inhabitant of the village called Bonielles, related to me the following:

"At the beginning of the affection, I was tormented by intolerable headaches with continual swooning, but without loss of sense or of reason. Then I felt a numbness all over the body, and a swelling, this swelling disappeared in a few days spontaneously, and then the cause was localized on the neck, without tumefaction but with great pain, that tormented me in a terrible manner in all parts, anterior, posterior, right, left, superior and inferior."

Then it happens that certain glands contiguous to the fauces may swell and make swallowing of food difficult. After feeling these symptoms the form of the little tumor was enlarged, taking on at the same time a light color, which was in truth the origin of the heat which, according to the same patient, flushed his face frequently. His tongue was coated with whitish sticky rust, and little by little suffered much heat and great pains. The nose and the lips were the seat of frequent pain and on them appeared little blisters, like those formed by boiling water. His legs were heavy, weak and feeble, so that it was difficult to walk, only when he began to exercise they became stronger. He had no appetite, but when beginning to eat, he did it without haste. His head trembled in such a way that with a single movement of his body, without holding to anything, he would fall on the floor without losing his senses. The bowel movements were difficult. He passed the nights sleeping very little and then his short dreams were stormy. All his body, especially the hands were blackish, scabby and terrible, from which I understood that he was suffering with the black *albarras,* complicated with the mal de la Rosa.

* * *

CONCERNING THE SYMPTOMS OF THIS DISEASE

1. From the stated facts, and many others which I have been able to deduce from mature reflection, the symptoms of this disease can be deduced, but as some of them are peculiar and characteristic of this disease and others are common to this disease and to other affections, we will discuss first the former.

2. The distinctive and inseparable symptoms of this disease are:

1^0 The constant trembling of the head, which although it is common to all patients, it is in many so lasting they are not a single moment without an irregular movement of the entire body. In the hospital of Santiago, of this city, I cured a little woman (and if necessary, I would swear it under oath) whose body, especially the upper half, was balanced like a swallow pushed by a varying wind; in order to hold herself steady, she had to move her legs very fast, to prevent herself from falling down to the ground at any moment.

2^0 The burning pain of the mouth, vesicles on the lips, and a coating on the tongue.

3^0 The distressing weakness of the stomach

and the weakness of the entire body, especially of the legs, and a strange laziness and carelessness.

4⁰ The crusts of the metacarpals and metatarsals and a sort of collar on the upper part of the neck.

5⁰ The scorching heat which torments them, especially in the chest.

6⁰ That smoothness or delicate fineness of the skin which does not resist either heat or cold; and

7⁰ The heaviness, which without any known cause, attacks them and causes them to give way to a sad crying, a phenomenon which by itself is a pathognomonic sign of the affection.

Francesco Frapolli

Francesco Frapolli graduated in 1757 at Pavia and began the practice of medicine in Milan under Dr. Guiseppe Biumi and twelve years after his graduation was appointed physician to the Ospitale Maggiore in Milan. Two years after his appointment, he published in 1771 his celebrated work on pellagra, a little volume of thirty pages written in Latin.

Frapolli regarded pellagra as essentially a skin disease, advising that the patients be shielded from the sunlight especially by wearing large straw hats, stockings and gloves, and that the skin be bathed and massaged frequently. He advised a starchy diet, the avoidance of meats and for the diarrhea prescribed ipecac, lemons, whey, wine and enemata. His work was neither profound nor very accurate but it had the great merit of focussing the attention of the medical profession upon pellagra. Frapolli died in 1773.

* * *

OBSERVATIONS ON THE DISEASE, COMMONLY CALLED "PELAGRA"*

There rages among the peasants of this our Lombardy a certain Disease, which because of a variety of symptoms by no means rarely fatal, and certainly because its newness to all, and particularly in the opinion of physicians, excites and rouses zeal in the highest degree for a careful and more penetrating study, so that more powerful remedies may be discovered for those in whom this may have occurred for the abundance of the People and of the fields, more fruitful harvests and for the public good that their precious well-being may be continually protected.

Now with the advent of harvest the rustics men & women, boys and girls, and everybody who has the proper age shares in the work with heavy and light duties, it happens very often, that the color of their skin is suddenly changed to a red, like erysipelas, and then red spots, (which the Rustics call *Rosas*) appear in the Epidermis, and on top very small tubercles of varied colors rise up

close together: then the skin dries, the adjacent teguments burst, the corroded skin turns into white scales or scurfs; especially the hands, feet, chest, but rarely the face, and the other parts of the Body exposed to the Sun are badly disfigured. Again, this remarkable series indeed of external affections, which we have thus far touched upon lightly constitute this disease which they popularly call *Pelagra*. But whence comes a disease of this character? With the passing of the summer season, everything is restored to its former state; the normal state of the skin returns, & unless worse troubles appear, the Peasants disregard the *Pelagra,* nor hereafter do they suffer any ill. However, often & more commonly the disease continues even then but not to the point where the skin desquamates, but is wrinkled, or indeed calloused, and full of fissures. Now the Patients first begin to suffer in the head, anxiety, depression, sleeplessness, dizziness, cloudiness of mind I may not say foolishness, hypochondriacal delirium, diarrhoea, & sometimes to suffer Mania. Man then failing in body

Whether Pelagra is a new Disease?

* Frapolli, Francesco, *Animadversiones in Morbum, vulgo Pelagram,* Milan, Galeatius, 1771, p. 7.

especially in the legs and thighs, and nearly losing the motion of these parts entirely, emaciated in the highest degree, seized with a debilitating diarrhoea most stubborn to all remedies, moreover Patients consumed by ghastly thinness expire at the end of day. See a brief added history of the disease with observations.

Concerning this disease I now proceed to make inquiries. 1st whether Pelagra be a new Disease? 2nd Whether contagious? 3rd what its cause is? 4th Always the same effect. 5th The attending Hygiene. 6th What also the cure? And thus the treatise proceeds in some order, and the whole thing itself in various parts becomes clearer.

Pelagra, if the name only is considered, is indeed judged a new disease; for no one, whom I know myself, has up to the present time written particularly concerning this affection of the skin, nor does any graphic account appear among the Ancients, whose skill in observing skin diseases was remarkable and in the highest degree astonishing. Resembling this disease are some symptoms of Impetigo, as hardness of the skin, dryness, harshness, and other things of this character, & which are observed in *Pelagra,* & have been described especially by Sennert *pract. lib.* 5 *part* 1. *cap.* 30 *de Impetig. fol.* 39. But this Disease is not the same, which fact, taking everything into consideration is as clear as the light of mid-day: but it does not interest me to carry this thing to a final judgment since the differences of other illnesses may not be clear to all physicians. What therefore? Truly a new disease? It is by no means easy to decide; when especially I found by chance a certain Order of the Venerable Head of the Hospital of greater Milan published in the Year 1578 the 6th day of March, which was as follows. *Fifth That those, who are suffering from Pellarella, Crusts, Gumma and Sores be received but having the Order countersigned as above.* Now the Learned should decide whether this term *Pellarella* designates our *Pelagra* or not. If they decide in the affirmative, then the disease is not modern: if in the negative then the matter is uncertain. Since however, the medical writers on this disease of the skin never describe it accurately, it is not possible at all to ascertain for certain whether a disease of this sort existed earlier. It is by no means impossible that the old Fathers of Medicine referred the same symptoms which the

Moderns now assign to *Pelagra,* to other Diseases & most especially of the Skin. Again with the same there is almost always a cause (as I will show later) producing it, for which reason was not then an effect? But we have had enough of this, I will leave this annoying question.

Meanwhile no one considers the sleep producing disease *Pelagra* to be contagious; indeed the contrary is most evident. Contagion is defined, as that Force or Activity which present in one Body excites the same condition in another and indeed either immediately & through bodily contact or mediately, & causes a series of external affects, nor it is possible that everyone would call that a contagious disease.

Whether contagious?

* * *

In fact there remains to me no other course to take except to describe the disease. I have retained the name *Pellagra* already employed to signify the entire disease, and have used the name *pellagrosa desquamazione* to designate the cutaneous disease symptoms. Pellagra than is called by me a chronic malady of the entire body, in which the most common symptoms are desquamation in the spring of the parts exposed to the sun, delirium, vertigo, tetanus, opisthotonos, emprosthotonos, pains in the spine and in the extremities, weakness of the lower parts, bulimia, etc. enumerating thus all those phenomena, which by their unusualness can most easily show us the presence of the disease. In spite of all these things I confess to not having known how to define Pellagra with precision; with my ignorance however I have taken a step towards knowing it, having demonstrated the error of my Predecessors who have located the malady either entirely or too essentially in the skin.

* * *

Also before these two Authors, Sig Odoardi already recognizes, that Pellarina owed its origin to a deficiency of diet. He says nothing of exposure to sun, but apparently decided, that the disease (with all its symptoms) arose *from a diet almost solely of polenta made from corn, and without salt, either mixed with barley, with buckwheat, or maize, and with sorghum or maize: of bread also of corn and more commonly mixed with rye, and the other mentioned cereals; of soup of green* beans, beans, chick peas, curds of goats' milk, of cheese, from passing in idleness the long winters after the continued labors of the other

the night in the stalls.

All then is in agreement in considering the bad food as the principal cause of the disease;

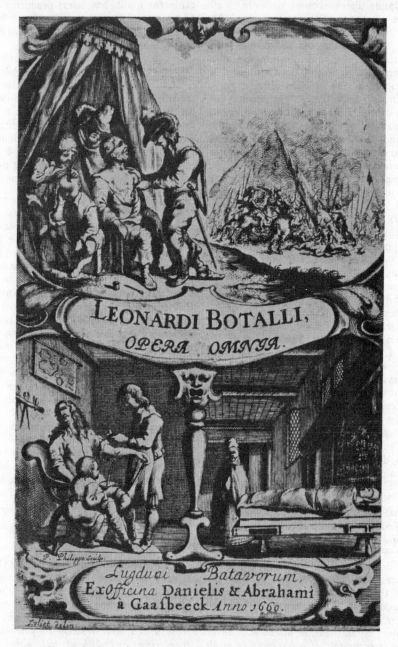

Frontispiece to Botalli's *Opera Omnia* (Leyden, 1660)

seasons; from living in rooms either poorly protected or on the ground, paved and damp; from passing a good part of the day, and of

and then each accuses something else in the disease according to the customs of his country.

OF THE NYCTALOPIA, OR NIGHT-BLINDNESS*

A MAN about thirty years old had in the spring a tertian fever, for which he took too small a quantity of bark, so that the returns of it were weakened without being entirely removed. He therefore went into the cold-bath, and after bathing twice he felt no more of his fever. Three days after his last fit, being then on board of a ship in the river, he observed at sunsetting, that all objects began to look blue, which blueness gradually thickened into a cloud; and not long after he became so blind, as hardly to perceive the light of a candle. The next morning about sunrising his sight was restored as perfectly as ever. When the next night came on, he lost his sight again in the same manner; and this continued for twelve days and nights. He then came ashore, where the disorder of his eyes gradually abated, and in three days was en-

tirely gone. A month after he went on board of another ship, and after three days stay in it, the night-blindness returned as before, and lasted all the time of his remaining in the ship, which was nine nights. He then left the ship; and his blindness did not return while he was upon land. Some little time afterwards, he went into another ship, in which he continued ten days, during which time the blindness returned only two nights, and never afterwards.

In the August following, he complained of loss of appetite, weakness, shortness of breath, and a cough: he fell away very fast, had frequent shiverings, pains in his loins, dysury, and vomitings; all which complaints increased upon him until the middle of November, when he died.

He had formerly been employed in lead-works, and had twice lost the use of his hands, as is usual among the workers in this metal.

* William Heberden, M.D., *Commentaries on the History and Cure of Diseases,* Boston, Wells and Lilly, 1818, pp. 269-270.

IX. ALLERGIC DISEASES

HAY-FEVER

Leonardo Botallo

Leonardo Botallo or Botallus was born in 1530 at Asti in Piedmont, studied medicine under Lanfranc, Trincavella, and Fallopia, graduated at Pavia and lived for a time in Paris. He became famous as an anatomist and his name has been known to successive generations for his description of the ductus arteriosus or duct of Botallo (ductus Botalli). He also achieved a great reputation through his treatise on gunshot wounds and his advocacy of bleeding as a remedy for practically every disease.

Botallo, in 1565, in his *Commentarioli duo,* described the condition to which we now apply the term allergy. His patient suffered from headache, sneezing, and itching of the nose when in the presence of roses. The following description of "rose catarrh" is translated from his *Opera Omnia* published at Leyden in 1660.

---

§25.* Now odors pleasant to physicians and agreeable to all men or to most can be used in moderation furthermore in patients themselves. For both heart and brain are made better by them, as well as the liver itself: for one of the five senses affects naturally the ordinary state of the body and the mind is soothed by Pleasant odors, they drive away unpleasant things. But sometimes, although they are pleasant to many, it happens that they may be unpleasant to one. I know men in health, who directly after the odor of roses have a severe reaction from this, so that they have a headache, or it causes sneezing, or induces such a troublesome itching in the nostrils that they can not, for a space of two days, restrain themselves from rubbing them. & I know women, who also have such an aversion to the odor of a calf that if they perceive one close by, they fall into a swoon or are provoked to vomit or have a heaviness of the head. For which reason the physician ought to avoid this, or any other odor which oppresses the patient, until he had cured the patient: not indeed as Quintus acted, who (as Galen narrates), smelling of wine drew near a rich and powerful patient, harassed by a severe fever. He commenced to ask Quintus if he would move a little farther away, so he would not then carry the odor of wine: Quintus instead then drew closer to him, said roughly. "Thou shouldst bear this odor of wine from me, for I tolerated the stench of fever from thee." This answer was certainly rude and boorish, which is not becoming to a physician, who has care of the health, not only of fine gentlemen but of other men as well.

Marginal notes:
How good odors are helpful to the Physicians

Some have aversion to the odor of roses

Others are affected by the odor of a calf

The rudeness of Quintus

* Botallo. Leonardo, *Opera Omnia,* Leyden. Gaasbeeck, 1660, p. 20.

Johann Nikolaus Binninger

Johann Nikolaus Binninger was born in 1628 at Montbéliard and studied medicine at Basle, Padua, and Montpellier. He received his M.D. degree at Basle in 1653, practised for several years in his native city, but removed to

Basle, where he taught in the medical school. A few years later he was appointed physician to the Duke of Württemberg and returned to Montbéliard, where he became Professor of Medicine in the newly founded University.

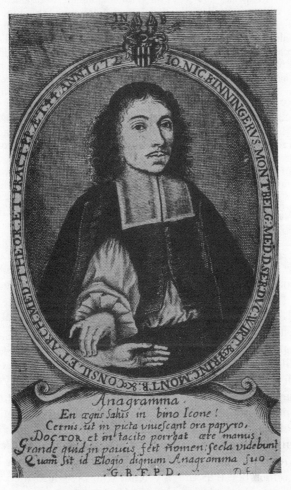

JOHANN NIKOLAUS BINNINGER (1628-1692)
From a portrait appearing in Binninger's *Observationum et curationum medicinalium* (Montbéliard, 1673)

Binninger's clinical experiences are detailed in his *Observationum et curationum medicinalium centuriae quinque*, which appeared at Montbéliard in 1673. This work, while unimportant as a medical work, contains many curious observations. Observation 86 in *Centuria secunda* describes a case of sensitiveness to roses, an early example of rose catarrh.

OBSERVATION LXXXVI

CONCERNING ODORS EXTRAORDINARILY AFFECTING & PURGING THE BODY*

L. B., student of Medicine, now a doctor, had an olefactory organ wonderfully constituted. For things emitting a pleasant odor he caught with his nostrils, in a very short time they disappeared, those on the contrary which smelled most foetid, persisted a long time, so that they remained many hours, dissipated by no arts. The worthy Matron *Ursula Falcisin,* Wife of that Illustrious Man, Master Jacob à Brun, Doctor of Medicine & Professor at Basle, of an ample and fleshy body, suffered from a Coryza many weeks at the season of roses, as I heard several times from the mouth of the Excellent Doctor. Now I wrote a work of Medicine in 1651, of an

*Binninger, J. K., *Observationum et curationum medicinalium,* Montbéliard, Hyppianis, 1673, Centuria secunda, p. 227.

inhabitant of Montpellier, a certain old person, morose & decrepit, of a hot dry temperament, melancholic, a Teacher, a neighbor in a wine-house (where I lived at that time), who as a joke we called Fellowguest & I, an Academician, suffered from an ordinary constipation. Since he suffered many days most badly from this affection & had fever, the Landlady asked would I be willing to give aid to the poor miserable sufferer: I showed him a soothing potion and a purge of senna equal parts, that same day he was cured, the illness leaving my friend of the Academy on the morrow. This man was never purged by any drug the rest of his life. From the smell alone of purgative drugs he was frequently aroused early in the morning, he remained in good health leaving off medicine.

John Bostock

John Bostock was born in Liverpool in 1773 and graduated in medicine at Edinburgh in 1794. He began soon after to practice in Liverpool but removed to London in 1817. Soon after this he gave up the practice of medicine to devote himself to science and to enjoy the company of his scientific friends.

He took a prominent part in the Geological Society, the Royal Society, the Linnaean, Zoölogical, Horticultural, and Medico-Chirurgical Societies, and in the Royal Society of Literature. "In a word," as the *Lancet* wrote in his obituary notice, "he may be said to have occupied a prominent position among those distinguished men who have united their powerful and efficient energies in the advancement of medical and physical science."

He wrote many articles in scientific publications and his *Elements of Physiology* was the first systematic treatise on the subject to appear in England. Today he is best remembered as the physician who first described hay-fever, being himself the patient. He died of cholera in 1846 at the age of seventy-three.

CASE
OF A
PERIODICAL AFFECTION
OF THE
EYES AND CHEST*

By John Bostock, M.D., F.R.S., & L.S.

Read March 10, 1819

The following case, it is presumed, will not be altogether uninteresting to the Society,

Med. Chir. Tr., London, 1819, x, 161-165.

as affording an example of an unusual train of symptoms, and it may perhaps be considered the more worthy of their attention, from its having occurred in the person of the narrator.

J. B., aet. 46, is of a spare and rather delicate habit, but capable of considerable exertion, and has no hereditary or constitutional affection, except various stomach complaints, probably connected with. or depend-

some time over the whole of the ball. At the commencement the external appearance of the eye is little affected, except that there is a slight degree of redness and a discharge of tears. This state gradually increases, until the sensation becomes converted into what may be characterized as a combination of the

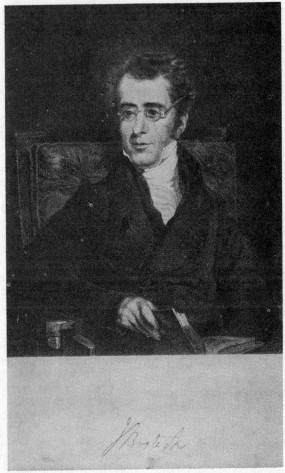

Courtesy of the Surgeon General's Library, Washington, D.C.

JOHN BOSTOCK (1773-1846)
From Jenkins' engraving of a portrait of
Bostock by Partridge

ing upon, a tendency to gout. About the beginning or middle of June in every year the following symptoms make their appearance, with a greater or less degree of violence. A sensation of heat and fullness is experienced in the eyes, first along the edges of the lids, and especially in the inner angles, but after

most acute itching and smarting, accompanied with a feeling of small points striking upon or darting into the ball, at the same time that the eyes become extremely inflamed, and discharge very copiously a thick mucous fluid. This state of the eyes comes on in paroxysms, at uncertain intervals, from about the second week in June to the middle of July. The eyes are seldom quite well for the whole of this period, but the violent paroxysms never occur more than two or three times daily, lasting an hour or two each time; but with respect to their frequency or duration there is the greatest uncertainty. Generally, but not always, their invasion may be distinctly traced to some exciting cause, of which the most certain is a close moist heat, also a bright glare of light, dust or other substances touching the eyes, and any circumstance which increases the temperature. After the violent inflammation and discharge have continued for some time, the pain and redness gradually go off, but a degree of stiffness generally remains during the day.

After this state of the eyes has subsided for a week or ten days, a general fulness is experienced in the head, and particularly about the fore part; to this succeeds irritation of the nose, producing sneezing, which occurs in fits of extreme violence, coming on at uncertain intervals. To the sneezings are added a farther sensation of tightness of the chest, and a difficulty of breathing, with a general irritation of the fauces and trachea. There is no absolute pain in any part of the chest, but a feeling of want of room to receive the air necessary for respiration, a huskiness of the voice, and an incapacity of speaking aloud for any time without inconvenience. To these local symptoms, are at length added a degree of general indisposition, a great degree of languor, and incapacity for muscular exertion, loss of appetite, emaciation, restless nights, often attended with profuse perspirations, the extremities, however, being generally cold. The pulse is permanently quickened, from 80, the average standard, to about 100, and upon any considerable exertion it rises to 120 or more.

This is an account of the complaint in its worst state, which, however, it does not assume in every season, and indeed its violence is generally less than is here described. The affection of the eyes is recollected to have occurred when the patient was eight years old, and there has been more or less of it every year since; the sneezings came on nearly at the same period, but the first attack of the test was at the age of sixteen or seventeen. Generally speaking, the complaints have increased for the last twenty years, although not progressively. All the acute symptoms disappear about the end of July, but a considerable degree of weakness and languor is left, which remains a month or six weeks longer. It has happened that the most severe summer complaints have been experienced, after the patient had enjoyed the best health during the preceding spring. On the contrary, it has been thought that after a severe summer attack, the patient has more completely and more rapidly regained his usual state of health and strength in the autumn.

The remedies employed have been various, and they have been persevered in with an unusual degree of steadiness. Topical bleeding, purging, blisters, spare diet, bark and various other tonics, steel, opium, alterative courses of mercury, cold bathing, digitalis, and a number of topical applications to the eyes, have been very fully tried, but it is doubtful whether any distinct or permanent benefit has been derived from any of them. The complaint once seemed to be decidedly stopped by a journey, but in other instances it has existed while the patient was travelling. By using every means for obtaining fresh air, without much exertion, and by carefully avoiding a moist and close atmosphere, the symptoms may in some measure be kept off, but they have frequently appeared under circumstances that seemed the least likely to have produced them.

It may form an important addition to the narrative to state, that during the last summer the patient was so situated as to be able to avoid almost every degree of bodily exertion; he remained confined to the house for about six weeks, and the result was that, notwithstanding the unusual warmth of the season, he experienced much less of the affection than he had done for several years before.

ALLERGY IN INFECTIOUS DISEASES

Edward Jenner

Edward Jenner, the discoverer of vaccination against smallpox, was born in the vicarage at Berkeley in 1749. His father was the Rev. Stephen Jenner, vicar of Berkeley and his mother was the daughter of the Rev. Mr. Head, former vicar of Berkeley. Edward Jenner, at the age of thirteen, began his professional education under Mr. Daniel Ludlow of Sodbury and then entered as a student of medicine at St. George's Hospital, London in 1770. The same

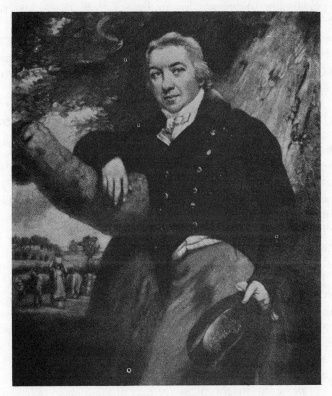

EDWARD JENNER (1749-1823)
From a portrait by J. R. Smith, 1801

year he went as a house pupil to John Hunter. Jenner soon became Hunter's favorite pupil, and a friendship and affection sprang up between them which lasted until Hunter's death.

In 1773 Jenner returned to Berkeley and began the practice of a country doctor. He kept up a constant correspondence with John Hunter, who stimulated his young pupil to continue his investigations in natural history. Many of these letters have been preserved and are quite amusing. In 1778 Jenner was crossed in love and received a letter from Hunter saying, "let her go, never mind her. I shall employ you with hedgehogs" (referring to his investigations on the heat of animals and vegetables). Ten years later Jenner married and upon the birth of his first-born Hunter wrote "sooner than the brat should not be a Christian, I will stand godfather, for I should be unhappy if the poor little thing should go to the devil because I would not stand godfather."

Jenner obtained the degree of M.D. from St. Andrews in 1792 and gave up general practice the same year. In 1796 he performed his first inoculation with cowpox on James Phipps, a boy of eight. This subject had interested him ever since he was a pupil at Sodbury when he asked a young girl about smallpox and she answered "I cannot take that disease for I have had cowpox." Jenner continued his inoculations for two years, and in 1798 applied to the Royal Society for permission to present his findings before them. His request was refused with the advice that "he ought not to risk his reputation by presenting to the learned body anything which appeared so much at variance with established knowledge, and withal so incredible." Undaunted, Jenner published his *Inquiry* describing his great discovery. Vaccination spread rapidly and Jenner's fame became world-wide.

In 1813, during the war with France, Jenner's relative, Captain Milman, was captured by the French and imprisoned at Verdun. Jenner wrote a letter to Napoleon requesting his release. Napoleon on reading the letter said "Ah! c'est Jenner, je ne puis rien refuser à Jenner," ("Ah, it's Jenner! I can refuse Jenner nothing.") and ordered his release. Jenner was not so successful in inducing the British authorities to release Captain Husson, brother of Dr. Husson one of the chief exponents of smallpox vaccination in France, who was a prisoner of war in England.

The English parliament in 1802 voted Jenner a grant of 10,000 pounds for his discovery. In 1813, Oxford conferred upon him the degree of Doctor of Physic. He died in 1823 and was buried in the chancel of Berkeley Church.

Jenner's personal appearance was described most vividly by his friend, Edward Gardner. "When I first saw him it was on Frampton Green. I was somewhat his junior in years, and had heard so much of Mr. Jenner, of Berkeley, that I had no small curiosity to see him. He was dressed in a blue coat, and yellow buttons, buckskins, well-polished jockey boots with handsome silver spurs, and he carried a smart whip with a silver handle. His hair, after the fashion of the times, was done up in a club, and he wore a broad-brimmed hat."

Jenner's *Inquiry* contains a typical account of an allergic reaction to cowpox virus, as pointed out by Professor Ludvig Hektoen.

CASE IV.*

MARY BARGE, of Woodford, in this parish, was inoculated with variolous matter in the year 1791. An efflorescence of a palish red colour soon appeared about the parts where the matter was inserted, and spread itself rather extensively, but died away in a few days without producing any variolous symptoms.† She has since been repeatedly employed as a nurse to Small-pox patients, with-

* Jenner, Edward. *An Inquiry into the Causes and Effects of the Variolae Vaccinae*, London, Law, 1798, p. 13.

† It is remarkable that variolous matter, when the system is disposed to reject it, should excite inflammation on the part to which it is applied more speedily than when it produces the Small Pox. Indeed it becomes almost a criterion by which we can determine whether the infection will be received or not. It seems as if a change, which endures through life, had been produced in the action, or disposition to action, in the ves-

out experiencing any ill consequences. This woman had the Cow Pox when she lived in the service of a Farmer in this parish thirty-one years before.

ANGIONEUROTIC EDEMA

Angioneurotic edema was first carefully studied by Heinrich Quincke although it had been previously observed by Graves and mentioned in his Clinical Lectures in the first edition of 1843.

Robert Graves

*"One of the most remarkable instances of fugitive inflammation affecting various parts of the body, which has come under my notice, occurred in the person of a gentleman lately under my care. I shall not go through the whole history of his disease, of which he has favoured me with a very minute account, but shall merely state that he is of a gouty habit, has had an attack of gout in the stomach, and is at present subject to a gouty affection of a very extraordinary character. After labouring for some time under langour and weakness, accompanied by spasms, pain and sense of weight in the stomach, the pain of the stomach ceases, and his face begins to swell at various points, generally commencing on the forehead, and involving the cheek and eye so as to close up the latter. He first feels as if a small current of air was directed on the face; then, as it were the fillip of a finger, or the bite of a gnat; and on looking in the glass, he suddenly perceives a tumor rising on the forehead, which in the space of half an hour, be-

comes as large as a pigeon's egg, and, as he expresses it, moves down until it closes the eye. Sometimes it attacks his lips, and other parts of his face, but never affects his nose. These tumors have also appeared on various parts of his body; and he observes in his letter to me, that he is sometimes led to think that they attack his stomach also. Before and during an attack of the face, which generally occurs on the left side, the discharge from the nostril of the affected side ceases.

But what is chiefly remarkable in this case is the singular character of the local affection. The tumors arise, run through the course, and disappear in the space of a few hours, and on the following day there is no trace of their existence. Sometimes the lips inside of the mouth, palate, and uvula are attacked, giving rise to a very considerable inconvenience. Were such tumors to occur in the neighbourhood of the glottis, I need not say that they would be pregnant with danger of no ordinary character. I may observe that this gentleman has derived great benefit from the use of hydriodate of patash, and from decoction of sarsaparilla with nitric acid, and that his health is at present much improved. His case presents a very curious example of transient local inflammation depending on the gouty diathesis."

sels of the skin; and it is remarkable too, that whether this change has been effected by the Small Pox, or the Cow Pox, that the disposition to sudden cuticular inflammation is the same on the application of variolous matter.

* Graves, Robert J., *Clinical Lectures on the Practice of Medicine*, II Edition, London, New Sydenham Soc., 1884, p. 531.

Heinrich Quincke

Heinrich Quincke was born at Frankfort-on-Oder in 1842, the son of a highly respected and capable physician. The family later moved to Berlin, where Heinrich finished the Gymnasium in 1858. He studied medicine at Berlin, Würzburg, and Heidelberg, having as teachers such celebrated men as Virchow, Kölliker, Frerichs, Helmholtz, Bunsen, Traube, and Scanzoni. Quincke took his degree at Berlin in 1863, became assistant to Frerichs in 1867, and in 1873 became professor of internal medicine at Berne. In 1878 he went to Kiel as professor of medicine, where he was active for thirty years. While at **Kiel** he declined calls to Königsberg and to Vienna, and retired in 1908. He died in 1922 at the age of eighty.

Quincke's entrance into medicine was "during the morning twilight of a new day in German medicine." In the clinics new chemical and microscopic methods of studying disease were appearing almost daily, and new problems were presented to the enthusiastic workers. Quincke found himself in a congenial atmosphere and threw himself into the work.

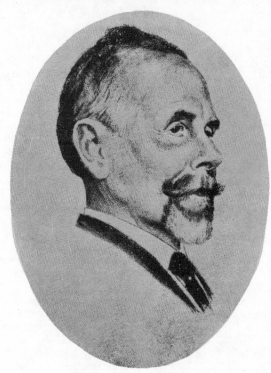

HEINRICH QUINCKE (1842-1922)

Quincke was the first to study carefully the phenomenon seen in aortic insufficiency which we now call the capillary pulse. He described with great precision a new disease complex, angioneurotic edema, or Quincke's disease, and was the first to note poikilocytosis in pernicious anemia. He is widely known for his initiative in introducing lumbar puncture as a therapeutic and diagnostic measure.

CONCERNING THE ACUTE LOCALIZED OEDEMA OF THE SKIN

By H Quincke*

With the name in the above title, I wish to label a skin disease which does not seem to be very rare; however, only a few cases of it have been described, principally as

*Monatsh. Prakt. Dermat., 1882, I, pp. 129-131.

curiosities. Dr. E. Dinkelacker, in his dissertation. *Über akutes Ödem.*, Kiel, 1882, described several of the cases we observed and presented a picture of the disease from the cases described up to that time.

This disease manifests itself in the appearance of oedematous swellings of the skin and the subcutaneous tissue in localized spots from 2 to 10 and even more centimeters in diameter. These swellings are present most commonly on the buttocks and in the face, here particularly on the lips and eyelids. The swollen parts of the skin are not so sharply separated from the surrounding skin, also the same color as the latter or even pale and translucent, more seldom a little reddened. Usually the patients have a sensation of tension, seldom of itching.—The mucous membranes may at the same time be affected by these small swellings, for example on the lips, the uvula, the entrance to the pharynx and larynx, indeed to such a degree that a severe asphyxia appears. Such localized swellings also appear in the gastric and intestinal mucosa, which produce gastro-intestinal symptoms.—In one case, also, there were repeated serous effusions in the joints.

These swellings appear suddenly, usually in several places at the same time. They reach, in one to a few hours, their maximum and then vanish very quickly after they have lasted several hours or a day. While the eruptions disappear in one place, new eruptions may appear at very distant spots, so that the disease in this manner may last several days or even weeks.

The general condition is usually not disturbed; in some cases there were besides prodromal subjective symptoms, also during the eruption, a general malaise, a slight headache, chills and a diminution in amount of the urine. An elevation of temperature was never observed.

When an individual had once had this acute oedema, it very often came back in new attacks and usually localized in the same places. Such new attacks came sometimes at irregular intervals, and at other times in regular weekly attacks, repeated for years.

Occasionally a cooling off of the skin, catching cold, or physical strain, could be demonstrated as active causative factors. The disease seems to appear more often in men than in women. The individuals attacked are otherwise healthy, some of them are rather irritable. In one of them in whom the attacks came at fairly regular intervals, the disease was transmitted to his son and appeared in his son during his first year of life.

Externally, and in its method of appearance, acute and localized oedema has a certain similarity to erythema multiforme, also to urticaria and there are also transitional types.

The true examples are distinguished, aside from their frequent involvement of the mucous membranes, by a slight reddening and a marked swelling in the subcutaneous connective tissue, by the different points of attack and (generally) the absence of itching, as opposed to erythema multiforme; there is also the tendency to spread in patchy distribution (not uniform). Compared with erysipelas, the eruption is more transitory and there is an absence of marked fever.

Erythema nodosum differs from acute localized oedema because of its preference for the lower extremities and the longer duration of the individual swellings.

Because of its manner of appearance, acute localized oedema of the skin and mucous membranes should be considered as an angioneurosis. Certainly it cannot be explained entirely from pure motor effect upon the vasomotors, but is probably caused by a change in the permeability of the vessel walls caused by a nervous influence—which makes the process seem a little more closely related to true inflammation. As analogous to acute localized oedema of the skin, I wish to call attention to the frequent menstrual oedemas, intermittent oedema after malarial fever and the so-called typical joint swellings.

For the treatment of this condition, which by frequent repetition may become a troublesome disease, in some cases, the regulation of the manner of life, especially of the digestion, has a prophylactic value. The individual attacks can be frequently shortened by rest, foot baths and cathartics. Atropin, also, seems to be of value. Oedema at the entrance of the larynx sometimes calls for scarification.

X. DISEASES OF THE DIGESTIVE TRACT

Diseases of the digestive tract have a long and at times very obscure history. Malignant tumors of the stomach, liver, and intestines were unquestionably known to the ancients but the accounts are so commonly inaccurate and so uncertain that they have been omitted in this section.

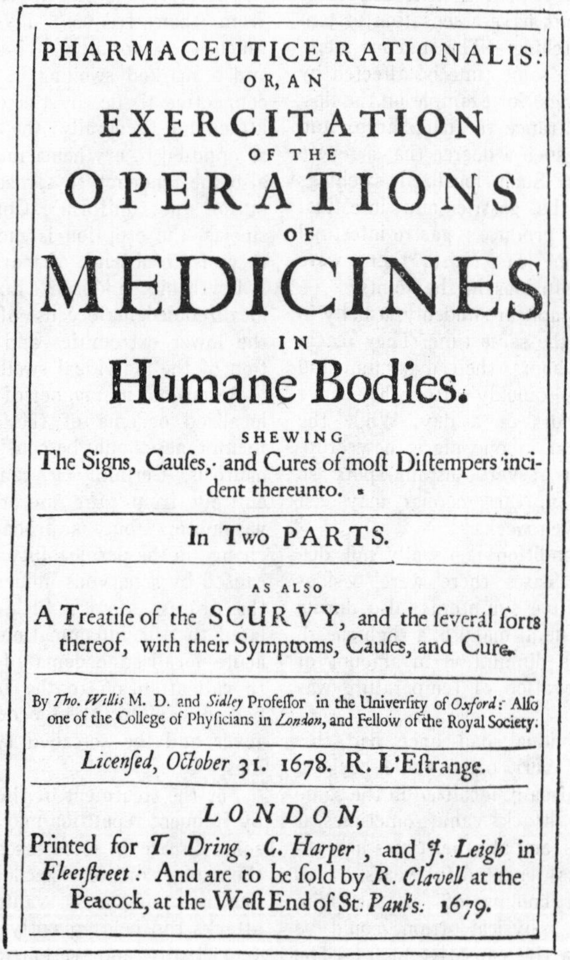

PHARMACEUTICE RATIONALIS:
OR, AN
EXERCITATION
OF THE
OPERATIONS
OF
MEDICINES
IN
Humane Bodies.
SHEWING
The Signs, Cauſes, and Cures of moſt Diſtempers incident thereunto.
In Two PARTS.
AS ALSO
A Treatiſe of the SCURVY, and the ſeveral ſorts thereof, with their Symptoms, Cauſes, and Cure.
By *Tho. Willis* M. D. and *Sidley* Profeſſor in the Univerſity of *Oxford*: Alſo one of the College of Phyſicians in *London*, and Fellow of the Royal Society.
Licenſed, October 31. 1678. R. L'Eſtrange.
LONDON,
Printed for *T. Dring*, *C. Harper*, and *J. Leigh* in *Fleetſtreet*: And are to be ſold by *R. Clavell* at the Peacock, at the Weſt End of St. *Paul's*. 1679.

Title page of *Pharmaceutice rationalis*, by
Thomas Willis (London, 1679)

Thomas Willis unquestionably described cardiospasm and was a pioneer in the method of treating this condition with dilatation. Cruveilhier gave us a masterful description of hemetemesis and gastric ulcer and from his time on the diagnosis of lienitis as a cause of bleeding from the stomach, becomes less frequent. The term "scirrhus of the liver" is often encountered in the medical literature of two and three centuries ago and, at times, may have referred to cirrhosis. The modern term "cirrhosis of the liver" dates from Laënnec although the condition had been described long before his time. Morgagni gives an excellent account of a patient suffering from this disease who showed a fluid wave on tapping the abdomen and he described the characteristic pathological findings in the liver at autopsy. Morgagni also refers to five previous observations collected in the *Sepulchretum* of Bonetus; those of Postius, Wepfer, Ruysch, Brown, and Hartmann. The association of ascites with disease of the liver was recognized by the ancients. Celsus relates that Erasistratus of Alexandria (300 B.C.) believed ascites always arose from disease of the liver. Hippocrates, Aretaeus, and Paul of Ægina refer to disease of the liver as a cause of ascites.

Stones in the bladder were known from the most ancient times as the reference to cutting for a stone in the Hippocratic oath shows. Gall stones, however, seem to have escaped the notice of physicians until the thirteenth century, when they were described by Gentile da Foligno. As public dissections and post-mortem examinations became more common, references to gall stones appear with increasing frequency. Benivieni, regarded by many as the father of pathology, described gall stones as a pathological finding at necropsy and Colombo has left us in his *De re anatomica* an account of an autopsy on the body of Ignatius of Loyola in whom he saw gall stones. The succeeding selections show how gall stones were found in the following centuries by physicians in various lands. One of the best of these descriptions is that of Fernel who, endowed with remarkable powers of observation, a wide clinical experience, and a lucid, logical mind, paints the picture of gall stone disease with an accuracy unapproached by any of his contemporaries and by but a few of his successors. Hildanus enlivens his description with a sketch in which the laminated structure of the gall stone is clearly shown. Morgagni in the course of his pathological investigation quite naturally found gall stones and his account is characteristic not only for its clearness and accuracy but also for its engaging and interesting mode of presentation. Morgagni's medical writings reveal the most unusual combination of scientific exactness with the absorbing style of an accomplished raconteur.

The history of appendicitis contains certain controversial points. Fernel may have seen a case of appendicitis or instead a case of intestinal obstruction with perforation. Heister's autopsy report is an unmistakable account of the pathological findings in appendicitis, although he did not see the patient during life. Mestivier, de la Motte, Parkinson, and Hodgkin all saw the disease in its acute stage and studied it carefully, but the disease was first christened appendicitis and delineated as a sharply defined, unmistakable picture by Fitz.

CARDIOSPASM
Thomas Willis
OF VOMITING*

Vomiting from the Mouth of the Ventricle being affected

No less will a very rare case of a certain Man of *Oxford* shew, an almost perpetual Vomiting to be stirred up by the shutting up of the left Orifice. A strong Man, and otherwise healthful enough, labouring for a long time with often Vomiting, he was wont, very often, though not always, presently to cast up whatsoever he had eaten. At length the Disease having overcome all remedies, he was brought into that condition, that growing hungry he would

A notable case of this Vomiting

eat until the *Oesophagus* was filled up to the Throat, in the mean time nothing sliding down into the Ventricle, he cast up raw (or crude) whatsoever he had taken in: when that no Medicines could help and he

* Willis, Thomas, *Pharmaceutice Rationalis*, London, Dring, Harper and Leigh, 1679, p. 23.

languished away for hunger, and every Day was in danger of Death, I prepared an instrument for him like a Rod, of a whale Bone, with a little round Button of Sponge fixed to the top of it; the sick Man having taken down meat and drink into his Throat, presently putting this down in the *Oesophagus,* he did thrust down into the Ventricle, its Orifice being opened, the Food which otherwise would have come back again; and by this means he hath daily taken his sustenance for fifteen Years and doth yet use the same Machine, and is yet alive, and well, who would otherwise perish for want of Food. Without doubt in this case the Mouth of the Stomach being always closed, either by a Tumour or Palsie, nothing could be admitted into the Ventricle unless it were violently opened.

PEPTIC ULCER
Jean Cruveilhier

Jean Cruveilhier was born at Limoges, Frances, in 1791, the son of an army surgeon. Cruveilhier in early life wished to enter the Church but at the command of his father proceeded to Paris in 1810 to study medicine. The first autopsies he witnessed filled him with such a distaste for the study of medicine that he fled from the medical school and giving way to his old desire to become a priest, entered the Seminary Sulpice of St. Sulpice, as a candidate for holy orders. His domineering father, however, hastened from Limoges to Paris and compelled his disobedient son to re-enter the medical school.

Cruveilhier took his doctor's degree at Paris in 1816 and soon afterwards returned to Limoges, where he married and began to practice. In 1823, through the influence of Dupuytren, he obtained the professorship of surgery at Montpellier. In 1825 he was appointed professor of descriptive anatomy at Paris and in 1836 was appointed to the newly created chair of pathological anatomy. He held this position for thirty years and published a series of remarkable books on pathological anatomy. He died in 1874 in his eighty-third year.

Cruveilhier is best remembered for his *Anatomie pathologique du corps humain, Paris,* 1830-1842. This work is a vast storehouse of pathological anatomy and from the artistic standpoint is the most beautiful and magnificent pathological atlas ever published. In this work Cruveilhier describes and pictures several cases of gastric ulcer—still called by the French "la maladie de Cruveilhier."

DISEASES OF THE STOMACH*

Concerning simple chronic ulcers of the stomach. Confused in practice sometimes with chronic gastritis, sometimes and more commonly with cancer, simple chronic ulcer of the stomach does not appear to me to have spontaneous loss of substance, ordinarily circular, with the margins cut perpendicularly, the bottom gashed and thick and of variable dimensions. Almost always single, the ulcer is situated most commonly either on the small

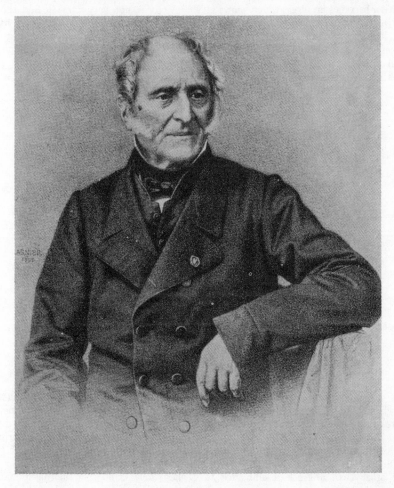

JEAN CRUVEILHIER (1791-1874)
From an engraving by Lasnier, 1865

attracted the attention of observers as a special disease. I will consider myself fortunate if plates 5 and 6 and the discussion which accompany them could fill in part of the gap which exists in this respect.

I. Anatomically considered, the simple chronic ulcer of the stomach consists of a

curvature or upon the posterior wall of the stomach. Sometimes it invades the pylorus, and then it takes the form of a circular zone; its advance is slow and progressive, it spreads out on the surface, but especially it excavates deeply; and if helpful adhesions do not oppose, sooner or later the stomach is perforated and the contents are scattered through out the peritoneal cavity.

* Cruveilhier, Jean, *Anatomie pathologique du corps humain*, Paris, Baillière, 1829-1842.

II. The simple ulcer of the stomach presents the same characteristics as the cutaneous ulcers produced by general internal causes or by a local disease. There is first an erosion of the mucosa as a result of the morbid process which Hunter has so ingeniously named ulcerative inflammation; the erosion or inflammation becomes an ulcer, which shows all the attributes of a syphilitic ulcer. Nevertheless, it has never been demonstrated that the ulcer of the stomach could have the venereal virus as a cause, and in this, the stomach does not deviate from that remark-

ulcer of the stomach is surrounded in profound obscurity or rather, this disease has all the causes of a gastritis. But why a single place in the stomach is deeply affected and all the other parts of the organ are in a state of perfect integrity? That indeed appears very difficult to explain.

V. It is not very rare to find the simple ulcer of the stomach in the body of an individual who has never had during his life any symptoms in this organ; but more commonly the distress in the stomach is part of a series of symptoms of more or less impor-

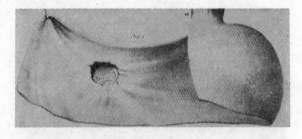

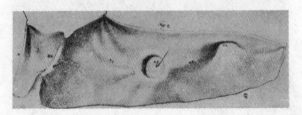

Illustrations of ulcer of the stomach. From Cruveilhier's
Anatomie pathologique du corps humain, Paris, 1835-1842

able law by which parts of the mucous membrane which border upon the natural openings are very commonly invaded by the venereal virus, while the mucous membranes deeply situated are immune to it.

III. Simple ulcer of the stomach does not present other than a gross resemblance to cancerous ulcer with which however it has always been confused. The base of it does not show any of the characteristics of either a hard cancer or a soft cancer, one does not find the circumscribed hypertrophy which practically always accompanies cancer and which has been taken so often for a cancerous degeneration itself. The best proof, however, that these ulcerations are not cancerous is their curability by a very simple, treatment, ineffectual in internal cancer as well as in external cancer.

IV. The history of the cause of the simple

tance. The principle symptoms are the following: loss of appetite or bizarre appetite, insurmountable distress, difficult digestion, nausea or heavy pains in the epigastrium, and sometimes epigastric pain extremely sharp during the process of digestion or indeed when there is no food in the stomach. The epigastric pain, or rather the xyphoid or substernal pain, is referred sometimes to a corresponding place on the spine, and I have seen many patients complain more of a spinal point than of an epigastric point of tenderness. The more or less rapid loss of weight, constipation, nausea, vomiting after the digestion of food, finally the hemorrhagic or black vomiting, are the ensemble of symptoms which individuals affected with simple ulcers of the stomach present; and it is easy to see that these symptoms are not always signs of pathognomonic. Among these morbid phenomena, the things that are common to a simple ulcer and a chronic gastritis, are at the same time present in a simple ulcer and a cancer. I have cared for a lady age sixty-eight, who for four or five months had very severe attacks which were attributed to cancer of the stomach; and indeed vomiting similar to coffee grounds; epigastric pain, sometimes extremely acute; a horror for every kind of food, the stomach unable to stand anything; rapid loss of weight, jaundiced appearance of the face, all leading one to think we had to do with malignant disease such was the opinion of the practicioners who had been consulted. My diagnosis was this: "Cancer of the stomach, if moreover this is not a simple ulcer." As a result, my prognosis was grave, but less desperate than my confieres. I had the satisfaction of seeing her recovery, after six months of care; and certainly I am far from thinking that the simple treatment that I had employed could heal the cancer. I do not see any difference between simple ulcer and cancer of the stomach. However, although in general, in the ulcer the patient has the sensation of an enemy who is always present, and it would take very little for his disease to conquer him, while in cancer, he can overcome this sensation and follow the occupation of an exacting profession. The absence of an epigastric tumor, the additional circumstances, and especially of the first effects of the regime can still point out the correct diagnosis.

VI. Pathological anatomy accounts fully for the bloody and black vomiting which often accompanies ulcer of the stomach: if we examine indeed, under layers of water with a naked eye or strong lens, the surface of the ulcer, we see masses of vascular orifices obliterated, the others not obliterated. We conclude then that when the erosion is not accompanied by the obliteration, the hemorrhage is naturally proportional to the caliber of the vessel; then hemorrhages more or less frequently; and as, the blood remains a longer or shorter time in the stomach, and is in contact with the acid of the gastric juice, it becomes a black color or the color of soot which had been noted by all observers. Besides, this color is common to all vomiting of blood which does not follow immediately after it appears in the stomach cavity. This was noted by one observer in cancer as well as in hemorrhages of the mucus gastritis. The black vomiting of yellow fever is due to the same mechanism.

VII. When an ulcer meeting, so to say, during its progress a vessel of considerable caliber, there results vomiting as well as bloody stools which recur at intervals more or less frequent, and sometimes produce death by hemorrhage. This termination appears to me more frequent in ulcer than in cancer of the stomach. The arterial tissue, which escapes because of a lowered vitality so many organic lesions and even cancer, escape the ulcerous process. It is not rare to find a simple ulcer of the stomach perfectly cicatrised, except at the point where the vessel is located. Thus, a break in the continuity of the vessels cannot heal firmly except by obliteration; it can happen, if this obliteration has not taken place the clot is released and it ceases to act as an obturator, and the hemorrhage reappears causing death almost immediately.

* * *

Ulcer occurring in the small part of the stomach. First hemorrhage healed; second hemorrhage fatal. Opening of the coronary artery of the stomach.

Little fellow, twenty-nine years, carpenter, sanguine temperment, muscular, since childhood given to the use of liquor. Five years ago he had large hemorrhages every evening for eight days which yielded to astringents. Two months of repose in bed were necessary for the patient to recover. His strength returned to him, he went back to his labor and again to his bad habit without his health appearing to suffer noticeably.

April 15, 1830, burning and pain in the epigastrium; loss of appetite. He was able however to continue his work until the evening of the 30th when general malaise forced him to go to bed. Immediately afterwards, vomiting of blood in a quantity perhaps of five or six pints. Carried to the Charité he showed a small pulse, compressible, on anemia almost complete which prohibited the idea of bleeding; we gave him then sinapisms to the feet.

The first of May, the patient vomited only once a small amount of blood, his pulse revived with his strength. (Twenty leeches to the epigastrium, sinapisms to the calves, rice mixed with eau de Kabel and syrup of quince; emulsion with the syrup of diacodium; diet.) In the evening, a large hematemesis.

The second of May, same condition, no stools. (Twenty leeches to the anus, sinapisms; same drink.) At five in the evening, hematemesis more marked than the preceding ones, extreme prostration; death at ten o'clock.

Opening of the Body—Skin discolored, marked adiposity. The abdomen opened, we are struck by the purplish red color of the large intestine, which contrasts with the pallor of the stomach and of the small intestine. The stomach contains a bloody fluid in which several clots swim. At the level of the lesser curvature P. C. Fig. 2 (Plate 6) there is a deep ulceration. circular. six lines in diameter, circumscribed by a very dense margin.

The edge and floor of the ulcer are cicatrised, excepting at the point A.P., where there is a clot of blood elevated like a nipple; a stylet introduced into the coronary artery of the stomach and directed towards the end of the vessel, pushes the clot out and enters the cavity of the stomach; but on withdrawing the stylet a little, and pushing it in the same direction, it can be made to reenter the vessel which was not completely severed but only cut about three-quarters of its circumference. The mucous fold which forms a circle around the pylorous O.P. is perforated partly on its adherent side. The external surface of the stomach is represented (Fig. 2) at the level of the ulcer. The wrinkled surface of the walls at the level of the ulcer has been perfectly reproduced.

CIRRHOSIS OF THE LIVER

John Brown

John Brown or Browne was born in Norwich, England, in 1642. He came of a family in which there were many surgeons, for he tells us that he was "conversant with chirurgery almost from my cradle, being the sixth generation of my own relations, all eminent masters of our profession." He was a friend of Sir Thomas Browne of Norwich, the immortal author of the *Religio Medici,* but apparently was not related to him. Brown studied at St. Thomas's Hospital, London, and, after serving a year in the navy, settled at Norwich. In 1677 he published his *Treatise of Preternatural Tumours* and the same year migrated to London, where he was appointed surgeon to Charles II. A vacancy occurring at St. Thomas's Hospital, the King sent a letter to the governors of the hospital recommending Brown most highly. The governors immediately elected Brown "in all humble submission to his majesty's letter." The entire hospital staff including Brown were dismissed in 1691 and he was never reinstated. He continued, however, to be in favor at Court and was surgeon to William III. He died probably in 1700.

Brown was a good surgeon, a well-educated man, and the author of two notable books, *Adenochoiradelogia: or An Anatomick-Chirurgical Treatise of Glandules & Strumaes, or Kings-Evil-swellings* and *Myographia nova.* The latter work contains elaborate pictures of muscles with the names printed directly upon the muscle, probably the first example of this method of labeling them in England. The *Philosophical Transactions of the Royal Society* contain an interesting communication made to them on December 1, 1685, by "Mr. John Brown, Surgeon of St. Thomas's Hospital in Southwark" in which he describes and pictures a typical example of cirrhosis of the liver.

II.* I send you here the Figure of the *Liver* of an *hydropical* Person. He was about 25 Years of Age, a Soldier in one of his Majesty's Regiments here in Town, who contracted his Distemper by drinking much Water, when he could not stir from his Duty, and catching Cold at Nights in being upon the Guard. He was under the

A Liver appearing Glanduous to the Eye, by Mr. J. Brown, n. 178, p. 1266

here the like Success, his Swellings returning upon him as before; so that there was nothing more now to be thought of but a *Paracenthesis;* which Operation however we judged very hazardous, by Reason of the Time of the Year, and for that the Patient was very much emaciated; yet he being so much swelled that it was uneasy to him to lie in his Bed, he importuned us very often, and with great Earnestness that the Operation

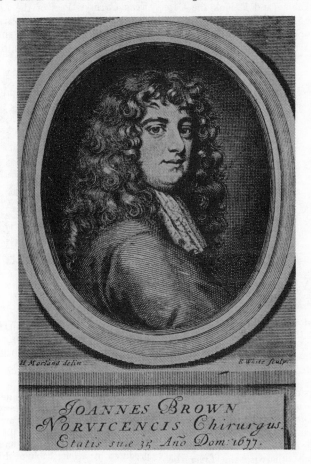

H. Morland delin   *R. White sculp*

JOANNES BROWN NORVICENCIS Chirurgus. Etatis sue 35 Año Dom: 1677.

JOHN BROWN (1642-1700)
Brown at the age of thirty-five. The frontispiece to *A complete treatise of preternatural tumours* (London, 1678)

Care of our Physicians in St. *Thomas's* Hospital for some Time, by whose Directions his Swellings did by Times abate: but afterwards it was observed, that the Method which had been beneficial to others, had not

might be performed. Hereupon a *Paracenthesis,* by the Physicians' Consent and Directions, was made by me, *Nov.* 14, 1685, whereby we drew from the Patient about 3 Pints of brinish Liquor, and within 4 Days after as much more; the next Morning he died; and his Death, as was found upon

* *Phil. Tr. Roy. Soc.*, London, 1685, III, 248.

Dissection, was partly occasioned by a Mortification upon his *Scrotum* and *Penis*. Upon Opening of the Body, I believe I took out about 24 Quarts of Water; he had a large inflammation upon the *Peritonaeum;* all his other inward Parts not much disaffected, except the *Liver*, which now I am going to describe to you.

Its Magnitude was not extraordinary, but rather seemed less than usual. But that which was very remarkable (and I think the Case scarce ever observed by any Author) and seems much to confirm the Opinion of the learned *Malpighius*,

Fig. 12

Explication of the Figures

of the *Liver*, as it was divided. DDDDD are several black Specks that appear infected in those *Glands*, which were probably from the Divarications of the Vessels being divided upon opening this *Lobe*. E, the *Vesicula Fellis*, which was of a greenish colour. F, the *Vena Porta* tied up with the *Ductus Biliarius*, &c. G, a particular Set of *Glands*, lodged between the same and the *Vena Cava*. H, the *Vena Cava*. I, Part of the *Ligamentum Suspensorium*. The convex Part of the *Liver* was, in every respect, the same with the concave Part of both *Lobes* as to its Glands here described.

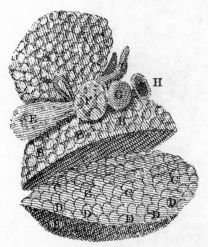

An illustration of cirrhosis of the liver from Brown's article in the *Philosophical Transactions of the Royal Society*, London, 1685

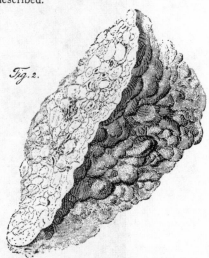

Fig. 2.

MATTHEW BAILLIE
CIRRHOSIS OF THE LIVER
A plate from Matthew Baillie's *Morbid Anatomy**

is this: It consisted, in its concave, convex, and inward Parts of *Glands*, which (with the Vessels) made up the whole Substance thereof. These *Glands* contained a yellowish *Ichor*, like so many *Pustles*, and was, I suppose, Part of the *bilious* Humour lodged in the same; though otherwise the *Liver*, between the *Glands*, was of its usual reddish Colour. In the Bladder of the *Gall* we found a soft friable Stone, but otherwise nothing considerable in that Part.

AAA describes the *Glands* in the concave Part of the lesser *Lobe* of the Liver. BBB, the *glands* in the concave Part of the greater *Lobe* of the *Liver*, which were of different Magnitudes, though in general they were much less in the Lesser than in the Greater. CCCC, the inward Part of the greater *Lobe*

PLATE II*

This Plate is intended to illustrate the most common kind of tubercles formed in the liver. The process by which they are formed is very slow, although it varies in this respect a good deal in different individuals, and it is commonly produced by a long habit of drinking spirituous liquors. When the liver has undergone this change, it is commonly said to be scirrhous, but the morbid appearance is very different from what is observed in the genuine scirrhus of other glands. It should rather be considered as a disease *sui generis*.

FIG. I

Represents a considerable portion of the liver studded with tubercles.

* Baillie. Matthew, *The Morbid Anatomy of some of the most important parts of the Human Body*, London, Bulmer, 1812, p. 101.

A. A part of the anterior surface of the liver, rendered very uneven from the irregular elevation of the tubercles.

B. A part of the suspensory ligament of the liver.

C. A section of the ligamentum teres, which, before birth, constituted a part of the umbilical vein. Although it has got the name ligament, yet it does not change into a true ligamentous substance, but retains very much the original structure of a vein, the cavity only being obliterated.

D. The lower end of the deep fissue which separates the right and the left lobe of the liver from each other.

From Mr. Heaviside's Museum

Fig. II

Represents a smaller section of the liver affected with the same disease. It is intended to shew that the tubercles are not merely formed near the surface of the liver, but throughout the whole of its substance, as may be distinctly perceived through the whole extent of its cut edge. In the cut edge may also be seen a few round cavities, which are sections of veins. The liver in this disease is not enlarged in its size, but is, on the contrary, somewhat diminished.

From the Author's Collection

René-Théophile-Hyacinthe Laënnec

OBS. XXXV. HEMORRHAGIC PLEURISY OF THE LEFT SIDE WITH ASCITES AND ORGANIC DISEASES OF THE LIVER*

The liver, reduced to a third of its ordinary size, was, so to say, hidden in the region it occupied; its external surface, lightly mamellated and wrinkled, showed a greyish yellow tint; indented, it seemed entirely composed of a multitude of small grains, round or ovoid in form, the size of which varied from that of a millet seed to that of a hemp seed. These grains, easy to separate one from the other, showed between them no place in which one could still distinguish any remnant of liver tissue itself: their color was fawn or a yellowish russet, bordering on greenish; their tissue, rather moist, opaque,

* Laënnec, R.-T.-H. *Traité de l'auscultation médiate*, Paris, Chaudé, 1826, ii, p. 196.

was flabby to the touch rather than soft, and on pressing the grains between the fingers, one could not mash but a small portion: the rest gave to the touch the sensation of a piece of soft leather.*

* This type of growth belongs to the group of those which are confused under the name of *scirrhus*. I believe we ought to designate it with the name of *cirrhosis*, because of its color. Its development in the liver is one of the most common causes of ascites, and has the pecliarity that as the cirrhosis develops, the tissue of the liver is absorbed, and it ends often, as in the subject, by disappearing entirely; and that, in all the cases, a liver which has cirrhosis becomes smaller in volume instead of increasing all the more. This type of growth develops also in other organs, and finishes by softening like all morbid growths

---

GALLSTONES

Gentile da Foligno

The first physician to describe gallstones was apparently Gentile da Foligno, who was born at Foligno in the latter part of the thirteenth century. He studied at Bologna and later was professor there. In 1337 he was called to Padua and while there carried out public dissections and performed autopsies. According to Tosoni, he performed at Padua in 1341, the earliest autopsy on record, finding upon this occasion a gallstone. In 1345 he removed to Perugia, where he died three years later of the plague. Gentile was one of the most learned physicians of his time and the author of numerous works. His published works apparently contain no account of gallstones but his classic observation is referred to by Marcellus Donato. The following extract is from Donato's *de medica historia Mirabili,* a work which passed through many editions and is noteworthy for its praise of autopsies as a means of controlling clinical observations.

In the gall bladder many stones were seen, Gentile himself testifies, in a certain woman, whose viscera were removed, so that the body could be embalmed they found in the duct of the gall bladder at its mouth, a stone tending to green, from which the moderns with right remark that there was jaundice present.*

* Donatus, Marcellus, *De medica historia mirabili libri sex*, Mantua, Parsius. 1586, p. 269.

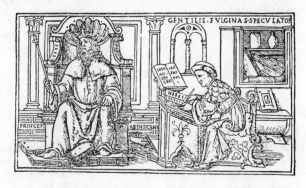

Picture of Gentile da Foligno from Avicenna's *Canonis libri,*
Venice, 1520

Antonio di Pagolo Benivieni

During the troublous and colorful times of Lorenzo de Medici, Savonarola, and Machiavelli in Florence, a physician, one Antonio Benivieni, was practising the profession öf medicine. Few details of his life have been preserved for us. He was born at Florence in 1443 of an ancient and noble Florentine family and was the eldest of five sons. One of his brothers, Domenico, called lo Scotino (the little Duns Scotus), became a well known professor of theology at Pisa. Another brother, Gerolamo, was a famous poet and writer. Antonio Benivieni studied medicine at Pisa and Siena and upon his return to Florence soon became a prominent physician, numbering among his patients the Medici, the Guicciardini and the Strozzi. He also became physician to the Hospital of Santa Maria Nuova and to the monastery of San Marco whose prior, the famous Savonarola, was both his patient and his friend. Benivieni was elevated to the rank of of a "signori" in 1494 and died in 1502, leaving a large patrimony to his children.

Osler's comments on Benivieni are of interest. "Benivieni, a shrewd and accurate observed, had formed the good habit of making brief notes of his important cases, and after his death these were found by his brother Jerome and published at Florence in 1507. The special interest of the work is that here, for the first time in modern literature, we have reports of postmortem examinations made specifically with a view of finding out the exact cause of death." According to Professor Bindo de Vecchi, who has investigated with great care the life and labors of Benivieni, his *De abditis causis morborum* was published by his brother Gerolamo in 1505, three years after the death of its author and is only a fragment of a larger work, which he had planned but whose completion was prevented by his death. The manuscript of forty-seven additional observations, not included in this work, was subsequently discovered by the historian Puccinotti. The observations of Benivieni, as de Vecchi remarks, differ from the writings of every previous writer in both form and substance.

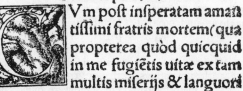

ANTONII [193]

BENIVENII DE ABDITIS
nōnullis ac mirandis morborũ
& fanationũ caufis liber.

HIERONYMVS BENIVENIVS
Ioanni Rofato, Medico &
Philofopho, S.

Vm poft infperatam amāt
tiffimi fratris mortem(quā
propterea quòd quicquid
in me fugiētis uitæ ex tam
multis miferijs & languori
bus fupererat, uno illo niteretur, nihil
mihi in terris potuit accidere grauius)
eius perquàm fanè honeftam, & omni
doctrinarum genere locupletem biblio
thecā euoluerem, incidi in pleraqʒ eius
ingenij monumenta:quæ ille,ut erat uir
doctrina & ætate prouectior, ac multa
rum rerum ufu & experientia pollens,
cudebat quotidie. Lectitāti igitur ea mi
hi, ac fæpius ob memoriam illius reuol
uenti,obtulit fefe interea libellus quidā,
in quo uir fummo & ftudio & diligētia
præditus, quæcunqʒ trigefimū fupra fea

Introduction to Benivieni's *de abditis* (Basle, 1529)

"Measured and exact in the exposition of the history and the symptoms of the patient, using a clear and fluent Latin, omitting every useless citation of Greek or Arabian authors, without discussions of philosophy or of alchemy or of astrology—although he was versed in such studies as was customary in a learned man of that epoch—Antonio works out the diagnosis relying solely on the meaning and the value of the symptoms, where possible discussing the prognosis, emphasizing a simple and sensible medical treatment, or when possible surgical. But above all he understands on every occasion to complete and control his clinical observation by investigations of the dead body." "With him for the first time . . . the physician considers the problems of the causes of disease and death and seeks their explanation in the dead body. No one had thought thus before him, and after him the physicians of the entire world should have had the same thought." Benivieni described stones in the gallbladder, fibrinous pericarditis, abscess of the hip-joint, senile gangrene, and noted the transmission of syphilis from the mother to the fetus. Many regard him as the father of pathological anatomy, but as Garrison remarks "It may be doubted if so slender a performance as Benivieni's (it consists of only 54 pages) can enter into comparison with the vast array of pathologic findings and descriptions of new diseases in Morgagni's majestic treatise. For such pioneer work as Benivieni's the time was hardly ripe."

STONES FOUND IN THE LINING OF THE LIVER. III*

A noble woman who was troubled many times during the day with a pain arising in the neighborhood of the liver, and on that account had consulted very many doctors, moreover by no aid could she escape this malady. Wherefore she was pleased to test out our ability together with the others. Therefore we met together with many physicians & and what could have been the hidden causes of the disease we discussed from that time on in many conversations. Indeed as is apt to happen commonly in obscure conditions, we did not reach a decision. For some declared it an abscess of the liver, others a

*Benivieni, Antonio, *De abditis nonnullis ac mirandis morborum & sanationum causis liber,* Basle, Crantander, 1529, p. 291.

bad humor: we indeed believed the disease to be in the hidden lining. And when after certain signs with general agreement, she departed this life, we took care to open the body of the dead. And in the sloping membraneous part of the liver stones of different shapes & colors were found collected. For some were round: others angular: others quadrate, according as posture & chance had worked, also marked with red, yellow and white spots. These formed by their weight from the lining a sac the length of ones palm with a breadth indeed of two fingers. Now this pronounced the cause of death we considered it vain & useless to dispute concerning obscure things.

* * *

CALCULUS IN THE WALL OF THE GALL BLADDER. xciiij

There died during these days a noble woman. Diamantes by name, with the prostrating pain of a stone: but since no injury had been perceived from this earlier, it seemed advisable to the physician to open the body of the dead, & a great many stones were found, not only in the bladder, as was thought, besides one, which was contained in the wall of the gall bladder of a black color

& the size of a dried chestnut, all the others in the lining, by which the liver is covered, from which besides they had formed a little bag, as it were, in a dependent skin. Now we believing this the cause of death, have considered the advice of a wise man to be, to hold for certain nothing whatever concerning uncertain & hidden diseases.

Matteo Realdo Colombo

The following reference to gallstones is found in the anatomy of Matteo Realdo Colombo, the celebrated anatomist, one of the discoverers of the pulmonary circulation. Colombo was born in Cremona, probably in 1516, and after practising in Venice, was called to Padua in 1544 as the successor of Vesalius in the chair of anatomy. Two years later he accepted a professorship in Pisa and in 1549 went to Rome as physician to Pope Paul IV. He died in 1559. In 1556 he was present at the autopsy on the body of St. Ignatius of Loyola, the founder of the Society of Jesus. The account of this autopsy is found in Colombo's *De re anatomica libri XV*, in the *Book Fifteen Concerning those things which are rarely found in anatomy*. This work appeared first in 1559. The following translation is from the edition of 1572.

Moreover I have taken out innumerable stones with my own hands, with various colors found in the kidneys, in the lungs, in the liver, in the portal vein as you saw with your own eyes with Jacob Bonus in the Venerable Ignatius, General of the congregation of Jesus. For I saw stones in the ureters, in the bladder, in the colon of the intestine, in the hemorrhoidal veins as well as in the umbilicus. Also in the gall bladder which he removed, I found stones of various shapes and of various colors & very many in some others.

Jean Fernel
SOME DISEASES IN THE GALL BLADDER. CHAPTER V*

Obstruction, calculus, fullness & emptiness attack the gall bladder. The obstruction is either of the duct by which the bile is led away from the liver, or of that by which it is discharged from the gall bladder into the intestine. In both, the bowels ore obstinate and sluggish, feces whitish, the urine is reddish and thick so that it frequently becomes dark, the bile diffused with the blood throughout the whole body disfigures the skin with jaundice. In the former moreover, the gall bladder is entirely empty: in the latter it is distended by the large amount of bile, and is oppressed by various symptoms of great importance.

A black calculus commonly forms in the gall bladder, but nevertheless is light & when immersed in water floats, but on the contrary that which is removed from the kidneys or bladder sinks. The origin of it is from the yellow bile which confined in a special receptacle for a long time neither at the right time emptied, nor renewed by a new influx, hardens in a remarkable manner. This moreover happens especially when both bile ducts are obstructed. Indeed neither signs nor evidence of this are present, but grave symptoms from these things can easily be seen. Moreover it should be suspected in those in whom the jaundice was severe & continued. A certain decrepid old man very prone to anger, after death was found without bile and without gall bladder in whose place a large calculus had formed. Indeed after continued jaundice with the appearance of diarrhoea, we detect commonly, innumerable calculi of this nature expelled like peas or barley grains.

Again, the bile belonging to the gall bladder sometimes is so greatly in excess that it distends to an enormous size. And when indeed it is attacked by the misfortune of sickness, by pressure, pain, and suffocation, with vomiting, heat, thirst, irascibility & if at any time it putrefies with intermittent fevers. Hence the most grave ills are produced, nor indeed is it milder when this appears.

Nor when the gall bladder is at once entirely emptied; he belches out his bile, or it causes bilious vomiting, or cholera morbus, or diarrhoea, or dysentery, or sudden jaundice in the entire body, or a thin flow of urine at first, then thick & imbued with the color of saffron, or other like symptoms. Many die, in whom no other cause of destruction exists, than that the sac is deprived of all of its bile.

* Fernel, Jean, *Io. Fernelii ambiani, universa medicina,* Frankfort, Wechelus, 1581, p. 577.

Felix Platter*

Calculus and sand in the Liver and its bladder are the cause of severe dull pains in the hypochondrium

From a *calculus* or *tophus* arising in the *liver*, or its gall bladder, or indeed from the sand & gravel collected and retained there in large amounts, a *distress* also from the same reason, as was said of *tumors*, unquestionably is felt. Which can happen, as shown to me and to others by *autopsy*, was common: and from the expelled sand intensely red & even *bloody*, which are seen to be produced in *large* amounts in *affections* of the *liver*. Thus while we find *calculi* frequently in the *liver* of *animals*, in *man* also this can happen, from whom we collect them easily. When these things happen both this *trouble* arises from them, and other *symptoms* besides: for such proceed from obstruction of the liver, we shall explain in these cases, by its location Which, indeed when it happens in the spleen, and if from this, although *calculi* can arise throughout the *whole body*, is formed in another manner, however as we have not yet seen this, nor do we remember to have gleaned it from the observation of others, we do not think this thing demonstrated as a fact.

* Platter, Felix, *Praxeos. Tomus secundus, de doloribus*, Basle, King, 1646, p. 477.

Wilhelm Fabry

Wilhelm Fabry, "the father of Germany surgery," was born in Hilden near Düsseldorf, Germany, in 1560. Early in his professional life he latinized his name, according to the custom of the times, calling himself Guilhelmus Fabricius Hildanus, by which name he is commonly known. His father, who was a respected clerk in one of the courts and, according to Hildanus, a "homo literatus," died when the son was but a year old. Hildanus as a boy was befriended

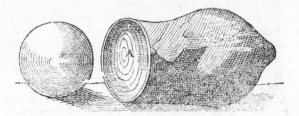

Illustrations of gallstones from Guilhelmi Fabricii Hildani
*Opera Observationum et Curationum Medico-Chirurgicarum
Quae Extant omnia*, Francofurto MDCLXXXII

by the poet Utenhof, who sent him to school in Cologne and urged him to study medicine. When fifteen years of age he was apprenticed to one Dumgens, a surgeon of Neusi. Four years later he entered the service of the Duke of Cleve as a surgeon and then began a series of wanderings. He practised successively at Metz, Cologne, Lausanne, Payern, and Berne. In Cologne he wrote his treatise on gangrene, in Basle his monograph on lithotomy, but his most important work was his *Centuries of Surgical Cases*, published at various times between 1606 and 1646. He died in 1634 at the age of seventy-four.

Hildanus was very conservative in theory, but in practice a bold and accomplished operator. He carried out the first successful amputation of the thigh, devised an ingenious tourniquet for use in amputations, extracted an iron splinter from the eye with a magnet, and devised an instrument for extracting foreign bodies from the esophagus. His *Centuries of Surgical Cases* was the authoritative surgical text of its day and contains an interesting illustrated account of gallstones.

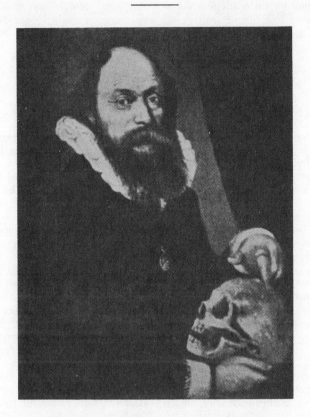

WILHELM FABRICIUS VON HILDEN (1560-1634)

OBSERVATION XLIV*
CONCERNING TWO STONES OF ENORMOUS SIZE, FOUND IN THE GALL BLADDER

On the 11 of February 1612, two stones of enormous size were shown to me by the most distinguished and learned Masters of Cologne, Johann Fabricius & Henry Stapedius, Doctors of Medicine, long renowned, which Master Fabricius removed from the gall bladder of a certain Comrade of seventy. One was oblong, the other quite round, moreover for their size they were not very heavy. The larger fourteen drachms, the smaller weighed only just four drachms & a

* Fabry, William, *Opera quae extant omnia. Observationum Centuria IV,* Frankfurt, Dufour, 1682, p. 320.

half, since they were spongy & formed in layers: but Master Fabricius asserts that they were in the beginning much heavier but not very hard & which moreover in these stones, especially in the larger is beautifully shown. For in it, cracks are seen here and there (as there is apt to be in mud, when it is dried by the sun). The color in some places is yellow, but in other places it inclines to black. I give a picture of those stones made from life the illustrious Master Stapedius, my especial friend, presented to me, which is seen added here.

The larger stone is of one piece, noted

here A, much indented, so that it may have lost nearly a third, it is certain that it was rubbed off from the continual friction of one against the other. The said Comrade was healthy throughout his entire life, nor did he scarcely ever suffer from illness (neither did he suffer from any jaundice); towards the

seventieth year of his age Master Fabricius states that he died with a continued malignant fever. For many years, as often as in its bed it moved from one place to the other, the large troublesome mass, slipping from one place to the other could be perceived in the region of the liver.

Daniel Sennert

CHAPTER VI†

CONCERNING CALCULI, WORMS & HYDATIDS ARISING IN THE LIVER

Not only humors are made hard in the liver & often indeed are changed into stones, & calculi are found in the dissection of cadavers, as Fallopius, Columbus & others have proved. So Kentmann reports in the *book concerning calculi,* to have found in the liver of a certain young Nobleman three stones, one of which equalled in size half that of a pigeon's egg. Also Antonio Benivieni in his *de albditis causis morborum,* chapter 3 relates he found in a certain woman of the nobility very many stones in the more sloping membraneous portion of the liver, differing in size & color. And Vesalius, in the *epistle de China to Joachin* relates that he saw in many who suffered from jaundice & from the jaundice developed ascites, the livers hard & full of stones, so that they were not able to remove them with a knife. And indeed Belloarmatus Senesis to have considered the liver whitish superficially, not on the left but to a great degree unequal, & rough with smooth tubercles, indeed its anterior surface & the whole left side to have been hard with stones. Caellius Rodiginus in his *book* 4 *antique lect. chapter* 17 & Cardanus *de rerum varietate book* 8 *chapter* 14 writes, on opening the body of Augustinus

† Sennert, Daniel, *Medicinae practicae,* Venice, Junta and Herty, 1650, p. 747.

Doge of Venice from the race of Barbodica, to have found a stone in the gall bladder, the size of a large olive, the color of serpent tending to blackness. Rondeletius saw a stone formed in an abscess of the liver, as he relates in *Chapter* 44 (method of curing diseases.) Matthiolus writes in his *Epistle to Jacob Camenicenus,* that he found a stone the size of an almond in the liver of a certain virgin. Gabriel Fallopius of Padua found five stones the size of a pea in a youth who had been hanged, as Dominicus Leonus relates. Felix Platter found also much gravel, calculi & trophi in the liver.

The *Causes* moreover & the modo of formation is the same, as in other organs, especially in the kidneys, concerning which will be treated in *its place.*

Moreover calculi in the liver are with difficulty & rarely completely recognized, nor after death in section of cadavers. And the signs are quite the same as in scirrhus of the liver. Also the pain is greater, if the calculus extends towards the membrane, which it presses & nips, and this daily.

Moreover the *Cure* of calculus in the liver is difficult, & if the hope of a cure survives, those medicaments, which are employed in scirrhus of the liver & in stone of the kidneys, can be administered.

Francis Glisson

Calculi in the biliary tract
Moreover* peculiar swellings are found in the biliary tract; in which it may happen that its tunic appears six times thicker than normal, its substance withers, and becomes less firm, & dissected becomes quite

* Glisson, Francis, *Anatomia hepatis,* London, Du Gardi, 1654, p. 88.

like a kind of soft cheese. These kinds of swellings are often found in the excised liver (especially in the ox). Frequently in various parts of the branches a stone is present which perforates the substance, and this either at the site of the swelling, or at least in its neighborhood. This stony substance, inside the vessels (in which it remains) looks like a pipe. About the time of lent, or of Easter, indeed before, I have often seen in the livers of oxen these sort of tubules, of such length, that (if they can be removed whole) they form many branches of the biliary tract with a continued series of stones (like corals): moreover now they are coalesced firmly in the ducts, so that, before the rupture of these, they can be separated with difficulty from the stones (for they are both very friable). These stones, which are found in the gall bladder, are clearly of the same kind as these & the shapes alone differ.

I knew very many, who expelled fragments of these kinds of stones in great quantities through the intestines: the place of whose origin I considered to be not other than the biliary tract, in which a stony tubule of this sort was by chance formed, & crumbling in small pieces, descended by the biliary passages into the intestine, and thence could be excreted through the bowel. In which opinion I agree more willingly, since I saw oxen in winter time (when they are fed with hay or straw) to be full of this kind of stony material, so that the liver is found completely filled with the same; moreover in spring time (when they are fed with fresh grass) this is more rarely found. Indeed they are dissolved, & these stones are driven away by the juice of fresh grass; so that it can be formed only by the bowel and by no other method.

Lorenz Heister

OBSERVATION IX*

OF A MORTAL WOUND OF THE HEAD FROM A BLOW, AT THE PUBLIC EXAMINATION OF WHICH, UPON OPENING THE ABDOMEN, MANY ANGULAR STONES WERE FOUND IN THE GALL BLADDER

The before-mentioned Dr. Möller, on account of his skill and eminence in the practice of physic, was called to Wetzler, where he read courses of medical lectures. He had not been there long before he was sent for into the country, upon the following accident: two country fellows having fought a long time with their fists, at last one of them, getting hold of the leg of a stool, struck the other with such violence on the head, that he fell down and died immediately on the spot: whether he received more blows than one, I cannot tell.

At the public judicial dissection of this body, the doctor took me and two or three more pupils along with him: the skull, on one side, was found so much beaten inwards, that it had penetrated the brain, and entirely destroyed its texture; and hence arose the cause of his death.

Hereupon, as is customary at such examinations, the abdomen and thorax were opened, and all the viscera found perfectly sound; but, as I was feeling under the liver for the gall-bladder and its ducts, I observed an hardness and inequality of the bladder, and a rattling; and being curious to know the cause, I opened the vesica fellea, and found

contained therein nineteen angular stones, some of a blackish, others of a green and yellow colour like marble: every one present took some of these stones, and those which I brought away I have ever since preserved in my cabinet.

We understand from the bystanders, that this man had always been a troublesome, hasty, passionate fellow, quarelling and fighting for very trifles; till at last, meeting with his match, he lost his life.

Note. It is difficult to determine whether these concretions, frequently found in the gall-bladder and its ducts, upon the dissection of choleric persons, are formed from a drying up, or too great heat of gall, and so become like stones; or whether they derive their origin from other causes, afterwards irritating the gall-ducts, and bringing on an increased motion and perturbation of the blood. But since that time, I have frequently met with these gall-stones in my dissections of a great number of bodies, in Holland and the Netherlands, during the five years I remained in those countries. I have also seen them at Altorff, where I was professor of anatomy, and here in Helmstadt. I have sometimes found them resembling a rough piece of gum-arabic, and one, particularly, quite round. But of the formation of these stones I cannot say any thing satisfactory.

* Heister, Laurence, *Medical Chirurgical and Anatomical Cases and Observations.* Translated by George Wirgman, London, Reeves, 1755, p. 10.

Giovanni Battista Morgagni

15.† Since, therefore, in this great infirmity, and intemperance, of human life, so many causes, which must be readily granted, are at hand to favour the production of cystic calculi, there is not the least reason to wonder that they have been so often found, both by the ancients, and by moderns. For after Gentilis[s] and Nicolus,[t] had testified their having seen concretions of this kind, the latter in the gall-bladder, and the former in the meatus thereof. Benivenius,[u] Vesalius,[x] Curtius,[y] Falloppius,[z] Fernelius,[*] Stephanus,[a] Columbus[b] and Coiterus,[c] to take no notice of authors of less note, produc'd their observations to the same effect: and from the time that human bodies began to be more frequently dissected, even to this very day, no writer in anatomical, or medical, matters has had occasion to speak pretty fully of that vesicle, but he has made mention of calculi being seen by him there; so that it is with justice the celebrated professor Fabricius[d] says, that calculi of the gall-bladder have, in general been more frequently observ'd than those of the urinary bladder; and it is shown by the illustrious Haller[e] that they are even to be met with more frequently in some countries.

Wherefore I would not have you be surpriz'd, if I say, that while I write this present letter, I have before my eyes, at least two hundred observations of this kind, nineteen of which are my own; but I would rather have you wonder that I have not read, or do not remember, a great many more. Yet those, of which I have spoken, are not so few in number, but that I may from them venture to answer your inquiry, as to what occurs more frequently, or more rarely, in cystic calculi, and that without seeming to answer too hastily, or rashly. You may make this inquiry first of all, in what kind of bodies they are most frequently found? For *Carolus Stephanus*[f] has asserted, that they have been seen by him, chiefly, in women, who were pretty "far advanc'd in life:" and, in this age, Frederick Hoffmann[g] has said, that they are found very rarely in men, who are in the flourishing time "of life, but more frequently in old men, and still more frequently in women than in men." The first thing pronounc'd by Hoffmann, therefore, is much more true than the last. For I see in the observations spoken of, that the number of males and females is nearly equal. But although I find old people, promiscuously, of both sexes, to the number of sixty-one, whose ages are particularly pointed out by the observators, I find no more than eight who are said to be young: and among these there is no infant, and but one child; and the least age, amongst these eight, is that of twelve years, the greatest nine and twenty.

Without doubt, in a flourishing time of life the juices are thinner, more briskly agitated, and less prone to concretion, than in the decline of life, or as Hoffmann particularly saw, than in the less laborious life of very old men, especially, and women. For which reason Haller, whom I have already commended, accounts for "the frequent calculi of the gall-bladder, which he found in criminals, who had bee long confin'd to prison," from the want of muscular action.[h] And to the same cause, you must refer what the illustrious Van Swieten[i] found to happen in bile, which was not agitated. For, "having left it to putrify in a pure glass vessel, he found calculous coagula in the bottom of the vessel." Yet the middle age, although it is an active season of life, has not juices to be compar'd with the flourishing prime of our age, for which reason it happens, that this time of life cannot equally resist the injuries of intemperance, and of the passions, to both of which it is still more liable than old age. If you add to this, that a great part of the women in the lower classes of the people, do not lead a very sedentary life: and if you compare all these things

† Morgagni, J. B., *The Seats and Causes of Disease*, Translated by Benjamin Alexander, M.D., London, Millar and Cadell, 1769, II, 225. Letter xxxvii.
[s] Apud Donat. de Med. Hist. Mir. 14 c30
[t] Ibid.
[u] Cit. supra. ad n. 13.
[x] Ibid.
[y] Comment. in Mundin. Anat. ubi de hepate in fin.
[z] Obs. Anat.
* Cit. ad n. 14.
[a] De dissect. part. corp. hum. l. 3, c. 42.
[b] De re anat. l. utt.
[c] Obs. Anat.
[d] Propempt. ad Dissert. Jo. Bart. Hoffmann.
[e] Opusc. pathol. obs. 33.

[f] C. 42. modo cit.
[g] Medit. rat. t. 4, n. 2, s. 2, c. 3 § 12.
[h] Experim. Anat. de Sang. mat c. 6.
[i] Comment, in Boehaav. aph. § 950.

with those which are said above[a] upon the causes that produce calculi of the gall-bladder; you will, of course, easily perceive that the observations are consonant to reason.

* * *

28. A poor old woman had receiv'd a violent blow upon her head, by a fall: of which alone were all her complaints as long as she liv'd; and she liv'd not a few days, till at length she gradually sunk away and died. This patient had no inequality of the pulse, no traces of a jaundice. And the reason of my making this remark will appear, when I tell you what I observ'd in the heart, and the gall-bladder, while I was busied in pursuits of quite a different nature. For I did not even dissect the body, that I might know what detriment she had receiv'd from her fall.

The body was fat, and yet the skin very hard. In the thorax nothing occur'd to me that was worthy of remark; for to some of those who were present, it seem'd otherwise, in regard to a polypous concretion, that we found in the right auricle of the heart, which was whitish, and if you attempted to dissolve it with your hand, gave considerable resistance, as if we did not frequently see a crust of this kind lying on the surface of the blood, which has been taken from a vein, and coagulated, or, as if this woman had been subject to an inequality of pulse, which they are so fond of attributing to polypi of the heart.

In the belly, the stomach appear'd to be almost double, so suddenly was that cavity contracted, before it came to the antrum pylori.

The gall-bladder was half-full of bile, and, being of a bright yellow like orpiment, had ting'd all the neighbouring parts with the same colour. In this bile were ten calculi, of an unequal magnitude, among themselves, but none of them small. Other circumstances which relate to them, you will read in the letter to Schroeckius;[b] for this is that woman of whom I there spoke in the third place, showing where, and at what time, I dissected her.

And from thence you may also learn, in like manner, what relates to another woman, the remaining part of whose history I shall

immediately add: for it is she who is spoken of, in the first place, in that letter.

29. A woman somewhat younger than the former, yet almost sixty years of age, who was not far from having an icteric colour, but endow'd with a very good complexion, was much given to drinking, and had been seven times married: this woman having complain'd of no other disorder, but of an inflammation of the thorax, of which she died, was dissected by me, not on account of her disease, but in order to examine into the abdominal viscera, and had some appearances in the genitals, but still more in the gall-bladder, which are not unworthy of being transcrib'd here.

The uterus had a tubercle externally, on the upper part of its fundus, of the figure, and magnitude, of a small filbert, partly prominent, and partly latent within the substance of the uterus, of a scirrhus hardness, of a white colour, both internally, and externally, and consisting of many different small parts which, in some measure, resembled cells contracted into themselves. And within the cavity of the uterus, from the middle and anterior part of the fundus, rose up a soft, and almost gelatinous excrescence. But although the testes, as was to be suppos'd from her age, were much shrivell'd and very narrow, yet the cervix uteri, and vagina, appear'd differently from what you would have expected in the wife of seven men. For in the latter part, were still a great number of rugae, prominent, even to half the extent of it, longitudinally; and in the former, the figure approaching to that of a virgin-cervix, and the valves, which were preserv'd on one side, made me suppose, that she had been the mother of very few children, which was also confirmed by the slender rugae, in the lower part of the abdomen.

But as to the gall-bladder, although it was much shorter than in proportion to the magnitude of the liver, (which was, in other respects, of its usual sound appearance) for it did not reach, with its fundus, so low as the edge of the liver, but was distant therefrom by almost two inches; it nevertheless contain'd together with a small quantity of bile, at least three hundred and thirty calculi, which were chiefly very small, as the shortness of the cyst, that I have describ'd would of itself argue. As to the other remarks I made upon these calculi, I have said just now,[f] where they may be met with: although in that letter, not only many typographical errors are admitted, but in the part, in particular, to which I refer, more than one whole line is omitted. Besides the great number of calculi which I have mentioned, and which occupied the cavity of the cyst, I discover'd one with the knife that lay hid be-

[f] N. 28.

tween the coats of this vesicle, which, in the blackness of its colour, and the smallness of its size, was very much like those that I took notice of above,[g] as having been found in the glands of the cyst, at other times; yet the orifice of the gland was not so evidently laid open here.

[g] N. 21.

APPENDICITIS

Jean Fernel

Jean Fernel, or Ioannes Fernelius, was born probably at Montdidier in 1497, although there is some uncertainty both in regard to the place and to the exact date of his birth. He describes himself as Ioannes Fernelius Ambianus, or of Amiens. However, the evidence points to Montdidier as the place of his birth, and Montdidier belonged to the Diocese of Amiens. He attended a school at Clermont and in 1516 he entered the College of Sainte-Barbe at Paris, where he studied philosophy and eloquence. He obtained the degree of Master of Arts in 1519 and shortly afterwards took up the study of mathematics and, in 1526, began the study of medicine. While studying medicine, he carried out his famous experiments in which he made the first exact measurement of a degree of the meridian.

In 1530, at the age of thirty-three, he took his degree in medicine, but apparently had no thought of practising his profession. Shortly afterwards he married and continued his mathematical and astronomical researches, but finally, in 1535, at the insistence of his family, which he was unable to support by his researches in pure science, he began the practice of medicine at the age of thirty-eight.

Fernel quickly achieved a great reputation in the practice of medicine, patients flocked to him and it was said that no poor man asked help of him and failed to get it. The Dauphin of France made him his chief physician, courtiers appealed to him, but he refused to live at court. When the Dauphin became King Henry II, Fernel was appointed first court physician and gained the friendship of Catherine de Medici, who believed that his skill saved her from a state of childlessness. On the birth of her first child, she paid him a fee of ten thousand ecus (*circa* $10,000) and ordered that the same fee be paid him upon the birth of each succeeding child. Fernel was plunged into despair at the death of his wife and died a few months later in 1558.

Fernel's best known works are his *Universa Medicina,* which was published in 1554, and his *Therapeutices Universalis,* which appeared in 1569. Both of these works passed through numerous editions.

The following selection from his *Universa Medicina* is believed by many to be the first description of a case of acute appendicitis with perforation. The decision as to whether he is describing a case of appendicitis rests largely upon the question whether the term "caecum intestinum" refers to the appendix or the caecum. Many anatomists of his time unquestionably used this term to describe the appendix, while others employed it to designate the caecum.

This description of the "memorable example" is found in Book VI, Chapter IX of *The Causes and Signs of Disease of the Intestines.*

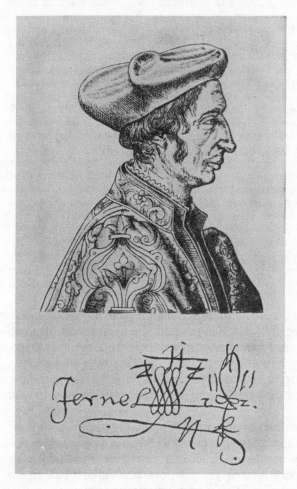

JEAN FERNEL (1497?-1558)
From his *Therapeutices Universalis* (Frankfort, 1581)

CAUSES & SIGNS OF DISEASES OF THE INTESTINES
CHAPTER IX*

Closely related to obstruction is coarction & narrowing of the intestine. This moreover may arise from the action of those things which are ingested: whether they be foods like bad quince, whether astringent clysters. Often from an impinging intestinal tumor of the mesentery or viscera: and this moreover is common. And it happens from an enterocele, when the intestine descends into the

* Fernel, Jean, *Universa Medicina. De partium morbis et symptomis. Liber VI,* Frankfort, Wechelus, 1581, p. 592.

scrotum and is constricted there as if by a band. And one of these cases is produced by the intestine itself, not by any other visible causes. It will not be out of order to mention in this place a memorable example.

A girl of seven afflicted with diarrhoea, passed for many days from the bowels a white, putrid and foul material, with no pain. The grandmother was tired of this daily flowing and to stop it took counsel with some other old women. In this case a quince as large as one's hand was secured and this the patient devoured, with the result that the stools were suppressed so that during the day and the following night nothing was passed. But with violent, most severe pains and cramps in the belly she swelled up until the swelling suddenly became putrid. A physician came, who, suspecting the true state of affairs tried first injections of mild clysters and then more severe ones to dislodge the noxious stinking material from the intestines and to ease the pain with fomentations: but in vain. Indeed with increasingly severe pains, repeated loss of consciousness and moreover with vomiting of a fecal liquid she died miserably in two days. On opening the body the caecum intestinum [appendix?] was narrowed and constricted; also the quince was found adherent to the inside and stopping up the lumen, so that it absolutely could not pass through any other way: whence it happened that this acrid and corrupt material prevented from passing; the obstacle overflowing opened up itself an unusual route into the abdominal cavity, by a necrosis and perforation a little above the obstructed place; from whence in the gut just as by the outlet & the passage escaping it filled up the abdomen to its entire capacity. Hence the suffering of most severe pains, hence distension, hence loss of consciousness, the most cruel death following shortly the appearance of foul vomiting. The history will be of value to those who in an excessive flow of abundant and toxic fluid from whatsoever cause, hasten intemperately to stop & subdue it to the greatest misfortune to the patient.

Lorenz Heister

Lorenz Heister or Laurentius Heisterus was born at Frankfort-on-the-Main in 1683, studied first at Giessen, and then served an apprenticeship of four years at Wetzlar. From there he proceeded to Holland, where he studied five years, devoting himself particularly to the study of anatomy. He became a docent in Amsterdam and gave courses in surgery on cadavers. In 1708 he received his doctor's degree at Harderwyk and entered the Dutch army as a surgeon.

Heister remained in the army a year, then studied in London, Paris, and Strassburg and, in 1710, was called to Altdorf as professor of surgery. Altdorf was a small university in Franconia and later united with Erlangen. He remained at Atldorf for ten years before accepting a call to the University of Helmstedt, founded in 1575, a very important university in 1720, but closed in 1810. Here Heister led a most active life, grew steadily in reputation, and declined professorships at St. Petersburg, Würzburg, Kiel, and Göttingen. He died in 1758 at the age of seventy-five.

Lorenz Heister was an extraordinarily industrious man and an indefatigable student. He was well informed upon a variety of topics, the master of several languages and an enthusiastic botanist. His best-known works are his *Institutiones Chirurgicae* and his *Chirurgische Warnehmungen*. In the latter work Heister describes an appendix which was the seat of an acute inflammation and calls attention to the possible importance of such lesions.

The following selection describing the case of appendicitis is from an English translation of Heister with the title, *Medical, Chirurgical and Anatomical*

Cases and Observations by Laurence Heister, translated by George Wirgman and printed in London by J. Reeves, 1755.

OBSERVATION CX

OF AN ABSCESS IN THE VERMIFORM PROCESS OF THE CAECUM*

In the month of November 1711, as I was dissecting the body of a malefactor in the public theatre at Altdorff, I found the small than usual. As I now was about to separate it, by gently pulling it asunder, the membranes of this process broke, notwithstanding the

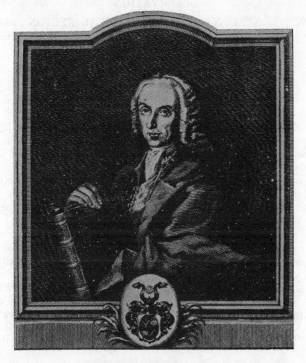

LORENZ HEISTER (1683-1758)
From the frontispiece to Heister's *Medicinische Chirurgische und Anatomische Wahrnehmungen* (Rostock, 1753)

guts very red and inflamed in several places, insomuch that the smallest vessels were as beautifully filled with blood, as if they had been injected with red wax, in the most skillful manner, after Ruysch's method. But, when I was about to demonstrate the situation of the great guts, I found the vermiform process of the caecum preternaturally black, adhering closer to the peritonæum

body was quite fresh, and discharged two or three spoonfuls of matter. This instance may stand as a proof of the possibility of inflammations arising, and abscesses forming, in the appendicula, as well as in other parts of the body, which I have not observed to be much noticed by other writers; and when, in practice, we meet with a burning and pain where this part is situated, we ought to give attention to it. It is probable that this person might have had some pain in the part; but of this I could get no information. In such cases, I look upon clysters prepared

*Heister, Laurence, *Medical, Chirurgical and Anatomical Cases and Observations,* translated by George Wirgman, London, Reeves, 1755, p. 136.

with emollient and discutient herbs, such as mallows, marsh-mallows, and camomile-flowers, and the like remedies against inflammations, boiled in milk and used frequently, to be of excellent use; as they reach the part, and may resolve the inflammation, or bring the abscess to a suppuration, partly by their warmth, partly by their resolving and discutient qualities, opening the abscess, that the matter may be discharged by stool, and the patient hereby may be saved; which. when the parts in the abdomen become corroded, can scarcely happen, but death must follow.

M. Mestivier

OBSERVATIONS

ON A TUMOR SITUATED NEAR THE UMBILICAL REGION ON THE RIGHT SIDE, PRODUCED BY A LARGE PIN FOUND IN THE VERMIFORM APPENDIX OF THE CAECUM

By M. Mestivier, Surgeon of Paris*

A man, aged about 45 years, of robust constitution, presented himself at the hospital St. André, Bordeaux, in the year 1757, to have himself treated for a tumor of considerable size, situated near the umbilical region on the right side. The surgeon of the said hospital, after having examined the tumour, noted there a considerable fluctuation; he believed he ought not to delay opening it up any longer, & did so; there escaped from it about a pint of pus of a very bad quality: the ulcer which resulted from the opening of this tumour could not be cleansed for a long time, but when he had every reason to hope that a cure was near, the patient died.

I opened his body in the presence of the surgeon.

I commenced by the caecum of the intes-

* *J. de med. chir. pharm.*, Paris, 1759, x, 441

tine, which showed nothing extraordinary; it was sprinkled with gangrenous sloughs; it was not the same, however, with his vermiform appendix: scarcely had I opened it, than we found here a large pin completely encrusted and so corroded in certain places that the least pressure would have broken it; which came not entirely from the humidity, but also from the acridity of the material enclosed within the vermiform appendix.

One will see easily, after what I have just said, in spite of the fact that the patient had never spoken of having swallowed a pin, that this pin, which forms the subject of this observation was enclosed for a long time in the vermiform appendix of the caecum and had irritated without ceasing the different tunics which form it, and caused here all the accidents of illness and death that followed.

Joubert de la Motte

OBSERVATIONS

MADE AT THE OPENING OF A BODY OF A PERSON DEAD OF TYMPANITES

By M. Joubert de la Motte, student of medicine at the University of Angers†

A man named Aleaume of the village of Bourg, died at the hospital of this city the 15th of September, of a flatulent colic, which tormented him for nine or ten months and degenerated finally into tympanites and caused him to suffer the most acute pains. The patient was so obstinate that he would not submit to any remedies; purgatives would

† *J. de med. chir. pharm.*, Paris, 1766, xxiv, 65-68.

not move him, enemas were returned as soon as he received them. The abdomen continued in the same condition, that is to say, hard and distended: finally having succumbed to the violence of the disease, we wished to see and to know the obstacle which opposed everything that art could do to relieve him: consequently it was decided to carry out a post-mortem examination and we proceeded in the accustomed manner. As the site of the malady was at the lower portion of the abdomen, we commenced by opening it. Having raised the skin and muscles and everything attached to it, we saw the peritoneum which showed nothing abnormal. After having examined it sufficiently, we opened it. We saw first the intestines in place, but so distended and of such a great volume, that one could not do better than to compare them to a balloon filled with air. After examining them most scrupulously and wishing to assure ourselves of the condition of the other viscera contained in the abdomen, we removed the epiploon, which was a little inflamed: as soon as this was elevated, we saw the stomach also distended & just as filled with air as the intestines. The liver and spleen were such as they ought to be in the natural state: nevertheless they were a little more elevated because of the distention of the colon and of the entire intestinal canal. The gall-bladder was also filled, as much as it possibly could be, with an extremely black bile; the communication of the cystic duct and of the hepatic duct, which by their junction, form the common duct, was free: the pancreas was entirely blocked off (obstructed): the kidneys, the ureters, the bladder, were very healthy. Finally, coming back to the affected part, we proceeded to consider with attention the intestines: they were so distended that the mesentery, the mesocolon, of which the glands were entirely obstructed, were also distended like the skin stretched tightly over a box. The size of the large intestine and the small was about the same: but the caecum was so large that it looked exactly like a

large bladder filled with air. The vermiform appendix, a good inch long, was much larger than the normal state. This fact appeared to me so extraordinary that I wished to assure myself of what this intestine might contain; I touched it, and I felt here a foreign body, as if petrified. But as we had decided to examine completely the entire intestinal tract, we proceeded to lift up the entire mass of the intestines in order to examine them most easily. This operation once done, we opened the stomach, which we found filled with air and with a yellowish material, liquid and extraordinarily foetid; the jejunum & ileum were the same. Coming to the caecum we found here in the beginning hard cherries; I say cherries, and not stones, the color of which was intensely black (observe that I write in September, and mark that the season for this fruit is past.) After having pressed out some faecal material, we extracted this hard body, which I had felt through the membranes of the intestine. It was the size of a large orange & resembled very much a potato a little flattened out, that is to say, much less elongated than they usually are. Its weight was 4 ounces, its color extraordinarily brownish, its substance like a fine floss firmly pressed together, its color inside a little like that of an ordinary sponge; it also appeared as solid as touch-wood.

We then examined the chest, in which we saw nothing abnormal except that the lungs were not filled out, the diaphragm having been pushed up into the thoracic cavity by the intestines whose volume was so much increased.

James Parkinson

Little seems to have been known regarding the life and labors of James Parkinson until the investigations of Rowntree unearthed many facts and incidents in the life of this physician. Parkinson was born in 1755, his family being one of culture and education, and his father a physician. We know little of his education but find that he was in active practice in 1785 and during this year attended John Hunter's lectures in surgery.

He lived during the American War of Independence and the French Revolution and was probably considered a dangerous individual by some of his neighbors, for he was himself a reformer, a radical, and a member of several secret political societies. He wrote several political pamphlets, one of which was entitled *Revolution without Bloodshed; or Reformation preferable to Revolt*, and attracted much attention. He wrote in 1802, *Hints for the Improvement of*

Trusses, which he says were "for the Use of the Labouring Poor, to whom this little tract is chiefly addressed." The following year he wrote *Medical Admonitions to Families,* a sort of Home Physician book, which went through several editions.

In 1817 his *Essay on Shaking Palsy* appeared. Had he not written it, his name would have died with him. The attitude, weakness, tremor, and gait of the patient are accurately described, but there is no mention of the "Parkinson mask." This, however, was not his sole contribution to medical science. His description of acute appendicitis, which appeared in 1816, ranks as one of the classic early accounts of this disease.

James Parkinson died in 1824.

CASE OF DISEASED APPENDIX VERMIFORMIS*

By John Parkinson, Esq., Surgeon. Communicated by James Parkinson, Esq.
Read January 21, 1812

A preparation of diseased appendix vermiformis in my possession, was removed from a boy about 5 years of age, who died under the following circumstances.

He had been observed for some time to decline in health, but made no particular complaint until two days before his death when he was suddenly seized with vomiting and great prostration of strength. The abdomen became very tumid and painful upon being pressed; his countenance pale and sunken, his pulse hardly perceptible. Death, preceded by extreme restlessness and delirium, took place with 24 hours.

Upon examination the whole surface of the peritoneum was found inflamed, and covered with a thin coat of coagulable lymph; and slight adhesions had taken place between the peritoneum covering the viscera, and the

parietes of the abdomen. The viscera independent of the inflammation of the peritoneal covering, appeared in a perfectly healthy state, excepting the appendix vermiformis of the coeum. No diseased appearance was seen in this part near to the coecum; but about an inch of its extremity was considerably enlarged and thickened, its internal surface ulcerated, and an opening from ulceration, which would have admitted a crow quill, was found at the commencement of the diseased part, about the middle of the appendix, through which it appeared, that a thin dark-coloured and highly fetid fluid, had escaped into the cavity of the abdomen.

Upon opening the appendix, a piece of hardened foeces was found impacted in that part of it which lay between the opening, and that portion of the appendix, which was not evidently marked by disease.

* *Med. Chir. Tr.,* London, 1812, III, p. 57.

Thomas Hodgkin

LECTURE VI*

The partial inflammation of the peritoneum, in the Iliac fossa, is sometimes set up by disease in the Appendix caeci. If this be inconsiderable, it may merely give rise to some very limited partial adhesions; at other times, the Appendix having been perforated by ulcerations, occasioned by the lodgement

* *Lectures on the Morbid Anatomy of the Serous and Mucous Membranes,* by Thomas Hodgkin, M.D., London, 1836.

of the faecal concretions in its cavity, extravasation takes place, and inflammation of a more severe and serious kind is originated. Even in these cases, nature sometimes succeeds in limiting the inflammation to a part of the right side; but it is at other times diffused over the whole abdomen, is accompanied by symptoms of the most serious nature, and quickly proves fatal.

Reginald Heber Fitz

Reginald Heber Fitz was born at Chelsea, Massachusetts, in 1843 and was educated at Harvard, receiving his M.D. degree in 1868. After two years of study in Europe, chiefly with Rokitansky and Skoda in Vienna, and with Virchow in Berlin, he returned to Boston, where at first his interest lay mainly in pathological studies. In 1879, he became professor of pathological anatomy at

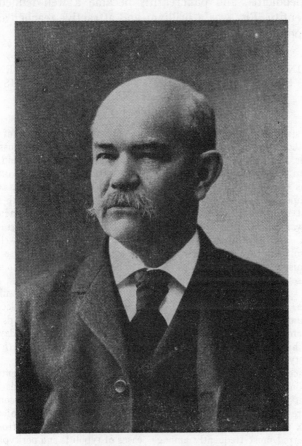

REGINALD H. FITZ (1843-1913)
From a photograph in the Library of the Jackson County
(Missouri) Medical Society

Harvard, but later his interest in clinical medicine increased and in 1892 he became professor of medicine at Harvard. In 1905 the degree of LL.D. was conferred upon him by Harvard and in 1908 he retired from his chair in the medical school. He died in 1913.

At the first meeting of the Association of American Physicians, in 1886, Fitz read a paper on perforative appendicitis which commanded instant attention by its clear, incisive statements and logical, orderly conclusions. Fitz pointed out that the frequent abscesses in the right iliac fossa "were not due to typhlitis, perityphlitis, paratyphlitis or epityphlitis but to perforation of the vermiform appendix." While Fitz did not discover or describe the condition for the first time, his paper aroused the interest of the medical profession in this disease. Fitz gave it the name of appendicitis, proved its origin in the appendix, pointed out its characteristic diagnostic features, and indicated the necessary treatment.

In 1889 Fitz performed for pancreatitis the same service he had previously rendered appendicitis, and pancreatitis became a well-defined clinical and pathological entity. Fitz was a brilliant and attractive teacher and left a deep impression upon his medical school and his pupils.

PERFORATING INFLAMMATION OF THE VERMIFORM APPENDIX, WITH SPECIAL REFERENCE TO ITS EARLY DIAGNOSIS AND TREATMENT†

By Reginald H. Fitz., M.D., of Boston

A historical statement was made of the origin of the terms typhlitis, perityphlitis, and perityphlitic abcess. The want of exact agreement as to what was understood by these terms was emphasized. Attention was called to the importance of bearing in mind that in the vast majority of cases, the primary disease was an inflammation of the caecal appendix. The term appendicitis was preferred to typhlitis, as avoiding the possibility of a misunderstanding, and as localizing the disease in its usual place of origin.

The paper was based upon an analysis of two hundred and fifty-seven cases of unquestionable perforating ulcer of the appendix, and of two hundred and nine cases diagnosticated as typhlitis, perityphlitis, and perityphlitic abscess. In the latter series, the diagnosis was clinical, not anatomical.

The important features in the etiology of appendicitis were considered, also the limitations as to sex and age. It was found that the disease occurred most frequently among previously healthy youths and young adults, especially males; that a faecal concretion or foreign body was present as a local cause in more than three-fifths of the cases. Attacks of indigestion and acts of violence, especially when indirect, were exciting causes in one-fifth of the cases. The action of these causes was favored by a constipated habit, or by congenial or acquired irregularities in the position and attachment of the appendix.

The first characteristic symptom of a perforating appendicitis was found to be a sudden, severe, abdominal pain. This occurred in eighty-four per cent of the cases, and usually in the right iliac fossa, where tenderness could always be found, even when the pain was referred to some other locality. The pain was attributed to the actual perforation or the detachment of fresh adhesions.

Fever was the next characteristic symptom, and occurred in the course of twenty-four hours. Finally came the swelling which made its appearance in the course of three days.

The chief source of danger from the appendicular peritonitis arose from its becoming generalized. Such a result followed most frequently between the second and fourth days. More than two-thirds of the patients died during the first eight days and two-thirds of these between the fourth and eight days, inclusive.

The question of a differential diagnosis was then discussed. The termination in resolution was referred to. It was considered to take place in about one-third of the cases as approximately determined from the recorded cases of typhlitis and perityphlitis. Even resolution might be undesirable since the number of cases of recurrent disease is considerable, and might have been prevented by appropriate treatment.

The reader recommended at the outset, the opium treatment with rest and a liquid diet, the food being given in small quantities, frequently repeated. If it became evident that general peritonitis was imminent at the end of twenty-four hours after the sudden intense pain the appendix should be exposed and removed. Usually the symptoms were not so urgent that the appearance of the swelling could not be awaited. Although Willard Parker advised that the abscess might be

† *Boston M. & S. J.*, 1886, cxv, 13.

opened as early as the fifth day, the practice has been to operate at a later date. Forty-seven per cent of the cases were operated upon in the second week and twenty-six per cent after the third week.

More favorable results in the future were to follow the earliest possible opening of the swelling. This in most instances was at the outset, a sac formed by a circumscribed peritonitis. It was usually present on the third day of the disease, dating from the pain, its first marked characteristic symptom. Negative results from a diagnostic puncture did not contraindicate the operation.

BIBLIOGRAPHY

Actuarius, Johannis
  Biographisches Lexikon der hervorragen-
    den Ärzte aller Zeiten und Völker,
    II Edition, Berlin, Urban & Schwarz-
    enberg, 1929, I, p. 23.
Adams, Robert
  Obituary: Lancet, 1875, I, 145.
Addison, Thomas
  Bettany, G. T.: Eminent Doctors, Lon-
    don, Hogg, 1885, II, p. 1.
  Long, Esmond R.: Thomas Addison and
    His Discovery of Idiopathic Anemia,
    Ann. M. Hist., 1935, N.S. VII, 130.
  Wicks, Samuel and Bettany, G. T.: A
    Biographical History of Guy's Hos-
    pital, London. Ward, Lock, Bowden
    & Co., 1892, p. 221.
Almenar, Juan
  Astruc, John: A Treatise of Venereal
    Diseases, London, W. Innys, 1754, p.
    154.
Aretaeus the Cappadocian
  Adams, Francis: The Extant Works of
    Aretaeus the Cappadocian, London,
    Sydenham Soc., 1856.
  Cordell, Eugene F.: Aretaeus the Cap-
    padocian, Bull. Johns Hopkins Hos-
    pital, 1909, XX, 371.
  Kussmann, R.: Wann lebte Aretaeus
    von Cappadocien?, München Med.
    Wchnschr., 1902, XLIX, 1265.
  Leopold, Eugene J.: Aretaeus the Cap-
    padocian, Ann. M. Hist., 1930, N.S.,
    II, 424.
Auenbrugger, Leopold
  Clar, Prof. Dr.: Leopold Auenbrugger,
    der Erfinder der Percussion des Brust-
    korbes, Graz, Lauscher & Lubensky,
    1867.
  Leopold Auenbrugger: Brit. M. J., 1909,
    I, 1191.
Baglivi, Giorgio
  Castiglioni, Arturo: Il Volto di Ippo-
    crate, Un Clinico del Secolo XVII
    (Giogio Baglivi), Milan, Unitas, 1925,
    p. 271.
Baillie, Matthew
  Macmichael, William: Lives of British
    Physicians, London, Murray, 1830, p.
    241.
  Macmichael, William: The Gold-Headed
    Cane, London, Murray, 1828, p. 236.

Baillou, Guillaume de
  Biographisches Lexikon der hervorragen-
    den Ärzte aller Zeiten und Völker,
    Berlin, Urban & Schwarzenberg, 1929,
    I, p. 292.
  Dictionnaire des sciences médicales: Bi-
    ographie Médicale, Paris, Panckoucke,
    1820, I, p. 502.
  Fiessinger, Ch.: La Therapeutique des
    Vieux Maitres, Paris, Soc. d'éditions
    scientifiques, 1897, p. 114.
Baker, Sir George
  Munk, William: The Roll of the Royal
    College of Physicians of London, Lon-
    don, 1878, II, p. 213.
Banting, Sir Frederick
  Hall, William E. B.: Sir Frederick Grant
    Banting (1891-1941), Arch. Path.,
    1941, XXXI, 657.
  King, E. J.: The Late Sir Frederick
    Banting, Lancet, 1941, I, 551.
  Obituary: Canada M. Assn. J., 1941,
    XLIV, 429.
  Obituary: J.A.M.A., 1941, CXVI, 1021.
Bard, Samuel
  White, J. P. & Gross, Samuel D.: Lives
    of Eminent American Physicians,
    Philadelphia, Lindsay & Blakiston.
    1861, p. 166.
Basedow, Carl A. von
  Sudhoff, Karl: Carl A. von Basedow,
    München Med. Wchnschr., 1910, LVII,
    749.
Bayle, Gaspard-Laurent
  Dictionnaire des sciences médicales: Bi-
    ographie Médicale, Paris, Panckoucke,
    1820, II, p. 75.
Benivieni, Antonio
  Major, Ralph H.: Antonio di Pagolo
    Benivieni, Bull. Inst. Hist. Med., 1935,
    III, 739.
  de Vecchi, Bindo: Il pensiero anatomico
    in medicina da Benivieni a Morgagni,
    Florence, 1939.
  de Vecchi, Bindo: La Vita e l'Opera di
    Maestro Antonio Benivieni-Fiorentino
    Atti della Società Colombario, Flo-
    rence, 1931.
Bennett, John Hughes
  Dr. John Hughes Bennett: Boston M.
    & S. J., 1875, XCIII, 509.

John Hughes Bennett: *Brit. M. J.*, 1875, II, 473.

Bertin, R. J. H.
Brown, Lawrason: *The Story of Clinical Pulmonary Tuberculosis*, Baltimore, Williams & Wilkins, 1941.
Dictionnaire des Sciences Médicales: Biographie Médicale, Paris, Panckoucke, 1920, II, p. 204.

Béthencourt, Jacques de
Dictionnaire des Sciences Médicales: Biographie Médicale, Paris, Panckoucke, 1920, II, p. 220.

Binninger, Johann Nikolaus
Dictionnaire des Sciences Médicales: Biographie Médicale, Paris, Panckoucke, 1820, II, p. 264.

Blackall, John
Brit. M. J., 1860, I, 75.
Munk, William: *The Roll of the Royal College of Physicians of London*, London, 1878, III, p. 138.

Bontius, Jacobus
Van Andel, M. A.: *Opuscula Selecta Neerlandicorum de Arte*, *Medica* Amsterdam, 1931, X, p. 9.

Bostock, John
Hurwitz, Samuel H.: John Bostock, *California West M.*, 1929, XXXI, 137.
Munk, William: *The Roll of the Royal College of Physicians of London*, London, 1878, II, p. 286.
Obituary: *Lancet*, 1846, II, 222.

Botallo, Leonardo
Dictionnaire des Sciences Médicales: Biographie Médicale, Paris, Panckoucke, 1820, II, p. 433.

Bouillaud, Jean Baptiste
Herrick, James B.: Jean-Baptiste Bouillaud and his Contributions to Cardiology, *Bull. Soc. Med Hist.*, Chicago, 1940 V, 230.
Rolleston, J. D.: Jean Baptiste Bouillaud (1796-1881), A Pioneer in Cardiology and Neurology, *Proc. Roy. Soc. Med.*, 1930-31, XXIV, II, 1252.

Bouveret, L.
Mouisset, F.: L. Bouveret, *Presse Méd.*, 1929, XXV, 413.

Bravo, Francisco (de Orsuna)
Lejeune, Fritz: Die ersten fünfzig Jahre spanischer Medizin in Amerika, *Janus*, 1926, XXX, 201.

Bretonneau, Pierre
Triaire, Paul: *Bretonneau et ses correspondants*, Paris, Alcan, 1892.

Bright, Richard
Bettany, G. T.: *Eminent Doctors*, London, Hogg, 1885, II, p. 1.
Chance, Burton: Richard Bright, *Ann. M. Hist.*, 1927, IX, 332.
Garrison, Fielding H.: Richard Bright's Travels in Lower Hungary, *Bull. Johns Hopkins Hosp.*, 1912, XXIII, 173.
Rochester, De Lancey: Richard Bright of Guy's Hospital, *Ann. M. Hist.*, 1923, V, 301.
Thayer, William S.: *Osler and Other Papers*, Baltimore, Johns Hopkins Press, 1931, p. 318.
Wilks, Samuel and Bettany, G. T.: *A Biographical History of Guy's Hospital*, London, Ward, Lock, Bowder & Company, 1892, p. 212.

Broadbent, Sir William
Broadbent, M. E.: *Life of Sir William Broadbent*, London, Murray, 1909.
Obituary: *Brit. M. J.*, 1907, II, 177.

Brown, John
Parsons, F. G.: *The History of St. Thomas' Hospital*, London, Methuen. 1934, II, p. 130.

Buerger, Leo
Obituary: *J.A.M.A.*, 1943, CXXIII, 500.

Burnett, Sir William
Obituary: *Lancet*, 1861, I, 200.
Walsh, James G.: The Irish School of Medicine, *Bull. Johns Hopkins Hosp.*, 1906, XVII, 301.

Cadwalader, Thomas
Dulles, Charles W.: Dr. Thomas Cadwalader's "Essay": A Hunt for a Historical Error, *Med. Libr. & Hist. J.*, 1903, I, 181.
Kelly, H. A.: *Cyclopaedia of American Medical Biography*, Philadelphia. Saunders, 1912, I, p. 181.
Krumbhaar, Edward B.: The Early History of Anatomy in the United States, *Ann. M. Hist.*, 1922, IV, 154.

Caius, John
Macmichael, William: *Lives of British Physicians*, London, Murray, 1830, p. 15.
Rolleston, Sir Humphry: *The Cambridge Medical School*, Cambridge University Press, 1932, p. 190.
Venn, John: *John Caius*, Cambridge University Press, 1910.

Cardan, Jerome
Dana, Charles L.: The Story of a Great

Consultation, *Ann. M. Hist.*, 1921, III, 122.

Jerome Cardan: *The Book of My Life*, Translated by Jean Stoner, New York, E. P. Dutton & Co., n.d.

Morley, Henry: *Jerome Cardan*, London, Chapman and Hall, 1854.

Waters, W. G.: *Jerome Cardan*, London Lawrence & Bullen, 1898.

Carey, Mathew
Kelly, H. A.: *Cyclopedia of American Medical Biography*, Philadelphia, Saunders, 1921, I, p. 161.

Cartier, Jacques
Bref récit et succincte narration de la Navigation faite, en MDXXXV et MDXXXVI par le capitaine Jacques. Réimpression figurée de l'édition originale rarissime de MDXLV, Paris, Tross, 1863.

Casál, Gaspar
Biographisches Lexikon hervorragender Ärzte aller Zeiten und Völker, II Edition, Berlin, Urban & Schwarzenberg, 1921, I, p. 847.

Canella y Secades, Don Fermin: Noticias Biográficas de Don Gaspar Casal in *Memorias historia natural y médica de Asturias por el Doctor Don Gaspar Casal*. Oviedo Escuela Topografica del Hospicio, 1900.

Major, Ralph H.: Don Gaspar Casál, Francois Thiéry and Pellagra, *Bull. Hist. Med.*, 1944, XVI, 351.

Morejon, D. Antonio Hernandez: *Historia bibliografica de la medicina española*, Madrid, 1852, Tomo VII, p. 252.

Celsus, Aulus Cornelius
Castiglioni, Arturo: Aulus Cornelius Celsus as a Historian of Medicine, *Bull. Hist. Med.*, 1940, VIII, 857.

Wellman, A.: A. Cornelius Celsus, *Arch. f. Gesch. d. Med.*, 1925, XVI, 209.

Chauliac, Guy de
Astruc, Jean: *Mémoires pour servir à l'histoire de la Faculté de Médicine de Montpellier*, Paris, Cavelier, 1767, 185.

von Brunn, alter: Die Stellung des Guy de Chauliac in der Chirurgie des Mittelalters, *Arch. f. Gesch. d. Med.*, 1921, XIII, 65.

Cheyne, John
Ormsby, Lambert H.: *Medical History of the Meath Hospital*, Dublin, Fannin & Co., 1888, p. 112.

Çitois, Francois
Astruc, Jean: *Mémoires pour servir à l'histoire de la Faculté de Médicine de Montpellier*, Paris, Cavelier, 1767, p. 368.

Clarke, John
Munk, William: *The Roll of the Royal College of Physicians of London*, London, 1878, II, p. 369.

Cober, Tobias
Biographisches Lexikon der hervorragenden Ärzte aller Zeiten und Völker, Berlin, Urban & Schwarzenberg, 1931, III, 564.

Collin, V.
Brown, Lawrason: *The Story of Clinical Pulmonary Tuberculosis*, Baltimore, Williams & Wilkins Co., 1941.

Colombo, Matteo Realdo
Capparoni, Pietro: *Profili Bio-Bibliografici di medici e naturalisti celebri italiani dal sec. XV al sec. XVIII°, Vol. II Instituto naz. med. farmacolog.*, Serono, Rome, 1928, p. 32.

Combe, James Scarth
Obituary: *Edinburgh M. J.*, 1883, XVII, 862.

Corrigan, Sir Dominic John
Dock, George: Dominic John Corrigan: His Place in the Development of our Knowledge of Cardiac Diseases, *Ann. M. Hist.*, 34, N.S., VI, 381.

Hancock, J. Duffy: The Irish School of Medicine, *Ann. M. Hist.*, 1930, N.S., II, 196.

Riesman, David: The Dublin Medical School and Its Influence Upon Medicine in America, *Ann. M. Hist.*, 1922, IV, 86.

Williamson, R. T.: Sir Dominic Corrigan, *Ann. M. Hist.*, 1925, VII, 354.

Corvisart, Jean Nicholas
Beeson, B. Barker: Corvisart, His Life and Works, *Ann. M. Hist.*, 1930, N.S., II, 297.

Cotton, Richard
Obituary: *Med. Times & Gaz.*, 1878, I, 24.

Cotugno, Domenico
Biographical Sketch of Cotugnius, *Lancet*, 1824, IV, 155.

Levinson, Abraham: Domenico Cotugno, *Ann. M. Hist.*, 1936, N.S., VIII, 1.

Cowper, William
Archaeologica Medica: William Cowper, The Anatomist, *Brit. M. J.*, 1898, I, 160.

Cruveilhier, Jean
Roussy, G.: Eloge de Jean Cruveilhier, *Presse Méd.*, 1926, XXXIV, 1643.

Curling, Thomas Blizard
Obituary: *Lancet*, 1888, I, 550.

Da Costa, Jacob M.
Clarke, Mary A.: Memoir of J. M. Da Costa, *Am. J. M. Sc.*, 1903, CXXV, 318.
Oppenheimer, B. S.: Neurocirculatory Asthenia and Related Problems in Military Medicine, *Bull. New York Acad. Med.*, 1942, XVIII, 367.

Defoe, Daniel
Nicholson, Watson: *The Historical Sources of Defoe's Journal of the Plague Year*, Boston, Stratford, 1919.

Dekkers, Frederik
Baumann, E. D.: Frederik Dekkers *Janus*, 1919, xxiv: 233.
Dock, William: Some Early Observers of Albuminuria, *Ann. M. Hist.*, 1922, IV, 287.

Devèze, Jean
Lane, John E.: Jean Devèze, *Ann. M. Hist.*, 1936, N.S., VIII, 202.

Dickinson, William H.
Obituary: *Brit. M. J.*, 1913, I, 141.
Rolleston, Sir Humphry: Reminiscences of St. George's Forty Years Ago, Reprinted from *St. George's Hospital Gazette*, March and June, 1931, London, John Bale Sons & Danielsson, 1931.

Dobson, Matthew
Launders, F. W.: *The Life of Matthew Dobson*, Liverpool, M-Chir. J., 1916, XXXVI, 127.

Duroziez, Paul-Louis
Helfenbein, F.: *Duroziez et son oeuvre. Thèse de Paris*, Paris, Librairie le François, 1922.

Ebers, Papyrus
Bryan, Cyril P.: *The Papyrus Ebers*, New York, D. Appleton, 1931.
Ebbel, B.: *The Papyrus Ebers*, Copenhagen, Levin & Minksgaard, 1937.
Major, Ralph H.: The Papyrus Ebers, *Ann. M. Hist.*, 1930, N.S., II, 470.

Fabry, Wilhelm (See Gullielmus Fabricius Hildanus)

Fauvel, S. A.
Bergeron: Décès de M. Fauvel. *Bull. d l'acad de méd.*, 1884. XLVIII, 1607.
Décès de M. Fauvel: *Rev. D'hyg.*, 1894, VI, 1030.
Obituary: *Lancet*, 1884, II, 893.

Fernel, Jean
Biography in *Le Meilleur Traitement du Mal Venerien* traduction de L. Le Pileur, Paris, Masson, 1879.
Capitaine, P. A.: *Un grand médecin du XVI siécle, Jean Fernel*, Paris, Librairie Le François, 1925.

Findlay, Carlos J.
Agramonte, Aristides: Dr. Carlos J. Findlay—A Biographical Sketch, *New Orleans M. & S. J.*, 1916, LXIX, 55.

Fitz, Reginald H.
Flick, Lawrence F.: *Development of Our Knowledge of Tuberculosis*, Philadelphia, 1925.
Morrison, Hyman: Reginald Heber Fitz. *Bull. Hist. Med.*, 1941, X, 250.

Flint, Austin
Austin Flint, Sr., M.D., LL.D.: *J.A.M.A.*, 1886, VI, 361.
Landis, H. R. M.: Austin Flint: His Contributions to the Art of Physical Diagnosis and the Study of Tuberculosis, *Bull. Johns Hopkins Hosp.*, 1912, XXIII, 182.
The Death of Dr. Austin Flint: *Lancet*, 1886, I, 556.

Foligno, Gentile da
Riesman, David: *The Story of Medicine in the Middle Ages*, New York, Hoeber, 1935.

Fothergill, John
Lettson, John Coakley: *Memoirs of John Fothergill M.D.* &c. London, C. Dilly, 1786.
Macmichael, William: *Lives of British Physicians*, London, Murray, 1830, p. 183.
Munk, William: *The Roll of the Royal College of Physicians of London*, London, 1878, II, p. 154.
Tuke, James H.: *A Sketch of the Life of John Fothergill, M.D., F.R.S.*, London, Harris, 1879.

Fracastorius, Hieronymus
Abraham, J. Johnston: *Introduction to Fracastor, Syphilis or the French Disease*. Translated by Heneage Wynne-Finch, London. Heinemann, 1935.
Fussel, Viktor: *Klassiker der Medizine*,

Drei Bücher von den Kontagien, den Kontagiösen Krankheiten und deren Behandlung, Leipzig, Barth, 1910, p. 5.

Montgomery, Douglas W.: Hieronymus Fracastorius, *Ann. M. Hist.,* 1930, N.S., II, 406.

Osler, William: Fracastorius, *Proc. Charaka Club,* New York, 1906, II, 5.

Singer, Charles and Dorothea: The Scientific Position of Girolamo Fracastoro, *Ann. M. Hist.,* 1917, I, 1.

Wright, William Cave: *Hieronymi Fracastorii de contagione et contagiosis morbis, etc.,* New York, Putnam, 1930.

Frapolli, Francesco

Verga, Andrea: Francesco Frapolli, *Gazz. med. ital. Lombardia,* 1871, XXXI, 361.

Freke, John

Moore, Norman: *The History of St. Bartholomews Hospital,* London, Pearson, 1918, II, 633.

Fröhlich, Alfred

Biographisches Lexikon der hervorragenden Ärzte der letzten fünfzig Jahre, Berlin, Urban & Schwarzenburg, 1932, I, p. 455.

Gerbezius, Marcus

Dictionnaire des Sciences Médicales: Biographie Médicale, Paris, Panckoucke, 1821, IV, p. 392.

Gerhard, William Wood

Middleton, W. S.: William Wood Gerhard, *Ann. M. Hist.,* 1935, N.S., VII, 1.

Glisson, Francis

Rolleston, Sir Humphry: *The Cambridge Medical School,* Cambridge University Press, 1932, p. 151.

Graefe, Albrecht von

Adler, Francis H.: Sketches from the Life of Albrecht von Graefe (1826-1870), *Ann. M. Hist.,* 1921, N.S., I, 284.

Graves, Robert James

Ormsby, Lambert H.: *Medical History of the Meath Hospital,* Dublin, Fannin & Co., 1888, p. 122.

Grévin, Jacques

Pinvert, Lucien: *Jacques Grévin,* Paris, Fontemiong, 1899.

Gull, Sir William

Acland, T. D.: Memoir in *Published Writings of William Withey Gull,* London, New Sydenham Soc., 1896.

Wilks, Samuel and Bettany, G. T.: *A Biographial History of Guy's Hospital,* London, Ward, Lock, Bowden & Co., 1892, p. 261.

Haller, Albrecht von

Pettigrew, Thomas J.: *Biographical Memoirs of the Most Celebrated Physicians, Surgeons, etc.,* London, Fisher, 1838, I.

Reed, Charles Bert.: Albrecht von Haller, *Bull. Soc. Med. Hist.,* Chicago, 1911-16, I, 23.

Sterling, William: *Some Apostles of Physiology,* London, Waterlow, 1902, p. 55.

Hammer, Adam

Ball, James M.: Dr. Adam Hammer, Surgeon and Apostle of Higher Medical Education, *J. Missouri M. A.,* 1909, VI, 155.

Harley, George

Obituary: *Brit. M. S.,* 1896, II, 1354.

Haygarth, John

Weaver, George H.: John Haygarth, *Bull. Soc. Med. Hist.,* Chicago, 1930, IV, 156, 1933, IV, 264.

Heberden, William

Davidson, Percy D.: William Heberden, M.D., F.R.S., *Ann. M. Hist.,* 1922, IV, 336.

Macmichael, William: *Lives of British Physicians,* London, Murray, 1830, 198.

Rolleston, Sir Humphry: The Two Heberdens, *Ann. M. Hist.,* 1933, N.S., V, 409, 566.

Heister, Lorenz

Dictionnaire des sciences médicales: Biographie Médicale, Paris, Panckoucke, 1822, V, p. 131.

Gerster, Arpad G.: Laurentius H. Heister—A Sketch, *Proc. Charaka Club,* New York, 1906, II, 131.

Henoch, Edward

Henoch, Edward: *München Med. Wchnschr.,* 1910, LVII, 1504.

Hering, H. E.

Lullies, H.: Zum 70 Geburtstag von H. E. Hering, *München Med. Wchnschr.,* 1936, LXXXIII, 777.

Herrick, James B.

Herrick, James B.: *A Short History of Cardiology,* Springfield, Thomas, 1942.

Hildanus, Guilhelmus Fabricius

Platt, Walter D.: Fabricius Guilhelmus Hildanus: The Father of German Surgery, *Bull. Johns Hopkins Hospital,* 1905, XVI, 7.

Schäfer, Rom. Joh.: Wilhelm Fabricius von Hilden, *Janus*, 1910, XV, 65.

Sudhoff, Karl: Guilhelmus Fabricius Hildanus, *München Med. Wchnschr.*, 1910, LVII, 1401.

Hillary, William

Creighton, Charles: *Dict. Nat. Biog.*, 1891, XXVI, 429.

Hippocrates

Adams, Francis: *The Genuine Works of Hippocrates*, New York, Wm. Wood, I, 3.

Baissette, Gaston: *Hippocrate*, Paris, Grasset, 1931.

Beck, Theodor: Hippokrates Erkenntnisse, Jena, Diederichs, 1907, Einleitung, p. 1.

Clifton, Francis: *Hippocrates upon Air, Water and Situation*, London, Whiston & White, 1752.
The Life of Hippocrates from Soranus, no pagination.

Dacier, André: Les Oeuvres d'Hippocrate, *Paris, Compagnie des Libraires*, 1697, 2 Vols., Vol. 1, La vie d'Hippocrate.

Daremberg, Ch.: *Oeuvres Choisies d'Hippocrate*, Paris, Labé, 1855, Introduction, p. XXII.

Grimm, J. F. C.: *Hippocrates Werke revidirt und mit Anmerkungen versehen von Dr. L. Lilienhain*, Glogau Prausnitz, 1837, Vol. 1, p. 1.

Littré, E.: *Oeuvres Completes d'Hippocrate*, 10 Vol., Paris, Baillière, 1839-1861, Vie d'Hippocrate, Vol. I, p. 26.

Moorman, Lewis J.: Francis Adams of Banchory, *Southern M. J.*, 1936, XXIX, 435.

Packard, Francis R.: Emile Littré, *Ann. M. Hist.*, 1927, IX, 411.

Petrequin, J. E.: *Chirurgie d'Hippocrate*, Paris Imprimerie Nationale, 1877, Discours preliminaire, Vol. 1, p. 1.

Sigerist, Henry E.: On Hippocrates, *Bull. Inst. Hist. Med.*, 1934, LIV, 190.

Singer, Charles: A Great Country Doctor: Francis Adams of Banchory (1796-1861). *Bull. Hist. Med.*, 1942, XII, 1.

Hodgkin, Thomas

Rosenbloom, Jacob: An Interesting Friendship—Thomas Hodgkin, M.D. and Sir Moses Montefiore Bart., *Ann. M. Hist.*, 1921, III, 381.

Wilks, Samuel and Bettany, G. T.: *A*

Biographical History of Guy's Hospital, London, Ward, Lock, Bowden & Co., 1892, 380.

Hoefer, Wolfgang

Dictionnaire des sciences médicales: Biographie Médicale, Paris, Panckoucke, 1822, v, p. 235.

Home, Francis

Hume, Edgar E.: Francis Home, *Bull. Inst. Hist. Med.*, 1942, XI, 48.

Hope, James

Hope, Mrs. James: *A Memoir of the Late James Hope, M.D.*, London. Hatchard, 1848.

Hunter, John

Bettany, G. T.: *Eminent Doctors*, London, Hogg, 1885, I, 119.

Home, Everard: A Short Account of the Life of the Author in a *Treatise on the Blood, Inflammation and Gunshot Wounds by the late John Hunter*, Philadelphia, Bradford, 1796.

McCrae, Thomas: William and John Hunter, *Ann. M. Hist.*, 1922, IV, 175.

Paget, Stephen: *John Hunter*, London, Unwin, 1897.

Peachey, George C.: *A Memoir of William and John Hunter*, Plymouth. Brendon, 1924.

Rohrer, C. W. G.: John Hunter: His Life and Labors, *Bull. Johns Hopkins Hospital*, 1914, XXV, 10.

Hutchinson, Sir Jonathan

Klauder, Joseph V.: Sir Jonathan Hutchinson, *Med. Life*, 1923, XLI, 313.

Sir Jonathan Hutchinson: *Brit. M. J.*, 1913, I, 1398.

The Versatility and Encyclopaedic Knowledge of the Late Sir Jonathan Hutchinson, *Brit. M. J.*, 1913, II, 1632.

Hutten, Ulrich von

Lane, John E.: Daniel Turner, *Ann. M. Hist.*, 1919, II, 367.

Sticker, George: Ulrich Von Huttens Buch über die Franzosenseuche als heimlicher Canon fur die Syphilistherapie im 16 Jahrhundert, *Arch. f. Gesch. d. Med.*, 1910, III, 197.

Strauss, Davis Friedrich: *Ulrich von Hutten*, Leipzig, Insel Verlag, 1927.

Zimmermann, Ernest L.: The French Pox of that Great Clerke of Almayne, Ulrich Hutten. Knyght, *Janus*, 1932, XXXV, 17.

Huxham, John
Macmichael, William: *Lives of British Physicians*, London, Murray, 1830, 168.
Moore, Norman: John Huxham, *Dict. Nat. Biog.*, London, 1891, XXVIII, 363.
Vogeler, William J.: John Huxham of Devonshire (1692-1768), *Bull. Johns Hopkins Hospital*, 1906, XVII, 308.

Jenner, Edward
Baron, John: *The Life of Edward Jenner, M.D., L.L.S., F.R.S.*, London, Colburn, 1838.
Bettany, G. T.: *Eminent Doctors*, London, Hogg, 1885, I, p. 252.
Fosbroke, Thomas D.: *Biographical Anecdotes of Edward Jenner in Berkeley Manuscripts*, London, Nichols, 1821.

Joubert, Laurent
Astruc, Jean: *Mémoires pour servir à l'histoire de la Faculté de Médicine de Montpellier*, Paris, Cavelier, 1767, p. 243.

King, Alfred Freeman Africanus
Album of Fellows of the American Gynecological Society, Philadelphia, Dornan, 1930, p. 342.
Fry, Henry D.: Alfred Freeman Africanus King, *Washington M. Ann.*, 1915, XIV, 89.
Haggis, A. W.: Fundamental Errors in the Early History of Cinchona, *Bull. Hist. Med.*, 1941, X, 417-568.
Howard, L. O.: Alfred Freeman Africanus King, *Washington M. Ann.*, 1915, XIV, 89.
Hurst, Barton Cooke: Alfred Freeman Africanus King, *Washington M. Ann.*, 1915, XIV, 89.
Shands, A. R.: Alfred Freeman Africanus King, *Washington M. Ann.*, 1915, XIV, 89.

Kircher, Athanasius
Erman, A.. Athanasius Kircher, *Allgem. Deutsch. Biograph.*, Leipzig, 1882, XVI, p. 1.
Major, Ralph H.: Athanasius Kircher, *Ann. M. Hist.*, 1939, III, Ser. 1, 105.
Seng, N.: *Selbstbiographie des P. Athanasius Kircher aus der Gesellschaft, Jesu*, Fulda, 1901.

Kirkes, William Senhouse
Obituary: *Lancet*, 1864, II, 674.

Knutsson, Bengt
Klebs, Arnold C. & Sudhoff, Karl: *Die ersten gedruckten Pestschriften*, München, Münchner Drucke, 1926, 19.
Sudhoff, Karl: Pestschriften aus den ersten 150 Jahren nach der Epidemie des "Schwarzen Todes" 1348, *Arch. f. Gesch. d. Med.*, 1912, V, 56.

Koplik, Henry
Obituary: *Am. J. Dis. Children*, 1927, XXXIII, 979.

Kussmaul, Adolf
Bast, Theodore: *The Life and Time of Adolf Kussmaul*, New York, Hoeber, 1926.
Kussmaul, Adolf: *Jugenderinnerungen eines alten Arztes*, Stuttgart, Bonz, 1899.
Kussmaul, Adolf: *Aus meiner Dozentenzeit in Heidelberg*, Stuttgart, Bonz, 1908.

Laënnec, René-Théophile-Hyacinthe
Saintignon, Henri: *Laënnec, sa vie et son oeuvre*, Paris, J. B. Baillière, 1904.
Thayer, William S.: Laënnec—One Hundred Years After, In His *Osler and Other Papers*, Baltimore, Johns Hopkins Press, 1931, p. 247.
Webb, Gerald B.: René-Théophile-Hyacinthe Laënnec, *Ann. M. Hist.*, 1927, IX, 27.

Lancisi, Giovanni Maria
Dictionnaire des sciences médicales: Biographie Médicale, Paris, Panckoucke, 1820, V, p. 499.

Lange, Johannes
Fossel, Viktor: Aus den medizinischen Briefen des pfalzgräflichen Leibarztes, Johannes Lange, *Arch. f. Gesch. d. Med.*, 1914, VII, 238.

Laveran, Charles Alphonse
Franchini, Joseph: Chas. Alphonse Laveran (1845-1922), His Life and Works, *Ann. Med. Hist.*, 1931, III, N.S., 280.

Leoniceno, Niccolo
Astruc, John: *A Treatise of Venereal Diseases*, London, W. Innys, 1754, p. 145.
Proksch, J. S.: *Die Geschichte der venerischen Krankheiten*, Bonn, Honstein, 1896, p. 307.
Streeter, Edward C.: Leoniceno and the School of Ferrara, *Bull. Soc. Med. Hist.*, Chicago, 1911-16, I, 18.

Lind, James
Stockman, Ralph: James Lind and Scurvy, *Edinburgh M. J.*, 1926, p. 329.

Louis, Pierre Charles Alexandre
Klebs, A. C.: Osler at the Tomb of Louis, *J.A.M.A.*, 1906, XLVI, 1716.
Sewall, Henry: The Influence of Louis on American Medicine, *Colorado Med.*, 1926, XXIII, 269.

Lower, Richard
Franklin, K. J.: Richard Lower (1631-1691) and His "De Corde," London, 1669, *Ann. M. Hist.*, 1931, N.S., III, 599.
Hollingsworth, Merril W.: Blood Transfusion by Richard Lower in 1665, *Ann. M. Hist.*, 1928, X, 213.
Wood, Anthony: *Athenae Oxoniensis*, London, Knoplock, Midwinter & Tonson, 1721, II, p. 957.

Lusitanus, Amatus
Friedenwald, Harry: Amatus Lusitanus, *Bull. Inst. Hist. Med.*, 1937, V, 603.

Mackenzie, James
Wilson, R. MacNair: *The Beloved Physician, Sir James Mackenzie*, New York, Macmillan, 1927.

Marie, Pierre
Guillain, Georges: Pierre Marie, *Bull. de l'Acad. d. Med.*, 1940, CIV, 524.

Minkowski, Oskar
Death of Prof. Minkowski: *Lancet*, 1931, I, 151.
Umber, F.: Oscar Minkowski zum 70. Geburtstag, *Deutsche Med. Wchnschr.*, 1928, LIV, 69.

Mitchell, S. Weir
Burr, Anna Robeson: *Weir Mitchell, His Life and Letters*, New York, Duffield, 1929.

Morgagni, Giovanni Battista
Adams, Edward W.: Giovanni Battista-Morgagni, *Med. Libr. & Hist. J.*, 1903, I, 270.
Capparoni, Pietro: Profili Bio-Bibliografici di medici e naturalisti celebri italini dal sec XV° al sec XVIII°, Rome *Istituto naz. med. farmacolog. "Serono,"* 1932, 106.
Pettigrew, Thomas J.: *Biographical Memoirs of the Most Celebrated Physicians, Surgeons, etc.*, London, Fisher, 1838, I.
Richardson, Sir Benjamin: *Disciples of Aesculapius*, London, Hutchinson, 1900, I, p. 283.
Sigerist, Henry E.: *The Great Doctors*, New York, Norton, 1933, p. 229.
Virchow, Rudolf: Morgagni and the Ana-

tomical Concept, *Bull. Hist. Med.*, 1939, VII, 975.

Morton, Richard
Osler, William: The "Phthisiologia" of Richard Morton, M.D., *Med. Libr. & Hist. J.*, 1904, II, 1.
Porter, B.: Richard Morton, *Dict. Nat. Biog.*, London, 1894, XXXIX, p. 157.

Murray, George R.
George Redmayne Murray: *Brit. M. J.*, 1939, II, 707.
George Redmayne Murray: *Lancet*, 1939, II, 767.

Nicolle, Charles
Annal. de l'inst. Pasteur, 1936, LVI, 353.
Mesnie, P.: Charles Nicolle, *Presse Méd.*, 1936, p. 594.

North, Elisha
Pleadwell, F. L.: A New View of Elisha North and His Treatise on Spotted Fever, *Ann. M. Hist.*, 1924, VI, 245.
Steiner, W. R.: Dr. Elisha North, One of Connecticut's Most Eminent Medical Practitioners, *Bull. Johns Hopkins Hospital*, 1908, XIX, 301.

Nott, Dr. J. C.
Hott, William Leland: Josiah Clark Nott of Mobile, *M. Life*, 1928, XXXV, 487.
Wilson, Robert: Dr. J. C. Nott and the Transmission of Yellow Fever, *Ann. M. Hist.*, 1931, N.S., III, 515.

Osler, William
Cushing, Harvey: *The Life of Sir William Osler*, Oxford, Clarendon Press, 1925.
Cushing, Harvey: William Osler, The Man, *Ann. M. Hist.*, 1919, II, 157.
Sir William Osler Bart., Baltimore, Johns Hopkins Press, 1920.

Otto, John C.
Kelly, Howard A. & Burrage, Walter L.: *American Medical Biographies*, Baltimore, Norman Remington, 1920, p. 869.

Paget, Sir James
Paget, Stephen: *Memoirs and Letters of Sir James Paget*, London, Longmans Green, 1901.

Paracelsus
Hartmann, Franz: *The Life of Philippus Theophrastus, Bombast von Hohenheim known by the name of Paracelsus*, London, Redway, 1887.
Liénard, René-Albert: *Paracelse, sa vie, son oeuvre*, Lyon, Bosc. & Riou, 1932.

Netzhammer, Raymund: *Theophrastus Paracelsus*, Einsiedeln, Benziger, 1901.

Sigerist, Henry: The Word "Bombastic," *Bull. Hist. Med.*, 1941, x, 688.

Stillman, John Maxson: *Paracelsus*, Chicago, Open Court, 1920.

Stoddart, Anna M.: *The Life of Paracelsus Theophrastus von Hohenheim*, Philadelphia, McKay, n.d.

Paré, Ambroise

Paget, Stephen: *Ambroise Paré and His Times*, New York, Putnam, 1897.

Packard, Francis: *Life and Times of Ambroise Paré*, New York, Hoeber, 1926.

Singer, Dorothy W.: *Selections from the Works of Ambroise Paré with Short Biography*, New York, Wm. Wood, 1924.

Parkinson, James

Rowntree, L. G.: James Parkinson, *Bull. Johns Hopkins Hospital*, 1912, XXIII, 33.

Parry, Caleb Hillier

Macmichael, William: *Lives of British Physicians*, London, Murray, 1830, p. 275.

Rolleston, Sir Humphry: Caleb Hillier Parry, *Ann. M. Hist.*, 1925, VII, 205.

Platter, Felix

Cumston, Charles Greene: A Brief Notice of Felix Platter, *Bull. Johns Hopkins Hospital*, 1912, XXIII, 105.

Potain, Pierre-Carl

Beeson, B. Barker: Potain: His Life and Works, *Bull. Soc. Med. Hist.*, Chicago, 1930, IV, 142.

Vaquez, Henri: Pierre-Carl Potain, eloge prononcé à l'academie de médicine dans la séance annuelle du 13 decembre 1927, *Bull. l'acad. de Med.*, 1927, XCVIII, 569.

Quincke, Heinrich

Hechhaus, H.: Heinrich Quincke zum 70. Geburtstag, *Deutsch. Med. Wchnschr.*, 1912, XXXVIII, 1605.

Külbs, Fr.: Heinrich Quincke, *Deutsch. Arch. fur Klin. Med.*, 1922, CXXXIX, 380, I.

Raynaud, Maurice

Dr. Fereol: *Brit. M. J.*, 188, II, 268.

M. Peter: Maurice Raynaud, *Bull. de L'Acad. de méd. Par.* 1881, x, 865.

Maurice Raynaud: *Progrès med.*, 1881, IX, 552.

Monro, Thomas K.: *Raynaud's Disease*

(*Biographical note*), Glasgow, Madehose, p. 1899.

The Works of the late Prof. Raynaud: *Brit. M. J.*, 1881, II, 92.

Reed, Walter

Kelly, Howard A.: *Walter Reed and Yellow Fever*, New York, McClure, Phillips & Co., 1907.

Rhazes

Opitz, Karl: *Klassiker der Medizin, Ueber die Pocken und die Masern*, Leipzig, Barth, 1911.

Sigerist, Henry E.: *The Great Doctors*, New York, Norton, 1933, p. 78.

Riverius, Lazarus

Astruc, Jean: *Mémoires pour servir à l'histoire de la Faculté de Médicine de Montpellier*, Paris, Cavelier, 1767, p. 259.

Ross, Sir Ronald

Megroz, R. L.: *Ronald Ross, Discoverer and Creator*, London, Allen & Unwin, 1932.

Rotch, Thomas

Thomas Morgan Rotch: *Boston M. & S. J.*, 1914, CLXX, 596.

Rufus of Ephesus

Daremberg Ch. et Ruelle, Ch. Emile: *Oeuvres de Rufus d'Ephesus*, Paris, Imprimerie Nationale, 1879, II.

Rush, Benjamin

Flexner, James T.: *Doctors on Horseback*, New York, Garden City, 1939, 57.

Lloyd, James Hendrie: Benjamin Rush and His Critics, *Ann. M. Hist.*, 1930, N.S., II, 470.

Richardson, Sir Benjamin: *Disciples of Aesculapius*, London, Hutchinson, 1900, I, 62.

Webster, Henry G.: A Sketch of Benjamin Rush. *Med. Libr. & Hist. J.*, 1906, IV, 240.

Rutty, John

Sharpless, William, T. S.: Dr. John Rutty of Dublin, *Ann M. Hist.*, 1926, x, 249.

Salicetti, Guglielmo

Pifteau, Paul: *Chirurgie de Guillaume de Salicet*, Toulouse, Imprimerie Saint-Cyprien, 1898, XXV.

Puccinotti: *Storia della Medicina*, Livorno, Wagner, 1859, II, Part III, p. 532.

Schönlein, Johann Lukas

Virchow, Rudolf: *Gedächtnissrede auf Joh. Lucas Schönlein*, Berlin, Hirschwald, 1865.

Sennert, Daniel
Allgemeine Deutsche Biographie, Leipzig, Duncker & Humblot, 1892, XXXIV, p. 34.
Fiessinger, Ch.: La Thérapeutique des Vieux Mâitres, Paris, Soc. d'éditions scientifiques, 1897, 120.

Skoda, Josef
Neuburger, Max: Masters of the Vienna Clinic in the Nineteenth Century, Med. Life, 1923, XLI, 208.
Sternberg, Maximilian: Josef Skoda, Vienna, Spring, 1924.

Soemmerring, Samuel Thomas von
Bast, Theodore H.: The Life and Work of Samuel Thomas von Soemmerring, Ann. M. Hist., 1924, VI, 369.
Stricker, Wilhelm: Samuel Thomas von Soemmerring, Frankfurt, Osterrieth, 1862.

Spens, Thomas
Dickson, T. Graeme: The Identity of Dr. Thomas Spens, Lancet, 1913, II, 1357.
Lea, C. Edgar: Dr. Thomas Spens. The First Describer of the Stokes-Adams Syndrome, Edinburgh M. J., 1914, N.S., XIII, 51.

Steell, Graham
Obituary: Lancet, 1942, I, 157.

Stokes, William
Ormsby, Lambert H.: Medical History of the Meath Hospital, Dublin, Fannin & Co., 1888, 129.
Stokes, William: William Stokes, His Life and Work, London, Unwin, 1898.

Sydenham, Thomas
Bettany, G. T.: Eminent Doctors, London, Hogg, 1885, Vol. I, p. 52.
Chaplin, Arnold: Thomas Sydenham, His Work and Character, Brit. M. J., 1924, II, 917.
Latham, R. G.: The Life of Sydenham in the Works of Thomas Sydenham, M.D., London, Sydenham Soc., 1848, p. 11.
Macmichael, William: Lives of British Physicians, London, 1830, p. 84.
Payne, J. F.: Thomas Sydenham, London, Unwin, 1900.
Riesman, David: Thomas Sydenham, Clinician, Ann. M. Hist., 1925, VII, 171.
Rolleston, Sir Humphry: Sydenham, Father of Clinical Medicine in Brittain, Brit. M. J., 1924, II, 919.

Sylvius, Franciscus
Jelliffe, Smith Ely: Franciscus Sylvius, Proc. Charaka Club, 1910, III, 14.

Talbor, Sir Robert
Dock, George: Robert Talbor, Madame de Sevigne and the Introduction of Cinchona, Ann. M. Hist., 1922, IV, 241.
Rolleston, Sir Humphry: History of Cinchona and Its Derivatives, Ann. M. Hist., 1931, N.S., III, 261.

Thiéry, François
Larousse: Grand Dictionnaire universel du XIX° Siècle, Paris, 1876, XV, p. 125.

Traube, Ludwig
Haberling, W.: Zum hundertsten Geburtstag Ludwig Traubes, Deutsch Med. Wchnschr., 1918, XLIV, 21.
Morrison, Hyman: Ludwig Traube, Boston M. & S. J., 1927, CXCVI, 1097.

Tronchin, Théodore
Geyle, A.: Dr. Théodore Tronchin, Paris, Plon-Nourrit, 1906.

Tulp, Nicholas
Fiessinger, Ch.: La Therapeutique des Vieux Maitres, Paris, Soc. d'editions scientifiques, 1896, p. 147.
Scolten, Adrian: The Work of Nicholas Tulp, Med. Life, 1928, XXXV, 381; 1929, XXXVI, 394; 1932, XXXIX, 297.

Vaquez, Henri
Clerc, A.: Henri Vaquez, La Presse Méd., 1936, 1041.
Laubry, Charles: Henri Vaquez, Arch. d. med. d. coeur, 1936, IX, 293.

Vieussens, Raymond
Astruc, Jean: Mémoires pour servir à l'histoire de la Faculté de Médicine de Montpellier, Paris, Cavelier, 1767, p. 389.
Blumer, George: Vieussens, Albany M. Ann., 1907, XXVIII, 625.
Major, Ralph H.: Raymond Vieussens and His Treatise on the Heart, Ann. M. Hist., 1931, N.S., IV, 147.
Sachs, B.: Raymond de Vieussens, Proc. Charaka Club, 1910, III, 99.

Vigo, Giovanni di
Astruc, John: A Treatise of Venereal Diseases, London, W. Innys, 1754, p. 156.
Pilcher, Lewis Stephen: A Surgeon to the Pope, Proc. Charaka Club, 1910, III, 106.

Villalobos, Franciso Lopez de
Dennie, Charles C.: *The Gift of Columbus*, Kansas City, Brown-White, 1936, p. 13.
Friedenwald, Harry: Francisco Lopez de Villalobos, *Bull. Hist. Med.*, 1939, VII, 1129.
Gaskoin, George: *The Medical Works of Francisco Lopez de Villalobos*, London, Churchill, 1870, p. 1.

Villemin, Jean-Antoine
Obituary: *Brit. M. J.*, 1892, II, 1091.

Virchow, Rudolf
Pagel, J.: *Rudolf v. Virchow*, Leipzig, Feuer Verlag, n.d.

Warren, Richard
Munk, William: *The Roll of the Royal College of Physicians of London*, London, 1878, II, p. 242.

Wells, William Charles
Pleadwell, Frank L.: That Remarkable Philosopher and Physician, Wells of Charleston, *Ann. M. Hist.*, 1934, N.S., VI, 128.

Wepfer, Johann Jakob
Brunner, Conrad and v. Muralt, Wilhelm: *Aus den Briefen hervorragender Schweizer Aerzte des 17 Jahrhunderts*, Basle, Benno Schwabe, 1919, p. 81.

Werlhof, Paul Gottlieb
Dictionnaire des sciences médicales: Biographie médicale, Paris, Pańckoucke, 1825, p. 493.
Pagel, J.: *Allgemeine Deutsche Biographie*, Leipzig, Duncker & Humblot, 1897, XLII, 16.

Whistler, Daniel
Munk, William: *Roll of the Royal College of Physicians of London*, London, 1878, I, p. 249.
Still, George Frederic: *The History of Paediatrics*, London, Oxford, 1931, p. 199.

Wilks, Sir Samuel
Obituary: *Brit. M. J.*, 1911, II. 1384.
Obituary: *Lancet*, 1911, II, 1441.

Willis, Thomas
Adams, Edward W.: Thomas Willis, *Med. Libr. & Hist. J.*, 1903, I, 265.
Miller, W. S.: Thomas Willis and his Phthisi Pulmonari, *Am. Rev. Tuberc.*, 1922, V, 934.
Munk, William: *The Roll of the Royal College of Physicians of London*, London, 1878, I, p. 338.
Rolleston, Sir Humphry: Thomas Willis, *Med. Life*, 1934, XLI, 177.
Viets, Henry: A Patronal Festival for Thomas Willis (1621-1675) with Remarks by Sir William Osler Bart., F.R.S., *Ann. Med. Hist.*, 1917, I, 118.
Wood, Anthony: *Athena Oxoniensis*, London, Laplock, Midwinter & Tonson, 1721, II, p. 550.

Winge, E. F. H.
Biographisches Lexikon der hervorragenden Ärzte aller Zeiten und Völker, Berlin, Urban & Schwarzenberg, 1934, V, p. 959.

Winterbottom, Thomas
Obituary: *Lancet*, 1859, II, 76.

Wiseman, Richard
Power, D'A.: Richard Wiseman, *Dict. Nat. Biog.*, London, 1900, LXII, p. 246.
Richardson, Sir Benjamin: *Disciples of Aesculapius*, London, Hutchinson, 1900, I, 158.

Withering, William
Moorman, L. J.: William Withering: His Work, His Health, His Friends, *Bull. Hist. Med.*, 1942, XII, 355.
Roddis, Louis H.: William Withering and the Introduction of Digitalis into Medical Practice, *Ann. M. Hist.*, 1936, N.S., VIII, 93, 185.
Withering, W.: *A Memoir of the Life, Character and Writings of W. Withering, M.D., F.R.S.*, in the *Miscellaneous Tracts of the Late William Withering, M.D., F.R.S.*, London, Longman. 1822.

Index

INDEX

A

Achondroplasia: 297
Acosta, Joseph: 553
Acromegaly: 305
Actuarius, Johannes: **540**
  on hemoglobinuria, 541
Adams, Francis: 4
Adams, Robert: **332**
  on heart-block, 333
Addison, Thomas: 245
  on anemia, 291
  on disease of suprarenal capsules, 291
  description of xanthomata, 245
Addison's disease: 290
Agramonte, Aristide: 131
Albuminuria: 528, 529, 531
Allergy: 616
  in infectious diseases, 621
Almenar, Juan: **19**
  description of syphilis, 20
Anemia, pernicious: 290
  description of Addison, 291
  description of Combe, 490
  treatment by Minot, 492
Anemia, sickle-cell: 494
Aneurysm: 443
  description of Corvisart, 455
  description of Fernel, 443
  description of Lancisi, 450
  description of Morgagni, 450
  description of Oliver, 457
  description of Paré, 445
  description of Wiseman, 447
Angina pectoris: 416
  description of Clarendon, 416
  description of Fothergill, 422
  description of Heberden, 420
  description of Hunter, 423
Angioneurotic edema: 623
  Graves on, 623
  Quincke on, 624
Aortic insufficiency: 339
  description of Corrigan, 354
  description of Cowper, 340
  description of Duroziez, 364
  description of Flint, 359
  description of Hodgkin, 348
  description of Hope, 351
  description of Morgagni, 346
  description of Quincke, 361
  description of Vieussens, 345

Aortic stenosis: 380
  description of Hope, 380
  description of Stokes, 380
Apoplexy: 474
  description of Baglivi, 476
  description of Wepfer, 474
Appendicitis: 646
  Fernel on, 647
  Fitz on, 654
  Heister on, 649
  Hodgkin on, 652
  Joubert de la Motte on, 650
  Mestivier on, 650
  Parkinson on, 652
Aretaeus: 134, 136, **235**
  on asthma, 576
  on diabetes, 236
  on diphtheria, 136
  on lobar pneumonia, 562
  on pleurisy, 569
  on sprue, 600
  on tetany, 134
Aristophanes, on malaria: 95
Asthma: 576
  Aretaeus on, 576
  Willis on, 577
Auenbrugger, Leopold: **563**
  on lobar pneumonia, 564
  on pericarditis, 408
  on pleurisy with effusion, 573
Auricular fibrillation: 390
  description of Hope, 380
  description of Stokes, 380

B

Baglivi, George: 476
Baillie, Matthew: **582**
  description of cirrhosis of liver, 634
  description of emphysema, 582
Baillou, Guillaume de: **137**
  on diphtheria, 138
  on pericarditis, 404
  on rheumatic fever, 212
  on whooping cough, 210
Baker, Sir George: **320**
  on Devonshire colic, 322
Ballonius: see Baillou
Banting, Sir Frederick: **256**
  discovery of insulin, 257
Bard, Samuel: **153**
  on diphtheria, 155

Basedow, C. A. von: 282
    on hyperthyroidism, 283
Bayle, Gaspard-Laurent: 64
    on tuberculosis, 64
Beck, Theodor: 134
Benivieni, Antonio: 636
    on gallstones, 638
Bennett, John H.: 505
    on leukemia, 506
Beriberi: 604
    Bontius on, 605
    Tulp on, 606
Bertin, R. J. H.: 372
    on mitral stenosis, 373
Best, C. H.: 256
Béthencourt, Jacques de: 35
    description of syphilis, 36
Binninger, Johann Nikolaus: 616
    on hay-fever, 618
Blackall, John: 530
    on albuminuria, 531
Boccaccio, Giovanni: 80
    description of plague, 80
Bontius, Jacobus: 604
    on beriberi, 605
Bostock, John: 618
    on hay-fever, 618
Botallo, Leonardo: 616
    on hay-fever, 616
Bouillaud, Jean: 220
    on endocarditis, 222, 460
    on pericarditis, 222
    on rheumatic fever, 221
Bouveret, Leon: 401
    on paroxysmal tachycardia, 401
Bouveret's disease: 401
Bravo, Francisco: 165
    on typhus fever, 165
Bretonneau, Pierre: 157
    on diphtheria, 159
    on typhoid fever, 182
Bright, Richard: 534
    on kidney disease, 535
Broadbent, Sir W. H.: 411
    on pericarditis, 412
Broadbent, Walter: 413
Broadbent's sign: 411
Bronchial cast: 555
    description of Tulp, 555
    description of Warren, 557
Brown, John: 632
    on cirrhosis of liver, 633
Buerger, Leo: 481
Buerger's disease: 481

Burnett, Sir William: 333
    on heart-block, 334
Burton, Henry: 324
    on lead line, 324

C

Cadwalader, Thomas: 299
    on osteomalacia, 301
Caius, John: 202
    on sweating fever, 204
Capillary pulse: 361
Cardan, Jerome: 161
    on typhus fever, 163
Cardiospasm: 628
Carey, Mathew: 114
    on yellow fever, 114
Carroll, James: 131
Cartier, Jacques: 587
    on scurvy, 587
Casál, Gaspar: 607
    on pellagra, 610
Celsus, Aulus Cornelius: 96
    on malaria, 96
Chauliac, Guy de: 77
    description of plague, 78
Cheyne, John: 548
    on Cheyne-Stokes respiration, 550
Cheyne-Stokes respiration: 548
    Cheyne on, 550
    Hippocrates on, 548
    Stokes on, 552
Chicken pox: 206
    description by Heberden, 206
Chlorosis: 487
    Lange's description, 488
Chrysippus: 4
Cirrhosis of liver: 632
    Baillie on, 634
    Brown on, 633
    Laënnec on, 635
Citois, François: 313
    on lead poisoning, 314
Clarendon, Earl of: 416
Clarke, John: 287
    on tetany, 287
Clowes, William: 20
Cober, Tobias: 166
    on typhus fever, 167
Coeliac affection: 600
Collin, V.: 409
Colombo, Matteo Realdo: 638
    on gallstones, 639
Combe, James S.: 490
    on anemia, 490

Contagion: 8
Coronary occlusion: 424
  Dock on, 428
  Hammer on, 426
  Herrick on, 435
  Osler on, 431
Corrigan, Sir Dominic John: 352
  on aortic insufficiency, 354
Corrigan pulse: 354
Corvisart, Jean Nicholas: 368
  on aneurysm, 455
  on mitral stenosis, 370
Cotton, R. P.: 398
  on paroxysmal tachycardia, 398
Cotugno, Domenico: 528
  on albuminuria, 528
Cowper, William: 339
  on aortic insufficiency, 340
Cruveilhier, Jean: 628
  on peptic ulcer, 629
Curling, Thomas B.: 266
  on myxedema, 267

D

DaCosta, J. M.: 381
  on irritable heart, 383
Darwin, Erasmus: 439
Deficiency diseases: 585
Defoe, Daniel: 91
  description of London plague, 92
Dekkers, Frederik: 527
  on albuminuria, 528
Devonshire colic: 316
Diabetes: 234
  description by Aretaeus, 236
  description by Dobson, 242
  description by Papyrus Ebers, 235
  description by Paracelsus, 237
  description by Willis, 240
  air hunger in, 247
  demonstration of sugar in, 243
  discovery of insulin, 254
  extirpation of pancreas produces, 250
  hyaline degeneration of islands of Langer-
    hans in, 254
  sweetness of urine in, 240
  xanthomata in, 245
Dickinson, William H.: 546
  on hemoglobinuria, 546
Dickson, Thomas: 302
Digestive tract, diseases of: 626
Digitalis: 437
  introduced by Withering, 440
  poem on, 439

Diphtheria: 135
  description by Aretaeus, 136
  description by Baillou, 138
  description by Bard, 155
  description by Bretonneau, 159
  description by Fothergill, 144
  description by Home, 149
  description by Huxham, 147
  description by Tulp, 141
Disease
  Bouveret's, 401
  Buerger's, 481
  Fröhlich's, 307
  Hodgkin's, 230
  Hungarian, 166
  Raynaud's, 479
  Schoenlein's, 226
  Weir Mitchell's, 485
Diseases of circulatory system: 326
Diseases, infectious: 7
Diseases of metabolism: 234
Dobson, Matthew: 242
  demonstrates sugar in urine of diabetic,
    242
Dock, George: 428
  on coronary occlusion, 428
Dressler: 542
Duroziez murmur: 364
Duroziez, Paul-Louis: 363
  on aortic insufficiency, 364

E

Ebers, Papyrus: 235
Emphysema: 582
  description of Baillie, 582
  description of Laënnec, 583
Empyema: 569
Endocarditis: 457
  Bouillaud on, 221
  description of Bouillaud, 460
  description of Kirkes, 464
  description of Morgagni, 459
  description of Riverius, 458
  description of Virchow, 461
  description of Wilkes, 469
  description of Winge, 472
  and rheumatic fever, 222
"Epilepsy with a slow pulse": 327
Erythromelalgia: 485
Evil, King's: 54
Extra-systoles: 397

F

Fabry, Wilhelm: 640
  on gallstones, 641

Fauvel, S. A.: **375**
  on mitral stenosis, 375
Fernel, Jean: **646**
  on aneurysm, 443
  on appendicitis, 647
  on gallstones, 639
Finlay, Carlos: **125**
  on yellow fever, 126
Fitz, Reginald H.: **653**
Fitz, Reginald, Jr.: **494**
Flint, Austin: **357**
  on cardiac murmurs, 359
Flint murmur: 359
Focal infection: 227, 229
Fothergill, John: **142**
  on angina pectoris, 422
  on diphtheria, 144
Fracastorius, Hieronymus: 7, **37**
  on contagion, 7
  poem on syphilis, 39
  on typhus fever, 164
Frapolli, Francesco: **612**
  on pellagra, 612
Freke, John: **303**
  on myositis ossificans, 304
"Frémissement cataire": 371
Fröhlich, Alfred: **307**
  on tumor of hypophysis cerebri, 307

G

Gallop rhythm: 386
Gallstones: 635
  Benivieni on, 638
  Colombo on, 639
  Fabry on, 641
  Fernel on, 639
  Gentile da Foligno on, 636
  Glisson on, 642
  Morgagni on, 644
  Platter on, 640
  Sennert on, 642
Gaskoin, George: 16
Gentile da Foligno: 635
  on gallstones, 636
Gerbezius, Marcus: **326**
  on heart-block, 326
Gerhard, William W.: **173**
  on typhus fever, 174
Glandular fever: 208
  description by Pfeiffer, 208
Glisson, Francis: **596**
  on gallstones, 642
  on rickets, 597
Gout: 288
  description of Sydenham, 288

Graefe, Albrecht von: **285**
  description of eyes in hyperthyroidism,
    286
Graves, Robert J.: **279**
  on angioneurotic edema, 623
  on hyperthyroidism, 280
Gull, Sir William: **268**
  on myxedema, 269

H

Haller, Albrecht von: 406
  on pericarditis, 408
Hammer, Adam: **424**
  on coronary occlusion, 426
Harley, George: **543**
  on hemoglobinuria, 545
Hay-fever: 616
  Bostock on, 618
  Botallo on, 616
  Binninger on, 618
Haygarth, John: **215**
  on rheumatic fever, 217
Heart
  Irritable, 383
  Rheumatism of, 219, 221
Heart-block: 326
  Adams on, 333
  Burnett on, 334
  Gerbezius on, 326
  Morgagni on, 327
  Spens on, 331
  Stokes on, 337
Heberden, William: 206, **418**
  on angina pectoris, 420
  on chicken pox, 206
  on nodes, 304
  on nyctalopia, 615
Heberden's nodes: 304
Heister, Lorenz: **648**
  on appendicitis, 649
Hemoglobinuria, paroxysmal: see paroxysmal
    hemoglobinuria
Hemophilia: 521
  Otto on, 522
Henoch, Eduard: **518**
  on purpura, 519
Hering: H. E.: **390**
  on pulsus irregularis perpetuus, 390
Herrick, J. B.: **434**
  on coronary occlusion, 435
  on sickle-cell anemia, 494
Hildanus, Guilhelmus Fabricius: **640**
Hillary, William: **603**
  on sprue, 603

Hippocrates: **3**, 4
  on Cheyne-Stokes respiration, 548
  on lobar pneumonia, 561
  on malaria, 94
  on mumps, 201
  on pleurisy, 568
  on tuberculosis, 52
Hippocratic succussion: 581
Hodges, Nathaniel: **85**
  on plague, 86
Hodgkin, Thomas: **230**
  on aortic insufficiency, 348
  on appendicitis, 652
Hodgkin's disease: 231
Hoefer, Wolfgang: **264**
  on myxedema, 264
Home, Francis: **149**
  on diphtheria, 149
Hope, James: **349**
  on aortic insufficiency, 351
  on aortic stenosis, 380
  on mitral stenosis, 374
  on pulmonary stenosis, 379
Hungarian disease: 166
Hunter, John: **42**
  on angina pectoris, 423
  on syphilis, 45
Hutchinson, Sir Jonathan: **46**
  on syphilis, 48
Hutchinson's teeth: 48
Hutten, Ulrich von: **28**
Huxham, John: **146**
  on Devonshire colic, 316
  on diphtheria, 147
  on scurvy, 592
Hyperthyroidism: 275
  description by Basedow, 283
  description by Graves, 280
  description by Parry, 276
  eyes in, von Graefe, 286

I

Infection, Theory of: 7
Influenza: 201
  description of Sydenham, 201
Insufficiency, aortic: see aortic insufficiency
Insulin, discovery of: 256
Irritable heart: 383

J

Jail distemper: 171
Jenner, Edward: **621**
  on allergy, 622
Joinville, Jean de: **586**
  on scurvy, 586
Joubert de la Motte: 650

K

Ketelaer, Vincent: **601**
Kidney diseases: 525
  Blackall on, 531
  Bright on, 535
  Cotugno on, 528
  Dekkers on, 528
  Salicetti on, 527
  Wells on, 529
King. A.F.A.: **103**
  mosquitoes and malaria, 104
King's evil: 54
Kircher, Athanasius: **9**
  description of plague, 11, 84
Kirkes, William S.: **462**
  on endocarditis, 464
Knutsson, Bengt: **82**
  on plague, 83
Koplik, Henry: **199**
  on measles, 199
Kussmaul, Adolf: **245**
  air hunger in diabetes, 247

L

Laënnec, R. T. H.: **68**
  on cirrhosis of liver, 635
  on emphysema, 583
  on lobar pneumonia, 565
  on mitral stenosis, 371
  on pleurisy, 574
  on pneumothorax, 580
  on tuberculosis, 70
Lancisi, Giovanni: **448**
  on aneurysm, 450
Lange, Johannes: **487**
  on chlorosis, 488
Laurenzi, Luciano: 4
Lazear, Jesse: 141
Lead line: 324
Lead poisoning: 311
  description of Sir George Baker, 322
  description of Henry Burton, 324
  description of François Citois, 314
  description of John Huxham, 316
  description of Nikander, 312
  description of Paul of Aegina, 313
  description of Théodore Tronchin, 319
Leoniceno, Nicolo: **13**
  description of syphilis, 15
Leukemia: 505
  Bennett on, 506
  Virchow on, 510
Lind, James: **589**
  on scurvy, 591
  on typhus fever, 171

Littré, Emile: 569
Liver, cirrhosis of: 632
Lobar pneumonia: 561
  Aretaeus on, 562
  Auenbrugger on, 564
  Hippocrates on, 561
  Laënnec on, 565
Louis, P. C. A.: 184
  on typhoid fever, 186
Lower, Richard: 404
  on pericarditis, 406
Loyola, Ignatius
  autopsy on, 639
Lusitanus, Amatus: 513
  on purpura, 514

M

Mackenzie, Sir James: 392
  on auricular fibrillation, 394
  on extra-systoles, 397
Mal de la Rosa: 608, 609
Malaria: 94
  Aristophanes on, 95
  Celsus on, 96
  Hippocrates on, 94
  King on, 104
  Mosquitoes in, 104, 110
  Pliny on, 97
  Ross on, 110
  Tabor on, 101
  Varro on, 96
Malpighi, Marcellus
  autopsy on, 476
Marie, Pierre: 305
  on acromegaly, 306
Measles: 196
  description of Koplik, 199
  description of Rhazes, 198
  description of Sydenham, 198
Meningitis, epidemic: 188
  description by North, 190
  description by Vieusseux, 188
Mestivier: 650
Metabolism, diseases of: 234
Michele di Piazza, 77
  on plague, 77
Minkowsky, Oskar: 249
  produced diabetes, 250
Minot, George R.: 492
  on anemia, 493
Mitchell, S. Weir: 483
  Weir Mitchell's disease, 485
Mitral stenosis: 364
  description of Bertin, 373
  description of Corvisart, 370

Mitral stenosis (Cont.)
  description of Fauvel, 375
  description of Hope, 374
  description of Laënnec, 371
  description of Morgagni, 367
  description of Steell, 377
  description of Vieussens, 364
Monroe, Robert D.: 494
Morbus maculosus Werlhofii: 518
Morgagni, Giovanni Battista: 327, 346
  on aneurysm, 450
  on aortic insufficiency, 346
  on endocarditis, 459
  on gallstones, 644
  on heart-block, 327
  on mitral stenosis, 367
Morton, Richard: 61
  on rheumatic fever, 214
  on tuberculosis, 62
Mosquitoes and malaria: 104, 110
Mosquitoes and yellow fever: 122, 126, 131
Mountain sickness: 553
Mumps: 201
Murmur
  Duroziez, 364
  Flint, 359
  Graham Steell, 377
Murphy, William P.: 493
Murray, George R.: 272
  treatment of myxedema, 272
Myositis ossificans: 303
Myxedema: 258
  description of Curling, 266
  description of Gull, 269
  description of Hoefer, 264
  description of Paracelsus, 260
  description of Platter, 264
  treatment by Murray, 272

N

Nicolle, Charles: 177
  on typhus fever, 178
Nikander: 312
  on lead poisoning, 312
Nodes, Heberden's: 304
North, Elisha: 189
  on meningitis, 190
Nott, Josiah C.: 121
  on yellow fever, 122
Nyctalopia: 615

O

Oliver, William S.: 456
  on aneurysm, 457
Opie, Eugene L.: 253
  on pathology of diabetes, 254

Osler, Sir William: **500**
  on coronary occlusion, 431
  on polycythemia, 502
Osteomalacia: 299
  Cadwalader on, 301
  Thomas on, 302
Otto, John C.: **521**
  on hemophilia, 522

P

Paget, Sir James: **294**
  Pulse, capillary, 361
  Pulse, Corrigan, 354
Paget's disease: 294
Papyrus Ebers: 235
Paracelsus: 237, **258**
  on diabetes, 237
  on myxedema, 260
Paré, Ambrose: 87, **443**
  description of aneurysm, 445
  description of plague, 87
  description of pleurisy, 570
Parkinson, James: **651**
  on appendicitis, 652
Parkinson, John: 652
Paroxysmal hemoglobinuria: 540
  Actuarius on, 541
  Dickinson on, 546
  Dressler on, 542
  Harley on, 545
Paroxysmal tachycardia: 397
  Bouveret on, 401
  Cotton on, 398
  Stokes on, 397
Parry, Caleb Hilliard: **275**
  on hyperthyroidism, 276
Paul of Ægina: **312**
  on lead poisoning, 313
Pectoris dolor: 420
Peliosis rheumatica: 226
Pellagra: 607
  Casál on, 610
  Frapolli on, 612
  Thiéry on, 608
Peptic ulcer: 629
Pericarditis: 404
  Auenbrugger on, 408
  Baillou on, 404
  Bouillaud on, 222
  Broadbent on, 412, 413
  Collin on, 409
  Haller on, 408
  Lower on, 406
  and rheumatic fever, 222
  Rotch on, 409

Pfeiffer, Emil: 208
  on glandular fever, 208
Plague: 71
  description of Bengt Knutsson, 83
  description of Boccaccio, 80
  description of Defoe, 92
  description of Guy de Chauliac, 78
  description of Hodges, 86
  observations of Kircher, 11, 84
  description of Michele di Piazza, 77
  description of Paré, 87
  description of Rufus, 76
  description of Thucydides, 73
Platter, Felix: **263**
  on gallstones, 640
  description of myxedema, 264
  on persistent thymus, 309
Pleurisy: 568
  Aretaeus on, 569
  Auenbrugger on, 573
  Hipprocrates on, 568
  Laënnec on, 574
  Paré on, 570
  Willis on, 571
Pliny the Elder, 97
  on malaria, 97
Pneumonia, lobar: see lobar pneumonia
Pneumothorax, 580
  Laënnec on, 580
Polycythemia, 497
  Osler on, 502
  Vaquez on, 497
Potain, P. C.: **386**
  on gallop rhythm, 388
Pulmonary stenosis: 379
  description of Hope, 379
Pulsus alternans: 385
Pulsus irregularis perpetuus: 390
Purpura: 513
  Amatus Lusitanus on, 514
  Henoch on, 519
  Riverius on, 516
  Werlhof on, 518

Q

Quincke, Heinrich: 361, **623**
  on angioneurotic edema, 624
  on capillary pulse, 361

R

Raynaud, Maurice: **478**
Raynaud's disease: 479
Reed, Walter: **130**
  on yellow fever, 131
Relapsing fever: 223

Rhazes: 196
    on measles and smallpox, 197
Rheumatic fever: 212
    description of Baillou, 212
    description of Haygarth, 215
    description of Morton, 214
    description of Sydenham, 213
    description of Wells, 218
Rheumatism of heart: 219, 221
    Bouillaud on, 221
    Wells on, 219
Rickets: 594
    description of Glisson, 597
    description of Whistler, 595
Riverius, Lazarus: 514
    on endocarditis, 458
    on purpura, 514
Ross, Sir Ronald: 108
    on malaria, 110
Rotch, T. M.: 409
    on pericarditis, 410
Rotch's sign: 409
Rufus of Ephesus: 76
    on the plague, 76
Rush, Benjamin: 227
    on focal infection, 229
    on yellow fever, 118
Rutty, John: 223
    on relapsing fever, 223

S

Saliceto, William de: 525
Salicetti, Guglielmo: 525
    on kidney disease, 527
Scarlet fever: 192
    description by Sennert, 193
    description by Sydenham, 196
Schoenlein, J. L.: 225
Schoenlein's disease: 225
Scurvy: 585
    described by Cartier, 587
    described by Huxham, 592
    described by de Joinville, 586
    described by Lind, 591
    described by de Vitry, 585
Sennert, Daniel: 192
    on gallstones, 642
    on scarlet fever, 193
Sickle-cell anemia: 494
Skoda, Josef: 558
Skodaic resonance: 560
Sleeping sickness: 224
Smallpox: 196
    description by Rhazes, 197

Soemerring, S. T.: 297
    on achondroplasia, 298
Spens, Thomas: 330
    on heart-block, 331
Sprue: 600
    described by Aretaeus, 600
    described by Hillary, 603
    described by Ketelaer, 601
Steell, Graham: 376
    on mitral stenosis, 377
Stenosis, mitral: see mitral stenosis
Stenosis, pulmonary: see pulmonary stenosis
Stokes, William: 335
    on aortic stenosis, 380
    on Cheyne-Stokes respiration, 552
    on heart-block, 337
    on paroxysmal tachycardia, 397
Succussion, Hippocratic: 581
Sweating fever: 202
Sydenham, Thomas: 194
    on gout, 288
    on influenza, 201
    on measles, 198
    on rheumatic fever, 213
    on scarlet fever, 196
Sylvius, Franciscus: 58
    on tuberculosis, 59
Syphilis: 12
    de Béthencourt's description, 36
    Fracastorius' poem, 39
    Hunter on, 45
    Hutchinson on, 48
    von Hutten's description, 31
    Leoniceno's description, 15
    di Vigo's description, 24
    Villalobos' description, 16

T

Tabor, Sir Robert: 100
    on malaria, 101
Tachycardia, paroxysmal: see paroxysmal
    tachycardia
Tate, Nahum: 39
Teeth, Hutchinson's: 48
Tetany: 287
Thiéry, François: 607
    on pellagra, 608
Thomas, Henry
    on osteomalacia, 302
Thrill in mitral stenosis: 371, 374
Thucydides: 73
Thymus, persistent: 309
Traube, Ludwig: 385
    on pulsus alternans, 385

Tronchin, Théodore: 317
  on lead poisoning, 319
Trousseau, Armand: 182
Tuberculosis: 51
  Bayle on, 64
  Hippocrates on, 52
  Laënnec on, 70
  Morton on, 61
  Sylvius on, 59
  Villemin on, 66
  Wiseman on, 53
Tulp, Nicholas: 140
  on beriberi, 606
  on bronchial cast, 553
  on diphtheria, 141
Turner, Daniel: 31
Typhoid fever: 179
  description by Bretonneau, 182
  description by Louis, 186
  description by Willis, 179
Typhus fever: 161
  description by Bravo, 165
  description by Cardan, 163
  description by Fracastorius, 164
  description by Gerhard, 173
  description by Lind, 171
  description by Tober, 167
  description by Willis, 169

U

Ulcer, peptic: 629

V

Vaquez, L. H.: 497
  on polycythemia, 497
Varro, Marcus Terentius
  on malaria, 96
Verbez: see Gerbezius
Vieussens, Raymond: 344
  on aortic insufficiency, 345
  on mitral stenosis, 364
Vieusseux, Gaspard: 188
  on meningitis, 188
Vigo, Giovanni di: 23
  description of syphilis, 24
Villalobos, Francisco Lopez de: 16
  poem on syphilis, 17
Villemin, Jean-Antoine: 66
  experiments on tuberculosis, 66

Virchow, Rudolf: 508
  on endocarditis, 461
  on leukemia, 510
Vitry, Jacques de: 585
  on scurvy, 585

W

Warren, Richard: 555
  on bronchial cast, 557
Weir Mitchell's disease: 485
Wells, William Charles: 218
  on albuminuria, 529
  on rheumatism of heart, 219
Wepfer, Johann J.: 474
  on apoplexy, 474
Werlhof, Paul G.: 517
  on purpura, 518
Whistler, Daniel: 594
  on rickets, 595
Whooping cough: 210
  description of Baillou, 210
Wilks, Sir Samuel: 467
  on endocarditis, 469
Willis, Thomas: 169, 170, 238
  on asthma, 577
  on cardiospasm, 628
  on diabetes, 240
  on pleurisy, 571
  on typhoid fever, 179
  on typhus fever, 169
Winge, E. F. H.: 471
  on endocarditis, 472
Winterbottom, Thomas: 224
  on sleeping sickness, 224
Wiseman, Richard: 53
  on aneurysm, 447
  on tuberculosis, 54
Withering, William: 437
  on digitalis, 440

Y

Yellow fever: 114
  Carey on, 114
  Finlay on, 126
  mosquitoes in, 122, 126
  Nott on, 122
  Reed on, 131
  Rush on, 118